Atlas of Transesophageal Echocardiography

Atlas of Transesophageal Echocardiography

Navin C. Nanda, MD
Professor of Medicine
Director, Heart Station/Echocardiography Laboratories
University of Alabama at Birmingham
Director, Echocardiography Laboratory
The Kirklin Clinic
Health Services Foundation
Birmingham, Alabama

Michael J. Domanski, MD
Head, Clinical Trials Group
National Heart, Lung, and Blood Institute
Washington, D.C.

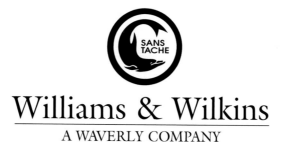

Williams & Wilkins
A WAVERLY COMPANY

BALTIMORE • PHILADELPHIA • LONDON • PARIS • BANGKOK
BUENOS AIRES • HONG KONG • MUNICH • SYDNEY • TOKYO • WROCLAW

Editor: Jonathan W. Pine, Jr
Managing Editor: Leah Ann Kiehne Hayes
Marketing Manager: Daniell T. Griffin
Production Coordinator: Carol Eckhart
Project Editor: Lisa J. Franko
Designer: Mario Fernandez
Illustration Planner: Wayne Hubbel
Cover Designer: Melissa Brown
Typesetter: Graphic World, Inc.
Printer and Binder: RR Donnelley & Sons Company

351 West Camden Street
Baltimore, Maryland 21201-2436 USA

Rose Tree Corporate Center
1400 North Providence Road
Building II, Suite 5025
Media, Pennsylvania 19063-2043 USA

Accurate indications, adverse reactions, and dosage schedules for drugs are provided in this book, but it is possible that they may change. The reader is urged to review the package information data of the manufacturers of the medications mentioned.

Printed in the United States of America

Library of Congress Cataloging-in-Publication Data

Nanda, Navin C. (Navin Chandar), 1937–
    Atlas of transesophageal echocardiography/Navin C. Nanda,
Michael J. Domanski. — 1st ed.
        p.   cm.
    Includes index.
    ISBN 0–683–06320–0
    1. Transesophageal echocardiography—Atlases.   I. Domanski,
Michael J. II. Title.
    [DNLM: 1. Echocardiography, Transesophageal—atlases.   2. Heart
Diseases—diagnosis—atlases.   WG 17 N176b 1998]
RC683.5.T83N36   1998
616.1′207543—dc21
DNLM/DLC
for Library of Congress

The publishers have made every effort to trace the copyright holders for borrowed material. If they have inadvertently overlooked any, they will be pleased to make the necessary arrangements at the first opportunity.

To purchase additional copies of this book, call our customer service department at (800) 638-0672 or fax orders to (800) 447-8438. For other book services, including chapter reprints and large quantity sales, ask for the Special Sales department.

Canadian customers should call (800) 665-1148, or fax (800) 665-0103. For all other calls originating outside of the United States, please call (410) 528-4223 or fax us at (410) 528-8550.

Visit Williams & Wilkins on the Internet: http://www.wwilkins.com or contact our customer service department at custserv@wwilkins.com. Williams & Wilkins customer service representatives are available from 8:30 am to 6:00 pm, EST, Monday through Friday, for telephone access.

                                          98 99 00 01 02
                                          2 3 4 5 6 7 8 9 10

Dedication

This book is dedicated to my late parents, Balwant Rai Nanda, MD, and Mrs. Maya Vati Nanda; my wife, Kanta Nanda, MD; and our children, Nitin, Anita, and Anil.

Navin C. Nanda, MD

I dedicate this book to my mother and father, Beatrice and Thaddeus Domanski, who made all things possible.

Michael Domanski, MD

Preface

The tremendous popularity and widespread application of transesophageal echocardiography in a large variety of cardiovascular disease entities provided the impetus for preparing this atlas for the use of physicians, technologists, and others interested in this exciting and innovative non-invasive diagnostic modality. It encompasses my experience with this technique since its first introduction in our Echocardiography Laboratories at the University of Alabama at Birmingham in 1988. The book provides a comprehensive, state-of-the-art review of this relatively new field in an atlas format to facilitate demonstration of the various findings observed in both acquired and congenital cardiac disease entities in a comprehensive manner.

The *Atlas* is organized into ten chapters. The first chapter is devoted to normal transesophageal echocardiographic findings. The introduction summarizes the various types of examination probes available and the technique of examination. This is followed by a large number of two-dimensional and conventional and color Doppler illustrations, which provide a comprehensive coverage of normal anatomy and physiology as delineated by transesophageal echocardiography. The second chapter deals with the mitral valve. Mitral stenosis, mitral regurgitation, balloon valvuloplasty, and various pathologies affecting the mitral valve, such as myxomatous degeneration and endocarditis, are illustrated. The next chapter deals with the aortic valve and the aorta. The usefulness of transesophageal echocardiography in the assessment of etiology and severity of aortic regurgitation, aortic stenosis, endocarditis, and other pathologic conditions involving the aortic valve is described and illustrated. Aneurysms involving various portions of the aorta, aortic dissection, and aortic atherosclerotic plaques are also extensively covered in this section. Chapter 4 demonstrates disease entities affecting the tricuspid and pulmonary valves. Various prosthetic valves (both tissue and mechanical) and rings are covered in Chapter 5. A large number of illustrations demonstrates normal transesophageal echocardiographic findings in prosthetic valves, including "normal" regurgitation and pressure gradients, abnormal valvar and paravalvar leaks, infection, pannus formation, and thrombosis, as well as degeneration and calcification. The next chapter deals with ischemic heart disease and covers left ventricular dysfunction, ischemic mitral regurgitation, and complications of myocardial infarction such as left ventricular aneurysms and pseudoaneurysms, ventricular septal and cardiac free wall rupture, and both left and right ventricular papillary muscle rupture. The role of transesophageal echocardiography in the assessment of coronary artery stenosis, especially using newer, recently developed echocardiographic systems as well as contrast echocardiography also is detailed in this chapter. Both hypertrophic and dilated cardiomyopathies and ventricular assist devices are illustrated in the following chapter. Chapter 8, the largest section in this *Atlas*, illustrates transesophageal echocardiographic findings in a large variety of congenital cardiac disease entities. In this section of the *Atlas*, examples of common shunt lesions are shown first, then the obstructive lesions (both left-sided and right-sided), and then the more complex congenital pathologies. Two sections specially written by Dr. Jesus Vargas Barron and his colleagues are included at the end of this section to supplement the material shown and provide an enhanced understanding of the role of transesophageal echocardiography in the evaluation of congenital cardiac lesions. Their excellent contributions to this *Atlas* are most gratefully acknowledged. Chapter 9 is devoted to tumors and other mass lesions. Not only relatively common tumors such as myxomas but other rare lesions as well, such as lipomas, fibroelastomas, leiomyosarcomas, and sclerosing mediastinitis, are illustrated. In addition, postoperative hematomas, intracardiac thrombi, and other tumor mimics are shown. The last chapter deals with miscellaneous lesions such as pericardial effusion, pericardial cysts, pleural effusions, intracardiac catheters, and pacemakers, as well as de-airing and other contrast effects during cardiac surgery.

Each section of the *Atlas* begins with a brief introduction that delineates and explains the transesophageal echocardiographic findings of the lesions covered in that section. The numerous transesophageal illustrations are supplemented by detailed anatomic drawings and tissue specimens. The illustrations exemplify fine points in technique and diagnosis as well as pitfalls to avoid during a transesophageal examination. A special attempt has been made to make the figure legends as comprehensive as possible. The Suggested Readings listed at the end of each section should provide additional background reading material for the reader and acknowledge the work of many investigators who have contributed to the advancement of transesophageal echocardiography.

In 1995, Dr. Michael J. Domanski graciously agreed to assist me by helping me in the writing of the figure legends and the introductions at the beginning of each chapter of this *Atlas*. I am grateful to him for this help and for kindly agreeing to be listed as coauthor of the *Atlas*.

This *Atlas*, with over 2100 illustrations from several commercially available machines, represents the most detailed, definitive and comprehensive work in this field to date. I selected nearly all of the illustrations used in this *Atlas* after thoroughly reviewing the videotapes of all transesophageal cases done at the University of Alabama at Birmingham since 1988. Many of the selected studies were performed by me or under my supervision. Care was taken to write the text in an easy to understand, uniform style, using simple language and a direct, straightforward, and concise approach. The book should therefore benefit the beginner as well as the more experienced echocardiographer. The *Atlas* also will be useful to our Preceptorship Teaching Program in transesophageal echocardiography. This program, begun in 1989, has been of use to several hundred physicians and echocardiographers from all over the world.

I must thank several individuals in the University of Alabama at Birmingham Hospital who have contributed directly or indirectly to the growth and development of our Echocardiography Laboratories. First and foremost, I am grateful to all the present and past members of the Division of Cardiovascular Disease for providing us full clinical support and facilitating access to hemodynamic data for correlation with transesophageal echocardiographic findings. The University of Alabama Hospital Administration have also taken an active interest and given us extraordinary support in terms of space, personnel, and equipment needs as our laboratories expanded rapidly over the past 8 years. Most of all, I am grateful to the Division of Cardiovascular Surgery, especially Dr. John W. Kirklin, Dr. Albert D. Pacifico, Dr. James K. Kirklin, Dr. George L. Zorn, Jr, Dr. William Holman, and Dr. David McGiffin, not only for facilitating the performance of intraoperative transesophageal echocardiography but also for providing us surgical correlation in the patients operated upon by them. Many other physicians at our medical center have referred their patients to us for transesophageal echocardiography, and I am grateful to them as well. The tremendous growth and expansion of our laboratories would not have been possible without the enthusiastic support and encouragement given by the above individuals.

Dr. Ricardo Ceballos, the late Professor of Pathology, and Dr. Benigno Soto, Professor of Radiology and Director of the Division of Cardiovascular Radiology, provided us with illustrations of pathological specimens for use in the *Atlas*. Most of the artwork for this *Atlas* was prepared by Dr. Luis Pinheiro de Melo Filho, who worked as a Fellow in our Echocardiography Laboratories. His extraordinary illustrations are a highlight of this *Atlas*. I most gratefully acknowledge his help and contributions to this work. I also thank my associate, Dr. PoHoey Fan, Assistant Professor of Medicine in the Division of Cardiovascular Disease, for his help and support in the preparation of this *Atlas*. I am thankful to Photography and Instructional Graphics of the University of Alabama at Birmingham, especially J. Michael Strawn and Steven W. Wood, for their support.

Fellows from the Heart Station/Echocardiography Laboratories and the Division of Cardiovascular Disease have actively assisted in our clinical as well as research efforts, and it is while teaching them that I became aware of the need for a book of this type. The present and former Clinical and Research Fellows, Echocardiographic Associates, and Observers who have helped, directly or indirectly, in the preparation of the *Atlas* are Drs. Sayed Mohammed Abd El-Rahman, Dipak Agrawal, Gopal Agrawal, Abdulgader Allam, Sudhir Bhatnagar, Claudia Truffa de Carvalho, Chung-Huo Chen, Sang-Man Chung, Francisco Edenio Regio Costa, Dina Krishna Das, Ashutosh Dwivedi, Miguel Espinal, PoHoey Fan (1986–1989), Ana Finch, Carlos Garcia del Rio, Ming Hsiung, Hans Jain, Farrukh Jamil, Mohammad Kamran, Gajendra Khatri, Kee-Sik Kim, Michal Kolda, Zhi-An Li, Ramesh R. Loungani, Sanjay Maheshwari, Sanjay Malhotra, Mohamed Moursi, Khidir Osman, Marcos Pariona, Luis Pinheiro, V.S. Punia, Punuru Reddy, Steven Rosenthal, Debasish Roychoudhury, Mariyappa Somashekhar, Rajat Sanyal, Marc S. Schwartz, Abhash Chandra Thakur, Conny Tirtaman, Tuong Van, and Guilherme Veri. I am particularly grateful to the following fellows who helped in the preparation of illustrations: Dipak Agrawal, Gopal Agrawal, Sudhir Bhatnagar, Sang-Man Chung, Ana Finch, Hans Jain, Farrukh Jamil, Mohammad Kamran, Gajendra Khatri, Kee-Sik Kim, Michal Kolda, Ramesh R. Loungani, Sanjay Malhotra, Mohamed Moursi, Khidir Osman, Steven Rosenthal, Debasish Roychoudhury, Rajat Sanyal, Marc S. Schwartz, Abhash Chandra Thakur, Conny Tirtaman, and Tuong Van. Lindy Chapman, my Administrative Assistant, and my wife, Kanta Nanda, MD, provided expert editorial assistance, and Vickie Carter, secretary, helped in the typing. It would not have been possible for me to complete this project were it not for the dedicated assistance and whole-hearted support given by the abovenamed individuals. Section 8.2 and 8.3 were contributed by the following individuals (in addition to myself): Jesus Vargas-Barron, Assistant Professor of Cardiology, Universidad Nacional Autonoma de Mexico, Head of the Department of Echocardiography, Instituto Nacional de Cardiologia "Ignacio Chavez," Mexico City, Mexico; Nilda Espinola Zavaleta, Associate Professor of Cardiology, Instituto Nacional de Cardiologia "Ignacio Chavez," Mexico City, Mexico; Angel Romero-Cárdenas, Associate Professor of Cardiology, Instituto Nacional de Cardiologia "Ignacio Chavez," Mexico City, Mexico; and Maria E.B. Rijlaarsdam, Pediatric Cardiologist, Department of Echocardiography, Instituto Nacional de Cardiologia "Ignacio Chavez," Mexico City, Mexico.

Finally, I am grateful to my family—my late mother, Mrs. Maya Vati Nanda, my wife Kanta, and our children, Nitin, Anita, and Anil, for their great patience and support during the innumerable hours I spent on this project in the evenings and on weekends for the past several years.

Contents

Preface .... *vii*
Abbreviations .... *xi*

1. Normal Anatomy 1

2. Mitral Valve 63

3. Aortic Valve and Aorta 103

4. Tricuspid and Pulmonary Valves 169

5. Prosthetic Valves and Rings 181

6. Ischemic Heart Disease 251

7. Cardiomyopathy 275

8. Congenital Heart Disease 295
    8.1 Overview of Congenital Heart Disease
    8.2 Transesophageal Sequential Analysis of Cardiovascular Segments in
        Diagnosis of Complex Congenital Heart Disease
        Jesus Vargas-Barron, Nilda Espinola Zavaleta, Angel Romero-Cárdenas,
        Maria Rijlaarsdam, Navin C. Nanda
    8.3 Transesophageal Echocardiography in Congenital Heart Disease
        Jesus Vargas Barron, Nilda Espinola Zavaleta, Angel Romero-Cárdenas,
        Maria Rijlaarsdam, Navin C. Nanda

9. Tumors and Other Mass Lesions 445

10. Miscellaneous Lesions 489

Index *507*

Abbreviations

AA = ascending aorta
AO = aorta
AR = aortic regurgitation
AV = aortic valve
CS = coronary sinus
DA = descending thoracic aorta
IVC = inferior vena cava
L = longitudinal plane
LA = left atrium
LAA = left atrial appendage
LLPV = left lower pulmonary vein
LPA = left pulmonary artery
LUPV = left upper pulmonary vein
LV = left ventricle
LVO, LVOT = left ventricular outflow tract
MPA = main pulmonary artery
MR = mitral regurgitation
MV = mitral valve
PA = pulmonary artery
PR = pulmonary regurgitation
PV = pulmonary valve

RA = right atrium
RAA = right atrial appendage
RLPV = right lower pulmonary vein
RPA = right pulmonary artery
RUPV = right upper pulmonary vein
RV = right ventricle
RVO, RVOT = right ventricular outflow tract
SVC = superior vena cava
T = transverse plane
TV = tricuspid valve
VS, IVS = ventricular septum

ORIENTATION SYMBOLS

A = anterior
I = inferior
L = left
P = posterior
R = right
S = superior

Normal Anatomy

1

The first probes used for transesophageal echocardiography provided imaging in only a single plane. The development of the biplane probe, which had an imaging plane orthogonal to the transverse view obtained with single-plane devices, added considerably to the diagnostic information that could be obtained. The currently available multiplane probes make imaging studies much more flexible by allowing visualization of the in-between planes. In fact, the monoplane probe should now be regarded as obsolete. Smaller probes that enhance patient comfort and increase safety have become available. Images obtained with the smaller probes usually are not as good in quality as those obtained with the larger probes, however, because the smaller probes have a smaller number of elements than do the larger probes.

Although the planes discussed usually refer to the orientation of the transducer relative to the esophagus, the terms also apply to the heart because the esophagus is located directly behind the heart. However, the exact relationship of the esophagus to the heart varies from individual to individual so that it is not always possible to obtain in a given individual all the planes and structures described in this chapter. The position and size of air-filled structures such as the trachea and the left and right main bronchi also determine the ability to image cardiovascular structures optimally in the upper chest. As in transthoracic echocardiography, the anatomic structures imaged by the transesophageal approach are identified by comparing them to known cardiovascular anatomy and, in some instances, by the use of contrast echocardiography. Transverse plane imaging (0° angle on the multiplane probe) generally provides transverse or horizontal sections of the heart, whereas longitudinal plane imaging gives longitudinal or vertical sections. During longitudinal plane examination, clockwise rotation of the probe shifts the vertical plane to the right so that right-sided structures such as the superior vena cava and the right pulmonary veins are brought into view, whereas counterclockwise rotation results in imaging of left-sided structures such as the left atrial appendage and the left pulmonary veins. Thus, obtaining transverse sections of the heart at various levels requires up-and-down movement of the probe; imaging of vertical sections, however, can be accomplished by mere rotation of the probe. The multiplane probe, like the biplane probe, can be moved up and down within the esophagus and also can be physically rotated in clockwise and counterclockwise directions to give both transverse and vertical sections. In addition, a manual switch on the handle rotates the transducer at the tip of the probe to provide oblique sections through the heart. Thus, a comprehensive examination of various cardiac structures can be performed using the multiplane probe.

There is no universally agreed upon transesophageal approach for examination of cardiac structures. In practice, however, one tends first to examine structures of immediate interest based on clinical indications and transthoracic echo findings. In the awake patient, it is best not to begin examination with the probe placed high up in the esophagus or in the stomach because this may result in gagging and increased patient discomfort. We often begin examination with the probe in mid-esophagus and proceed with examination of structures from a high esophageal or transgastric position only after the patient has relaxed, and frequently toward the end of the study. However, for the sake of simplicity and convenience, the anatomic findings in this section of the *Atlas* are shown as if the examination commenced in the upper esophagus, with the probe advanced gradually down the esophagus into the stomach. Thus, the great vessels and their branches or tributaries located at the base of the neck are displayed first, followed by the aortic valve and adjacent structures such as the coronary arteries and the pulmonary veins, then the cardiac chambers and the atrioventricular valves, then the descending thoracic aorta, and lastly, structures visualized from the transgastric approach.

Transesophageal examination with the probe positioned in the upper esophagus is useful in imaging the mid- and distal portions of the ascending aorta as well as the aortic arch and its branches. The innominate artery is the easiest branch to visualize, but other branches also can be imaged. Color Doppler–guided pulsed Doppler interrogation is useful in distinguishing an arterial branch from an accompanying vein. Flow signals from an artery are predominantly systolic, whereas the venous flow shows prominent systolic and diastolic components. Comprehensive evaluation of the aortic arch requires meticulous examination with a multiplane probe using transverse, longitudinal, and oblique planes. Because the aortic arch courses not only to the left but also posteriorly, the first, largest, and most anterior branch is the innominate artery; the left common carotid and the left subclavian arteries are identified arising more posteriorly. We have found longitudinal plane examination most useful in the identification of the aortic branch branches. Clockwise rotation with the probe set at an angulation of 90° moves the plane to the right, bringing the innominate artery origin into view. Counterclockwise rotation of the probe, on the other hand, moves the vertical plane to the left, which helps in locating and identifying the left common carotid and left subclavian arteries. The innominate artery also may be followed to its bifurcation into the right common carotid and the right subclavian branches. The vein most commonly imaged when examining the aortic arch is the left innominate vein, but other veins such as the right innominate and the subclavian veins may also be visualized. Venous valves occasionally may be imaged as linear, mobile echoes in the tributaries of the major veins and should not be mistaken for a dissection flap. The main pulmonary artery and its branches, especially the left pulmonary artery, are often imaged adjacent to the aortic arch, and the left pulmonary artery can be followed to its branching into lobar arteries. A small portion of the left atrium also may be imaged next to the aortic arch. Contrast echocardiography has proved useful in identifying anatomic structures imaged in this region.

Advancement and rotation of the probe from the position where the aortic arch and its branches are identified brings into view the ascending aorta in short axis during transverse plane (0°) examination. The main pulmonary artery and a long segment of the right pulmonary artery can be seen wrapping around the aorta in this view. The origin and proximal portion of the left pulmonary artery may also be imaged. To the right of the aorta, the superior vena cava is imaged in short axis. The superior branch of the right pulmonary artery and segments of the right pulmonary veins also may be visualized. Longitudinal plane examination images the ascending aorta in long axis and the right pulmonary artery in short axis posterior to it. Further advancement of the probe images the aortic root, with the left atrium located posteriorly and the right ventricular outflow tract and pulmonary valve located anteriorly and to the left. All three aortic leaflets and sinuses can be easily identified using a multiplane probe. This usually is best accomplished at a plane angulation between 30° and 60°. During transverse plane examination, slight adjustment of the probe with rotation to the left brings the left atrial appendage and the left pulmonary veins (usually the left upper) into view; rotation to the right is used to image the right upper pulmonary vein and its junction with the left atrium. Slight advancement of the transducer often images the right lower pulmonary vein and its junction with the left atrium. Minimal withdrawal of the probe from the aortic root position with rotation to the left and right is used to identify the origins and proximal segments of the left and right coronary arteries, respectively. Longitudinal plane (90°) examination is used to view the aortic root and the proximal ascending aorta in long axis. Counterclockwise (leftward) rotation of the probe from this position views the right ventricular outflow tract, the pulmonary valve and the proximal main pulmonary artery in long axis. The anterior and posterior (inferior) leaflets of the tricuspid valve may also be identified in this vertical section. Further counterclockwise rotation displays the two-chamber view, in which the inferior and anterior free walls of the left

ventricle are imaged together with the mitral valve, the left atrium, and the left atrial appendage. The left-sided pulmonary veins also can be imaged using this approach. Further counterclockwise rotation points the probe posteriorly and images the descending thoracic aorta in long axis. Clockwise (rightward) rotation of the probe from the aortic root position moves the vertical plane to the right, displaying the superior vena cava in long axis. The atrial septum and the fossa ovalis region also are often well visualized in this plane. Further clockwise rotation images the right upper pulmonary vein in long axis.

Advancement of the probe from the aortic root position during transverse plane (0°) examination usually displays the five-chamber view, in which the left ventricular outflow tract, aortic root, left atrium, mitral valve, right ventricle, and right atrium are imaged. Further advancement gives the four-chamber view, in which both the mitral (anterior and posterior leaflets) and tricuspid (anterior and septal leaflets) valves are imaged, in addition to the atrial septum, ventricular septum, both atria, and both ventricles. From this position, further advancement with some clockwise rotation during transverse plane (0°) imaging brings into view the openings of the inferior vena cava and coronary sinus into the right atrium, together with the eustachian and thebesian valves, the right atrial appendage, and the tricuspid inflow region. Leftward probe rotation may image the mitral valve in short axis. It is important to realize that at this point the transducer is close to the esophageal-gastric junction. Rotation of the probe with the transducer pointing posteriorly permits comprehensive examination of the descending thoracic aorta in long, short, and oblique axes, and at all levels by moving the transducer up and down the entire length of the esophagus. Azygos and hemiazygos veins and intercostal arteries and veins can be imaged. Higher up in the esophagus the intervertebral discs together with the spinal canal and the "pulsating" spinal cord within it also may be viewed.

The probe can then be advanced into the stomach to view both left and right ventricular cavities, the mitral and tricuspid valves, the chordae, and the papillary muscles in long, short, and oblique axes. The aortic root, proximal ascending aorta, right ventricular outflow tract, and pulmonary valve may also be imaged from the transgastric approach. The abdominal aorta and its branches, e.g., the celiac, superior mesenteric, and renal arteries and veins, as well as other abdominal structures, e.g., the kidneys, spleen, pancreas, liver, and stomach, have been imaged using the transgastric approach.

TRANSESOPHAGEAL ECHOCARDIOGRAPHIC EXAMINATION
Indications
Transesophageal echocardiographic examination (TEE) is indicated in the following circumstances: to determine the cardiac source of an embolism; to diagnose or rule out

suspected endocarditis; to check suspected prosthetic valve dysfunction; to assess for aortic dissection; to assess the severity of valvular regurgitation; to compensate for a poor acoustic window; and to detect congenital cardiac lesions.

Intraoperative Indications

TEE is used during surgery to assess the adequacy of a valve repair; to assess prosthetic valve or ring regurgitation; to monitor ventricular function; to evaluate removal of air from the heart; and to assess the adequacy of repair of congenital heart lesions.

Contraindications

TEE is contraindicated in the presence of esophageal tumor, stricture, diverticulum, fistulas, and previous esophageal surgery.

Esophageal varices and severe cervical spine problems are relative contraindications.

Complications

Complications are rare, but include esophageal bleeding, esophageal rupture, oropharyngeal injury, supraventricular tachycardia, laryngospasm, and problems related to oversedation.

PERFORMANCE OF TRANSESOPHAGEAL ECHOCARDIOGRAPHY

Transesophageal echocardiography is now a well-developed procedure. There is no substitute for adequate training under expert supervision. Our recommended approach to the performance of transesophageal echocardiography is described in the following paragraphs.

Prerequisites

The physician/cardiologist performing transesophageal echocardiography must have expertise in two-dimensional and conventional and color Doppler echocardiography. He or she also must be fully trained in intubating the esophagus.

Procedure Room Set-up

When performing TEE, the physician echocardiographer, a technologist echocardiographer or fellow, and a nurse are in attendance.

The procedure room is equipped with an examination table, an ultrasound machine, TEE probes, a bite guard, tongue depressors, gloves, a flashlight, a stethoscope, an intravenous (IV) setup, wall oxygen, suction apparatus, a fingertip oximeter, and a Dinamap (for blood pressure monitoring). CPR equipment and medications must be available. Sedatives and other medications must be on hand. Facilities for probe cleaning and sterilization are necessary.

Before Starting the Procedure

Before TEE is begun, discuss the case and the indications for the study with the referring physician. Ascertain that the probe has been sterilized as follows: (1) clean the probe with a mild cleansing agent and water; (2) immerse the probe in 2% glutaraldehyde (Cidex) or metricide for 20 minutes.

Remember: Transesophageal echocardiography is modestly invasive but is safe and feasible in 98% to 99% of patients. This procedure is well tolerated by critically ill patients and also by elderly patients.

Establish rapport with the patient. Explain the procedure fully, including its benefits and risks. Obtain informed consent. Verify that the patient has been fasting for the preceding 4 to 6 hours.

Question the patient closely about any dysphagia; esophageal problems (e.g., diverticula, strictures, rings, carcinoma); operations on the esophagus, throat, or chest, especially in childhood; any thoracic radiation; hematemesis; or allergies. If there is a question of dysphagia or the history is not clear-cut, perform a barium swallow to make sure the esophagus is normal.

Determine whether the patient has severe pulmonary disease, including chronic obstructive pulmonary disease (COPD) or bronchial asthma.

Perform a brief cardiovascular examination, check vital signs, and perform auscultation of the lungs. Check O_2 saturation with fingertip oximetry. Check the mouth and throat. Look for loose teeth and remove any dentures. If the patient's blood pressure (BP) is too high, nifedipine, 5 to 10 mg sublingually, can help bring it down.

Inspect the CPR equipment. Insert an IV line, or, if one is already in place, check its patency. Give prophylactic antibiotics if the patient has a prosthetic valve or any other internal device such as a defibrillator, if the patient is at increased risk for endocarditis (e.g., bad teeth or gums, previous history of endocarditis), or if the referring physician recommends them. Follow AHA guidelines for endoscopy procedures when giving antibiotics.

Prophylactic Antibiotics. The gastroenterology and infectious disease literature suggests no serious bacteremia or increased chances of endocarditis for endoscopy procedures without biopsy. No evidence has been adduced that mandates bacterial endocarditis prophylaxis for this procedure, and it is reasonable to use none. Nevertheless, many physicians prefer to employ antibiotics in an attempt to forestall endocarditis, particularly if the patient has a prosthetic valve. In this event, give ampicillin, 2 g intravenously in 50 ml of D5W or 0.9% NaCl, then gentamycin 1.5 mg/kg intravenously in the same manner after vigorously flushing the IV system, 30 minutes before the procedure. This may be repeated in 8 hours. If the patient is allergic to penicillin, give gentamycin first, flush the IV system vigorously, then give vancomycin 1 g intravenously over 60 minutes in 50 ml D5W or 0.9% NaCl. This may be repeated in 8 to 12 hours. For children, follow the same technique but adjust the dosages as follows: ampicillin 50 mg/kg, gentamicin 2.0 mg/kg, vancomycin 20 mg/kg.

Anesthesia and Sedation. Check the suction apparatus. Anesthetize the pharynx with 20% benzocaine spray to suppress the gag reflex and retching. Each spray should be 1 second in duration, and the patient should gargle for at least 1 minute before swallowing. Two or three sprays usually are sufficient to suppress the gag reflex, which should be tested using a tongue depressor following each spray. In some patients, the gag reflex is suppressed immediately after using the spray; in others the effect may be delayed for as long as 5 minutes. The duration of gag reflex suppression also varies from individual to individual, from a few minutes to several minutes. It is advisable not to use too much spray because potentially fatal methemoglobinemia resulting in oxygen desaturation and cyanosis may occur in susceptible patients. If necessary, give an anticholinergic agent such as glycopyrrolate, 0.2 mg intravenously, to reduce salivary and gastroenterologic secretions.

Give IV sedation if the patient is very apprehensive. Begin with low doses, and increase if necessary. If the patient has pulmonary disease or is elderly, give no or minimal sedation. No sedation should be given if the patient plans to drive home.

The most commonly used sedative is midazolam (Versed), 0.5 to 5 mg. This causes anterograde amnesia, but respiratory arrest can occur. The effect of midazolam can be reversed by flumazenil (Romazicon), 1.0 mg. Other commonly used sedatives are morphine, 1 to 4 mg; Phenergan, 12.5 to 25 mg; diazepam (Valium), 1 to 5 mg; and meperidine (Demerol), 12.5 to 50 mg. The effect of Demerol can be reversed by naloxone (Narcaine), 0.4 to 0.8 mg). More sedation is desirable to lower the patient's BP if aortic dissection is suspected, because BP often increases following benzocaine spray.

Final Preparations. Select the appropriate probe. Check for any breakage, and make sure the probe was sterilized. Check whether the transducers are operational and the echo system is in appropriate working condition. Unlock it if it is locked. Stop IV heparin at least 2 hours before the procedure.

Performance of the Procedure

Flex the patient's neck with the patient in the left lateral decubitus position. Place a bite guard in the patient's mouth. Apply gel liberally to the probe, up to at least 15 to 20 cm, flex it slightly, insert it in the patient's mouth through the bite guard, and ask the patient to swallow when he or she feels it at the back of the throat. If necessary, guide the probe by inserting one finger along the side of the bite guard. This prevents the patient from biting the operator's fingers or damaging the probe. An alternative approach is to ask the patient to open his or her mouth, grasp the probe near the transducer between the index and middle fingers, and direct it at the back of the pharynx, asking the patient to swallow it. A bite-block, previously placed on the probe, is then advanced into the mouth.

Remember that patient cooperation is required for swallowing the probe. If too much sedation is given, the patient may not be able to cooperate.

Gently advance the probe into the esophagus up to 30 or 35 cm. Then stop to let the patient get used to the probe for 1 to 3 minutes, especially if he or she is retching or gagging. Keeping the probe stationary allows any gagging to pass. It also allows the patient's heart rate and BP to revert toward baseline. Monitor the patient's vital signs and O_2 saturation with Dinamap, fingertip oximetry, and one-lead ECG on the echo monitor while the probe is being passed and afterward. Suction intermittently and as required. Give oxygen if needed.

Never advance the probe if any resistance is encountered. Warn the patient not to swallow secretions after probe passage and to signal if suctioning is needed. Withdrawing the probe into the esophagus is helpful if nausea or vomiting occurs when it is in the stomach. If a vasovagal episode or hypotension occurs, lower the head end of the table and give atropine, 0.5 to 1.0 mg intravenously, and run IV fluids and IV pressor agents.

Perform a multiplane examination of each chamber and structure using various angulations from 0° to 180°. A good approach is to begin by addressing the problem that precipitated the examination in case the patient is not able to tolerate the probe and the procedure has to be terminated early.

THE INTUBATED PATIENT

It may be difficult to pass a probe beyond an inflated endotracheal cuff in an intubated patient. In such a case, briefly deflate the cuff as the probe meets resistance from the cuff and then immediately reinflate it when the probe has passed beyond it. Extending the patient's neck often is helpful in passing the probe when the cuff is not deflated. A good rule is to keep the probe parallel and close to the endotracheal tube while advancing it. Some physicians also remove any nasogastric tube to facilitate probe passage. In the very uncooperative intubated patient, temporary pharmacologic paralysis may facilitate performance of the procedure.

AFTER THE PROCEDURE

Check the probe tip for any evidence of bleeding. Check the patient's mouth and pharynx for any abrasions or other trauma. Monitor vital signs for 20 to 30 minutes. The patient can leave with a caregiver once the sedative effect has worn off.

POSTPROCEDURE PRECAUTIONS FOR THE PATIENT

The patient should be given the following instructions after the procedure:

Do not swallow, eat, or drink for 1 to 2 hours after the procedure.

Do not drive or operate machinery for at least 12 hours after the procedure.

Have another person drive home if sedation was used.

Report to physician if sore throat persists for more than 2 days.

See a physician immediately if bleeding occurs from the mouth, the IV site becomes painful and inflamed, or fever or other symptoms develop.

Figure 1.1. **Transesophageal probes. A.** From left to right: pediatric, biplane, and monoplane probes, all from the same manufacturer, are displayed. At least one manufacturer has marketed an adult probe that is only slightly larger than the pediatric probe. The smaller probes produce less discomfort but sacrifice some image quality. **B.** The nasogastric tube (right) is only slightly smaller than the pediatric probe shown next to it. (Reproduced with permission from Helmcke F, Mahan EF III, Nanda NC, Cooper JW, Sanyal R. Use of the smaller pediatric transesophageal echocardiographic probe in adults. Echocardiography 1990;7:727–737.)

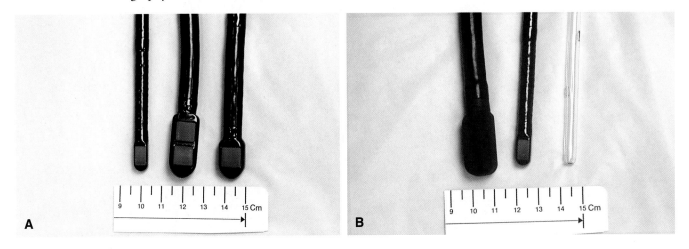

Figure 1.2. **Multiplane probe. A.** The multiplane probe shown here has a maximum width of 15.7 mm. A switch on the handle rotates the annular phased-array transducer, permitting multiplanar views. **B.** Various imaging planes can be obtained at the level of the aortic root with a multiplane probe, which can rotate the imaging plane through all of the angles from 0° to 180°. (Reproduced with permission from Nanda N, et al. Multiplane transesophageal echocardiographic imaging and three-dimensional reconstruction. Echocardiography 1992;9:667–676.)

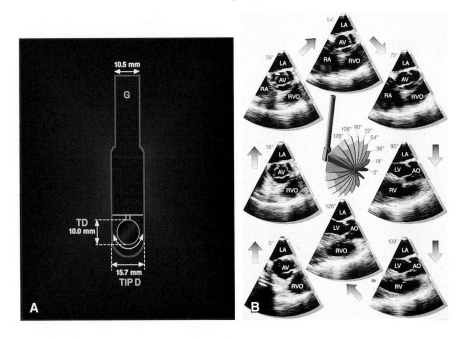

Figure 1.3. **Transverse and longitudinal imaging planes.** Examples of transverse imaging planes that can be obtained by moving the probe up and down the esophagus **(A)**. **B** shows both transverse (T) and longitudinal (L) planes. (**A** reproduced with permission from Nanda NC, Mahan EF III. Transesophageal echocardiography. AHA Council on Clinical Cardiology Newsletter 1990;Summer:3–22; **B** reproduced with permission from Nanda NC, Pinheiro L, Sanyal RS, Storey O. Transesophageal biplane echocardiographic imaging: technique, planes, and clinical usefulness. Echocardiography 1990;7:771–788.)

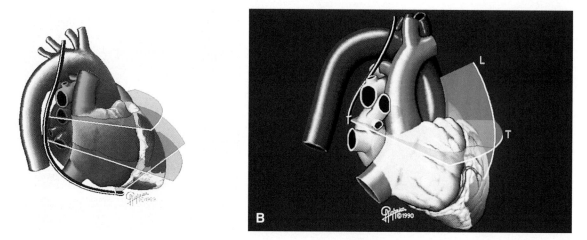

Figure 1.4. **Transverse sections.** **A** and **B** show sections obtained at the level of the sixth **(A)** and eighth **(B)** vertebral levels. *AZ*, azygos; *DA*, descending thoracic aorta; *E*, esophagus; *HAZ*, hemiazygos vein; *LAA*, left atrial appendage; *LPA*, left pulmonary artery; *LUPV*, left upper pulmonary vein; *PA*, main pulmonary artery; *RAA*, right atrial appendage; *RUPV*, right upper pulmonary vein; *SVC*, superior vena cava. (Reproduced with permission from Nanda NC, Pinheiro L, Sanyal RS, Storey O. Transesophageal biplane echocardiographic imaging: technique, planes, and clinical usefulness. Echocardiography 1990;7:771–788.)

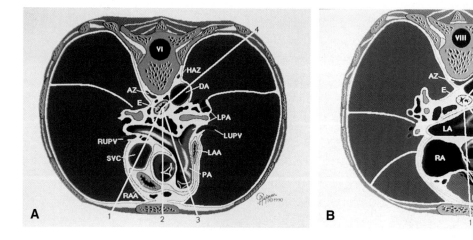

Figure 1.5. **Ascending aorta and pulmonary artery.** Transverse plane examination with the transducer in the upper esophagus. **A-C.** Schematics show an imaging plane passing through the ascending aorta and the adjacent pulmonary artery. The corresponding transesophageal images are shown in **D** and **E**.

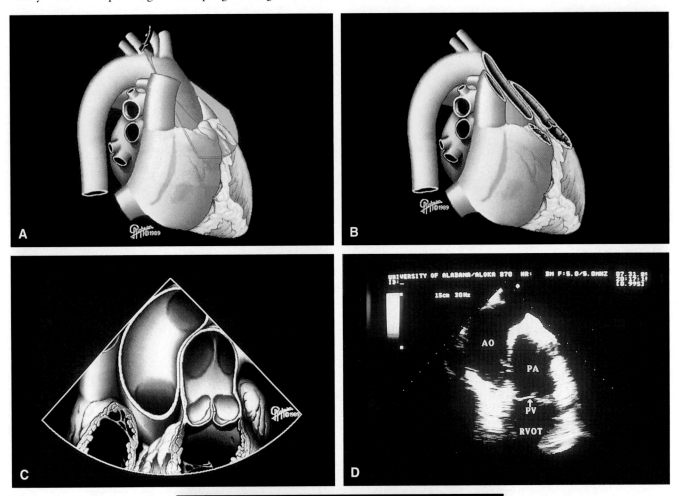

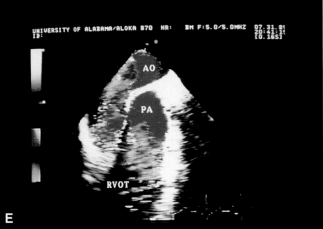

Figure 1.6. **Aortic arch.** Transverse plane examination with the transducer in the upper esophagus. **A,B.** The aortic arch (ACH) and the adjacent left innominate vein (IV) are shown. Note that the blood flow in these vessels is in opposite directions **(B)**. Pulsed Doppler interrogation of the aortic arch **(C)** shows predominantly systolic (arterial-type) flow signals in contrast to prominent systolic and diastolic (venous-type) flow signals **(D)** obtained from the innominate vein. Imaging of the left innominate vein next to the aortic arch may mimic aortic dissection. The pulsed Doppler examination rules out dissection by demonstrating venous-type flow in the innominate vein.

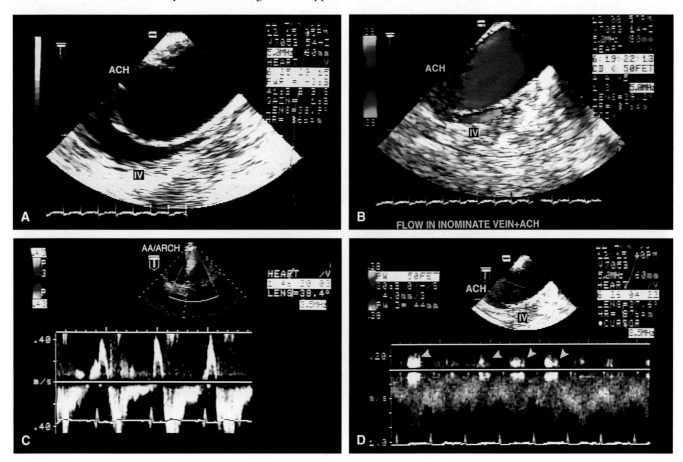

Figure 1.7.   **Aortic arch.** Longitudinal plane examination with the transducer in the upper esophagus. **A.** The aortic arch (ACH) and its relation to the adjacent main pulmonary artery and the left innominate vein (IV). The innominate artery (IA) can be seen arising from the aortic arch **(B,C).**

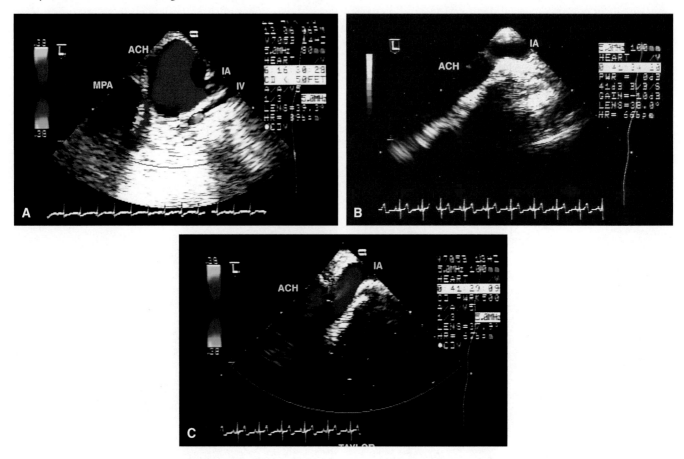

Figure 1.8.   **Ascending aorta and arch.** Transducer in the upper esophagus. Transverse plane examination shows flow signals anteriorly, representing an artifact (AF), not flow in a vascular structure. Such artifacts are fairly common but are easily recognized because they are not confined by any known anatomic structure. *AA,* ascending aorta.

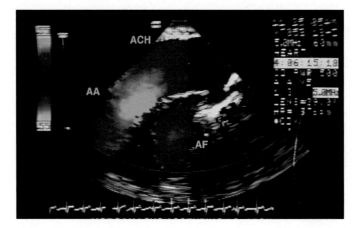

Figure 1.9.   **Identification of individual arch vessels**. **A.** Schematic representation of the technique used for identifying the aortic arch branches during longitudinal plane examination. *AA*, ascending aorta; *IA*, innominate artery; *LC*, left common carotid artery; *LPA*, left pulmonary artery; *LS*, left subclavian artery; *MPA*, main pulmonary artery; *RC*, right common carotid artery; *RPA*, right pulmonary artery; *RS*, right subclavian artery; *T*, transducer. **B-E.** All three arch vessels could be delineated in this patient using both transverse (T) and longitudinal (L) planes. *ACH*, aortic arch; *CA*, left common carotid artery; *SA*, left subclavian artery. **F-H.** Longitudinal plane examination in a different patient shows the innominate artery (IA) clearly arising from the aortic arch (ACH, **F**). The left common carotid (LCA) and left subclavian arteries (LSA) are located more posteriorly and were best visualized in this patient by counterclockwise rotation of the transducer, which resulted in the innominate artery becoming less prominent and less recognizable **(G).** In this patient also, all three arteries could be visualized in the transverse plane **(H).** *IV*, innominate vein. **I.** Another patient in whom all three arch vessels could be delineated in longitudinal plane examination. **J-M.** In another patient the innominate artery (IA) could be followed to its bifurcation into the right common carotid (CCA) and right subclavian (SCA) arteries. Color Doppler–guided pulsed Doppler interrogation of the innominate artery shows predominantly systolic, arterial-type flow signals (arrowhead, **M**). (Reproduced with permission from Agrawal G, LaMotte LC, Nanda NC. Identification of the aortic arch branches using transesophageal echocardiography. Echocardiography 1997;14:461–466.)

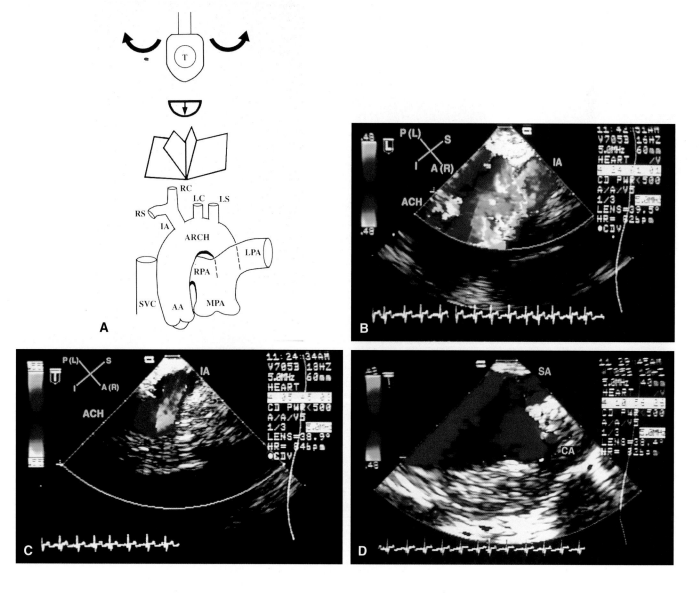

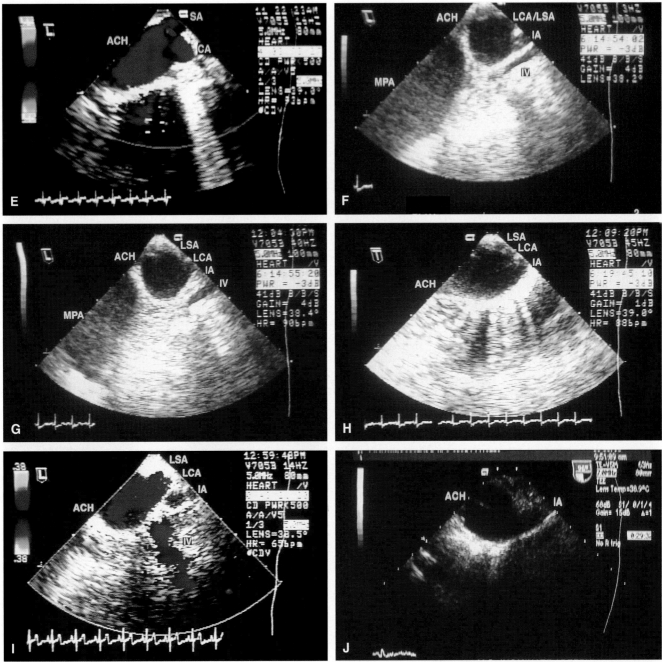

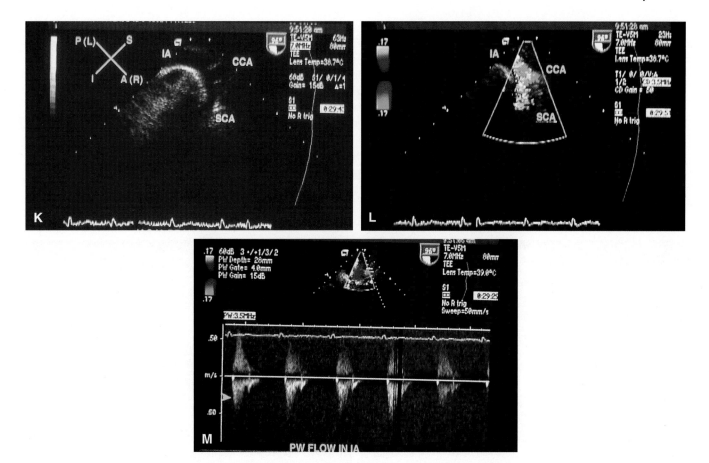

Figure 1.10. **Aortic arch and pulmonary artery.** Transducer in the upper esophagus. **A.** The appearance of contrast signals (black arrow) in the left innominate vein following an intravenous bolus of saline contrast. Contrast signals (arrowheads) also are noted in the main pulmonary artery. The small contrast-free space adjacent to the main pulmonary artery represents the LA, which is imaged anterior to the aortic arch (AO). **B.** The left subclavian (SA) and the left common carotid (CA) arteries arising from the aortic arch (ACH). The left subclavian vein (SCV) is imaged next to the left subclavian artery. Also seen are the LA and the main pulmonary artery. **C-G.** The LA is imaged anterior to the aortic arch (ARC). Injection of normal saline through a left atrial line resulted in the appearance of contrast (CON) echoes in the LA **(E).** Color Doppler–guided pulsed Doppler examination **(G)** demonstrates normal low-velocity phasic signals in the left atrium. Contrast echocardiography is useful in identifying structures adjacent to the aortic arch. *AA,* ascending aorta. **H.** Linear echo on the pulmonary valve (arrowhead) in another patient, consistent with Lambl's excrescence. This is a normal finding. *PV,* pulmonary valve. (**D** and **F** reproduced with permission from Agrawal GG, Parekh HH, Tirtaman C, Nanda NC. Transesophageal echocardiographic imaging of the left atrium behind the ascending aorta mimicking aortic dissection: validation by contrast echocardiography. Echocardiography 1997;14:411–415.)

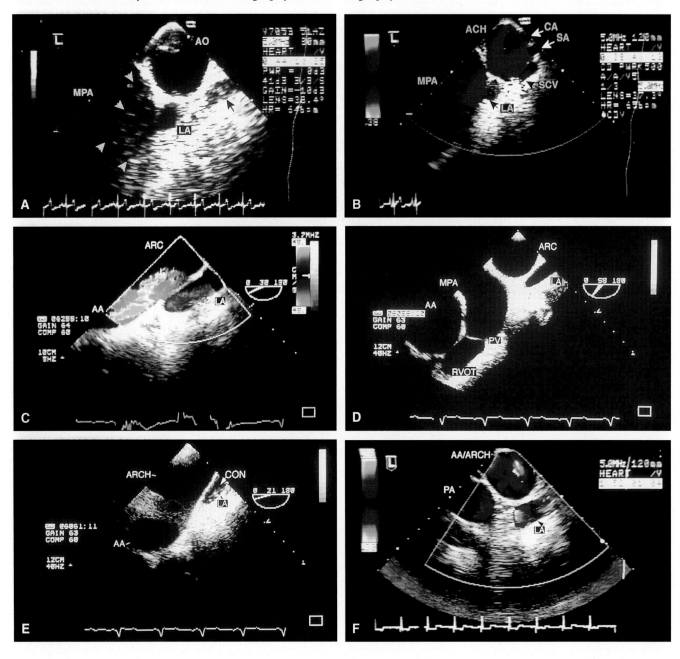

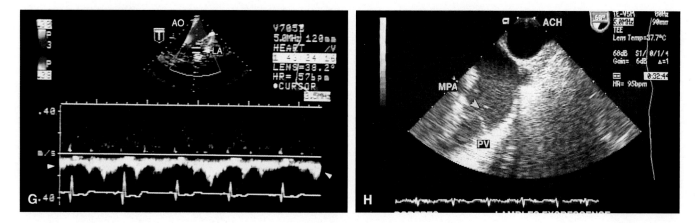

Figure 1.11. **Left pulmonary artery branches.** Transducer in the upper esophagus. Numbers 1 and 2 in **A** and **B** are branches of the left pulmonary artery (LPA). **C-E.** Multiple branches, some of them representing lobar arteries to upper and lower lobes of the left lung (arrowheads, numbers 1–4), in another patient. **F.** Pulsed Doppler interrogation of one of the branches demonstrates predominantly systolic flow signals (arrowhead).

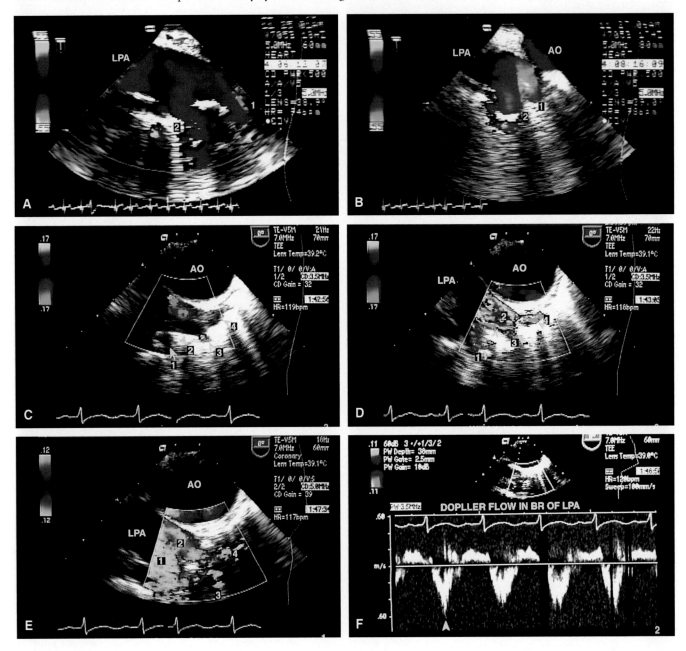

Figure 1.12. **Ascending aorta and pulmonary artery.** Transducer in the upper esophagus. **A-D.** Transverse plane examination shows the aorta in short axis with the main and right pulmonary arteries wrapping around it. The echo-free space to the right of the aorta is the superior vena cava (unlabeled in **D**). **D.** A catheter (C) is seen in the right pulmonary artery. **E.** A greater length of the left pulmonary artery is seen than in **D**. **F.** *Right panel:* The aorta and the SVC imaged in short axis using the transverse plane. The echo-free space anterior to the aorta is a pericardial effusion (PE). *Left panel:* Longitudinal plane examination of the SVC in the same patient. The pericardial effusion is seen anterior to the right atrium. **G.** The right pulmonary artery turns anteriorly after giving off the superior branch to the upper lobe. **H.** Longitudinal plane examination shows the ascending aorta (AO) in long axis and the right pulmonary artery (RPA) in short axis. (**E** reproduced with permission from Agrawal GG, Parekh HH, Tirtaman C, Nanda NC. Transesophageal echocardiographic imaging of the left atrium behind the ascending aorta mimicking aortic dissection: validation by contrast echocardiography. Echocardiography 1997;14:411–415.)

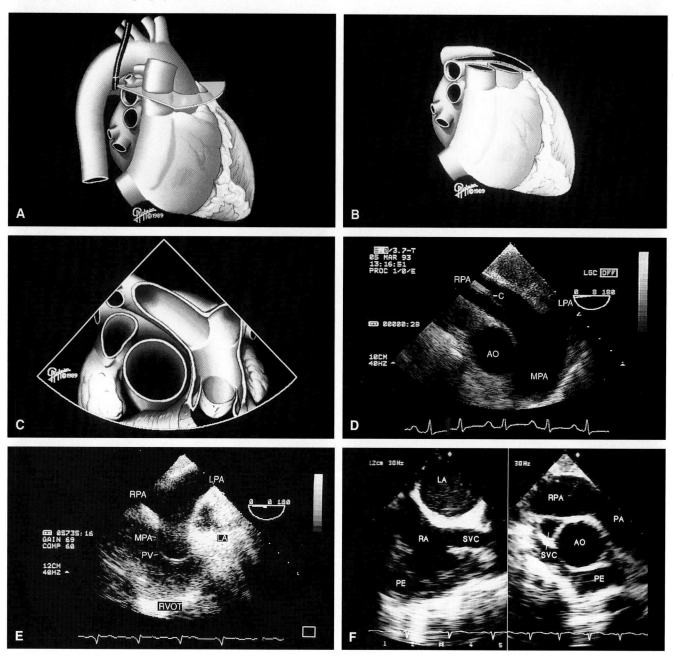

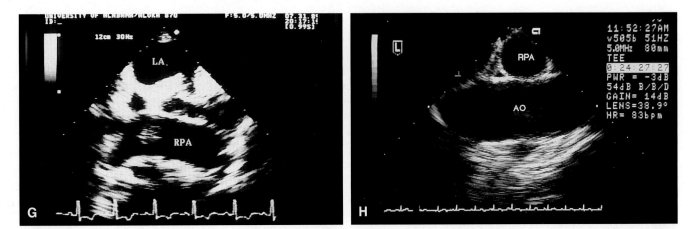

Figure 1.13. **Aortic root.** Advancement of the probe from the ascending aorta and arch position brings the aortic root into view. **A-E.** All three leaflets of the aortic valve (AV, AoV) are shown, open in systole and closed in diastole. *N*, noncoronary cusp; *L*, left coronary cusp; *R*, right coronary cusp. **F.** Aortic cusp (arrow) imaged in an oblique plane; this should not be mistaken for prolapse. In the true short-axis view (usually imaged at a plane angulation between 30° and 60° from the transverse plane, 0°) there was no cusp redundancy. (**A** reproduced with permission from Nanda NC, Pinheiro L, Sanyal RS, Storey O. Transesophageal biplane echocardiographic imaging: technique, planes, and clinical usefulness. Echocardiography 1990;7:771–788.)

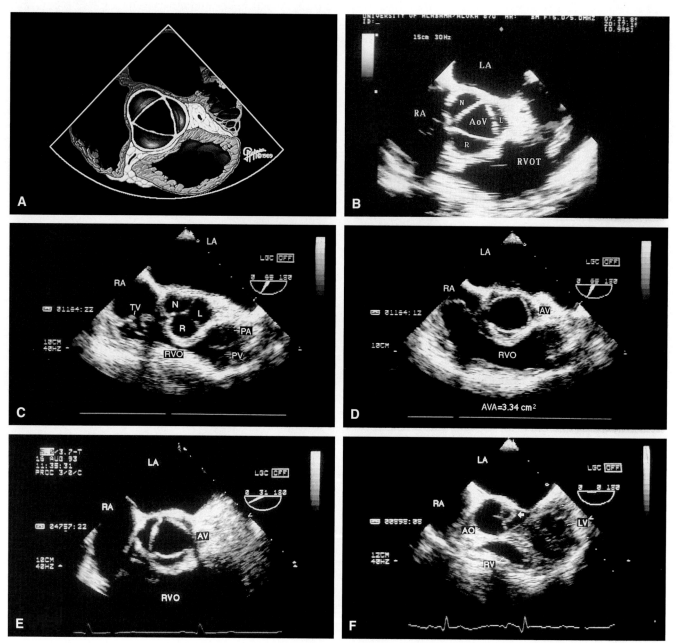

Figure 1.14. **A-G. Left atrial appendage.** The LAA should be imaged at various angulations with the multiplane probe to visualize all its lobes. **B.** Bilobed appendage (arrowheads). **C.** Pulsed Doppler interrogation of the LAA shows a prominent velocity waveform above the baseline following the P wave of the electrocardiogram, representing flow moving out of the LAA during atrial systole. This is followed immediately by a waveform recorded below the baseline, representing flow into the LAA in atrial diastole. With LAA dysfunction the velocities and waveform slopes are reduced. **D,E.** The pectinate muscles (arrows), which usually are transversely oriented and should not be mistaken for clot. The echo-free space lateral to the appendage most commonly indicates fat; however, the same picture is produced by a pericardial effusion. **F.** The echo density separating the appendage from the left upper pulmonary vein (LUPV) is a normal variant caused by nonspecific thickening. The arrow points to the left main coronary artery. **G.** Pectinate muscles in the LAA (arrowheads) in a patient with aortic dissection. The echo-free space lateral to the LAA is pericardial effusion. *F,* dissection flap; *FL,* false lumen; *TL,* true lumen.

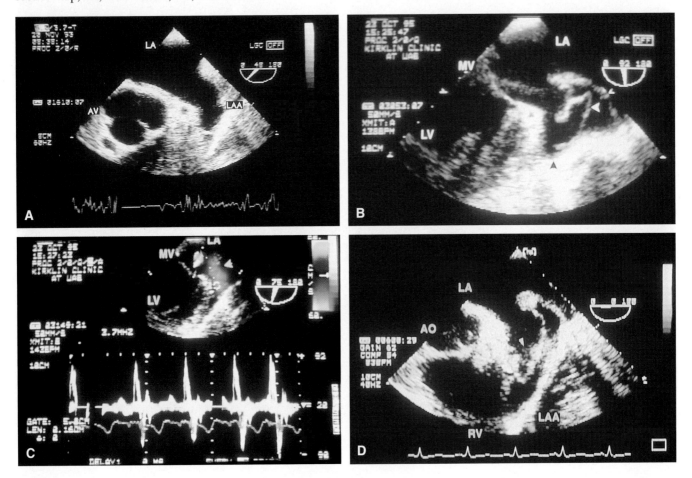

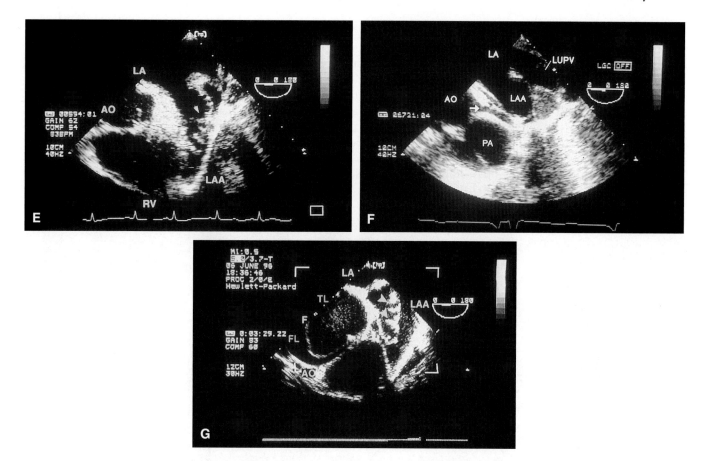

Figure 1.15. **A-C. Pulmonary valve**. All three leaflets of the pulmonary valve (left, anterior, and posterior cusps) are imaged in the closed position in diastole **(B)** and in the open position in systole **(C)**. Most commonly, only two cusps are seen **(A)**. **D-N. Coronary arteries. D.** The left main coronary artery (arrow) is seen originating from the aortic root and coursing laterally. The more distal anteriorly directed flow signals represent the left anterior descending branch. **E.** The left atrial branch (BLA) is well seen. *LM,* left main coronary artery. **F-I.** The left circumflex coronary artery (arrowheads) in the left atrioventricular groove in another patient. **J-L.** The first marginal branch of the left circumflex artery (Cx; arrowheads). **M.** Pulsed Doppler interrogation of the first marginal branch demonstrates predominantly diastolic flow signals (arrowheads). **N.** The right coronary artery is seen arising anteriorly from the aortic root between RA and RVO and coursing to the right toward the atrioventricular groove. **(F** and **K** reproduced with permission from Samdarshi T, et al. Usefulness and limitations of transesophageal echocardiography in the assessment of proximal coronary artery stenosis. J Am Coll Cardiol 1992;19:572–580.)

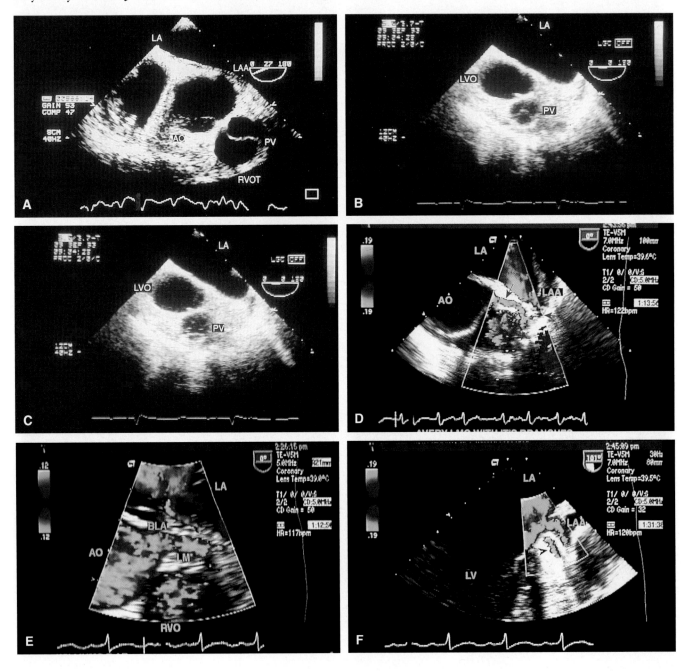

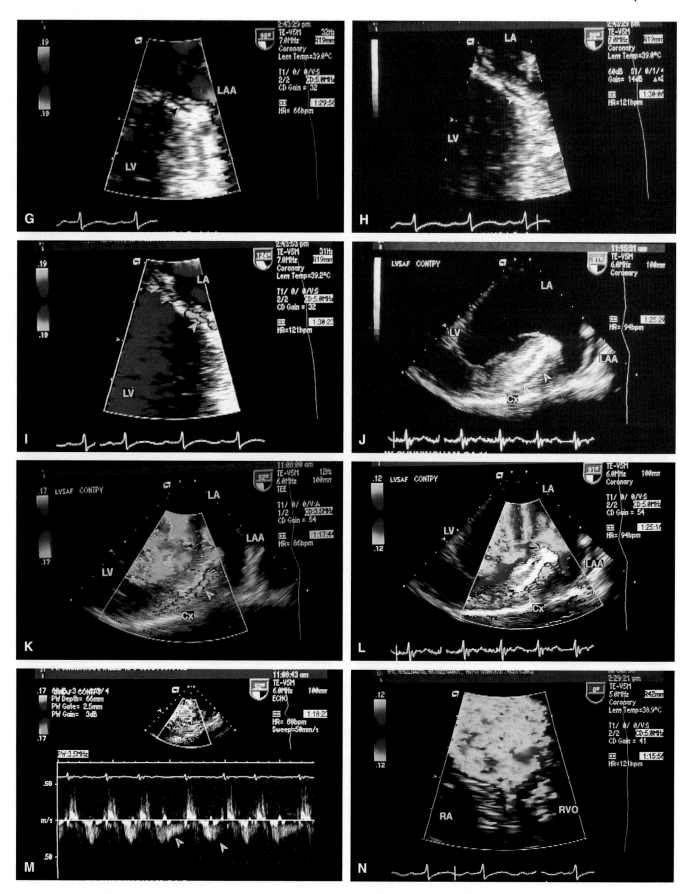

Figure 1.16. **Coronary arteries. A.** Slight withdrawal of the probe from the aortic root brings the sinuses of Valsalva into view. The left main (LM) coronary artery is seen arising from the left coronary sinus and the right coronary artery (RCA) from the right sinus. **B-F.** The entire course of the left main coronary artery (LM, LMCA) and its bifurcation into the left circumflex (CX, LCX) and left anterior descending (LAD) coronary arteries are shown. **G.** Pulsed Doppler examination of the LAD shows both systolic and diastolic flow signals. The diastolic flow signals have much higher velocity than the systolic signals. **H,I.** A long segment of the circumflex (CX) branch is seen coursing laterally. **J.** A long segment of the LAD courses anteriorly. **K.** The anterior (ANT) interventricular (I.V.) vein imaged next to the LAD. The flow in the vein is directed opposite to the LAD. This image was taken during rapid cardioplegia infusion, which reduced cardiac motion, thereby enhancing visualization of the vein. **L.** A ramus branch (br) is shown. **M.** The left main (LM), left circumflex (LCX), LAD, and a long segment of the first diagonal branch are all well seen. **N.** The left circumflex coronary artery (LCX CA) is shown in short axis next to the coronary sinus (CS) and the mitral valve. **O-R.** The right coronary artery (RCA, arrow) is seen originating anteriorly from the aorta and coursing to the right toward the right atrioventricular groove. **S,T.** Pulsed Doppler examination of the RCA demonstrates prominent systolic and diastolic signals. **T.** The systolic signals are more prominent than the diastolic signals in this patient. **U.** The posterior descending coronary artery (PDA) is visualized using the transgastric approach. (**F** and **K** reproduced with permission from Samdarshi T, et al. Usefulness and limitations of transesophageal echocardiography in the assessment of coronary artery stenosis. J Am Coll Cardiol 1992;19:572–580.)

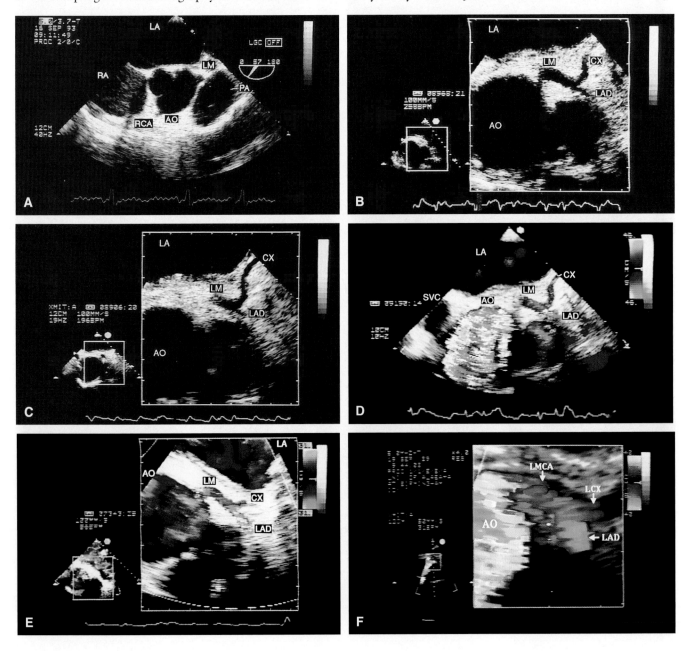

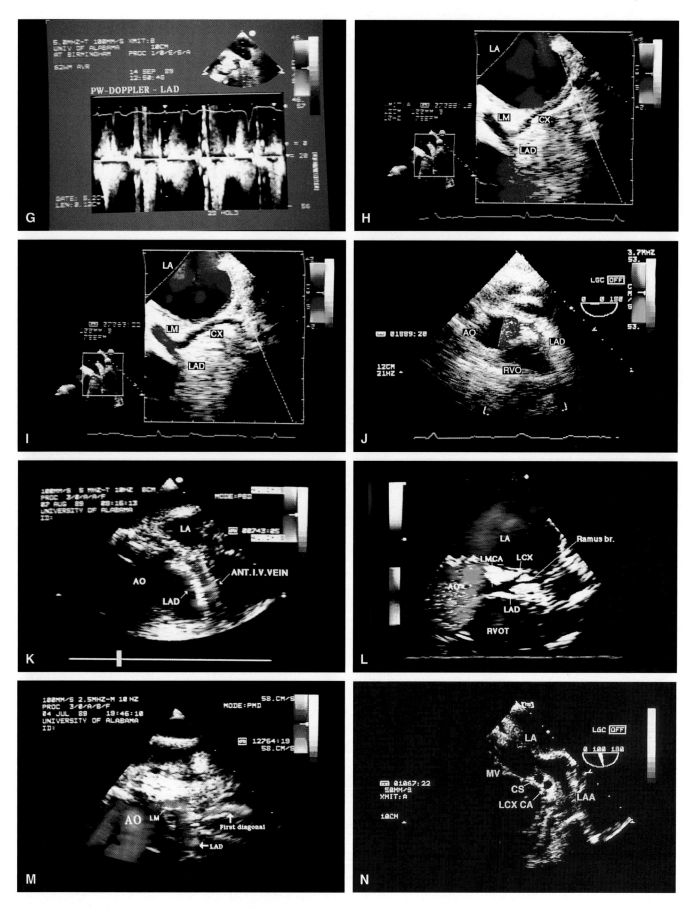

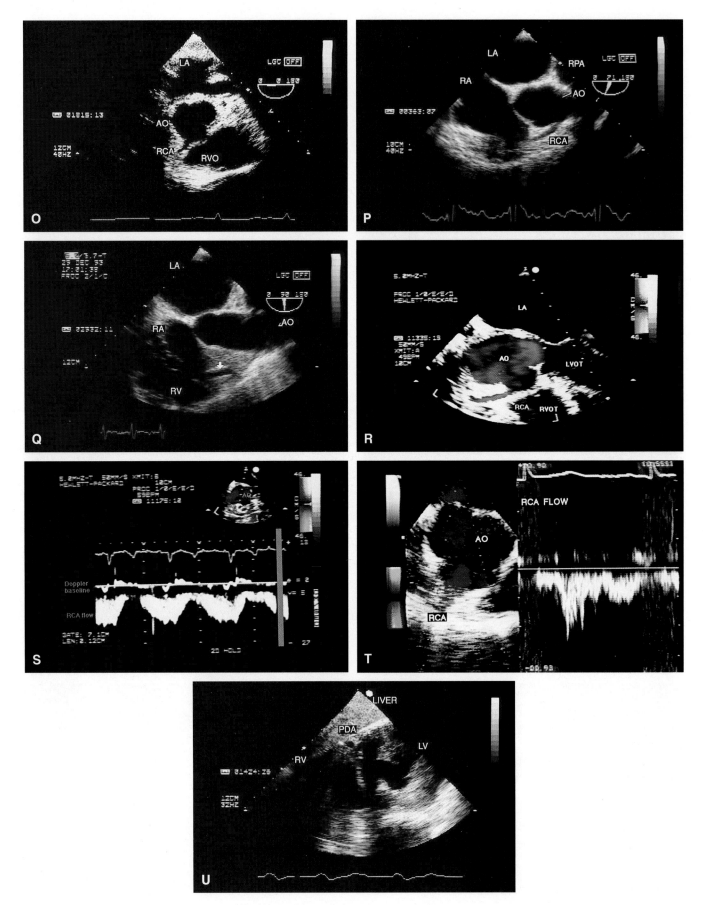

Figure 1.17. A-G. **Aortic root and ascending aorta.** Longitudinal plane examination shows the aortic root and the ascending aorta (AO) in long axis. **B.** The sinuses of Valsalva are well seen. Two other patients are shown, one in **E** and one in **F** and **G**. The linear echo (arrowheads in **F** and **G**) attached to the aortic valve on the side of the aorta is a Lambl's excrescence, which is a normal finding. (**A** and **B** reproduced with permission from Nanda NC, Pinheiro L, Sanyal RS, Storey O. Transesophageal biplane echocardiographic imaging: technique, planes, and clinical usefulness. Echocardiography 1990;7:771–788.)

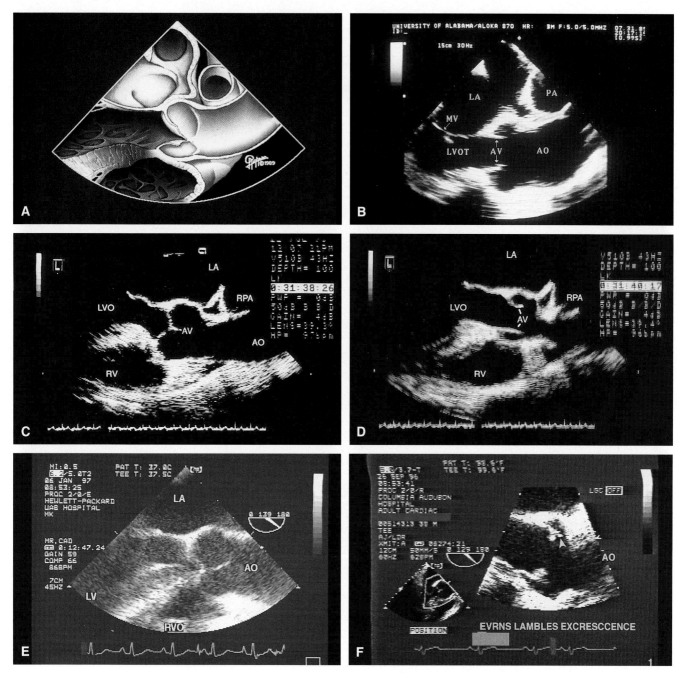

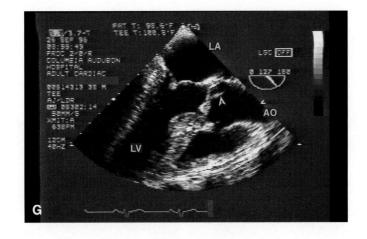

Figure 1.18. Pulmonary veins. A-O. A. Diagrammatic representation of the pulmonary veins. *Left:* Posterior view of the heart. The relationship of the pulmonary veins to the adjacent structures is shown. The arrows depict the spatial orientation of the pulmonary vein trunks. *Right*: Superior view of the heart. During longitudinal plane examination, imaging of the right and left pulmonary veins is accomplished by posterior displacement of the ultrasonic plane by rotation of the probe (T1) from the position used for viewing the right and left upper pulmonary veins. When the lower veins enter the left atrium in a posteroanterior direction rather than the frontal plane (as shown with the right lower pulmonary vein [RLPV]), successful imaging of their proximal portions is accomplished by first advancing the probe (from T1 to T2) and then rotating it. B. Diagrammatic representation of transverse (T) and longitudinal (L) plane examination of the upper and lower pulmonary veins (right-sided veins are used in this example). The RLPV is visualized by slight advancement (straight arrow) and clockwise rotation (curved arrows) of the probe. C. Composite image obtained by combining three consecutive transverse views shows the angle of entrance of the left upper pulmonary vein (LUPV) into the LA and its close relationship with the LAA and the descending thoracic aorta (DA). D-G. Sequence of frames from one patient demonstrates all four pulmonary veins using transverse and longitudinal plane examination. D. Transverse plane imaging of the left lower pulmonary vein (LLPV; left panel) and LUPV (right panel). E. Longitudinal plane imaging of the LLPV (left panel) and LUPV (right panel). The left pulmonary artery (LPA) is located superior to the LUPV. F. Transverse plane imaging of the RLPV (left panel) and right upper pulmonary vein (RUPV; right panel). Unlike the RUPV, the entrance of the RLPV is located at a considerable distance from the interatrial septum. The RUPV enters LA just posterior to the SVC. G. Longitudinal plane imaging of the RLPV (left panel) and RUPV (right panel). The right pulmonary artery (RPA) is seen in short axis just superior to RUPV. The insets show pulsed Doppler spectral traces from the respective pulmonary veins. H. Longitudinal plane imaging of the distal portion of the LUPV. Several tributaries (T) are seen joining the main trunk of LUPV (left panel). Slight counterclockwise rotation of the probe with further leftward displacement of the ultrasonic plane demonstrates branching of the left pulmonary artery (LPA) (arrows, right panel). I. Transverse plane examination of the LUPV and LLPV in another patient. Note that, unlike the LUPV, the lower vein is not related to the LAA. In this example, the lower vein is seen together with the posterior atrioventricular groove and the LV. Withdrawing the probe from this position to the level of the main pulmonary artery (PA) brought the LUPV into view in this patient. J. In the longitudinal plane examination (left) in this patient, the LUPV was imaged first. The transducer was then tilted to the left to include the lower vein. The probe was not rotated or advanced. In the transverse plane examination (right), the lower vein was delineated first, and the transducer then was tilted upward to image the upper vein. The two pulmonary veins are separated by a wide angle, but they converge to open into the left atrium (LA) not far from each other. K. In the transverse plane examination (left) in a different patient, the right upper and lower pulmonary veins are visualized simultaneously. The dotted line represents the level at which the longitudinal plane is taken (right panel). Although the RUPV is visualized in both examination modes, the transverse plane sections the lateral walls of the vein while the longitudinal plane cuts through the superior and inferior walls. *C*, catheter in right pulmonary artery. L. Composite image resulting from the combination of three consecutive transverse views, obtained by rotation of the probe. The presence of pleural effusion (PLE) in this patient permits delineation of the entire course of the RLPV from the hilum of the lung to its entrance into the left atrium (LA). M. Examination of the right pulmonary veins in an adult patient with sinus venosus atrial septal defect. The RUPV overrides the defect (arrowheads), and its flow is seen to enter both the RA and the LA (left panel). The RLPV enters LA normally (right panel). N-O. Separate (N) and simultaneous (O) examination of the RLPV and RUPV in another patient. As with the left-sided veins, the right-sided veins are separated from each other by a wide angle. This is more apparent when the veins are imaged separately rather than simultaneously. In this patient, the RUPV was imaged first and then the transducer was tilted to the right to view the RLPV simultaneously. **Left pulmonary veins. P-S.** The left upper pulmonary vein (LUPV, LPV) is imaged adjacent to the left atrial appendage. **T.** The left lower pulmonary vein is imaged at a plane angulation of 41°. When two left-sided veins are imaged, the one adjacent to the left atrial appendage usually is the left upper pulmonary vein, and the one not adjacent to the appendage is the left lower pulmonary vein. **Right pulmonary veins. U-Y.** Transverse plane examination (U) shows the RUPV imaged next to the SVC viewed in short axis. Pulsed Doppler examination shows a large systolic (S) wave, a smaller diastolic (D) wave, and a small atrial systolic A wave in the opposite direction representing flow from the LA into the vein. Longitudinal plane examination (V–X) shows the RUPV imaged adjacent to the right pulmonary artery (RPA). **Y.** The RUPV and RLPV are simultaneously visualized. The RLPV is imaged lateral and posterior to the RUPV (small vertical arrow). (A–O reproduced with permission from Pinheiro L, Nanda NC, Jain H, Sanyal R. Transesophageal echocardiographic imaging of the pulmonary veins. Echocardiography 1991;8:741–748.)

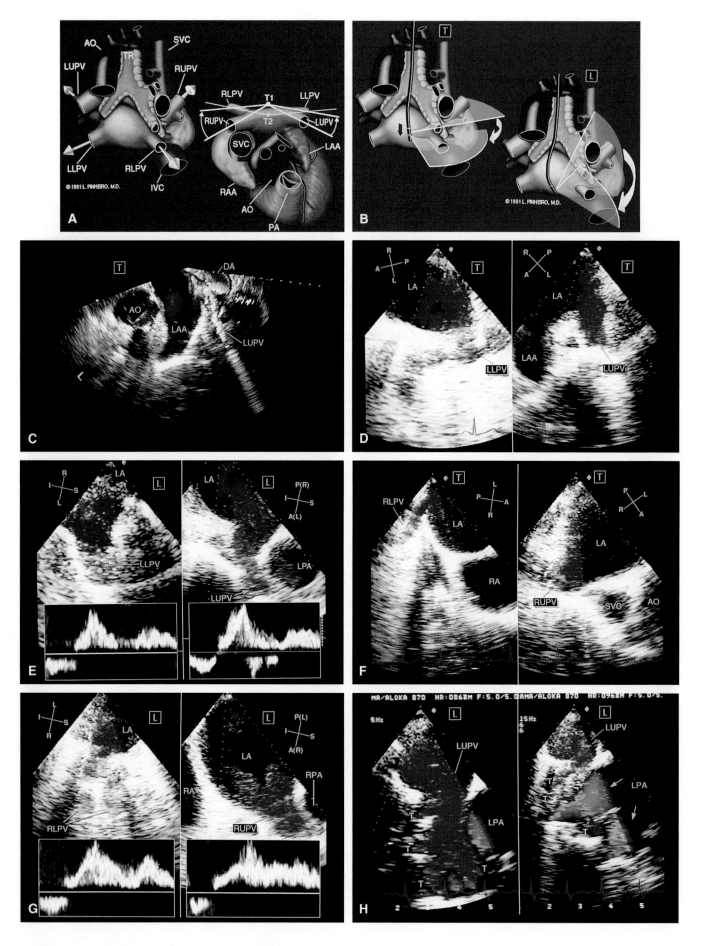

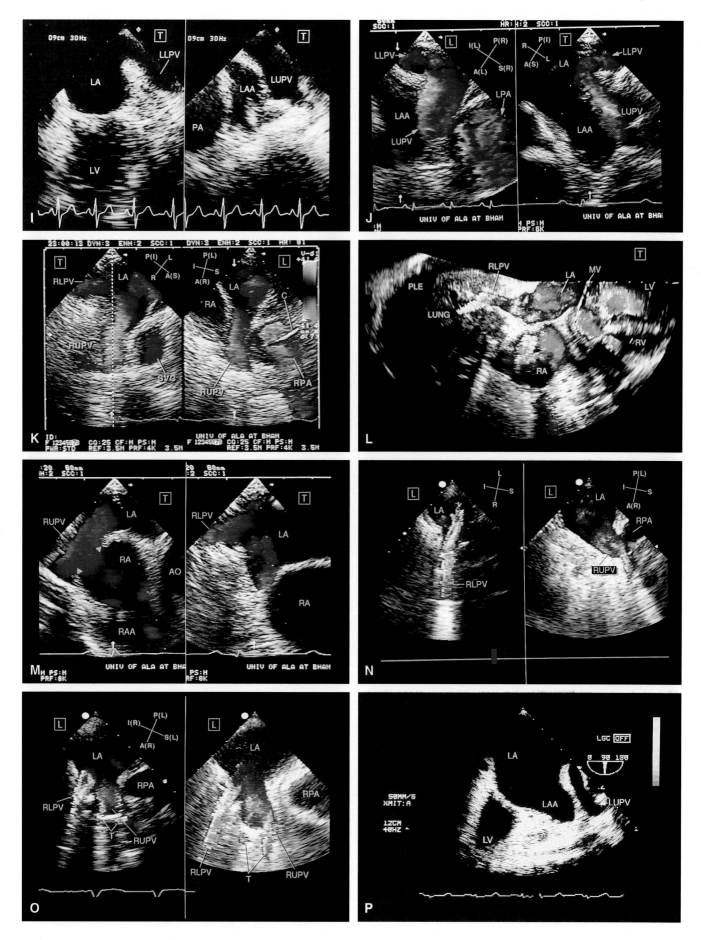

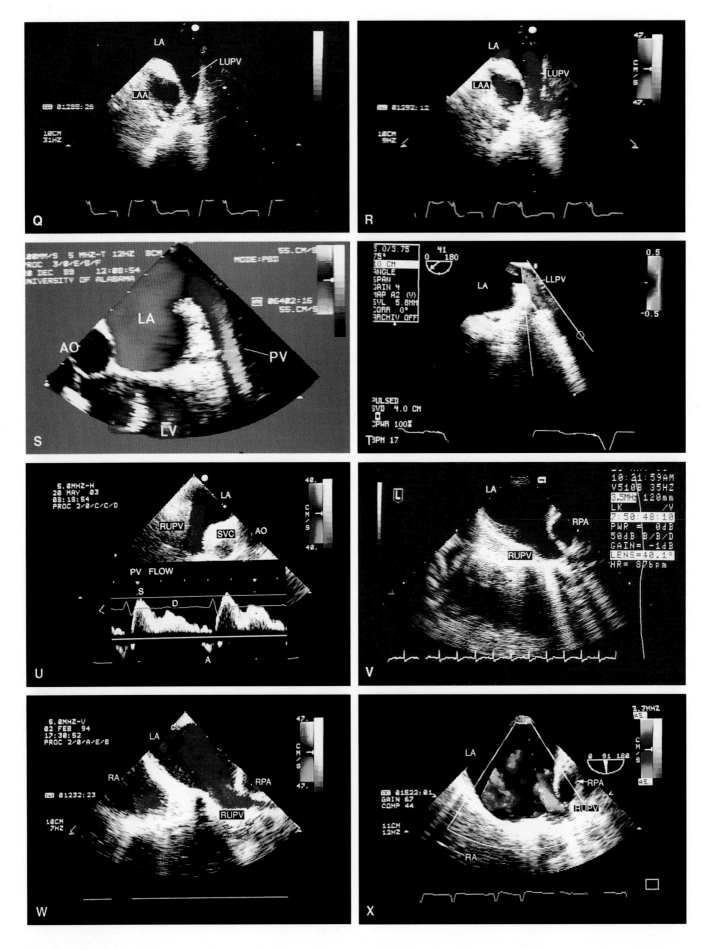

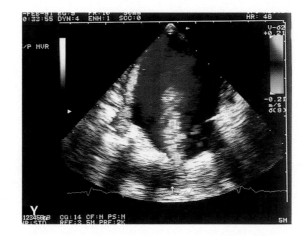

Figure 1.19. **A–K. Right ventricle and pulmonary valve.** The longitudinal plane examination demonstrates the right ventricular outflow tract (RVOT), the PV, and the proximal pulmonary artery in **A** through **G**, **I**, and **K**. Abnormalities of the RVOT and PV are often well seen in this plane. The TV leaflets are demonstrated in **B** and in **F** through **J**. **H.** The inferior posterior (P) and the anterior (A) leaflets of the TV are shown. **I,J.** All three leaflets of the tricuspid valve (*A*, *AL*, anterior; *P*, *PL*, posterior or inferior; *S*, *SL*, septal) can sometimes be imaged. The anterior and septal leaflets are separated by the anteroseptal commissure, the anterior and posterior leaflets by the anteroposterior commissure, and the posterior and septal leaflets by the posteroseptal commissure. *AZ*, azygos vein; *E*, esophagus; *LCC*, left coronary cusp; *NCC*, aortic noncoronary cusp; *RCC*, aortic right coronary cusp; *TC*, tricuspid valve cusps. **L–N. Ascending aorta.** Clockwise rotation of the probe from the position where one sees the RVOT and pulmonary artery brings the aortic root and ascending aorta (A) into view. The IVC and eustachian valve (EV) also are visualized in **N**. (**A** through **D**, **G**, and **K** reproduced with permission from Nanda NC, Pinheiro L, Sanyal RS, Storey O. Transesophageal biplane echocardiographic imaging: technique, planes, and clinical usefulness. Echocardiography 1990;7:771–788. **H** through **J** reproduced with permission from Maxted W, Nanda NC, Kim KS, et al. Transesophageal echocardiographic identification and validation of individual tricuspid valve leaflets. Echocardiography 1994;11:585–596.)

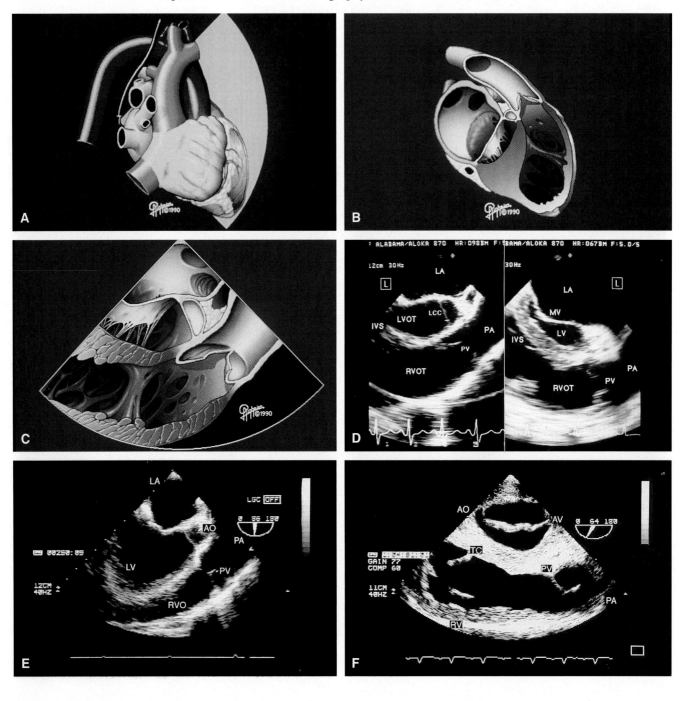

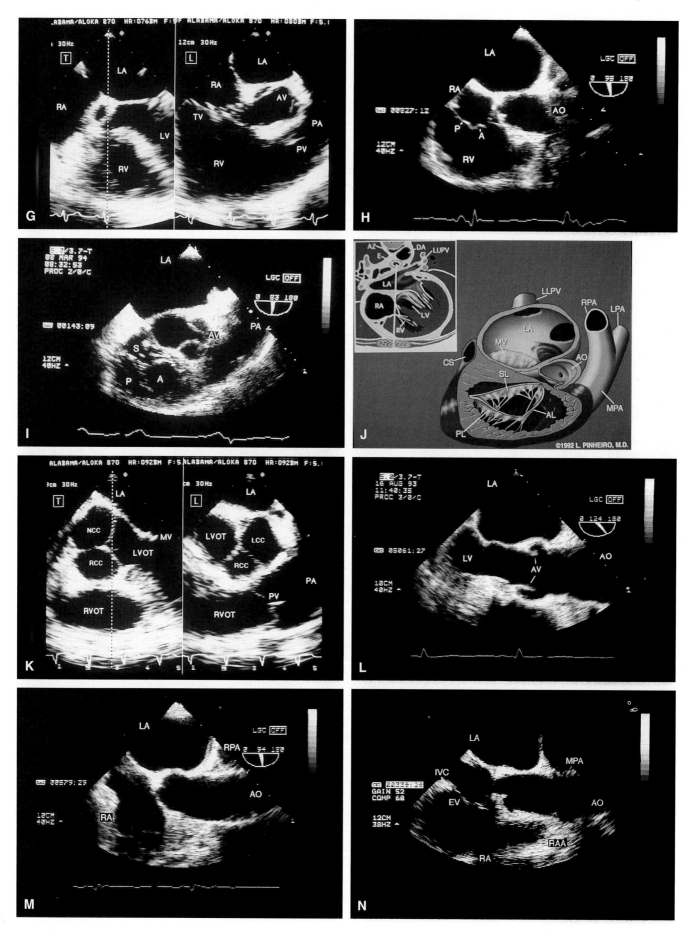

Figure 1.20. **A–N. Superior vena cava and right atrium.** Longitudinal (L) plane examination shows the SVC and its entry into the RA, viewed in long axis. **D.** The crista terminalis (arrow). **E.** A right pulmonary artery (RPA) bifurcation is seen. **F.** Normal trabeculation in the RA (arrowheads). **I–K.** Intravenous injection of normal saline results in the appearance of contrast echoes in the SVC, with subsequent filling of the RA. **L.** Intravenous normal saline injection results in the appearance of contrast echoes in the SVC (left panel), with subsequent filling of the right pulmonary artery (RPA; middle and right panels). The arrow in the left panel points to a catheter in the RPA). **M,N.** The azygos vein (closed arrow) is seen entering the right superior vena cava (RSVC). The open arrow represents the superior branch of the right pulmonary artery. Intravenous injection of normal saline results in the appearance of contrast echoes in the RSVC and RA. A few contrast signals are noted entering the azygos vein. A large thrombus (TH) with adjacent spontaneous contrast echoes is noted in the LA in this patient with mitral stenosis. (**A** through **D, G,** and **L** reproduced with permission from Nanda NC, Pinheiro L, Sanyal RS, Storey O. Transesophageal biplane echocardiographic imaging: technique, planes, and clinical usefulness. Echocardiography 1990;7:771–788. **M** and **N** reproduced with permission from Nanda NC, Pinheiro L, Sanyal R, et al. Transesophageal echocardiographic examination of left-sided superior vena cava and azygos and hemiazygos veins. Echocardiography 1991;8:731–739.)

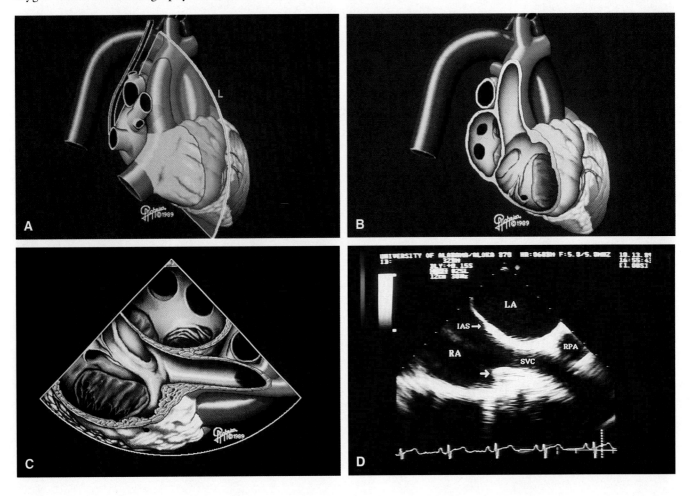

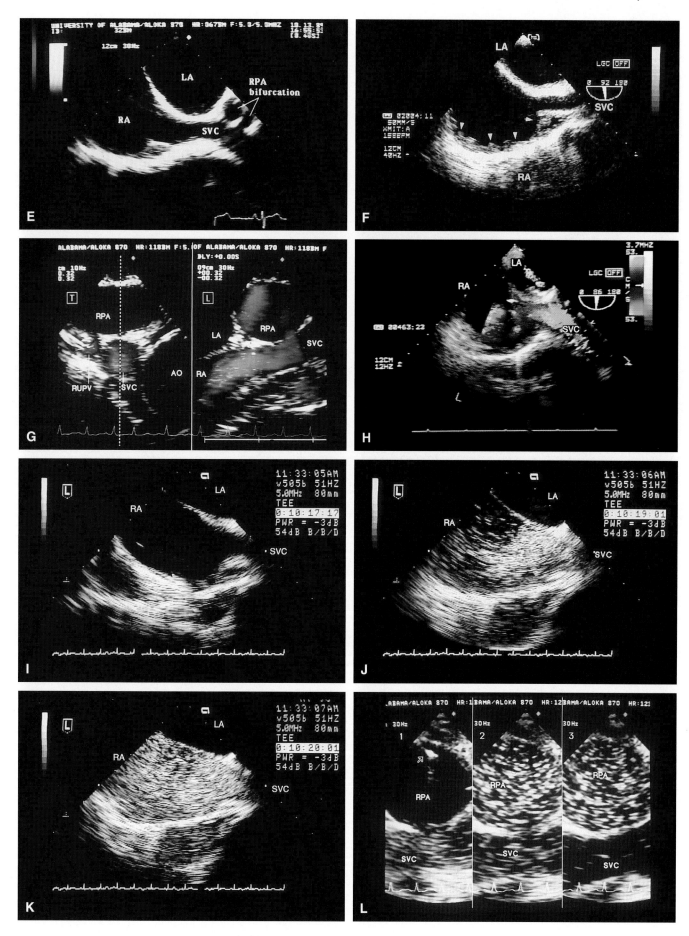

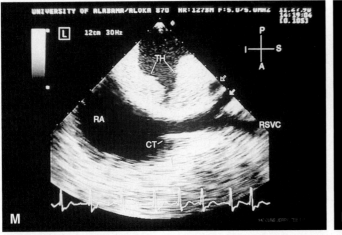

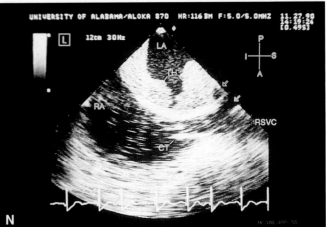

Figure 1.21. **A-I. Five-chamber view.** This view is obtained by further advancement of the probe from the aortic root position. In addition to imaging both atria and ventricles, this view shows the aortic root (AO in **E**). **H.** A plane angulation of 5° shows the noncoronary (N) and the right coronary (R) cusps of the aortic valve; plane angulation at 111° shows the left (L) and right (R) leaflets. **I.** Intravenous injection of normal saline results in the appearance of contrast echoes in the RA and the RVOT, but the left-sided structures are not opacified. (**C** reproduced with permission from Nanda NC, Mahan EF III. Transesophageal echocardiography. AHA Council on Clinical Cardiology Newsletter 1990;Summer:3–22.)

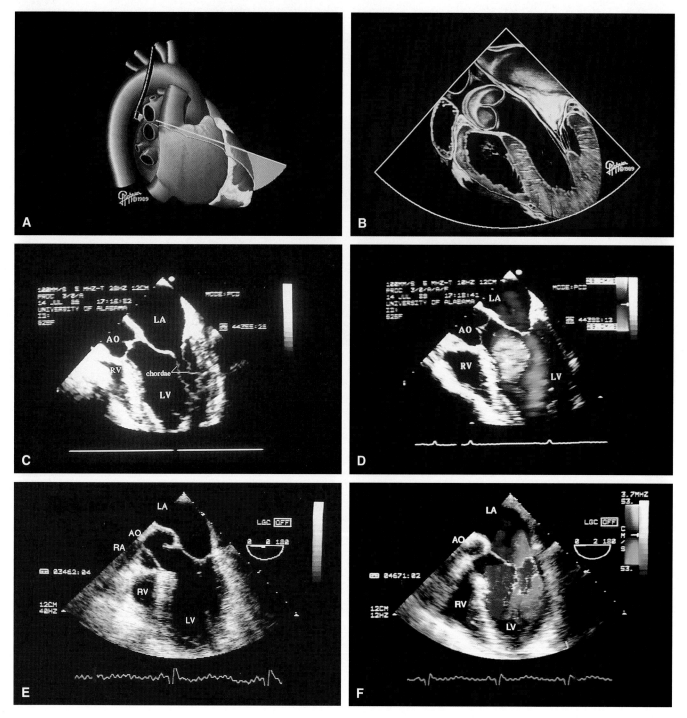

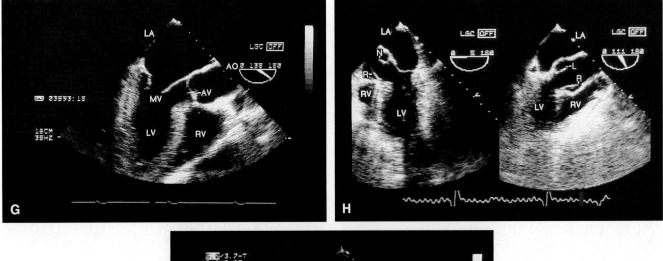

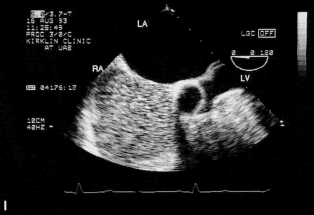

Figure 1.22. **A-I. Four-chamber view.** The four-chamber view is obtained by slight advancement of the probe from the five-chamber view. Both the atria and ventricles as well as the mitral (anterior [AML] and posterior [PML] leaflets) and tricuspid (anterior [A] and septal [S] leaflets) valves are seen. The VS and the LV posterolateral walls are seen in this view. In **C** the linear echo on the ventricular aspect of the MV represents a Lambl's excrescence. **G.** The valve of the foramen ovale (VFO) is shown. **H,I.** The atrial septum (arrowheads) bulging into the RA **(H)** and into the LA **(I)** during different phases of the cardiac cycle reflecting changing hemodynamics. The atrial septum bulges into the atrium with the lower pressure. (**B** reproduced with permission by Nanda NC, Pinheiro L, Sanyal RS, Storey O. Transesophageal biplane echocardiographic imaging: technique, planes, and clinical usefulness. Echocardiography 1990;7:771–788. **F** reproduced with permission from Maxted W, Nanda NC, Kim KS, et al. Transesophageal echocardiographic identification and validation of individual tricuspid valve leaflets. Echocardiography 1994;11:585–596.)

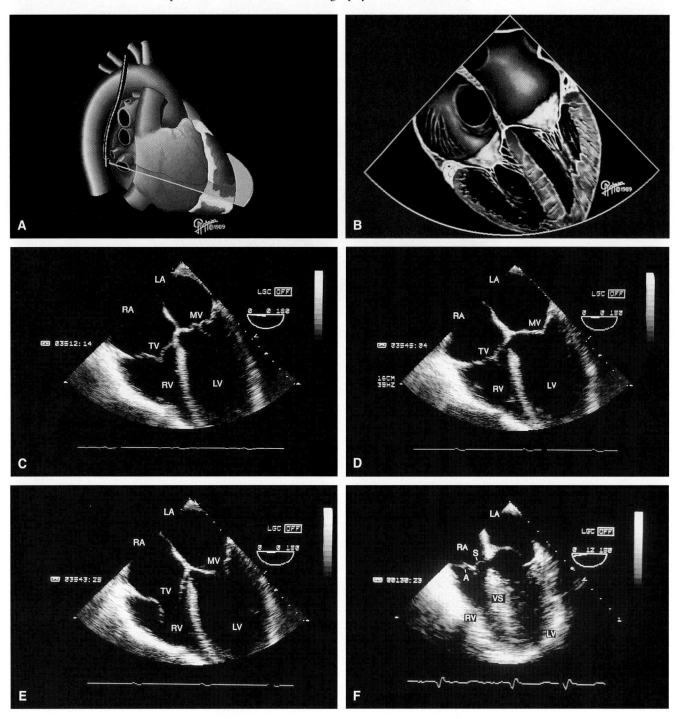

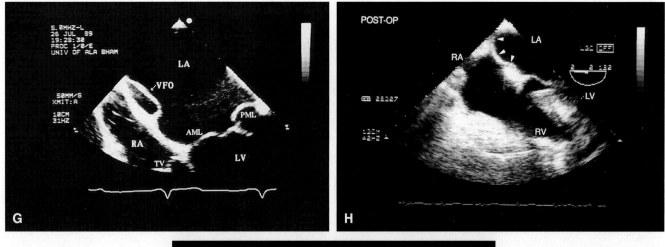

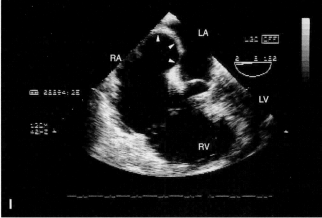

Figure 1.23. Two-chamber view. Angulation of the beam 90° from the four-chamber view demonstrates the orthogonal two-chamber view. In this view the inferior and anterior free walls of the LV are seen. The LAA is noted on the same side as the anterior free wall. *C*, chordae tendinae. (**A** and **E** reproduced with permission from Nanda NC, Pinheiro L, Sanyal RS, Storey O. Transesophageal biplane echocardiographic imaging: technique, planes, and clinical usefulness. Echocardiography 1990;7:771–788. **B** reproduced with permission from Nanda NC, Mahan EF III. Transesophageal echocardiography. AHA Council on Clinical Cardiology Newsletter 1990;Summer:3–22. **C** reproduced with permission from Mahan EF III, Nanda NC. Transesophageal echocardiography. In: Rackley CE, ed. Challenges in Cardiology I. Mount Kisco, NY: Futura, 1992:85–101.)

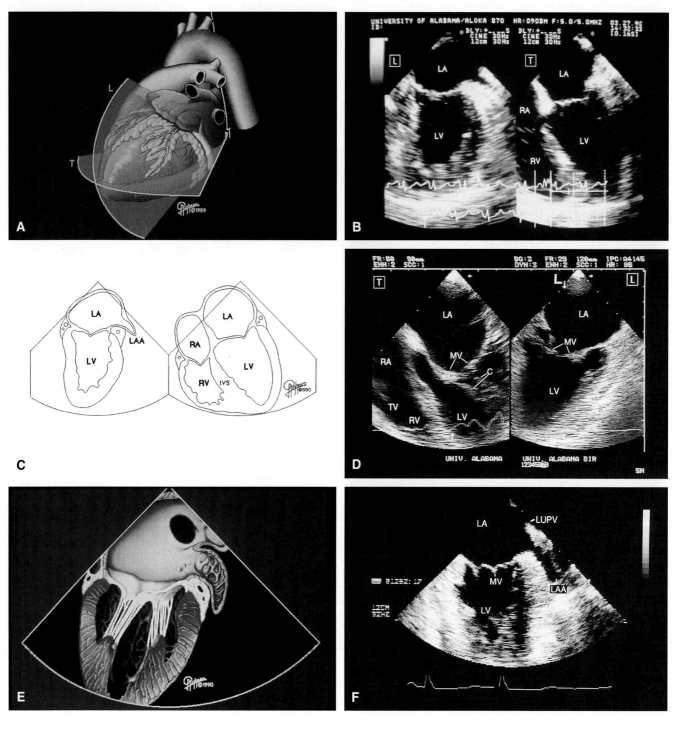

Figure 1.24. **Superior and inferior vena cava. A-J.** The SVC and IVC are shown simultaneously in **A** through **E** and **H** through **J**. The eustachian valve (EV) is noted at the IVC-RA junction in **E** through **G**. The region of the foramen ovale and the tricuspid valve may also be visualized.

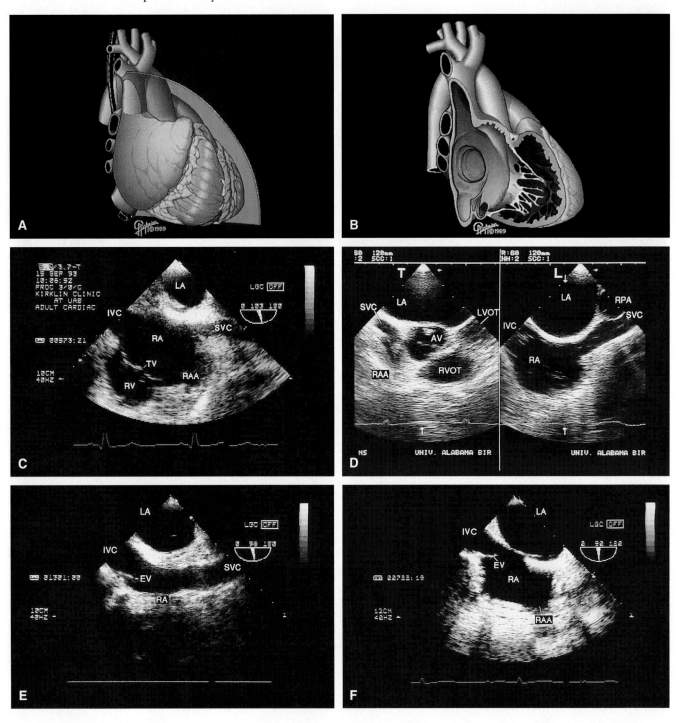

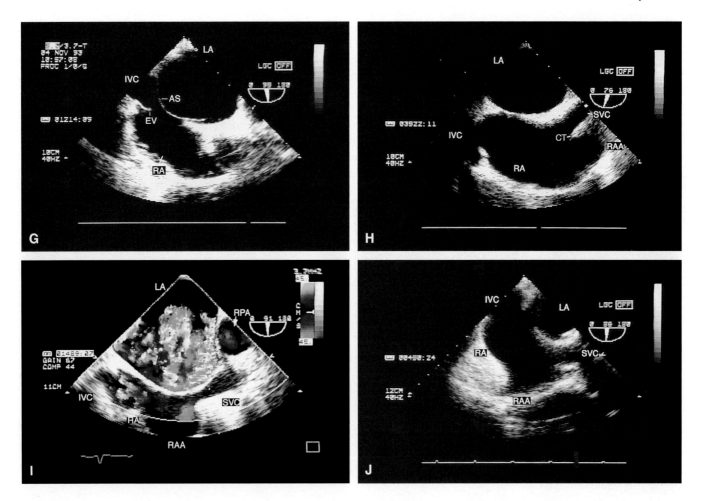

Figure 1.25. **A-M. Right atrial appendage and tricuspid valve.** Advancing the probe down the esophagus from the four-chamber view with slight rotation often brings the RAA into view. The coronary sinus (CS), IVC, and the anterior (A) and septal (S) leaflets of the tricuspid valve may also be well visualized. **D.** A pericardial effusion (PE) is present behind the RAA. **G.** A catheter (arrow) in the RV. The eustachian valve (EV), a normal vestigial structure, often is seen at the RA-IVC junction. **I,J.** A large, patulous eustachian valve with a fishnet appearance often is referred to as a Chiari network (C). It generally produces no obstruction or embolism but has been confused with RA tumor. **K.** The thebesian valve, another vestigial structure, often is seen at the coronary sinus-RA junction. **L.** SVC, IVC, and CS are imaged simultaneously. This corresponds to the schematic shown in **C. M.** Pulsed Doppler interrogation of the coronary sinus shows prominent systolic and diastolic flow signals. (**E** reproduced with permission from Maxted W, Nanda NC, Kim KS, et al. Transesophageal echocardiographic identification and validation of individual tricuspid valve leaflets. Echocardiography 1994;11:585–596.)

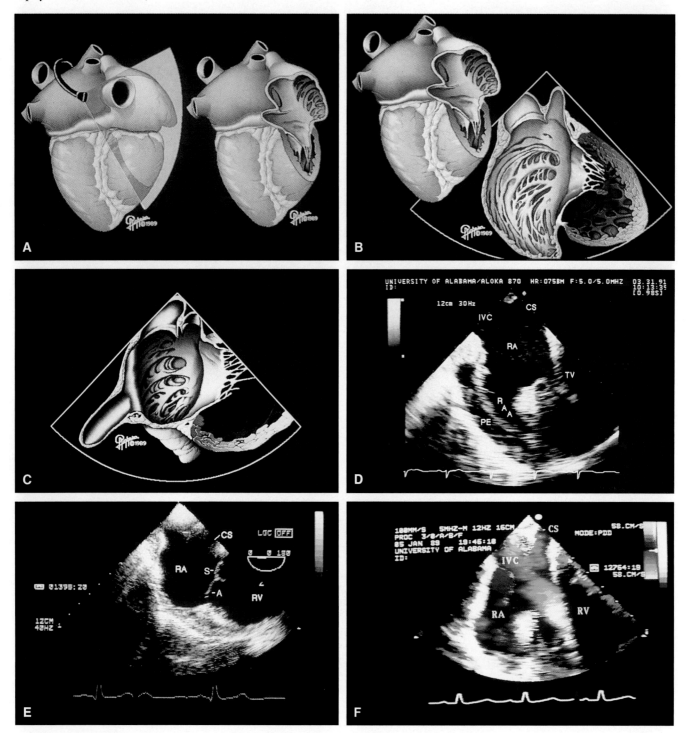

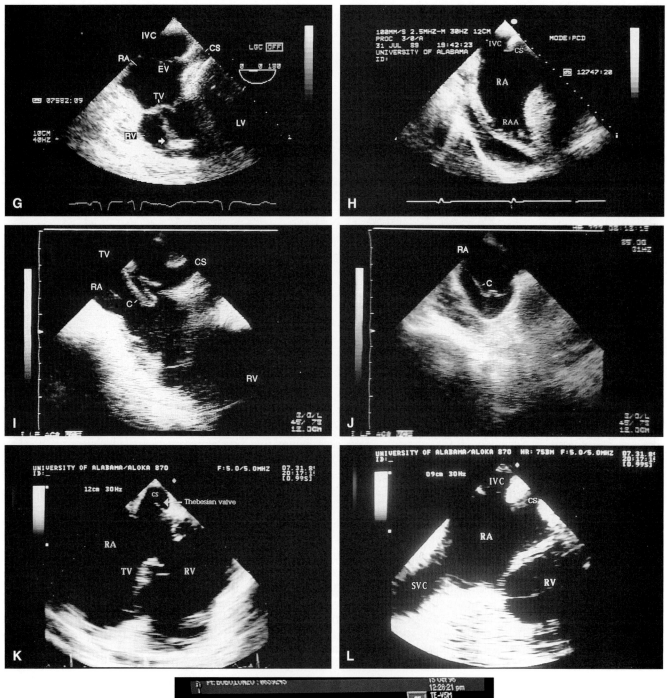

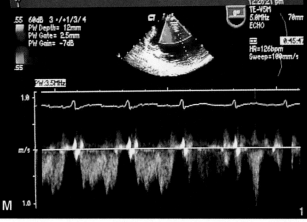

Figure 1.26. **Mitral valve.** The short-axis view of the mitral valve may be obtained with the transducer positioned close to the esophageal-gastric junction. *AMVL*, anterior mitral leaflet; *PMVL*, posterior mitral leaflet.

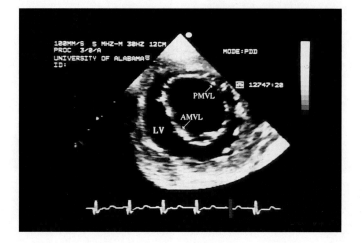

Figure 1.27. **A-S. Descending thoracic aorta and azygos and hemiazygos veins.** The entire extent of the descending thoracic aorta (AO) can be viewed in multiple planes by rotating the transducer posteriorly and moving it up and down the esophagus. **A.** Schematic. **B,C.** Echo-free spaces seen behind the aorta represent an artifact caused by the close proximity of the aorta to the transducer. The vertical echoes within this space are reverberation artifacts. **E.** An intercostal artery is well seen and should not be confused with aortic dissection. **F.** Pulsed Doppler interrogation of the intercostal artery shows both systolic and diastolic flow signals, typical of a low-resistance vessel. **G.** A large pleural effusion (PLE) is present behind the aorta. **H.** A large color artifact is present next to the descending aorta and should not be mistaken for a vascular structure. **I.** Flow signals are more prominent in the reverberation artifact (R) than in the descending aorta (AO) itself. **J- L.** The hemiazygos vein (HAZ) is noted joining the azygos vein (AZ) in the transverse plane examination **(J,K).** Both HAZ and AZ are located posterior to the descending thoracic aorta (DA). Pulsed Doppler interrogation of HAZ and AZ demonstrates low-velocity, continuous signals throughout the cardiac cycle, typical of venous flow **(K). L.** Both AZ and DA are imaged in long axis using the longitudinal plane examination. When AZ is prominently imaged, as in this patient, an erroneous diagnosis of aortic dissection may be made because the two vessels are in close contact with each other and their contiguous walls may be misinterpreted as a dissection flap separating the true and false lumens of a dissected aorta. Therefore, it is important to perform a pulsed Doppler examination, which will show continuous venous flow pattern throughout the cardiac cycle in AZ. **M.** An intercostal vein (ICV) is seen draining into the HAZ, which connects with the AZ. **N.** Anatomic illustration shows the relation of the AZ to the RSVC, the RPA, and the superior branch of RPA. **O–R.** Pulsed Doppler interrogation also helps to differentiate the veins of the azygos system from other vessels in the vicinity, e.g., intercostal and bronchial arteries. **O.** The right (RIC) and left (LIC) posterior intercostal arteries are noted adjacent to HAZ. Pulsed Doppler interrogation of RIC in this patient (P) shows arterial-type flow signals confined mainly to systole. **Q.** ICVs viewed adjacent to the DA imaged in long axis in the longitudinal plane examination. The inset shows venous-type flow signals obtained by color Doppler–guided pulsed Doppler interrogation of one of these veins. **R.** The relationship of a bronchial artery (BA) to the DA, the LPA, and its branches (arrows). The inset shows arterial-type flow signals obtained by color Doppler–guided pulsed Doppler interrogation of this vessel. The prominent flow signals in diastole reflect the flow resistance of the pulmonary vascular bed. *SP*, spine. **S.** An intervertebral disk (VB), as well as a "pulsating" spinal cord, may be visualized posteriorly from the upper esophagus. (**A** and **G** reproduced with permission from Nanda NC, Pinheiro L, Sanyal RS, Storey O. Transesophageal biplane echocardiographic imaging: technique, planes, and clinical usefulness. Echocardiography 1990;7:771–788. **D** reproduced with permission from Nanda N, et al. Innovations in echocardiography. Cardiology Trends 1990;10:1,22–23. **J–R** reproduced with permission from Nanda NC, Pinheiro L, Sanyal R, et al. Transesophageal echocardiographic examination of left-sided superior vena cava and azygos and hemiazygos veins. Echocardiography 1991;8:731–739.)

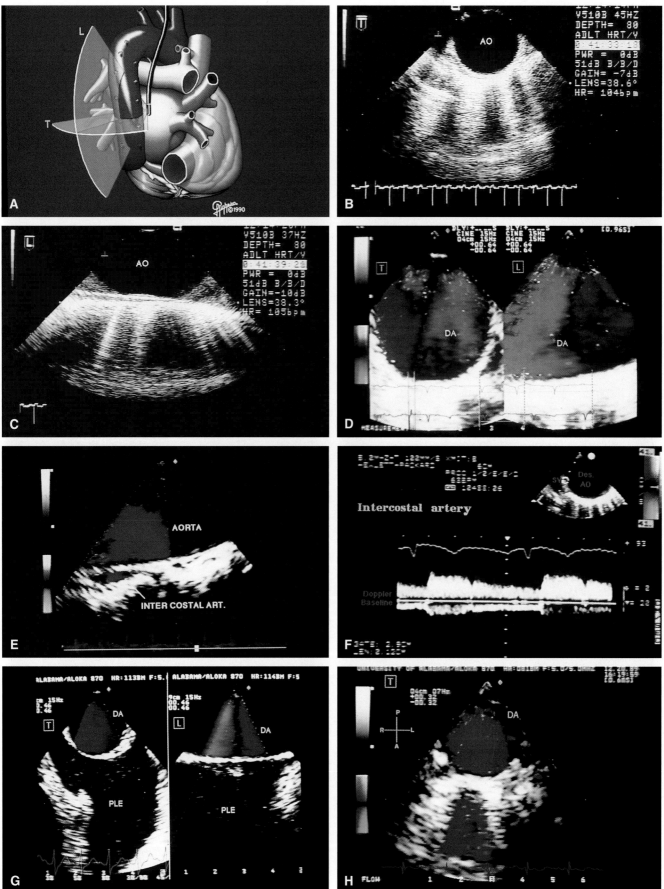

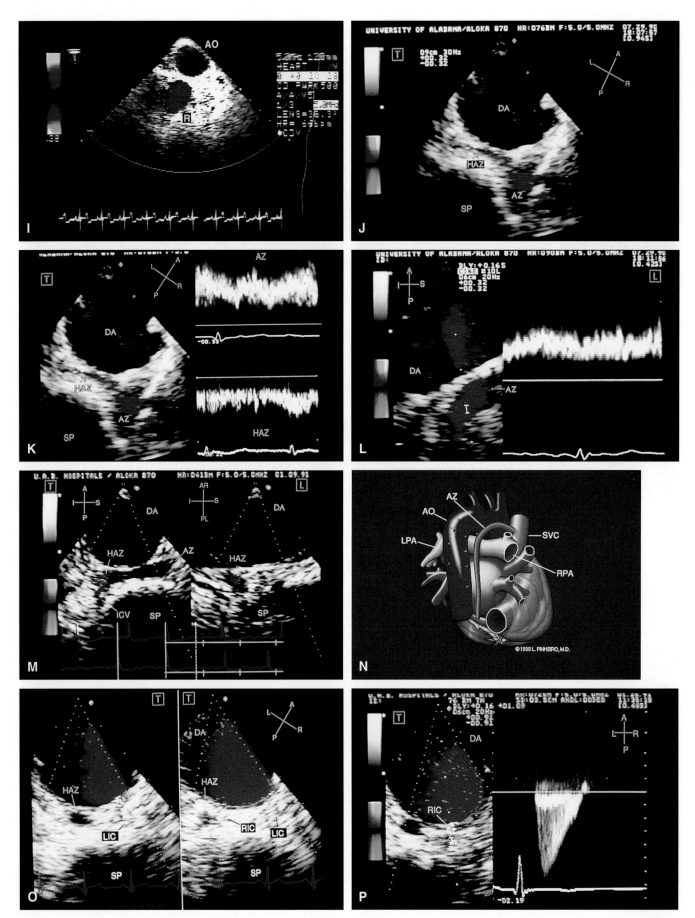

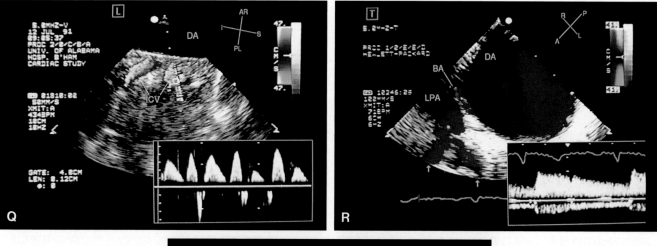

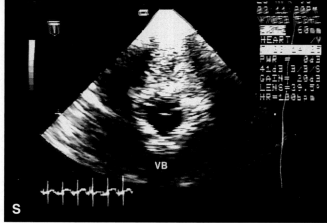

Figure 1.28. **Transgastric views.** The transducer is advanced into the stomach and is flexed when it abuts the gastric wall. In these views, the liver (L) is always in the near field. **A.** Schematic. **B–D.** The anterior (AML) and posterior (PML) leaflets of the mitral valve, together with chordae tendinae (C), are seen in short axis in the open and closed positions (transverse plane examination). The mitral valve commissures are well seen. **E.** LV endocardium (closed arrow) and trabeculated RV wall (open arrow). **F–L.** Minimal advancement from the mitral leaflets brings the papillary muscles into view. These can be imaged in both long and short axis. *S, VS,* ventricular septum; *A, AL, ALPM,* anterolateral papillary muscle; *P, PM, PMPM,* posteromedial papillary muscle; *ANT,* anterior LV wall; *INF,* inferior LV wall; *LAD,* lateral wall. **M,N.** A heavily trabeculated LV (arrowheads) imaged in the apical region. **O,P.** A hypertrophied LV imaged in long axis in diastole **(O)** and systole **(P)**. **Q.** Both papillary muscles (PM) and the chordae tendinae (CH) are well shown. **R,S.** Long-axis views from another patient showing the left ventricle in diastole **(R)** and systole **(S)**. Note the marked thickening of the LV walls in systole. **T–V.** LAA and left upper pulmonary vein (PV) imaged from the transgastric view. **W.** An intramyocardial coronary vessel (arrow) imaged using a high- resolution color Doppler system. (**F–H** and **U** reproduced with permission from Nanda NC, Pinheiro L, Sanyal RS, Storey O. Transesophageal biplane echocardiographic imaging: technique, planes, and clinical usefulness. Echocardiography 1990;7:771–788.)

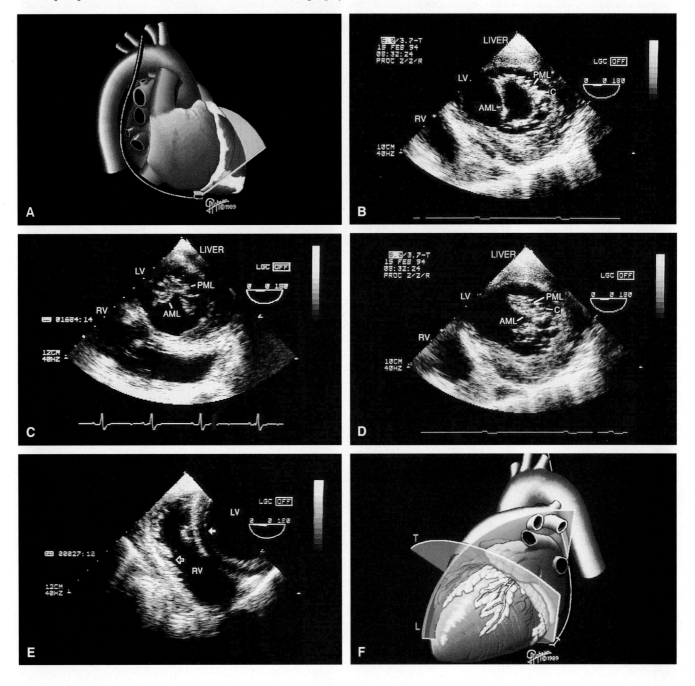

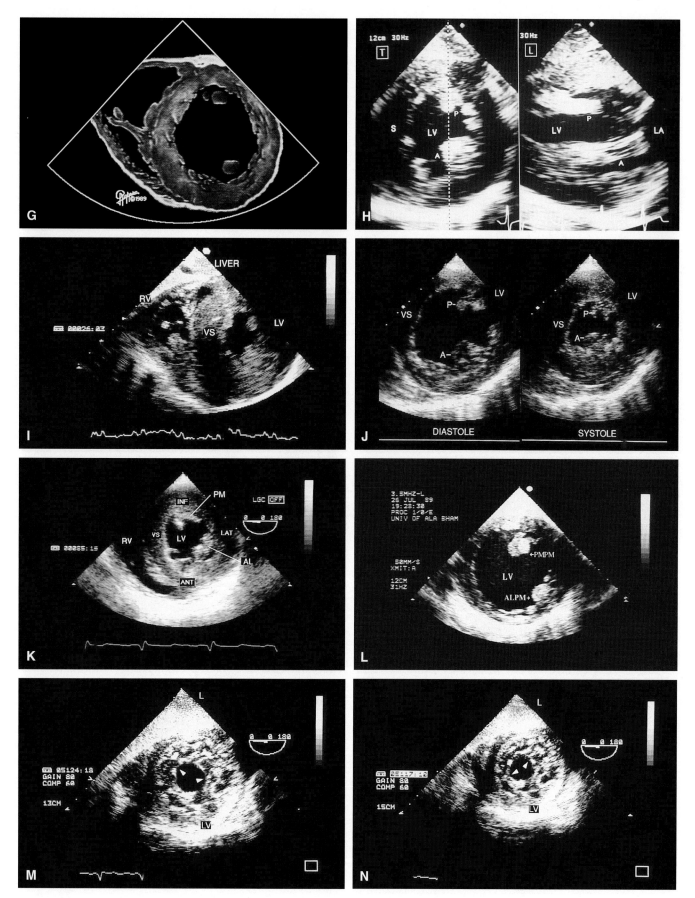

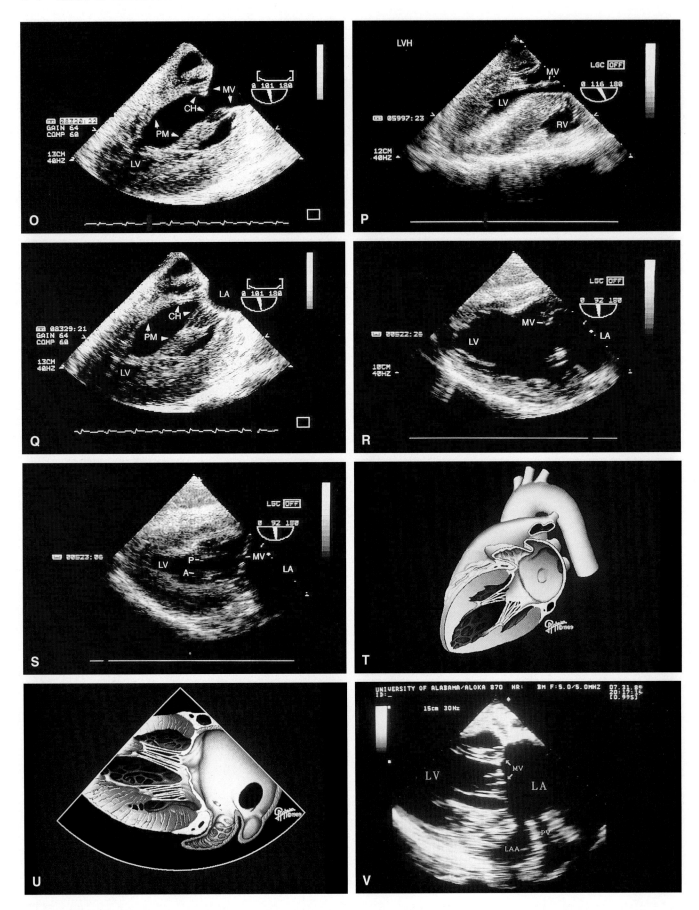

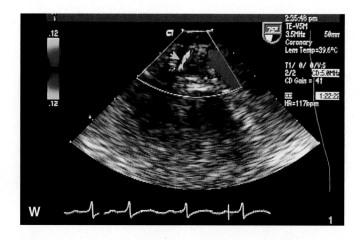

Figure 1.29. **A-F. Transgastric views.** Anterior angulation of the transducer often brings into view the aortic root (AO) surrounded by the RA, TV, RV, RVOT, PV, and PA. **E.** The SVC and RV apex also are visualized. **F.** Pulsed Doppler interrogation shows normal systolic flow signals from the main pulmonary artery (PA).

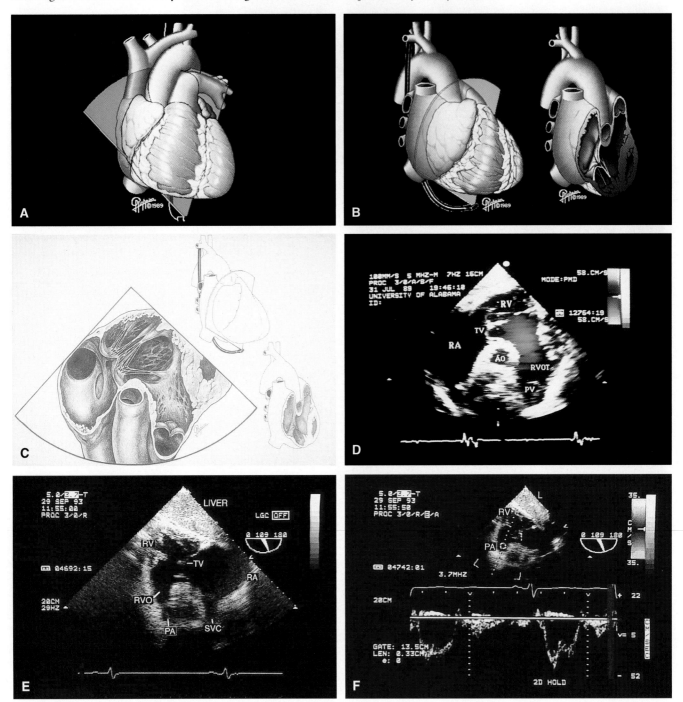

Figure 1.30. **A-G. Transgastric views.** The aortic root (AO) and the ascending aorta are viewed in long axis. Both LV and RV are well imaged. **G.** All three leaflets of the TV (*A*, anterior; *P*, posterior or inferior; *S*, septal) are imaged in systole adjacent to the aorta (AO). The normal TV in systole has a star-shaped appearance rather than the "smile" of a closed normal MV. (**G** reproduced with permission from Maxted W, Nanda NC, Kim KS, et al. Transesophageal echocardiographic identification and validation of individual tricuspid valve leaflets. Echocardiography 1994;11:585–596.)

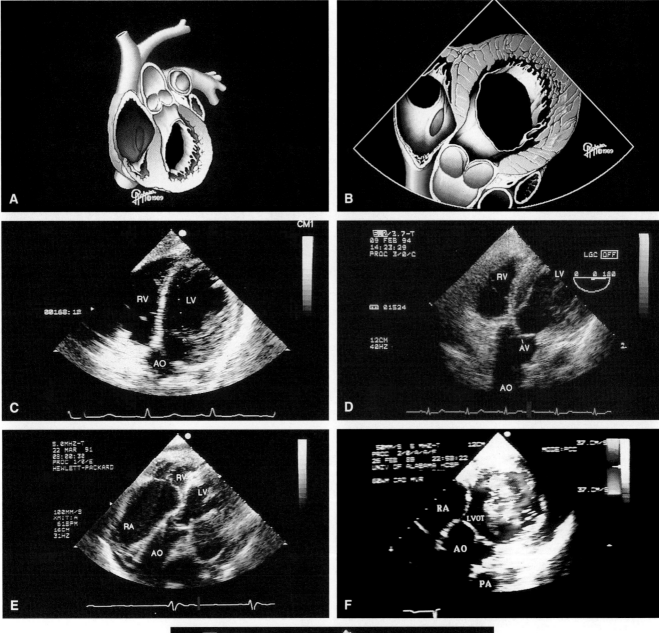

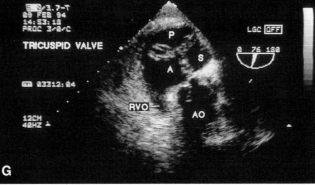

Figure 1.31. **Transgastric views**. A–J. Examination of superior mesenteric and renal vessels. **A–C.** Transverse plane imaging. **A.** Both the superior mesenteric (SMA) and the left renal (LRA) arteries are visualized arising from the abdominal aorta (AO). *Inset:* Pulsed Doppler spectral tracing obtained from the SMA. **B.** The left renal vein (LRV) is seen crossing anterior to the abdominal aorta (AO) to drain into the IVC. **C.** Color Doppler–guided pulsed Doppler interrogation of the LRV demonstrates low-velocity flow signals practically throughout the cardiac cycle. **D.** Schematic representation. **E-J.** Examination of the abdominal structures and vessels in another patient. **E.** Longitudinal and transverse plane imaging of the left kidney (LK). *C*, cortex; *M*, medulla. **F.** Visualization of the pancreas (PN) using transverse plane imaging. **G.** Transverse and longitudinal plane imaging of the splenic artery (SA) and vein (SV). **H.** Pulsed Doppler interrogation shows relatively high velocity pulsatile flow in the SA and lower-velocity continuous flow in the SV. **I.** Pulsed Doppler interrogation of the proximal LRA reveals a peak systolic velocity of 0.52 m/sec (not angled correct). The fairly prominent antegrade diastolic flow denotes a low-resistance vessel. **J.** Visualization of the intrarenal artery (RA) and vein (RV). Pulsed Doppler interrogation of the artery in this patient demonstrates pulsatile signals with prominent antegrade diastolic flow. *SMV,* superior mesenteric vein; *SP,* spleen. **K.** Multiple hepatic veins (HV) are seen entering the IVC. (**A** through **J** reproduced with permission from Chouinard MD, Pinheiro L, Nanda NC, Sanyal RS. Transgastric ultrasonography: a new approach for imaging the abdominal structures and vessels. Echocardiography 1991;8:397–403.)

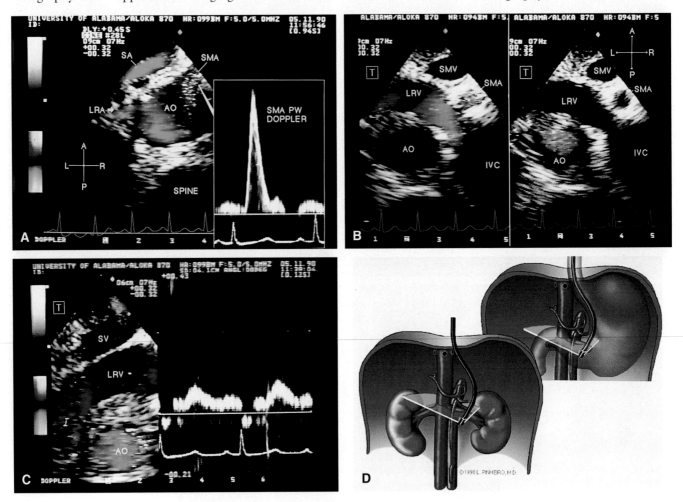

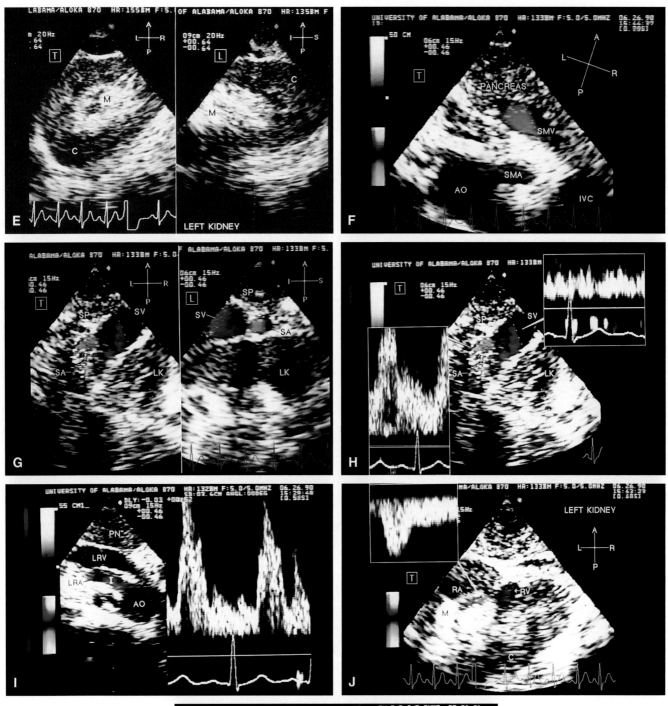

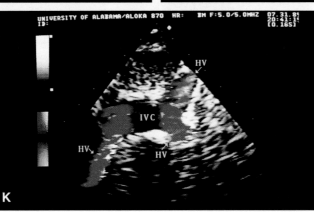

Figure 1.32. **A-D. Transgastric views.** The stomach is well seen. **B.** Rugae (arrowheads). **C,D.** Slow-moving contrast echoes (arrowheads) caused by the stomach contents.

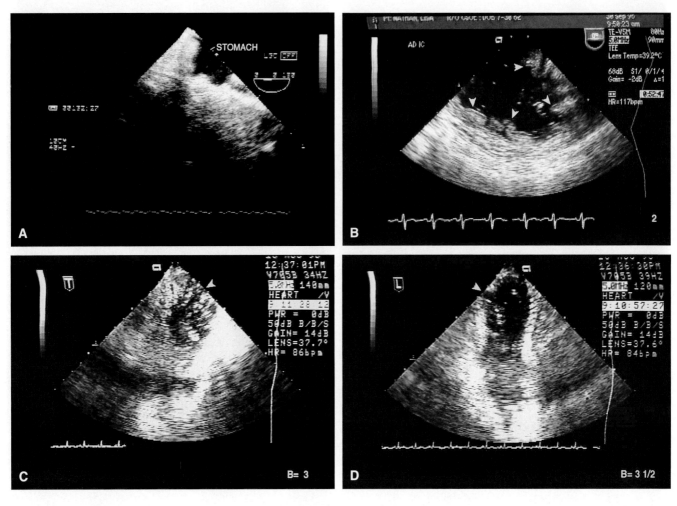

SUGGESTED READINGS

Agrawal G, LaMotte LC, Nanda NC. Identification of the aortic arch branches using transesophageal echocardiography. Echocardiography 1997;4:461–466.

Agrawal GG, Parekh HH, Tirtaman C, et al. Transesophageal echocardiographic imaging of the left atrium behind the ascending aorta mimicking aortic dissection: validation by contrast echocardiography. Echocardiography 1997;4:411–415.

Bansal RC, Shakudo M, Shah PM, et al. Biplane transesophageal echocardiography: technique, image orientation, and preliminary experience in 131 patients. J Am Soc Echocardiogr 1990;3:348–366.

Chan KL, Cohen GI, Sochowski RA, et al. Complications of transesophageal echocardiography in ambulatory adult patients: analysis of 1500 consecutive examinations. J Am Soc Echocardiogr 1991;4:577–582.

Cromme-Dijkhuis AH, Djoa KE, Bom N, et al. Pediatric transesophageal echocardiography by means of a minute 5-MHZ multiplane transducer. Echocardiography 1996;13:685–689.

Daniel WG, Erbel R, Kasper W, et al. Safety of transesophageal echocardiography: a multicenter survey of 10,419 examinations. Circulation 1991;83:817–821.

DeBelder MA, Leech G, Camm AJ. Transesophageal echocardiography in unsedated outpatients: technique and patient tolerance. J Am Soc Echocardiogr 1989;2:375.

Del Rio CG, Taylor GW, Nanda NC, et al. Color Doppler visualization of intramyocardial coronary arteries using a new echo system: effect of contrast enhancement and vasodilation. Echocardiography 1996;13:645–650.

Eichelberger JP. Antibiotic prophylaxis for endocarditis prevention during transesophageal echocardiography. Echocardiography 1996;13:459–462.

Erbel R, Khandheria BK, Brennecke R, et al, eds. Transesophageal Echocardiography: A New Window to the Heart. New York: Springer-Verlag, 1989.

Fisher EA, Stahl JA, Budd JH, et al. Transesophageal echocardiography: Procedures and clinical application. J Am Coll Cardiol 1991;18:1333.

Frazin L, Talano JV, Stephanides L, et al. Esophageal echocardiography. Circulation 1976;54:102–108.

Gilbert TB, Panico FG, McGill WA, et al. Bronchial obstruction by transesophageal echocardiography probe in a pediatric cardiac patient. Anesth Analg 1992;74:156–158.

Grauer SE, Giraud GD. Toxic methemoglobinemia after topical anesthesia for transesophageal echocardiography. J Am Soc Echocardiogr 1996;9:874–876.

Helmcke F, Mahan EF III, Nanda NC, et al. Use of the smaller pediatric transesophageal echocardiographic probe in adults. Echocardiography 1990;7:727–737.

Hopkins WE, Feinberg MS, Barzilai B. Initial clinical experience with a miniature biplane transesophageal echocardiographic probe in adults. Echocardiography 1996;11:165–172.

Katz ES, Konecky E, Tunick PA, et al. Visualization and identification of the left common carotid and left subclavian arteries: a transesophageal echocardiographic approach. J Am Soc Echocardiogr 1996;9:58–61.

Khandheria BK. The transesophageal echocardiographic examination: is it safe? Echocardiography 1994;11:55–63.

Khandheria BK. Prophylaxis or no prophylaxis before transesophageal echocardiography? [editorial]. J Am Soc Echocardiogr 1992;5:285–287.

Kharasch ED, Sivarajan M. Gastroesophageal perforation after intraoperative transesophageal echocardiography. Anesthesiology 1996;85:426–428.

Lightly GW Jr, Hare CL, Kaplan DS. Use of a mouth gag instrument to facilitate bite block insertion and prevent finger and probe bites during transesophageal echocardiography. Echocardiography 1992;9:485.

Mahan EF III, Nanda NC. Transesophageal echocardiography. In: Rackley CE, ed. Challenges in Cardiology I. Mount Kisco, NY: Futura, 1992:85–101.

Marcovitz PA, Williamson BD, Armstrong WF. Toxic methemoglobinemia caused by topical anesthetic given before transesophageal echocardiography. J Am Soc Echocardiogr 1991;4:615.

Maurer G, ed. Transesophageal Echocardiography. New York: McGraw-Hill, 1994.

Maxted W, Finch A, Nanda NC, et al. Multiplane transesophageal echocardiographic detection of sinus venosus atrial septal defect. Echocardiography 1995;12:139–143.

Maxted W, Nanda NC, Kim KS, et al. Transesophageal echocardiographic identification and validation of individual tricuspid valve leaflets. Echocardiography 1994;11:585–596.

Missri J. Transesophageal Echocardiography: Clinical and Intraoperative Applications. New York: Churchill Livingstone, 1993.

Nanda NC, Mahan EF III. Transesophageal echocardiography. AHA Council on Clinical Cardiology Newsletter 1990;Summer:3–22.

Nanda NC, Pinheiro L, Sanyal R, et al. Transesophageal echocardiographic examination of left-sided superior vena cava and azygos and hemiazygos veins. Echocardiography 1991;8:731–739.

Nanda NC, Pinheiro L, Sanyal RS, et al. Transesophageal biplane echocardiographic imaging: technique, planes, and clinical usefulness. Echocardiography 1990;7:771–788.

Ofili EO, Rich MW, Brown P, et al. Safety and usefulness of transesophageal echocardiography in persons aged greater than or equal to 70 years. Am J Cardiol 1990;66:1279.

Oh JK, Seward JB, Khandheria BK, et al. Transesophageal echocardiography in critically ill patients. Am J Cardiol 1990;66:1492–1495.

Omoto R, Kyo S, Matsumura M, et al. New direction of biplane transesophageal echocardiography with special emphasis on real-time biplane imaging and matrix phased-array biplane transducer. Echocardiography 1990;7:691–698.

Omoto R, Kyo S, Matsumura M, et al. Recent advances in transesophageal echocardiography: Development of biplane and pediatric transesophageal probes. Am J Cardiac Imaging 1990;4:207–214.

Orihashi K, Sueda T, Matsuura Y, et al. Buckling of transesophageal echocardiography probe: a pitfall at insertion in an anesthetized patient. Hiroshima J Med Sci 1993;42:155–157.

Orsinelli DA, Pearson AC. Usefulness of multiplane transesophageal echocardiography in differentiating left atrial appendage thrombus from pectinate muscles. Am Heart J 1996;131:616–618.

Osk Y, Goldiner PL, eds. Transesophageal Echocardiography. Philadelphia: JB Lippincott, 1992.

Pandian NG, Hsu TL, Schwartz SL, et al. Multiplane transesophageal echocardiography. Echocardiography 1992;9:649.

Pearson AP, Castello R, Labovitz AJ. Safety and utility of transesophageal echocardiography in the critically ill patient. Am Heart J 1990;119:1083.

Piel JE Jr, Lewandowksi RS, Lorraine PW, et al. 7.5-MHz pediatric phased array transesophageal endoscope. Echocardiography 1996;13:677–683.

Pinheiro L, Nanda NC, Jain H, et al. Transesophageal echocardiographic imaging of the pulmonary veins. Echocardiography 1991;8:741–748.

Rafferty TD. Basics of transesophageal echocardiography. New York: Churchill Livingstone, 1995.

Richardson SG, Weintraub AR, Schwartz SL, et al. Biplane transesophageal echocardiography utilizing transverse and sagittal imaging planes. Echocardiography 1991;8:293.

Ritter SB. Transesophageal echocardiographic imaging in infants and children: the elements of the plane truth. Echocardiography 1993;10:609–610.

Ritter SB, Thys D. Pediatric transesophageal color flow imaging: smaller probes for smaller hearts. Echocardiography 1989;6:431–440.

Roelandt JRTC, Thomson IR, Vletter WB, et al. Multiplane transesophageal echocardiography: latest evolution in an imaging revolution. J Am Soc Echocardiogr 1992;5:361–367.

Seward JB. Transesophageal echocardiographic anatomy. In: Freeman WK, Seward JB, Khandheria BK, Tajik AJ, eds. Transesophageal Echocardiography. Boston: Little, Brown, 1994:99.

Seward JB, Khandheria BK, Edwards WD, et al. Biplanar transesophageal echocardiography: anatomic correlations, image orientation, and clinical applications. Mayo Clin Proc 1990;65:1193–1213.

Seward JB, Khandheria BK, Freeman WK, et al. Multiplane transesophageal echocardiography: image orientation, examination technique, anatomic correlations, and clinical applications. Mayo Clin Proc 1993;68:523–551.

Seward JB, Khandheria BK, Oh JK, et al. Transesophageal echo: technique, anatomic correlations, implementation, and clinical applications. Mayo Clin Proc 1988;63:649–680.

Stoddard MF, Liddell NE, Longacker RA, et al. Transesophageal echocardiography: Normal variants and mimickers. Am Heart J 1992;124:1587.

Tardif JC, Vannon Ma, Pandian NG. Biplane and multiplane transesophageal echocardiography methodology and echo-anatomic correlations. Am J Cardiac Imaging 1995;9:87–99.

Mitral Valve

2

Transesophageal echocardiography is superior to the transthoracic approach for characterizing the anatomy and function of the mitral valve. It would completely replace transthoracic echocardiography for this purpose were it not that there is more discomfort, a small risk, and higher cost in both time and money when transesophageal echocardiography is used.

Transthoracic echocardiography is often adequate for the study of mitral stenosis. In patients with poor echocardiographic windows, or in whom transesophageal echocardiography is performed for other reasons, however, the cause and severity of mitral stenosis are almost always revealed by transesophageal echocardiography. Mitral stenosis produces clearly visible diastolic doming of the mitral valve. This doming is the result of fusion of the leaflet commissures with relatively greater mobility of the remainder of the leaflets. In adults with mitral stenosis the valve is usually thickened and calcified. Conventional Doppler examination allows the mean pressure gradient and the valve area to be calculated, the latter by the pressure half-time technique. Because of limitations imposed by the angle at which the mitral valve can be imaged, planimetry of the valve from the transesophageal approach usually is not very accurate. Color Doppler flow examination in patients with severe mitral stenosis reveals a narrow jet and a region of prominent proximal diastolic flow acceleration in the left atrium. Transesophageal echocardiography provides excellent imaging of the subvalvular apparatus, which can thicken and contribute to mitral outflow obstruction. Indeed, when the pressure half-time suggests stenosis more severe than that suggested by planimetry (from transthoracic echocardiography), the possibility of significant submitral obstruction should be considered.

The severity of mitral regurgitation cannot be assessed by comparing jet area to left atrial area, as is done in transthoracic echocardiography, because the entire left atrium is not visualized. Instead, a semiquantitative grading system based on total jet area may be used. A jet area smaller than 4 cm^2 indicates mild mitral regurgitation; an area 4 to 8 cm^2 indicates moderate regurgitation; and an area larger than 8 cm^2 indicates severe regurgitation. The entire area of jet flow, including low velocity flow, should be planimetered because the angle at which the flow is measured, which is nearly perpendicular at times, may cause the appearance of low velocity in a high velocity jet.

Sometimes the total jet area is misleading. In the case of eccentric jets (typically seen with mitral valve prolapse or flail mitral valve) or jets that strike a vegetation or course along a mitral leaflet or the atrial wall, momentum and jet energy are lost, less blood is entrained, and the jet size suggests less severe regurgitation than is actually the case. To determine the severity of mitral regurgitation, therefore, the entire study must be considered. Visible extension of the regurgitant flow into the left atrial appendage or any of the pulmonary veins indicates the presence of severe regurgitation. In such cases, pulse Doppler interrogation of a pulmonary vein near its entrance into the left atrium demonstrates systolic flow reversal that may be aliased. This typically occurs in midsystole or late systole because the jet has to traverse the whole length of the left atrium before it reaches the pulmonary vein. It is important to interrogate all the pulmonary veins by Doppler because systolic flow reversal may be found in only one of them. Reduction in the height of the systolic wave without flow reversal may be seen with moderate regurgitation, but this is not a specific finding. It may also occur in patients with left ventricular dysfunction without mitral regurgitation.

Prominent proximal flow acceleration also alerts the echocardiographer to the presence of significant mitral regurgitation in patients with small eccentric regurgitant jets. The size of this proximal flow convergence varies according to the Nyquist limit that has been set, with the best results usually obtained with a very low Nyquist limit. However, quantitation of regurgitant volume using proximal flow convergence is fraught with inaccuracies that make the qualitative approach more appropriate.

Prolapse of the mitral valve may be well seen by transesophageal echocardiography. The most convincing evidence of prolapse is seen when the prolapse is localized. The picture of the entire leaflet bulging into the left atrium may be an artifact produced by the imaging plane rather than true prolapse, especially in the four-chamber or five-chamber view. Multiple views help make the distinction. It is necessary to distinguish between the redundancy that is sometimes seen in these valves and vegetation.

Chordal rupture results in severe mitral prolapse and noncoaptation of the mitral leaflets. The ruptured chordae can be identified as linear echoes fluttering in the left atrium. These linear echoes must not be confused with Lambl's excrescences, which are small linear filaments that may normally be present on the mitral valve or any of the other valves. These filaments are best seen on transesophageal echocardiography. Rupture of primary chordae causes severe mitral regurgitation, whereas rupture of secondary or tertiary chordae may cause less severe insufficiency.

Transesophageal echocardiography is far more sensitive in identifying vegetations than is transthoracic echocardiography. For this reason, in the appropriate clinical setting, a negative transthoracic echocardiogram should lead to transesophageal echocardiography. Valve thickenings are most convincingly diagnosed as vegetations when they are mobile. They are most often seen on the proximal (low velocity) side of the valve, but they can be seen anywhere. The presence of a vegetation on one valve should prompt a search for vegetations on other valves. Serial echoes may be needed for the diagnosis, because vegetations may grow over time. The presence of calcification may make the vegetation appear larger.

Abscesses usually present as echo-free spaces, although echolucency may be diminished by the presence of thick pus in the abscess. Abscesses can rupture and produce fistulous connections to any structure. A common location for an abscess is in the annulus fibrosus, located at the junction of the mitral and aortic valves (mitral–aortic intervalvular fibrosa). The mitral valve may become aneurysmal and perforate, as may the fibrosa between the mitral and aortic valves. These aneurysms may become very large. Color-flow Doppler can demonstrate the to-and-fro flow of blood into and out of the aneurysm. Infection is the most common cause of such aneurysms, but they may also be caused by trauma, particularly surgical trauma.

Transesophageal echocardiography is useful in the performance of mitral valvuloplasty. A scoring system has been devised to help decide whether the procedure is feasible. Pliability, thickening, calcification, and subvalvular thickening are each scored on a scale from 0 to 4. A total score lower than 8 suggests that the valve structure is very suitable for the procedure. Transesophageal echocardiography also can be used to ensure that there are no clots in the left atrium (including the left atrial appendage), because the presence of a clot contraindicates the procedure. Transesophageal echocardiography can be used as a guide when performing the procedure, specifically the needle puncture of the interatrial septum. The septum can be seen to "pucker" when it is touched by the needle. In addition, the tip of the needle produces a prominent reverberation that helps to identify it. A rapid assessment for the presence of mitral regurgitation can be made following the procedure. The presence and size of atrial septal defects produced by the procedure can be assessed, although these usually close over time.

Figure 2.1. **Mitral stenosis. A.** Noncalcific mitral stenosis. There is diastolic doming of the valve and restricted leaflet motion, but the leaflets are only mildly thickened. The orifice appears small. Note the much enlarged LA. At surgery, the commissures were fused and there was a fixed, central orifice. **B,C.** Calcific mitral stenosis. In this patient the leaflets are much thicker than those seen in **A,** and they are calcified. The arrowheads point to the stenotic orifice. **D,E.** Calcific mitral stenosis. In this study, the leaflet tips are much thicker than the rest of the leaflets (arrowhead in **D**). TV (arrow in **D**) appears to open well. Color-flow Doppler in **E** shows flow acceleration (arrow) proximal to the valve in diastole and a very narrow orifice, indicating severe mitral stenosis. At surgery, the MV had severe rheumatic pathology with severe stenosis and a fixed, central orifice. **F,G.** Pathology specimens demonstrate severe mitral stenosis.

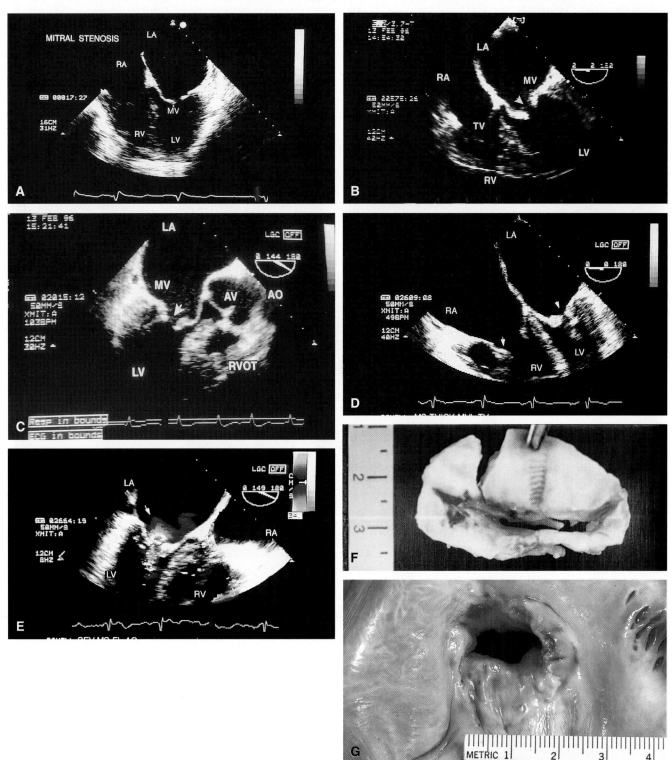

Figure 2.2. **Mitral stenosis: subvalvular thickening. A.** The closed arrow points to calcified mitral leaflets; the open arrow points to chordal thickening. **B,C.** The arrowheads point to calcified mitral leaflets with a markedly thickened subvalvular apparatus (arrow in **B**, lower arrowhead in **C**) in another patient. **D.** Color Doppler study in this patient shows prominent flow acceleration (arrow) and a narrow jet (arrowhead) consistent with mitral stenosis. **E.** Gross specimen from a different patient shows thickened and fused chordae with nodular leaflet calcification.

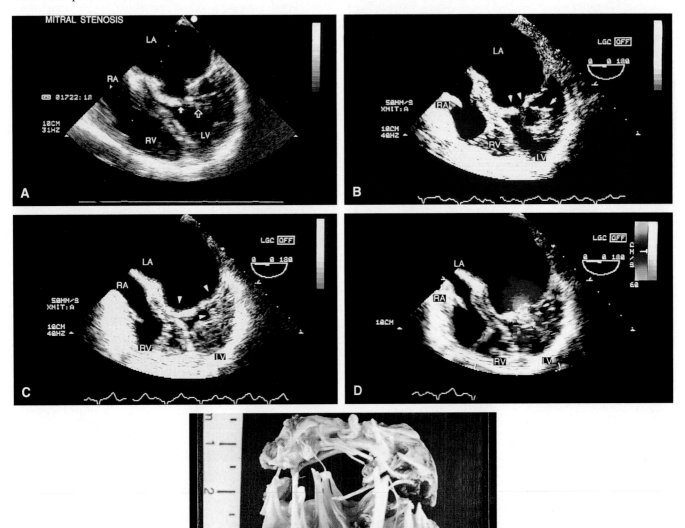

Figure 2.3. **Mitral stenosis with prolapse.** The open arrow in **A** and **B** points to thickened chordae. The closed arrows in **B** demonstrate systolic prolapse of both posterior and anterior leaflets. **C.** Doppler interrogation of a pulmonary vein in this patient demonstrates a large A wave typical of mitral stenosis. *D*, diastolic wave; *S*, systolic wave.

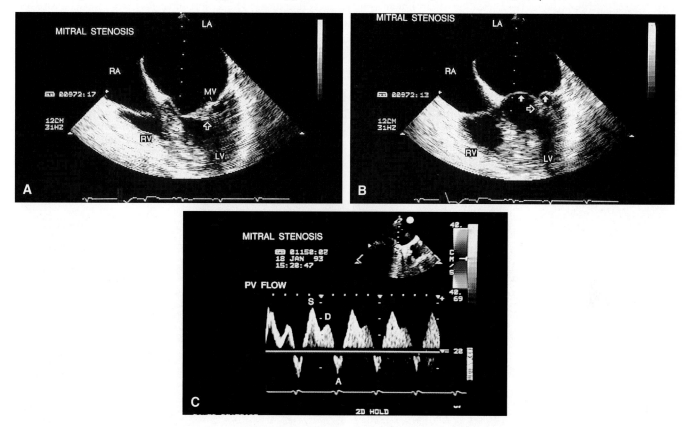

Figure 2.4. **Mitral stenosis: left atrial appendage flow. A.** Pulsed Doppler interrogation of LAA in this patient shows normal flow velocity of waveforms with rapid upslope and downslope that suggests normal LAA function. **B.** Patient with atrial fibrillation. Pulsed Doppler interrogation of LAA shows a spiking pattern often seen in atrial flutter and fibrillation.

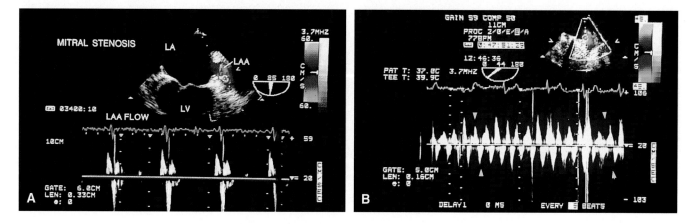

Figure 2.5. **Mitral stenosis: spontaneous contrast echoes and thrombus. A.** An M-mode examination shows spontaneous contrast echoes throughout the cardiac cycle in LA, consistent with stasis and low flow velocity. *Dias*, diastole; *Sys*, systole. **B.** Spontaneous contrast echoes (arrowheads) fill most of the LA. **C.** Pectinate muscles (arrows) in the LAA can be differentiated from clot by their linear transverse orientation. **D.** Thickening involves the MV tips of both mitral leaflets (arrows) in this patient. **E.** Clot (arrow) lines the lateral wall of the LAA in a 64-year-old woman with mitral stenosis (same patient as in **D**). **F.** A large clot in the LAA (arrow) is seen in another patient. **G.** In contrast, in this illustration the arrow points to nonspecific thickening between the LAA and the LUPV. In motion, it was clear that this structure was outside the LAA. **H-J.** A large nonmobile thrombus (TH) is seen in the body of the LA.

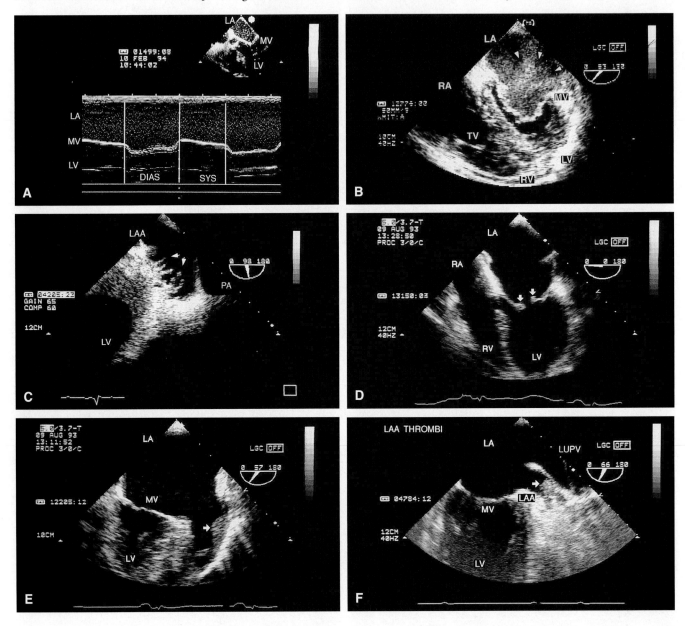

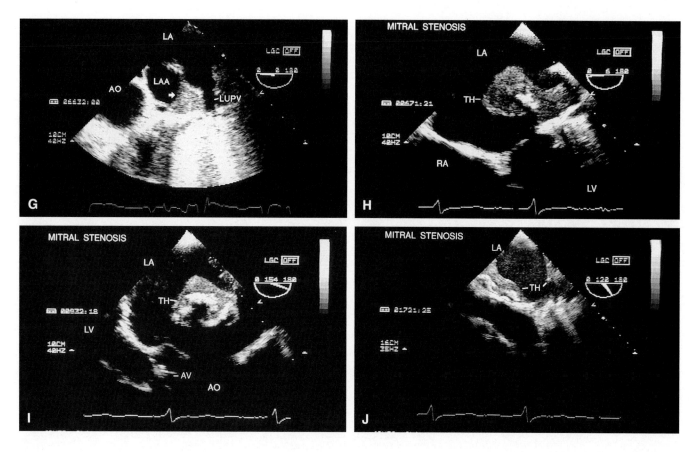

Figure 2.6. **Mitral stenosis and regurgitation. A,B.** A large region of flow acceleration on the atrial aspect of the stenosed MV (arrow) and turbulent flow signals in the LV are seen. **C.** A large jet of MR with a prominent region of flow acceleration on the ventricular aspect of the MV. **D.** The regurgitant jet can be seen to extend into the LUPV, indicating the presence of severe MR.

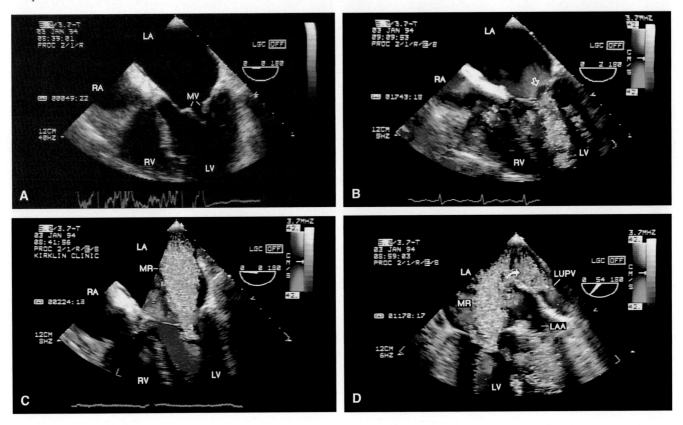

Figure 2.7. **Mitral and aortic stenosis.** The arrow points to the stenotic MV. The AV is thickened and, in other views, showed markedly restricted motion consistent with aortic stenosis.

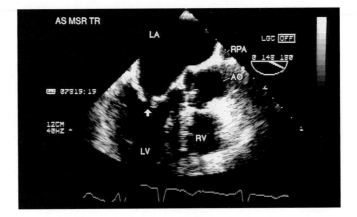

Figure 2.8. **Mitral stenosis and atrial septal defect. A.** The MV leaflets demonstrate thickening and calcification, diastolic doming, and a small orifice, all indicative of severe mitral stenosis. The TV leaflets are thin and open fully. Examination of the atrial septum **(B)** shows a large secundum atrial septal defect (D).

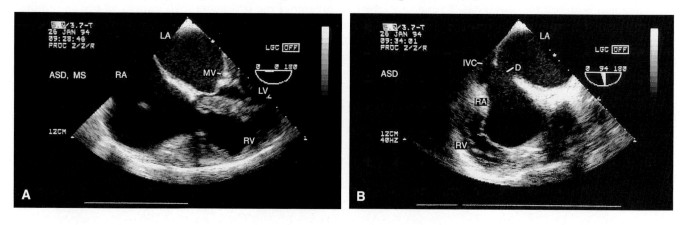

Figure 2.9. **Percutaneous mitral balloon valvuloplasty.** A Brockenbrough needle within a Mullins sheath and dilator, and then the Brockenbrough needle protruding from the Mullins sheath, were introduced separately into a water-filled plastic container and scanned with a 3.5-MHz transthoracic probe as well as a 5-MHz transesophageal probe. **A.** Prominent posterior reverberations (R) and side lobe (SL) artifact of the Brockenbrough transseptal needle (N) protruding from the sheath (S) and dilator (D) are demonstrated. **B.** The less prominent reverberation (R) of the needle within the sheath. **C.** Transesophageal echocardiography-guided atrial septal puncture. The transseptal needle (arrow) is in contact with the fossa ovalis and has a prominent reverberatory tail. **D.** The four-chamber view shows the transseptal needle (arrow) traversing the fossa ovalis into the LA. **E.** The Critikon catheter (arrow) is shown in the MV orifice. **F.** An eccentrically directed MR jet that developed after balloon dilation of the MV. (Reproduced with permission from Ballal RS, Mahan EF III, Nanda NC, Dean LS. Utility of transesophageal echocardiography in interatrial septal puncture during percutaneous mitral balloon commissurotomy. Am J Cardiol 1990;66:230–232.)

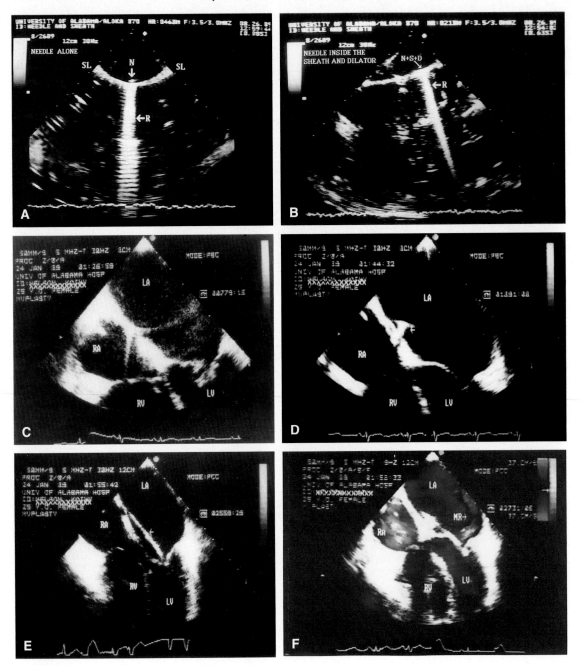

Figure 2.10. Mitral valve rupture following balloon mitral valvuloplasty. **A.** Four-chamber view during systole shows a large area of discontinuity or perforation (PR) in the midportion of the anterior MV leaflet (AML). The posterior MV leaflet (PML) is intact. **B.** Color Doppler flow imaging illustrates a large mosaic-colored MR jet that traverses the AML area of discontinuity and impinges upon and moves along the posterolateral wall of the LA. **C.** During diastole, color flow signals move from the LA into the LV through both the MV orifice and the AML tear. (Reproduced with permission from Mahan EF III, Ballal RS, Nanda NC. Mitral valve tear complicating percutaneous valvuloplasty: diagnosis by transesophageal Doppler color flow mapping. Am Heart J 1991;122:238–242.)

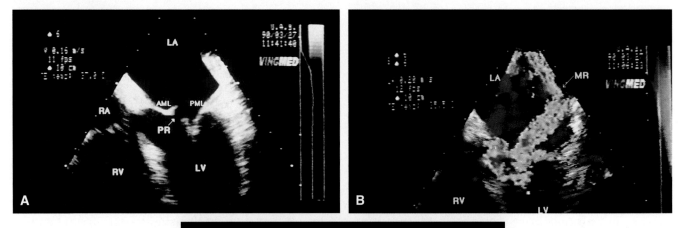

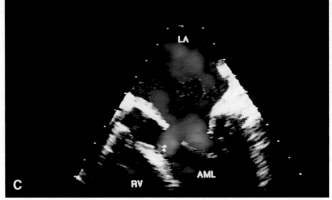

Figure 2.11. Mitral valve rupture following balloon valvuloplasty. **A.** A large rupture in the anterior mitral leaflet (arrowhead). **B.** Color Doppler examination demonstrates MR signals at the rupture site (arrowhead). *LI*, liver.

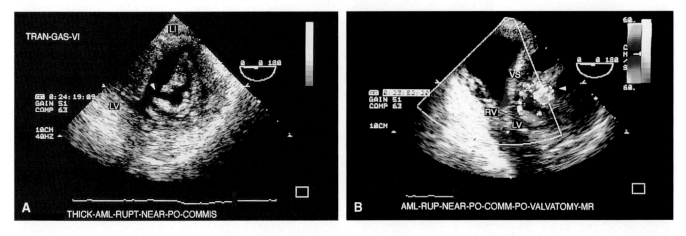

Figure 2.12. Atrial septal defect following balloon mitral valvuloplasty. **A.** Bidirectional shunting through a small atrial septal defect created by needle puncture and by the catheter crossing the atrial septum. Such atrial septal defects usually are hemodynamically insignificant and close over time. **B.** Left-to-right shunting through an ASD created during balloon mitral valvuloplasty and associated TR are shown.

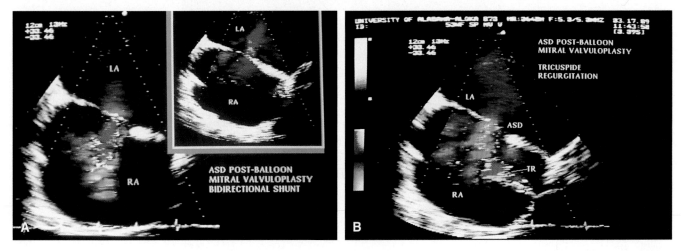

Figure 2.13. **Mitral regurgitation. A.** A small jet of MR consistent with mild MR. **B.** Color M-mode examination of another patient shows MR. In the second cardiac cycle, two MR jets are seen. **C.** Torrential MR with the flow signals filling the entire LA. The arrow points to a very large zone of flow acceleration on the ventricular side of the MV. **D-F.** Three jets of MR (numbered 1, 2, and 3) are seen moving through the anterior mitral leaflet, which prolapses into LA.

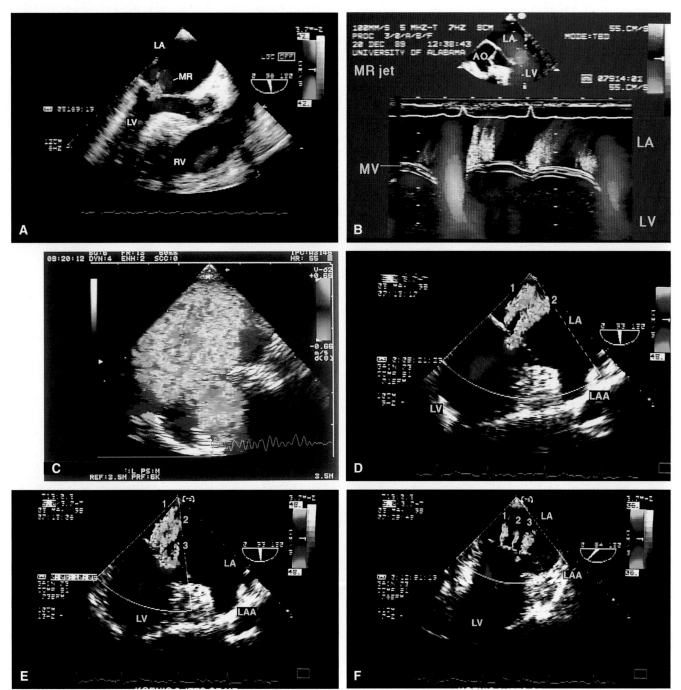

Figure 2.14. **Mitral valve prolapse. A.** Both leaflets of the MV prolapse (P) into the LA. The posterior leaflet prolapse appears to be more severe than the anterior leaflet. **B.** In another patient with MVP an eccentric MR jet directed laterally along the posterior leaflet and the lateral wall of the LA is seen. *LPV,* left upper pulmonary vein. **C,D.** Another patient with severe prolapse (arrows in **C**) of both anterior (AML) and posterior (PML) leaflets. The chordae tendinae are well seen. **D.** Color Doppler examination shows an eccentric MR jet that is directed laterally. Even though the jet appears small, a large zone of flow acceleration on the ventricular side of the mitral valve and systolic backflow in the pulmonary veins (which were seen in other views) allowed correct diagnosis of severe MR. (**D** reprinted with permission from Rosenthal SM, Nanda NC. Assessment of valvular regurgitation by transesophageal echocardiography. J Invasive Cardiol 1992;4:366–372.)

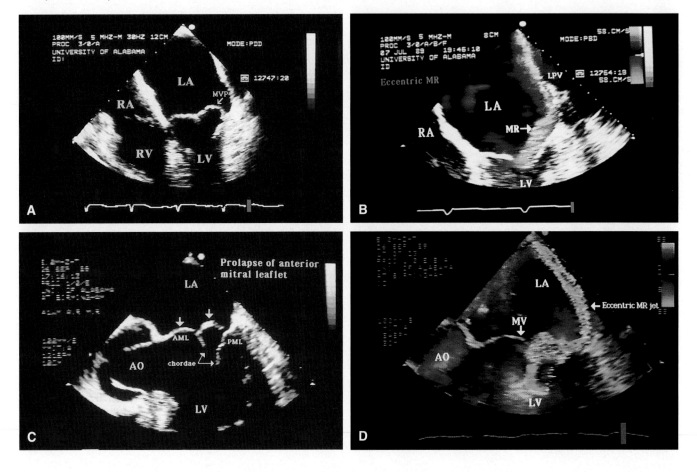

Figure 2.15. **Mitral valve prolapse. Transgastric short-axis views. A.** Redundancy of both the anterior (AML) and posterior (PML) mitral leaflets is shown in the semi-open position. **B-D.** Prominent redundancy of the middle scallop of the posterior mitral leaflet (arrowheads). This is best seen in the semi-open position. *L,* liver. **E.** Gross specimen shows redundancy and myxomatous degeneration of the mitral leaflets.

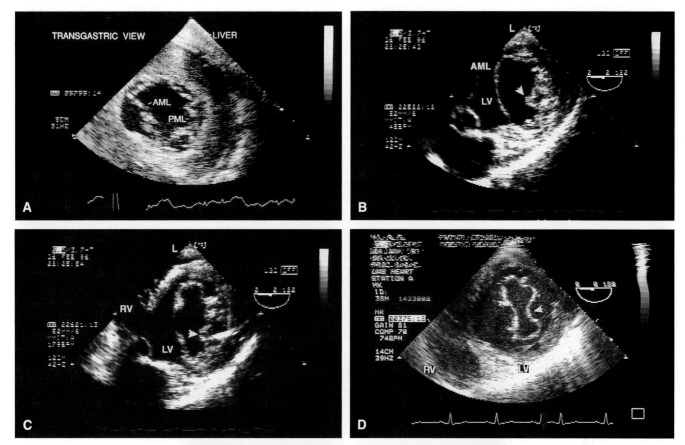

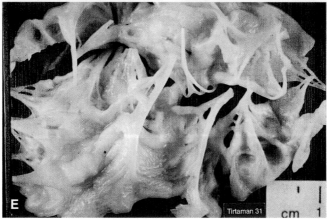

Figure 2.16. **Mitral regurgitation. A,B.** A small MR jet is imaged. The fact that the jet is seen only distally suggests that it is more extensive than is demonstrated on this study. This underscores the need for careful transducer angulation to find the full extent of the jet. **C.** Two MR jets (arrowheads) caused by a dilated mitral annulus secondary to reduced LV function are seen in this patient with coronary artery disease.

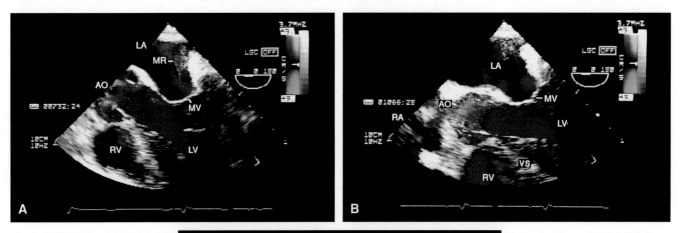

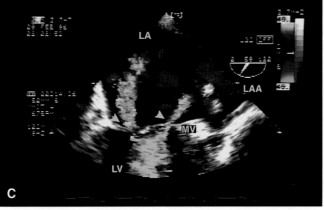

Figure 2.17. **Left atrial aneurysm. A,B.** A massively dilated LA in a patient with redundant mitral leaflets. **C.** Color Doppler examination demonstrates severe MR, which occupies almost the entire LA imaged in this frame. Note also the very large zone of proximal flow acceleration on the ventricular side of the MV. This patient underwent mitral annuloplasty. **D.** Postoperative study showed only mild residual MR.

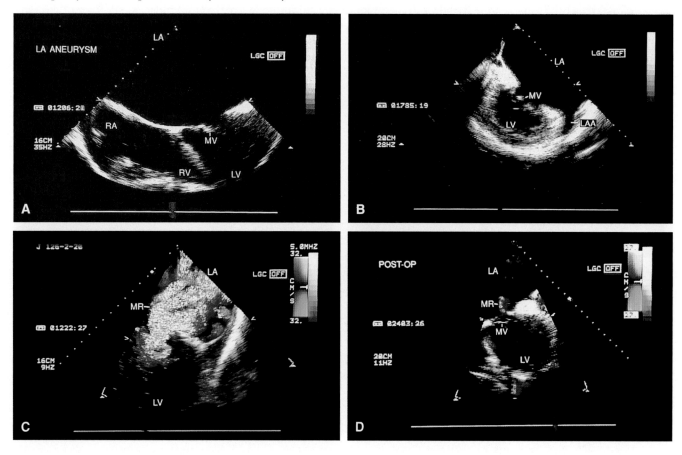

Figure 2.18. **Chordal rupture. A.** The posterior leaflet and one of its chordae are seen prolapsing dramatically into the LA and failing to coapt with the anterior leaflet, which shows only mild prolapse. **B-D.** A long segment of the ruptured chordae to posterior leaflet is seen prolapsing into the left atrium (arrowheads). **E.** Color Doppler examination demonstrates a small, narrow, eccentric MR jet directed along the atrial septum. However, the prominent region of flow acceleration (arrowhead) and systolic backflow in the pulmonary veins (seen in other views) indicates severe mitral regurgitation.

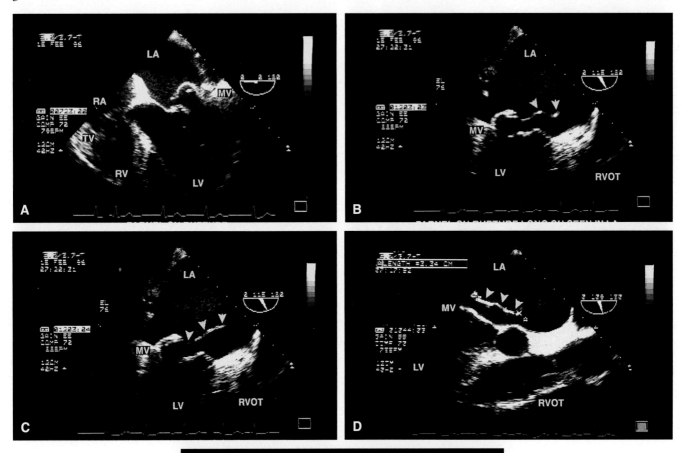

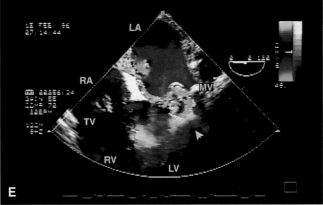

Figure 2.19. **Chordal rupture. A.** Severe prolapse of the posterior leaflet (arrow). There is only mild prolapse of the anterior leaflet. In this frame, there is no evidence to suggest rupture of the chordae, and both leaflets appear to coapt. **B.** A change in transducer angulation demonstrates both chordal rupture with chordae prolapse into the LA (arrow) and failure of coaptation with eccentric MR jet demonstrated by color flow Doppler **(C). D.** Even though the MR jet in **C** appears to be relatively small, Doppler interrogation of the LUPV shows aliased backflow in late systole (SBF), confirming the presence of severe MR. *A*, atrial systolic wave; *D*, diastolic wave; *S*, S wave.

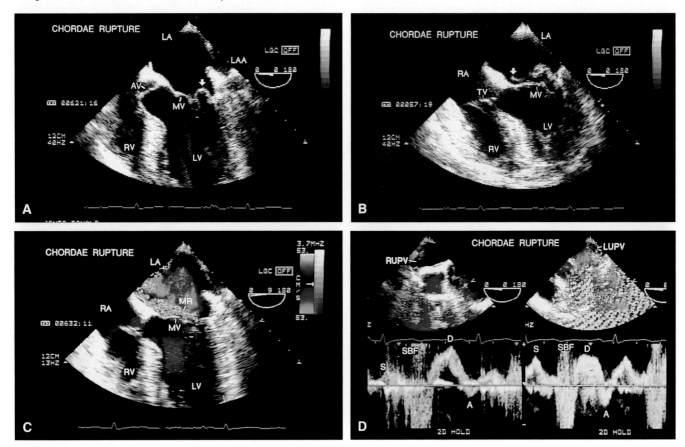

Figure 2.20. **Chordal rupture. A.** Marked prolapse of the posterior mitral leaflet (arrow) with its ruptured chordae (arrowhead) and noncoaptation. **B.** Color Doppler examination shows a large jet of medially directed, eccentric MR with a large zone of flow acceleration indicative of severe MR. This patient underwent mitral annuloplasty with a Duran ring (R). The postoperative study showed no evidence of annulus stenosis **(C)** or residual MR **(D),** indicating an excellent surgical result.

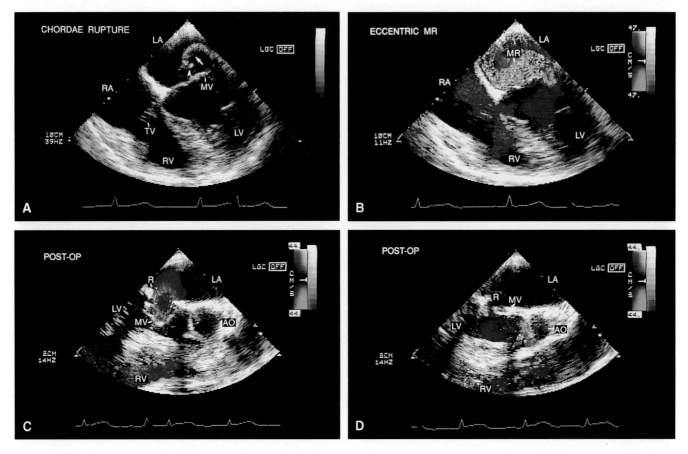

Figure 2.21. **Mitral valve prolapse. A.** Noncoaptation produced by prolapse of the posterior mitral leaflet into the LA (arrow). **B,C.** Color Doppler examination demonstrates an eccentric MR jet coursing medially along the anterior leaflet and the atrial septum. The arrow in **C** points to a large area of flow acceleration indicative of severe MR.

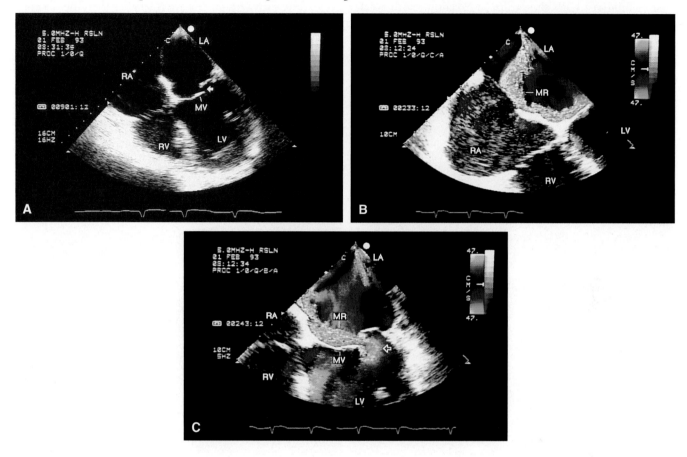

Figure 2.22. **Chordal rupture.** M-mode study demonstrates a ruptured chordae (CH) imaged as a linear echo recorded posterior to the MV.

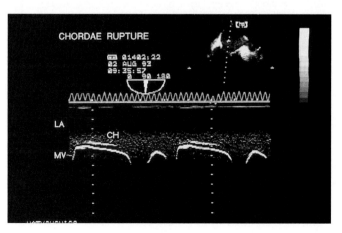

Figure 2.23. **Chordal rupture. A.** The ruptured chordae of both anterior and posterior leaflets of the MV are seen prolapsing dramatically into the LA (arrows). **B.** Diastolic frame shows a flail posterior leaflet with its chordae (arrow) prolapsing into the LA. **C.** Color Doppler examination demonstrates severe MR filling the entire LA. **D.** Pulsed Doppler examination of LUPV shows aliased backflow (SBF) in late systole. The early systolic S wave is smaller than the diastolic D wave. A small A wave caused by atrial systolic backflow into the LUPV is also seen. **E.** This patient underwent mitral annuloplasty. The postoperative study did not demonstrate any MR.

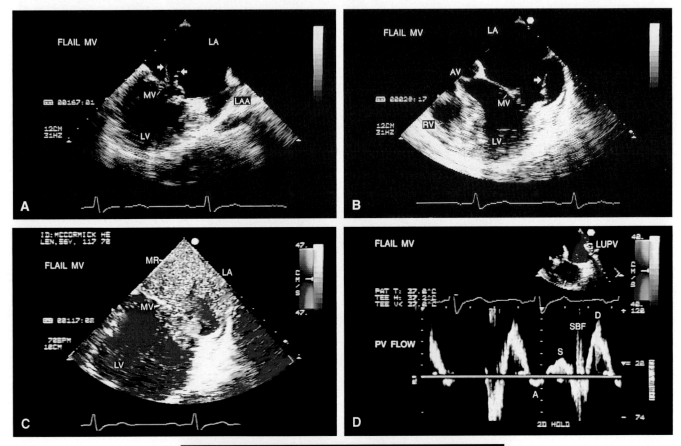

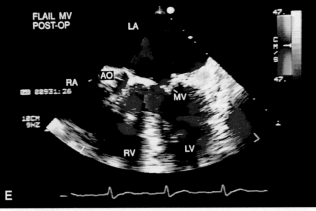

Figure 2.24. **Chordal rupture.** Chordal rupture of both anterior (AML) and posterior (PML) mitral leaflets with noncoaptation (arrows).

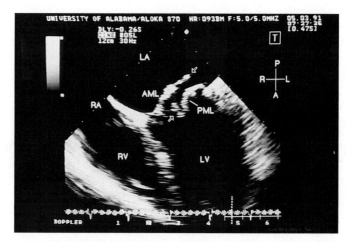

Figure 2.25. **Mitral regurgitation.** **A.** The large jet of eccentric, superiorly directed MR extends into the LAA. **B.** In the same patient, the MR jet entering the LUPV (closed arrow) and its extension into the LAA (open arrow) are seen. Both findings are indicative of severe MR. **C.** Pulsed Doppler interrogation in another patient with severe MR shows prominent aliased systolic backflow (SBF) in the LUPV. **D.** Another patient in whom reversed systolic flow (RSF) was recorded by placing the Doppler sample volume (SV) in the LUPV during surgery. A simultaneously recorded LA tracing shows a prominent V wave, also consistent with severe MR. **E.** Following surgery, systolic backflow is absent. Note the presence of normal A, S, and D waves. **F.** Study of another patient with moderate MR shows a small S wave compared to the D wave and no evidence of systolic backflow. These findings are consistent with moderate MR but may also be seen in patients with diminished LV function without MR. (**D** and **E** reproduced with permission from Rosenthal SM, Nanda NC. Assessment of valvular regurgitation by transesophageal echocardiography. J Invasive Cardiol 1992;4:366–372.)

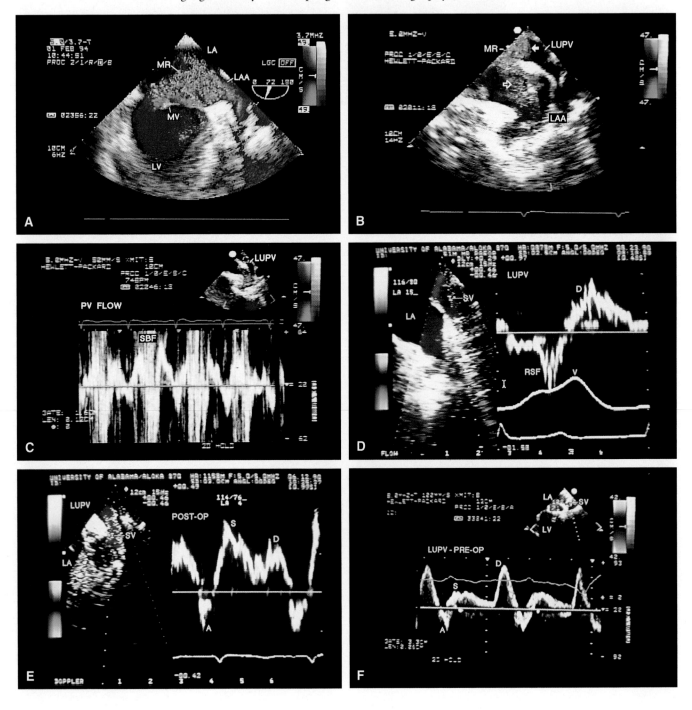

Figure 2.26. **Mitral annuloplasty. A.** A Duran ring (R, R) that was placed in the mitral annulus to reduce the severity of MR in this patient with MV prolapse, severe MR, and a huge LA. **B.** Following surgery two jets of only mild residual MR (arrows) are seen, indicating an excellent surgical result.

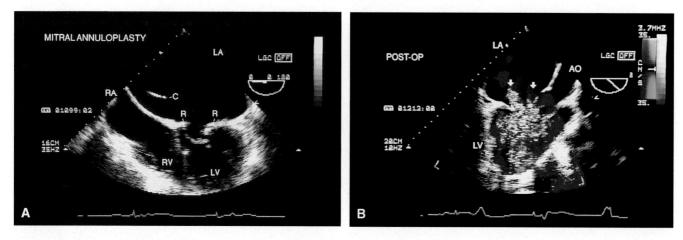

Figure 2.27. Vegetation. **A.** A large vegetation (V) is seen attached to the anterior mitral leaflet on the atrial side. **B,C.** Large vegetations (V) attached to the chordae tendinae in the same patient. *A*, anterior mitral leaflet; *P*, posterior mitral leaflet. **D.** Color Doppler examination shows an unimpressive MR jet. However, there is prominent flow acceleration, and in **E**, systolic backflow (SBF) is seen in RUPV during pulsed Doppler interrogation, indicative of severe MR.

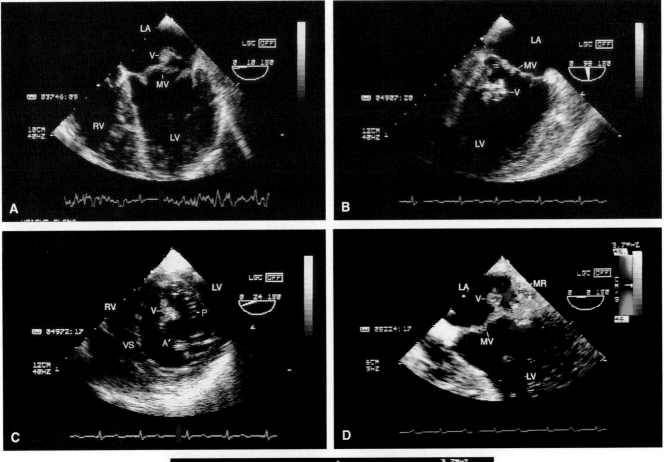

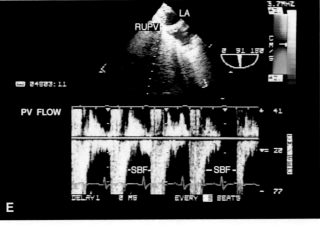

Figure 2.28. **Mitral valve vegetation.** A large vegetation (V) with a long linear, mobile component that has a high propensity to embolize is noted on the atrial side of the anterior leaflet of the mitral valve.

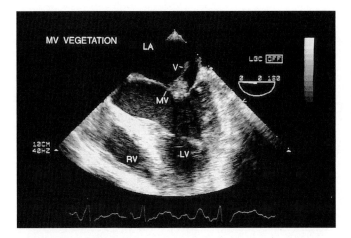

Figure 2.29. **Mitral valve vegetation.** Gross specimen of MV with vegetations.

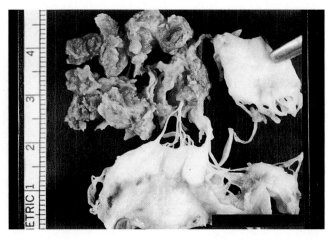

Figure 2.30. **Mitral valve vegetation.** A flail posterior leaflet with a large vegetation (arrowhead) that extends to involve the LV inferior wall (arrow) in this longitudinal plane examination. Another vegetation is present on the tip of the anterior leaflet.

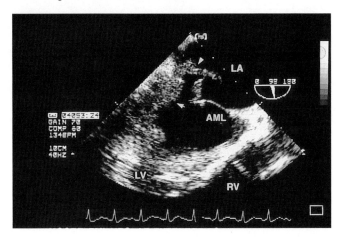

Figure 2.31. **Mitral and aortic vegetations.** An AV vegetation prolapsing into the LVOT (arrow). A much larger vegetation is seen on the atrial side of the MV.

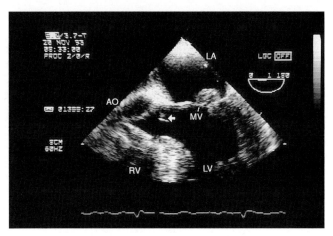

Figure 2.32. **Myxomatous changes. A,B.** A markedly thickened flail posterior leaflet prolapsing into the LA (arrows). The thickening that involves the anterior leaflet is less marked. Such degenerative myxomatous changes produce an image that may be indistinguishable from vegetation. The entire clinical picture must be taken into account to make the correct diagnosis. The diagnosis of myxomatous degeneration in this patient with a flail mitral valve was confirmed at surgery and pathology examination.

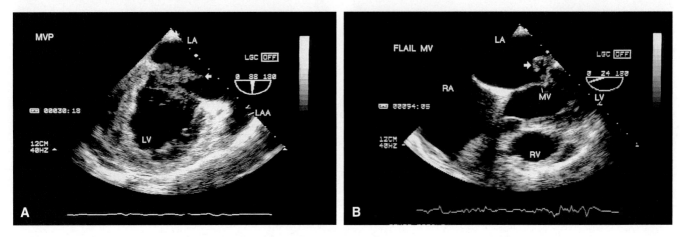

Figure 2.33. **Mitral and aortic valve endocarditis: perforation of the anterior mitral leaflet. A.** A large perforation (arrow) in the body of the anterior mitral leaflet, which is mildly thickened. Note the absence of coaptation of the anterior and posterior leaflets. **B.** A large MR jet (arrowhead) moving through the perforation into the LA. A second MR jet (arrow) is seen moving through the area of noncoaptation of the mitral leaflets. **C.** Color M-mode examination shows pansystolic mitral regurgitation as well as a pandiastolic jet of AR in the LVOT in this patient with endocarditis involving the aortic and mitral valves.

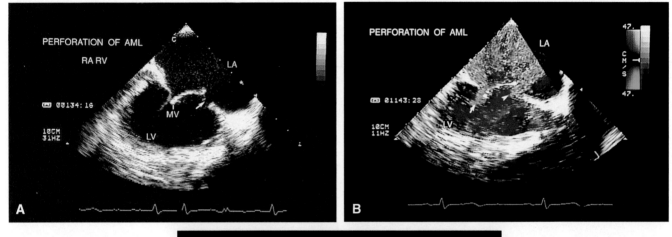

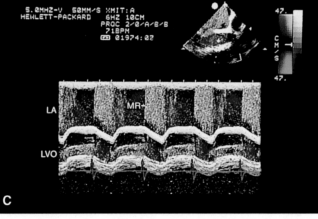

Figure 2.34. **Mitral and aortic valve endocarditis: perforation of mitral and aortic valves. A.** Five-chamber view during diastole demonstrates the anterior mitral leaflet (AML) perforation site, which measures 2.9 mm. AV perforation is also visualized. **B.** Four-chamber view during systole demonstrates significant MR, as indicated by the mosaic-colored flow signals that move through the AML perforation into the LA. The MR jet is directed posteriorly, and a localized area of increased flow velocity (flow acceleration) is seen on the ventricular aspect of the perforation. The defect size by color Doppler is 3.2 mm. **C.** Four-chamber view during diastole demonstrates severe AR, as indicated by the mosaic colored flow signals that occupy the entire proximal LVOT. There is a small mosaic colored jet traversing the perforation site of the AML and moving into the LA. This represents diastolic mitral regurgitation (DMR) that results from LV diastolic pressure being transiently higher than the LA pressure during late diastole. This finding is specific for severe aortic regurgitation in the absence of atrioventricular block. The PR interval was normal in this patient. **D.** The systolic four-chamber view following surgery demonstrates the patch used to repair the AML perforation. **E.** The five-chamber view during diastole shows severe AR, indicated by the mosaic colored flow signals that occupy the entire LVOT. **F.** The five-chamber view during diastole demonstrates a 3-mm left aortic cusp perforation (arrow) with prolapse (PR) of part of this aortic leaflet into the LVOT. (Reproduced with permission from Ballal RS, Mahan EF III, Nanda NC, Sanyal R. Aortic and mitral valve perforation: diagnosis by transesophageal echocardiography and Doppler color imaging. Am Heart J 1991;121:214–217.)

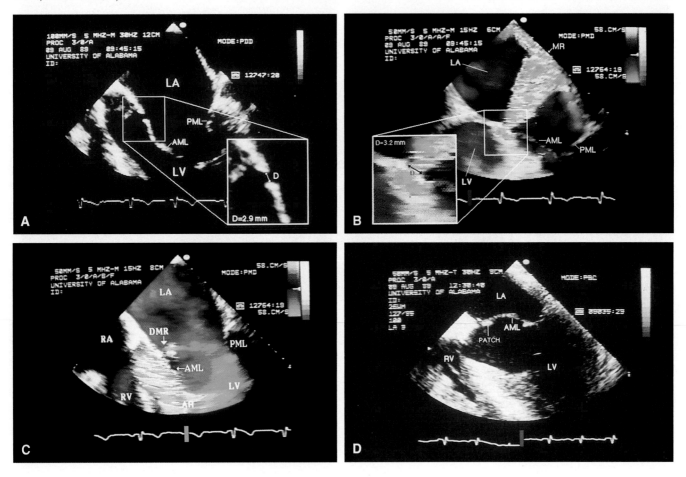

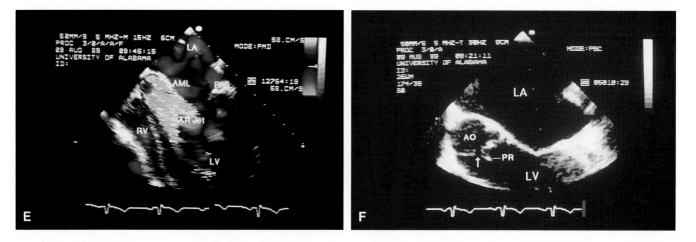

Figure 2.35. **Mitral valve endocarditis.** Gross specimen of an infected MV.

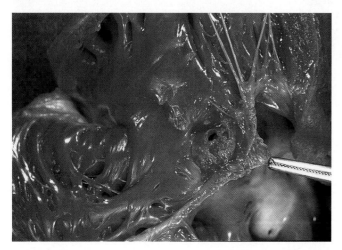

Figure 2.36. **Mitral valve abscess.** A rounded echolucency (arrow) in the infected mitral valve consistent with abscess formation.

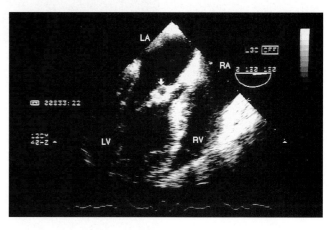

Figure 2.37. **Mitral valve endocarditis. A.** A large vegetation involving the posterior mitral leaflet (arrowhead) and an abscess (arrow) are seen. **B.** A large vegetation involving the posterior mitral leaflet (arrow) and infected chordae (arrowhead). **C.** An MR jet (arrowhead) moving through the vegetation into the LA.

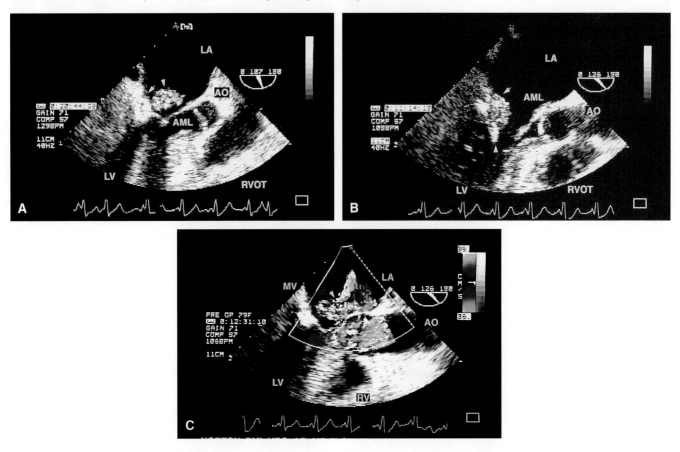

Figure 2.38. **Mitral valve endocarditis.** A round echolucency (arrow) within a large anterior mitral leaflet (AML) vegetation consistent with abscess formation.

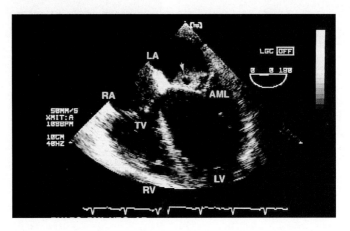

Figure 2.39. **Mitral valve vegetation. A.** *Left panel.* Four-chamber view illustrates a large vegetation (V) attached to the atrial aspect of the MV, which measured 6.71 cm² in maximum area. *Right panel.* Two-chamber view shows involvement of the LA free wall (arrow). **B.** Right ventricular inflow view of the RA illustrates the vegetation (V) on the RA portion of the pacemaker wire (W). **C.** *Left panel.* Intraoperative study before debridement illustrates the smaller size of the vegetation (3.82 cm² in maximum area) on the anterior mitral leaflet (AML), suggestive of embolization. *Right panel.* A pedunculated mass on the ventricular aspect of the AML that remained after debridement, suggestive of residual vegetation. **D.** *Left panel.* Two-chamber view on the 7th postoperative day shows echo-free spaces consistent with abscess (A) formation within the LA vegetation. *Right panel.* Color Doppler study shows MR. **E.** Four-chamber view illustrates abscess formation. **F.** MV vegetation during MV replacement operation. *Left panel.* Preoperative study illustrates rupture of the abscess (arrow) in the LA. *Right panel.* Color Doppler study reveals a sinus tract that communicates with the LV through a 6-mm perforation in the body of the AML. **G.** Postoperative study after replacement of the infected MV with a 27-mm Carpentier-Edwards heterograft shows the structurally normal appearance of the leaflets of the mitral prosthesis (MP) in the long-axis (left panel) and short-axis (right panel) views. **H.** Recurrence of the MV vegetation on the prosthetic valve 8 days after replacement. A large cystic mass consistent with redevelopment of the abscess (A) is seen on the medial aspect of the MP. This case—a 52-year-old man presenting with an MV vegetation—demonstrates the value of serial examinations. Abscess formation, embolization, leaflet perforation, and rupture of the abscess with formation of a sinus tract, as well as vegetations extending to involve the LA free wall and growing on a prosthetic valve and pacemaker lead, were seen in the same patient. (Reproduced with permission from Massey WM, Samdarshi TE, Nanda NC, et al. Serial documentation of changes in a mitral valve vegetation progressing to abscess rupture and fistula formation by transesophageal echocardiography. Am Heart J 1992;124:241–248.)

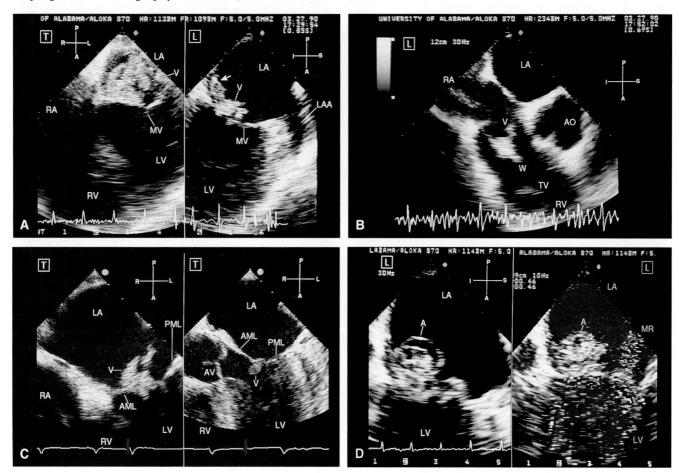

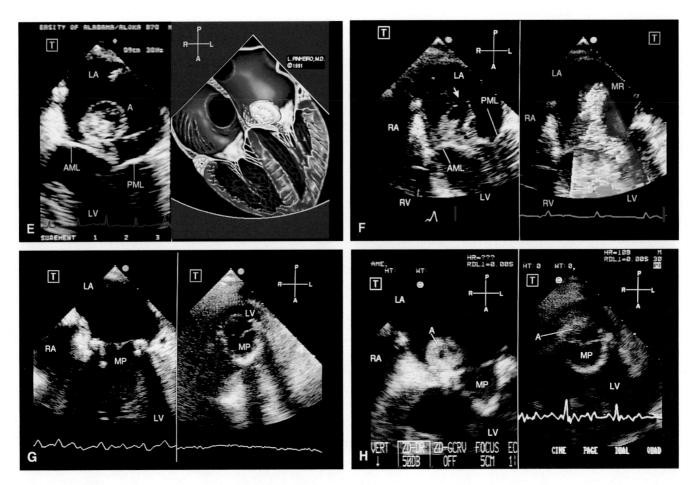

Figure 2.40.   **Mitral valve endocarditis. A,B.** A ruptured chordae (arrows) of an infected posterior mitral leaflet prolapsing into the LA. The large bounded echo-free space is an abscess cavity (AB) involving the mitral annulus. **B.** The MR jet is seen to extend all the way to the junction of the LUPV, indicative of severe MR. **C.** A diastolic frame shows the mitral leaflets in the open position and flow signals from the LAA and LUPV moving into the LA.

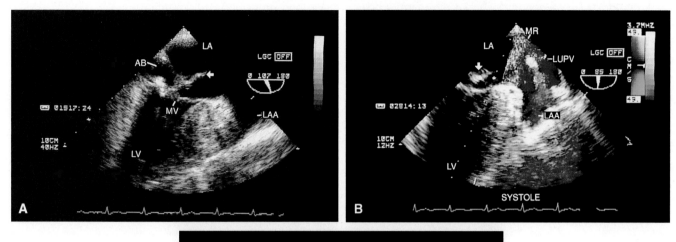

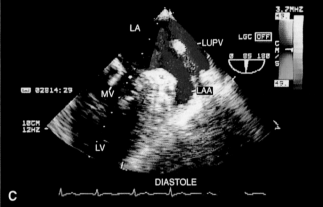

Figure 2.41. **Mitral and aortic valve endocarditis: aneurysm of the annulus fibrosa. A.** Aneurysm at the mitral–aortic junction (arrowhead). **B.** The full extent of the large aneurysm and a fistulous communication with the LA (arrow) are seen. **C.** Color Doppler examination shows flow signals moving from the aneurysm into the LA (arrow). A small MR jet is also seen passing through the region of coaptation of the mitral leaflets. This patient underwent homograft AV replacement and closure of the aneurysm communication using a pericardial patch.

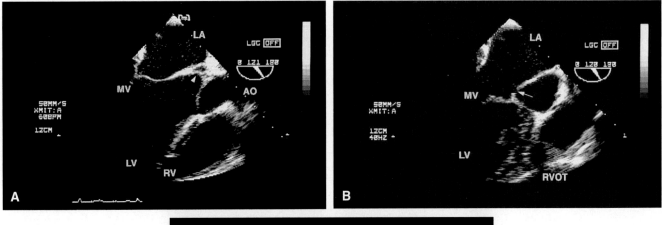

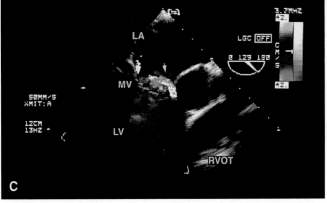

Figure 2.42. **Mitral and aortic valve endocarditis: aneurysm of the annulus fibrosa. A.** Flow signals (arrowhead) moving from the aneurysm (AN) into the LVOT. A small zone of flow acceleration is present on the side of the aneurysm. **B.** A large vegetation (VEG) involving the AV, which was bicuspid. **C,D.** Systolic frames demonstrate flow signals (arrowhead) moving from the LVOT into the aneurysm cavity. In **D,** a small MR jet is seen through the coaptation point. This patient underwent homograft AV replacement, debridement of the abscess cavity, and primary closure of the fistulous communication.

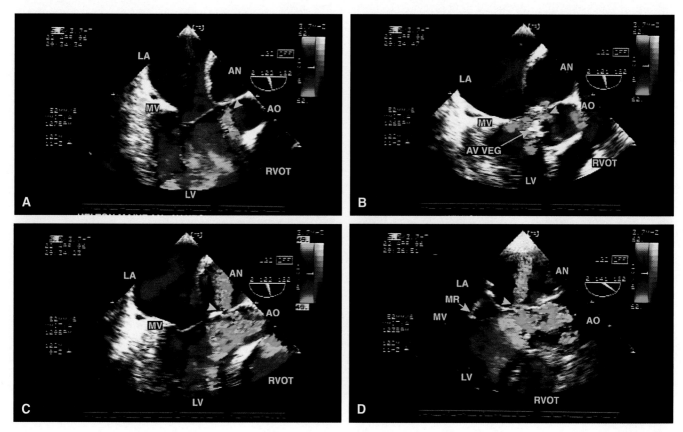

Figure 2.43. **Aneurysm of the annulus fibrosa. A.** A large communication (arrow) between a huge aneurysm (AN) at the mitral–aortic junction and the LVOT. **B.** Color Doppler study shows flow signals moving into the aneurysm from the LVOT. **C.** Color Doppler–guided pulsed Doppler examination shows to-and-fro flow signals moving into and out of the aneurysm sac. **D.** Large aneurysmal sac (AN) opened at surgery. **E.** Pericardial patch (arrows) used to close the opening of the aneurysm shown in the inset (arrowheads). The cause of the aneurysm was not clear in this patient. Three years previously he had undergone aortic valve and root replacement with a pulmonary autograft. There was no evidence of infection. It is possible that this aneurysm was related to his previous surgery.

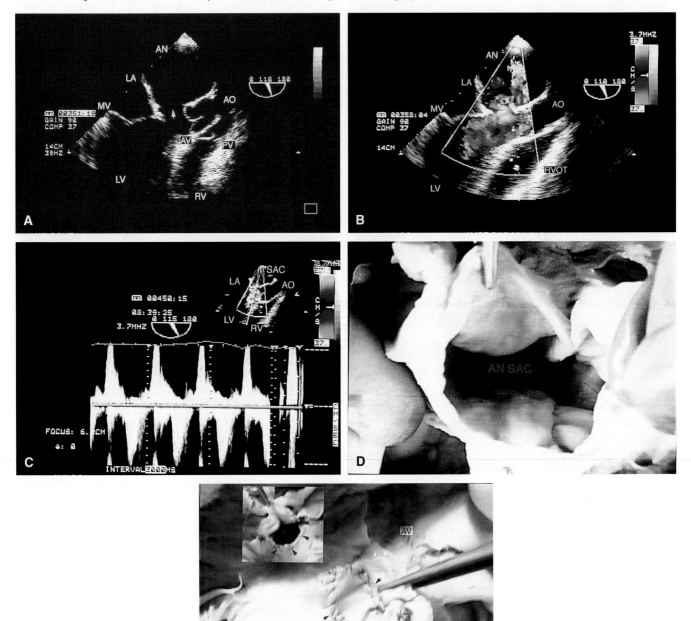

SUGGESTED READINGS

Amuchastegui LM, Cravero C, Salomone O, et al. Atrial mechanical function before and after electrical or amiodarone cardioversion in atrial fibrillation: assessment by transesophageal echocardiography and pulsed Doppler. Echocardiography 1996;13:123–129.

Anayiotos A, Perry GJ, Myers JG, et al. A numerical and experimental investigation of the flow acceleration region proximal to an orifice. Ultrasound Med Biol 1995;21:501–516.

Aschenberg W, Schluter M, Kremer P, et al. Transesophageal two-dimensional echocardiography for the detection of left atrial appendage thrombus. J Am Coll Cardiol 1986;7:163–166.

Bach DS, Deeb GM, Bolling SF. Accuracy of intraoperative transesophageal echocardiography for estimating the severity of functional mitral regurgitation. Am J Cardiol 1995;76:508–512.

Ballal RS, Mahan EF III, Nanda NC, et al. Utility of transesophageal echocardiography in interatrial septal puncture during percutaneous mitral balloon commissurotomy. Am J Cardiol 1990;66:230–232.

Ballal RS, Mahan III EF, Nanda NC, et al. Aortic and mitral valve perforation: diagnosis by transesophageal echocardiography and Doppler color imaging. Am Heart J 1991;121:214–217.

Bansal RC, Graham BM, Jutzy KR, et al. Left ventricular outflow tract to left atrial communication secondary to rupture of mitral-aortic intervalvular fibrosa in infective endocarditis; diagnosis by transesophageal echocardiography and color flow imaging. J Am Coll Cardiol 1990;15:499–504.

Birmingham GD, Rahko PS, Ballantyne F. Improved detection of infective endocarditis with transesophageal echocardiography. Am Heart J 1992;123:774–781.

Black IW, Hopkins AP, Lee LCL, et al. Left atrial spontaneous echo contrast: A clinical and echocardiographic analysis. J Am Coll Cardiol 1991;18:398–404.

Black IW, Stewart WJ. The role of echocardiography in the evaluation of cardiac source of embolism: left atrial spontaneous echo contrast. Echocardiography 1993;10:429–439.

Castello R, Fagan L, Jr, Lenzen P, et al. Comparison of transthoracic and transesophageal echocardiography for assessment of left-sided valvular regurgitation. Am J Cardiol 1991;68:1677–1680.

Chan KL, Marquis JF, Ascah C, et al. Role of transesophageal echocardiography in percutaneous balloon mitral valvuloplasty. Echocardiography 1990;7:115–123.

Currie PJ. Transesophageal echocardiography: intraoperative applications. Echocardiography 1989;6:403–414.

Daniel WG, Mugge A, Martin RP, et al. Improvement in the diagnosis of abscesses associated with endocarditis by transesophageal echocardiography. N Engl J Med 1991;324:795–800.

Daniel WG, Nellessen U, Schroder E, et al. Left atrial spontaneous echo contrast in mitral valve disease: an indicator for an increased thromboembolic risk. J Am Coll Cardiol 1988;11:1204–1211.

Daniel WG, Schroder E, Mugge A, et al. Transesophageal echocardiography in infective endocarditis. Am J Cardiac Imaging 1988;2:78–85.

Eicher JC, Falcon-Eicher S, Sota FX, et al. Mitral ring abscess caused by bacterial endocarditis on a heavily calcified mitral annulus fibrosus: diagnosis by multiplane transesophageal echocardiography. Am Heart J 1996;131:818–820.

Erbel R, Rohmann S, Drexler M, et al. Improved diagnostic value of echocardiography in patients with infective endocarditis by transesophageal approach. A prospective study. Eur Heart J 1988;9:43–53.

Fan PH, Anayiotos A, Nanda NC, et al. Intramachine and intermachine variability in transesophageal color Doppler images of pulsatile jets. In vitro studies. Circulation 1994;8:2141–2149.

Freeman WK, Schaff HV, Khandheria BK, et al. Intraoperative evaluation of mitral valve regurgitation and repair by transesophageal echocardiography: incidence and significance of systolic anterior motion. J Am Coll Cardiol 1992;20:509–609.

Hausmann D, Daniel WG, Heublein B, et al. Transesophageal echocardiography in candidates for percutaneous balloon mitral valvuloplasty. Echocardiography 1994;11:553–559.

Hellemans IM, Pieper EG, Ravelli AC, et al. Comparison of transthoracic and transesophageal echocardiography with surgical findings in mitral regurgitation. Am J Cardiol 1996;77:728–733.

Hozumi T, Yoshikawa J, Yoshida K, et al. Direct visualization of ruptured chordae tendineae by transesophageal two-dimensional echocardiography. J Am Coll Cardiol 1990;16:1315–1319.

Kamp O, Huitink H, van Eenige MJ, et al. Value of pulmonary venous flow characteristics in the assessment of severity of native mitral valve regurgitation: an angiographic correlated study. J Am Soc Echocardiogr 1992;5:239–246.

Klein AL, Obarski TP, Stewart WJ, et al. Transesophageal Doppler echocardiography of pulmonary venous flow: a new marker of mitral regurgitation severity. J Am Coll Cardiol 1991;18:518–526.

Liu F, Ge J, Kupferwasser I, et al. Has transesophageal echocardiography changed the approach to patients with suspected or known infective endocarditis? Echocardiography 1995;12:637–650.

Mahan EF III, Ballal RS, Nanda NC. Mitral valve tear complicating percutaneous valvuloplasty: diagnosis by transesophageal Doppler color flow mapping. Am Heart J 1991;122:238–242.

Manning WJ, Reis GJ, Douglas PS. Use of transesophageal echocardiography to detect left atrial thrombi before percutaneous balloon dilation of the mitral valve: a prospective study. Br Heart J 1992;67:170–173.

Massey WM, Samdarshi TE, Nanda NC, et al. Serial documentation of changes in a mitral valve vegetation progressing to abscess rupture and fistula formation by transesophageal echocardiography. Am Heart J 1992;124:241–248

Mugge A, Daniel WG. Echocardiographic assessment of vegetations in patients with infective endocarditis: prognostic implications. Echocardiography 1995;12:651–661.

Mugge A, Daniel WG, Frank G, et al. Echocardiography in infective endocarditis: reassessment of prognostic implications of vegetation size determined by the transthoracic and the transesophageal approach. J Am Coll Cardiol 1989;14:631–638.

Mugge A, Daniel WG, Hausmann D, et al. Diagnosis of left atrial appendage thrombi by transesophageal echocardiography: Clinical implications and follow-up. Am J Cardiac Imaging 1990;4:173–179.

Mugge A, Kuhn H, Daniel WG. The role of transesophageal echocardiography in the detection of left atrial thrombi. Echocardiography 1993;10:405–417.

Nomeir A-M, Downes TR, Cordell AR. Perforation of the anterior mitral leaflet caused by aortic valve endocarditis: diagnosis by two-dimensional, transesophageal echocardiography and color flow Doppler. J Am Soc Echocardiogr 1992;5:195–198.

Patel JJ, Ross JJ, Jr, Chandrasekaran K. A form fruste of Shone's complex diagnosed by transesophageal echocardiography. Echocardiography 1996;13:147–149.

Pearson AC. Transthoracic echocardiography versus transesophageal echocardiography in detecting cardiac sources of embolism. Echocardiography 1993;10:397–403.

Pieper EP, Hellemans IM, Hamer HP, et al. Value of systolic pulmonary venous flow reversal and color Doppler jet measurements assessed with transesophageal echocardiography in recognizing severe pure mitral regurgitation. Am J Cardiol 1996;78:444–450.

Pieper EP, Hellemans IM, Hamer HP, et al. Additional value of biplane transesophageal echocardiography in assessing the genesis of mitral regurgitation and the feasibility of valve repair. Am J Cardiol 1995;75:489–493.

Pollick C, Taylor D. Assessment of left atrial appendage function by transesophageal echocardiography. Implications for the development of thrombus. Circulation 1991;84:223.

Porte JM, Cormier B, Lung B, et al. Early assessment by transesophageal echocardiography of left atrial appendage function after percutaneous mitral commissurotomy. Am J Cardiol 1996;77:72–76.

Reichert SL, Visser CA, Moulijn AC, et al. Intraoperative transesophageal color-coded Doppler echocardiography for evaluation of residual regurgitation after mitral valve repair. J Thorac Cardiovasc Surg 1990;100:756–761.

Roberson DA, Arcilla RA, Sachsteder W, et al. Transesophageal echocardiographic diagnosis of intussusception of the left atrial appendage. Echocardiography 1993;10:619–622.

Roguin A, Rinkevich D, Milo S, et al. Diagnosis of mitral valve aneurysms by transesophageal echocardiography. Am Heart J 1996;132:689–691.

Rohmann S, Erbel R, Gorge G, et al. Clinical relevance of vegetation localization by transesophageal echocardiography in infective endocarditis. Eur Heart J 1992;13:446–452.

Rosenthal SM, Nanda NC. Assessment of valvular regurgitation by transesophageal echocardiography. J Invasive Cardiol 1992;4:366–372.

Sadoshima JI, Koyanagi S, Sugimachi M, et al. Evaluation of the severity of mitral regurgitation by transesophageal Doppler flow echocardiography. Am Heart J 1992;123:1245–1251.

Shively BK, Gurule FT, Roldan CA, et al. Diagnostic value of transesophageal compared with transthoracic echocardiography in infective endocarditis. J Am Coll Cardiol 1991;18:391–397.

Smith MD, Harrison MR, Pinton R, et al. Regurgitant jet size by transesophageal compared with transthoracic Doppler color flow imaging. Circulation 1991;83:79–86.

Stewart WJ, Griffin B, Thomas JD. Multiplane transesophageal echocardiographic evaluation of mitral valve disease. Am J Cardiac Imaging 1995;9:121–128.

Stoddard MF, Dawkins PR, Prince CR, et al. Left atrial appendage thrombus is not uncommon in patients with acute atrial fibrillation and a recent embolic event: a transesophageal echocardiographic study. J Am Coll Cardiol 1995;25:452–459.

Yoshida K, Yoshikawa J, Yamaura Y, et al. Assessment of mitral regurgitation by biplane transesophageal color Doppler flow mapping. Circulation 1990;82:1121–1126.

Aortic Valve and Aorta

3

Transesophageal echocardiography (TEE) has assumed a central role in the echocardiographic examination of the aortic valve because of the superior imaging detail that it provides compared to transthoracic echocardiography (TTE). Because the multiplane probe permits great flexibility in the selection of the imaging plane, it is far more effective than single and biplane probes in providing a complete study of a variety of lesions. TEE should be considered a complement to, but not a replacement for, transthoracic echocardiography.

A number of findings suggest or are consistent with aortic stenosis (AS). Thickening of the aortic valve is clearly seen on TEE; when limitation of motion also is present, this is consistent with AS. Color Doppler detection of a narrow (7 mm or less at its origin) systolic jet indicates severe stenosis.

Planimetry of the minimum orifice area in the short-axis view (usually best imaged at 30° to 60°) has been shown to correlate well with catheterization-derived aortic valve area. The stenotic valve often has the geometry of a truncated cone. It is important that the very top of this cone be studied, because it is the flow-limiting orifice. To ensure that the minimum orifice is imaged, the probe first is moved up the esophagus in the short-axis view until the aortic valve disappears. The probe is then advanced until the full perimeter of the valve just comes into view, which should demonstrate the minimum cross-sectional area (flow-limiting orifice). Gain must be carefully adjusted to minimize the "blooming" effect of the extensive calcium that is usually present in adults, and the probe must be manipulated to avoid acoustic shadowing by the calcium. In the presence of severe calcification it may be difficult to identify the orifice. When this difficulty arises, color Doppler is often helpful because the first signals appear in the orifice at the beginning of systole.

An attempt can be made to position the TEE image so that a pressure gradient can be measured between the left ventricle and the aorta using the transgastric view. If a high gradient is obtained, AS can be diagnosed. It is difficult to be certain that the maximum gradient has been measured, however, because TEE has limited capacity for looking for the maximum jet at multiple angles.

Left ventricular hypertrophy is well imaged by TEE and commonly accompanies aortic stenosis. It is particularly important to exclude the presence of coexisting hypertrophic cardiomyopathy (HCM), because the hypertrophied muscle can be resected at the time of aortic valve replacement. A narrow left ventricular outflow tract

(<20 mm) and hypertrophy out of proportion to what would be expected from the degree of aortic stenosis present alerts the echocardiographer to the possibility of coexisting HCM. Systolic anterior motion of the mitral valve may be absent in HCM patients with severe aortic stenosis.

An interesting lesion that can be identified by TEE is supravalvular AS. This lesion may be congenital, or it may be present in patients with atherosclerosis and very high cholesterol levels.

The morphologic data available from TEE allow detailed examination of the aortic valve. The multiplane probe is substantially more effective than are single or biplane probes. The mild thickening normally present at the points of leaflet coaptation (nodules of Arantius) also may be identified. TEE effectively defines the number of leaflets and the degree of commissural fusion present. The median raphe of a bicuspid valve can be clearly seen. The distinction between tricuspid and bicuspid aortic valve is important because of the difference in prognosis and the implications for valve repair versus valve replacement. The presence of valve redundancy, which may be confused with a vegetation on transthoracic echo, can be delineated. Eversion ("rolling up" of the edges) of the leaflets is also well demonstrated.

The cause of aortic regurgitation (AR), including thickening, eversion of the leaflets, infection, dilatation of the proximal aorta with loss of leaflet coaptation, and redundancy, can be delineated. Intermittent AR, caused by varying coaptation points resulting from valve redundancy (especially in a bicuspid valve), can also be detected. Small fenestrations as well as large holes and their exact location and size can be imaged.

TEE is of particular importance in the workup for endocarditis. TEE is far more sensitive for the assessment of vegetations than is TTE. For this reason, in the appropriate clinical setting, the absence of a vegetation on TTE should prompt the performance of TEE. Abscesses are also far more likely to be seen on TEE than TTE. Their anatomic location and extent are readily imaged, and their communication with other structures is diagnosed using color-flow Doppler.

Assessment of the severity of AR is based on semiquantitation using the fraction of the left ventricular outflow tract (LVOT) at the origin of the diastolic jet on the ventricular aspect of the aortic valve that is covered by the jet. The ratio of proximal jet width to LVOT diameter (taken at the same location) of <39% represents mild or moderate regurgitation; 39% to 74% represents moderately severe AR; and ≥75% represents severe AR. Two technical points are important. First, the assessment must be made at the origin of the jet. Second, the Nyquist limit is important. If it is set higher than 35 to 45 cm/sec, changes in the color filter result in loss of imaging of lower velocities and thus change the size of the proximal jet.

Defining aortic anatomy is another important application of TEE. The location and extent of aortic aneurysms are more effectively visualized using TEE than TTE. The ability of TEE to image the entire aorta is an important advantage over TTE. Evidence of rupture can be sought and the extent of associated AR can be assessed using color-flow Doppler. In many centers, TEE is the modality of choice for diagnosing aortic dissection because of its ability to rapidly and accurately make the diagnosis. This is important because these patients may die suddenly if surgery is not performed immediately.

The diagnosis of dissection is based on the demonstration of a flap that separates the true (TL) and false (FL) lumens. It is necessary to examine the aorta in multiple planes because the flap is not well seen in all views. The flap is usually, but not always, mobile, which aids in making the diagnosis. Flow in opposite directions on the different sides of the flap, if present, helps to confirm the diagnosis. A number of features aid in differentiating the TL from the FL and may help confirm the diagnosis of aortic dissection. Flow in the TL usually has higher velocity than flow in the FL; as a result, the signals are generally brighter. In addition, the TL expands in systole and the FL expands in diastole. When a clot is present it is usually in the FL. Communications between the TL and FL seen on color Doppler are helpful in confirming the diagnosis. Because the entire thoracic and proximal abdominal aorta can be imaged using the multiplane probe, the exact location and full extent of dissection can be delineated.

Dissections that involve the ascending aorta, arch, or both, and the descending aorta are DeBakey type I. Those that involve the ascending aorta, arch, or both (but not the descending aorta) are DeBakey type II, and those that involve only the descending aorta are Type III. In the Stanford classification, any dissection involving the ascending aorta, the arch, or both arch is type A, whereas dissection involving the descending aorta only is type B.

TEE is useful in assessing prognosis and making management decisions. A clotted false lumen has a better prognosis than a flow-filled false lumen because it acts as a buttress for the true lumen, thereby diminishing the chance of rupture. Assessment of the cause and severity of AR in dissection patients helps in making a decision regarding the necessity of resuspension or replacement of the aortic valve. Involvement of the coronary arteries in the dissection can also be diagnosed. Dissections that involve only the descending aorta do not require surgery unless there is evidence of impending rupture or compromise of organ flow, which occurs rarely.

Atherosclerotic plaques in the aorta are readily identified by TEE. The presentation varies from uniform intimal thickening to large mobile plaques protruding into the lumen. Atherosclerosis in the aorta is a risk factor for stroke and emboli to other parts of the body. The greater the mobility, the higher the risk of embolization. Fixed plaques protruding more than 5 mm into the lumen are also at high risk for embolization.

Figure 3.1. **Aortic stenosis. A,B.** The valve is mildly thickened and doming but opens well, consistent with mild aortic stenosis. **C-E.** Patient with severe calcific aortic stenosis. The valve is markedly thickened and calcified (arrows), and the opening of the valve is severely restricted. Flow acceleration (arrowheads) and turbulence in the aortic root, **(E)** are indicative of significant aortic stenosis. This patient underwent aortic valve replacement. **F.** The wide aortic jet (arrowheads) in another patient suggests an absence of significant aortic stenosis. **G.** The jet (arrowhead) shown in this illustration, on the other hand, is narrow (<7 mm) at its origin, indicative of severe aortic stenosis. Marked poststenotic dilatation of the aorta is present. It is important to assess jet width at its exit point from the aortic valve. At surgery, this patient was found to have a heavily calcified, severely stenotic aortic valve. He underwent CarboMedics aortic valve replacement.

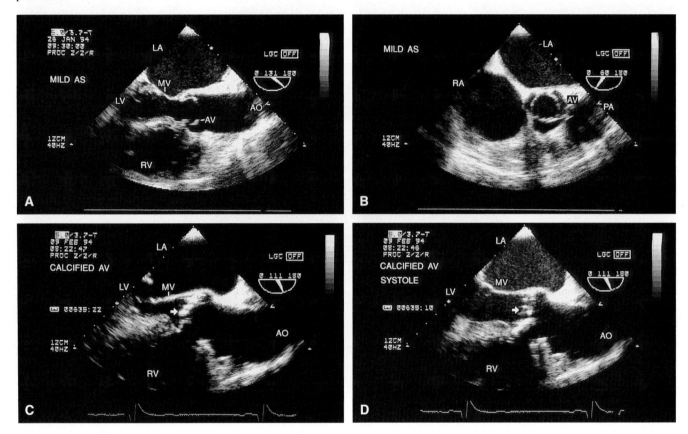

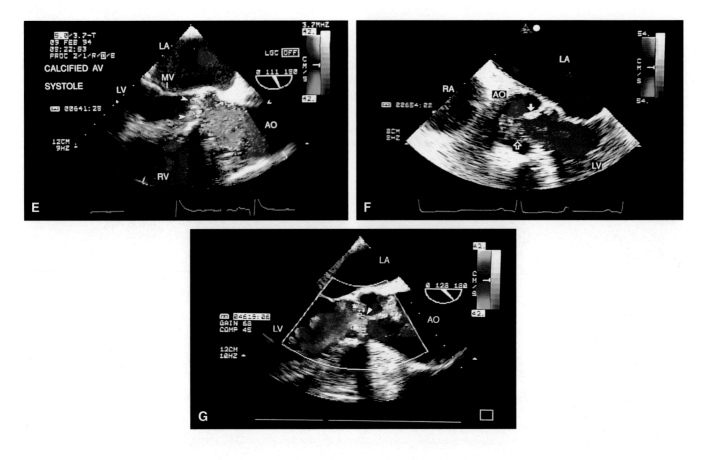

Figure 3.2. **Aortic stenosis. A,B.** A thickened aortic valve with markedly restricted opening (arrow). The inset in **B** shows the valve orifice imaged in short axis. **C.** Planimetry of the orifice of a thickened valve in the short-axis view is shown in another patient. An area of 0.74 cm² is found in this patient. The bottom inset in **C** demonstrates that color Doppler can help to identify the orifice; the top inset shows a narrow jet (arrowheads) consistent with severe stenosis. The probe must be moved carefully up and down the esophagus until the minimum cross-sectional area is found. This yields the flow-limiting orifice area. This point is emphasized in **D**, which shows that planimetry of the minimum area yields a valve area of 0.68 cm² whereas planimetry more proximally gives an area of 1.43 cm². **E-G.** Gross specimens of thickened tri-leaflet aortic valves show calcium in the cusps that restricts opening. (**C** reproduced with permission from Kim KS, Maxted W, Nanda NC, et al. Comparison of multiplane and biplane transesophageal echocardiography in the assessment of aortic stenosis. Am J Cardiol 1997;79:436–441.)

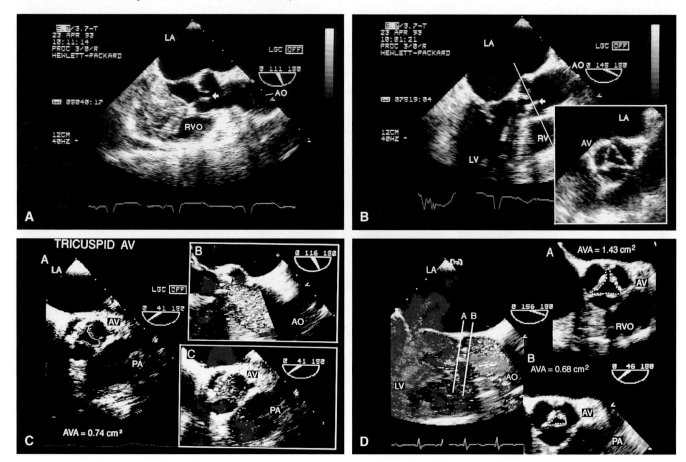

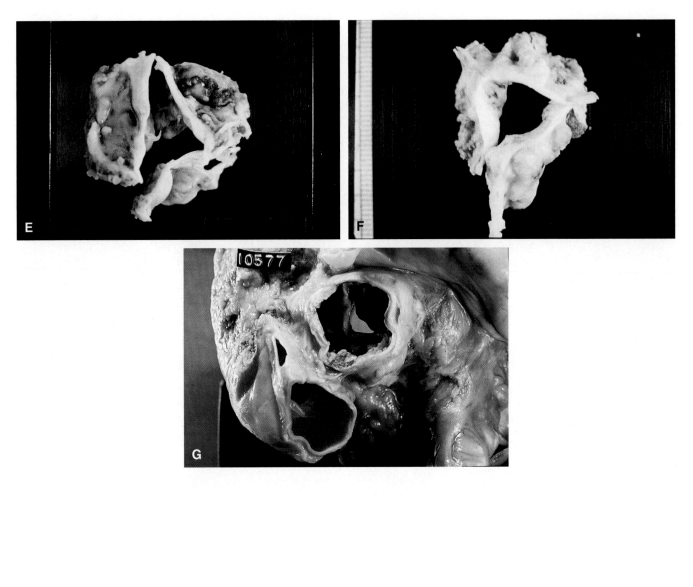

Figure 3.3. **Aortic stenosis. A.** Planimetry reveals severe bicuspid aortic stenosis with a valve area of 0.52 cm². *Upper inset panel*: A very narrow jet consistent with severe aortic stenosis. *Lower inset panel*: Acoustic shadowing that results in dropout of part of the image so that color does not fill the entire orifice. Careful positioning of the probe is necessary if the valve is to be accurately planimetered. **B.** Severe bicuspid aortic valve stenosis is seen in another patient. **C.** Gross specimen shows a thickened and calcified bicuspid aortic valve. (**A** reproduced with permission from Kim KS, Maxted W, Nanda NC, et al. Comparison of multiplane and biplane transesophageal echocardiography in the assessment of aortic stenosis. Am J Cardiol 1997;79:436–441.)

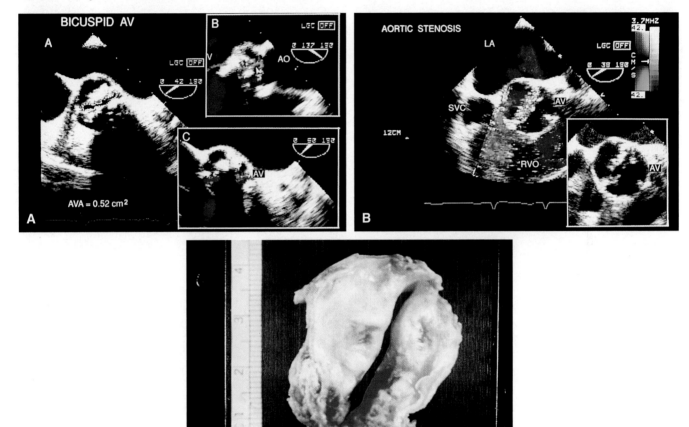

Figure 3.4. **Aortic stenosis. A,B.** A bicuspid valve mimicking a tricuspid aortic valve. Although the valve appears to have three leaflets, it was found to be tricuspid at surgery. **C,D.** This valve (arrowheads) appears to be bicuspid but was surgically shown to be tricuspid. **E.** The narrow jet (arrow) confirms the presence of severe stenosis in this patient. **F.** In another patient, color Doppler examination was helpful in identifying the eccentric severely stenotic orifice. This patient underwent aortic valve replacement. **G.** The surgically resected specimen from the patient in **F** shows a heavily calcified, severely stenotic bicuspid valve.

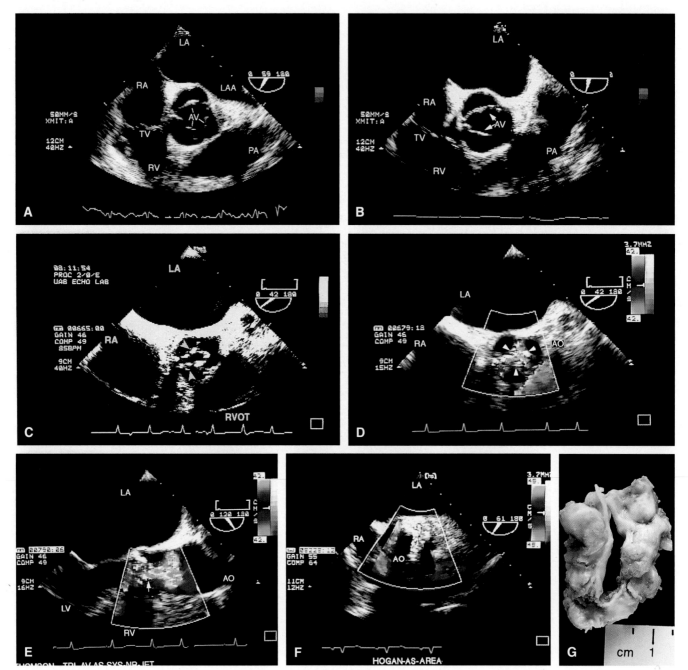

Figure 3.5. Aortic stenosis. Two patients with fixed stenotic orifices are shown. **A.** Size of the orifice (arrow), which measures 0.36 cm², does not change from diastole to systole. Color Doppler examination (inset) was helpful in delineating the orifice. **B-D.** Another patient with a fixed stenotic orifice (arrowheads), which does not change in size from diastole (**B**) to systole (**C**). In such cases, color Doppler examination is useful in identifying the orifice (**D**). (**A** reproduced with permission from Kim KS, Maxted W, Nanda NC, et al. Comparison of multiplane and biplane transesophageal echocardiography in the assessment of aortic stenosis. Am J Cardiol 1997;79:436–441.)

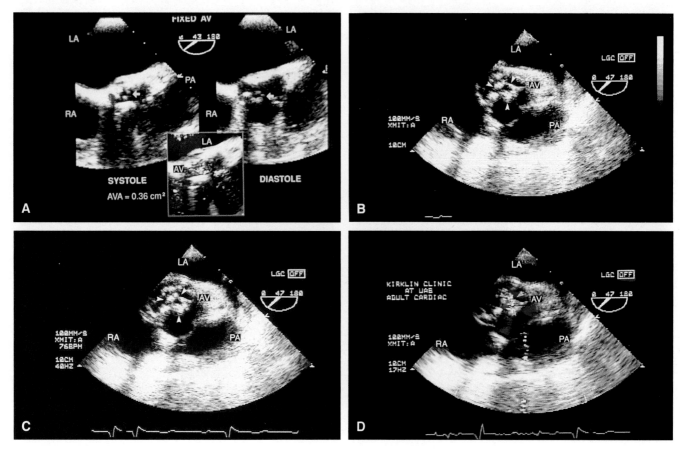

Figure 3.6. **Aortic stenosis.** Associated LV hypertrophy is shown in the transgastric view. **A.** The wall thickness measures more than 20 mm. **B,C.** Fibroelastosis developing in another patient with aortic stenosis. Note the thickened, hyper-refractile endocardium (arrowheads).

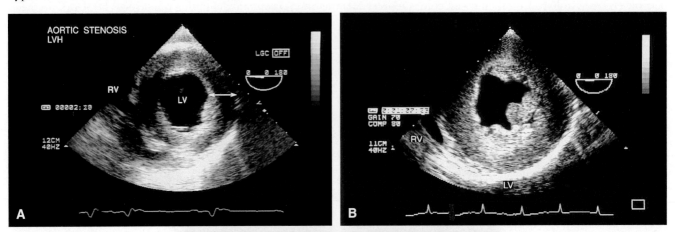

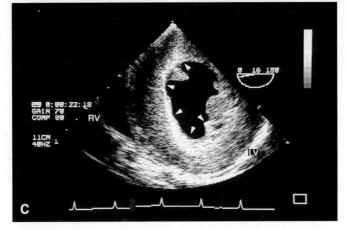

Figure 3.7. **Aortic stenosis. A.** Aortic stenosis coexisting with hypertrophic cardiomyopathy. A markedly thickened ventricular septum, narrow LVOT, systolic anterior motion (SAM) of the mitral valve, and aortic valve with restricted opening are seen. **B,C.** Another patient with SAM of the anterior mitral leaflet, hypertrophied ventricular septum, and a thickened aortic valve with marked restriction of opening. This patient underwent aortic valve replacement for severe stenosis and left ventricular septal myomectomy.

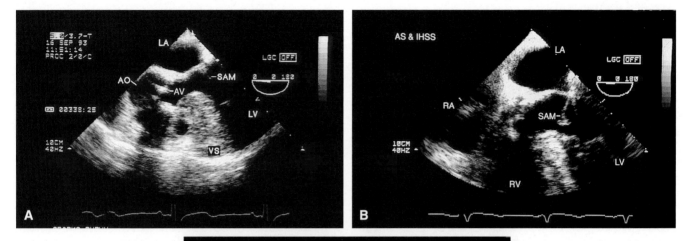

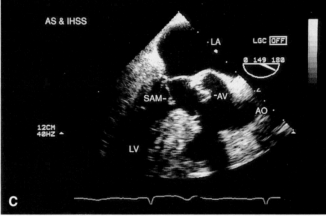

Figure 3.8. **Aortic valve thickening. A,B.** Localized thickenings (arrowheads) called nodules of Arantius are often seen in normal patients on the aortic valve at the points of leaflet coaptation. **C,D** Another patient with prominent localized thickening (arrow) of the right coronary cusp causing aortic regurgitation (arrow in **D**). **E.** Calcification results in mild narrowing of the aorta at the level of the sinotubular junction (arrows). Severe acquired supravalvular aortic stenosis can occur in patients with familial, homozygous hypercholesterolemia. **F.** Fibrotic thickening (arrowheads) is shown at the base of the aortic leaflets.

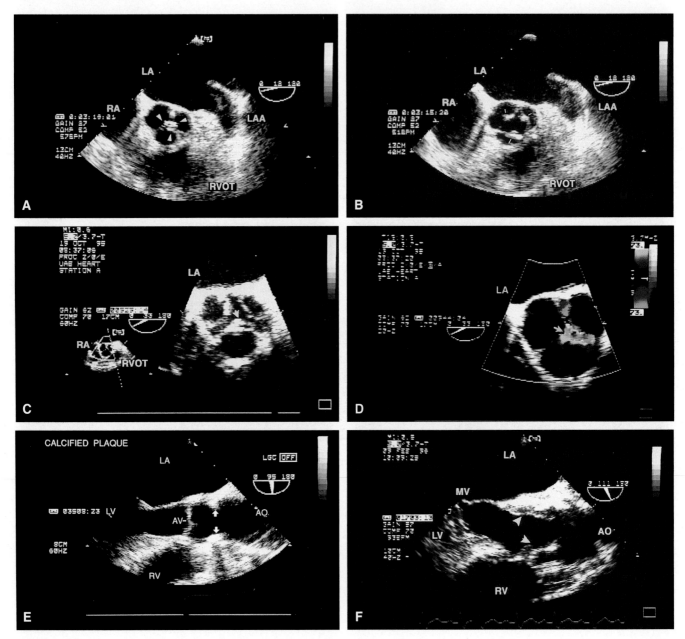

Figure 3.9. **Aortic regurgitation. A,B.** Mild aortic regurgitation (arrows). Note the narrow jet width at its origin. **C.** The aortic regurgitation jet is seen between the left and right aortic cusps. **D.** A color M-mode shows a narrow, eccentric, pandiastolic aortic regurgitation jet. **E,F.** Somewhat wider jets, suggesting more severe aortic regurgitation than in the earlier panels, are seen. **G.** The width of the jet at its origin occupies approximately 60% of the LVOT, indicating moderately severe (3/4) aortic regurgitation. **H-J.** The proximal regurgitant jet occupies the entire LVOT, indicative of severe aortic regurgitation (4/4). **K,L.** The effect of changing the Nyquist limit on the width of the regurgitant jet. At the lower Nyquist limit of 37 cm/sec (**L**) the jet width/LVOT width ratio is 81%, indicating severe aortic insufficiency, which was confirmed at cardiac catheterization. When the Nyquist limit is increased to 55 cm/sec (**K**), the ratio of jet width to LVOT width is reduced to 53%, consistent with moderately severe regurgitation. This illustrates that the Nyquist limit should be kept in the range of 35 to 45 cm/sec for accurate assessment of AR severity. The primary reason for the alteration in jet width with a change in the Nyquist limit is the associated change in the color filter.

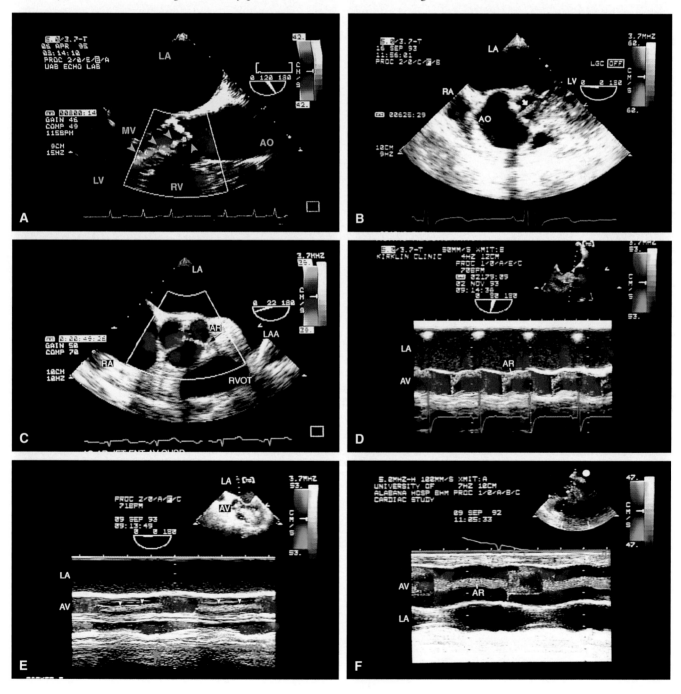

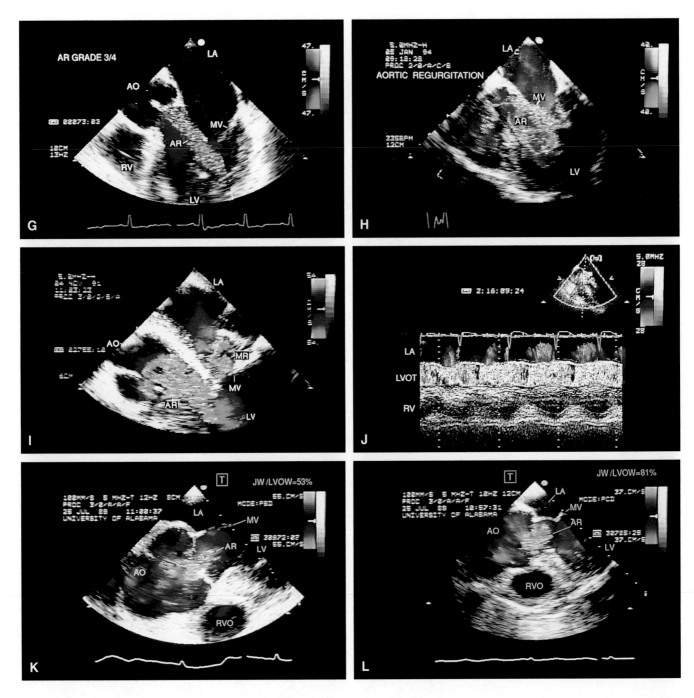

Figure 3.10. **Redundant aortic valve. A,B.** Redundant (arrowhead) right coronary cusp is shown with and without color Doppler. The other cusps do not appear to be redundant. **C,D.** In another patient the linear echo prolapsing into the LVOT (arrowhead) represents cusp redundancy. **E.** An M-mode study shows systolic fluttering of the aortic valve, which is a normal finding and is not necessarily related to the redundancy.

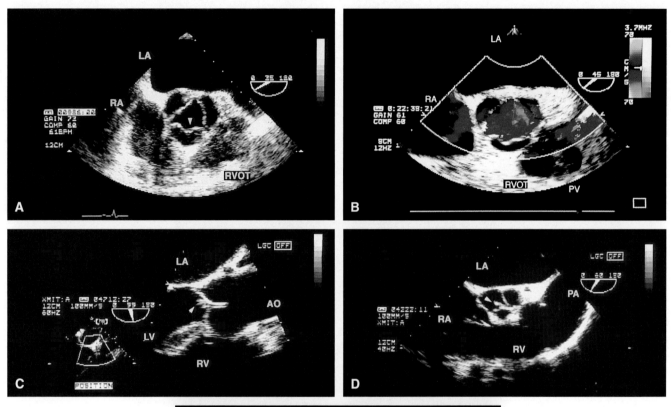

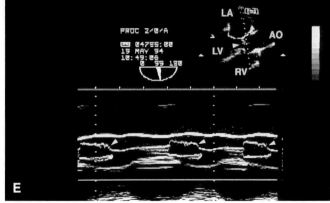

Figure 3.11. **Redundant aortic valve. A.** Redundant aortic valve (arrow) prolapsing into the LVOT. **B,C.** Eccentric jets of aortic regurgitation (arrows). In both patients the aortic regurgitation jet is directed posteriorly and abuts the mitral valve.

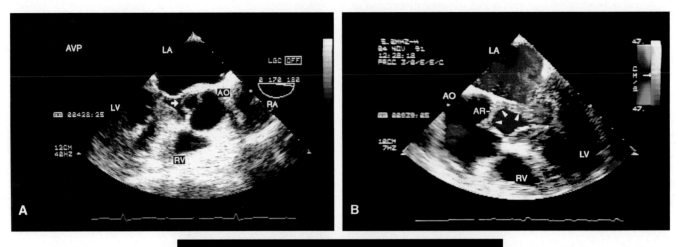

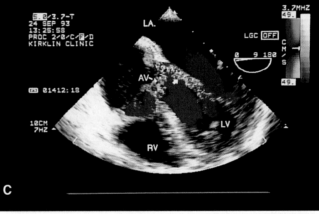

Figure 3.12.   **Redundant aortic valve.** The arrows show various components of a redundant, noninfected bicuspid aortic valve prolapsing into the LVOT **(A-D)** with a posteriorly directed regurgitant jet **(E,F).** The flow acceleration (FA) is large, indicating significant regurgitation even though the proximal jet width appears narrow. This is related to the eccentric geometry of the jet as well as to the high Nyquist limit of 49 cm/sec. **G.** Systolic frame in the same patient clearly shows a bicuspid aortic valve with a raphe (lower arrow). **H.** The diastolic frame mimics a tricuspid aortic valve, emphasizing the importance of examining the valve throughout the cardiac cycle. This patient underwent aortic valve annuloplasty.

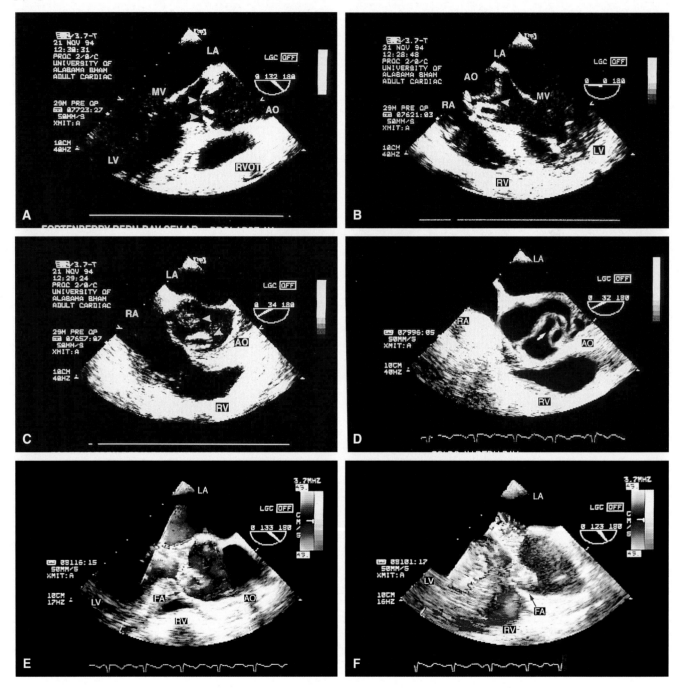

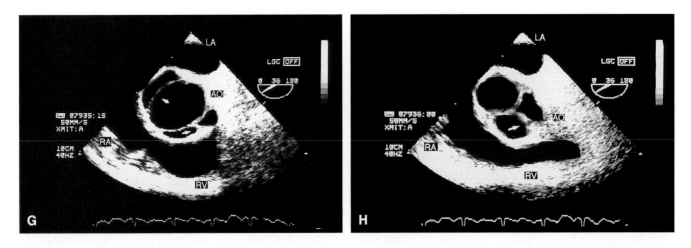

Figure 3.13. **Redundant aortic valve. A-C.** The diastolic frames show central noncoaptation (NC) of the aortic valve leaflets that results in aortic regurgitation (arrow in **C**). **D.** Cusp separation in diastole is also well seen in the M-mode study.

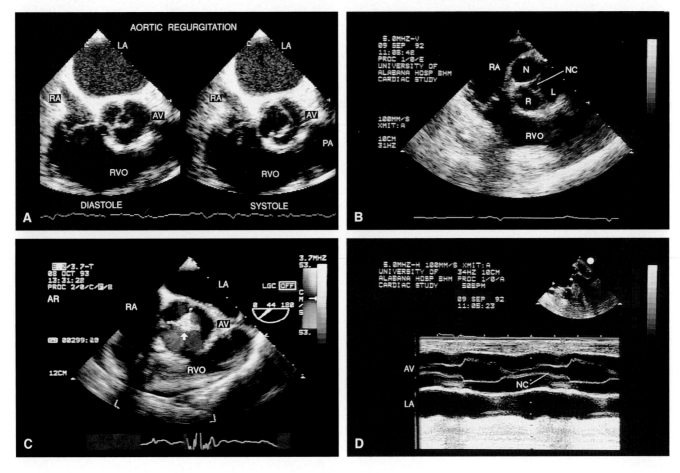

Figure 3.14. Redundant aortic valve with hole in right coronary cusp. **A,B.** A hole (arrows) in the right coronary cusp of the aortic valve, which prolapses into the LVOT. **C.** An area of noncoaptation (arrow) between the left and noncoronary cusps. **D.** Severe aortic regurgitation with a large flow acceleration (arrow).

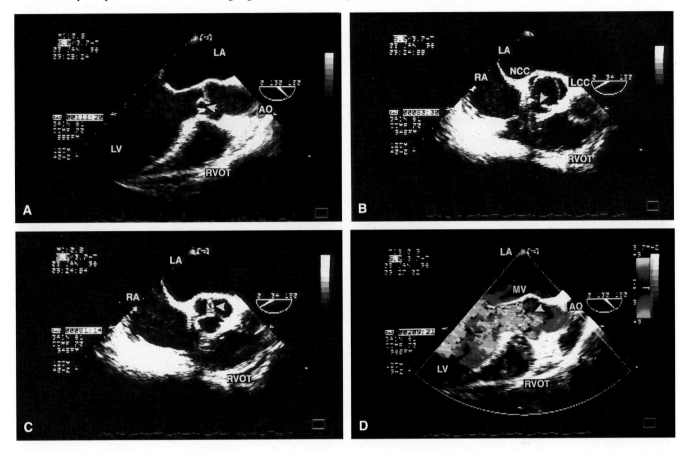

Figure 3.15. **Flail aortic valve. A-C.** A flail right coronary cusp (arrows) prolapsing into the LVOT in diastole, resulting in prominent diastolic noncoaptation seen in the long-axis views. **D.** High-frequency diastolic fluttering (arrow) indicative of a flail aortic valve (AV). There was no evidence of infection. **E.** Severe eccentric aortic regurgitation with a large flow acceleration. **F,G.** Systolic turbulence in LVOT was also seen in this patient and was due to associated hypertrophic cardiomyopathy (IHSS). At surgery, the right coronary leaflet was found torn from its attachment at the commissure between the right and left sinuses. A portion of autologous pericardium was used to reconstruct the right coronary cusp, and the annulus size was reduced from 24 mm to 18 mm in diameter by performance of a triple annuloplasty.

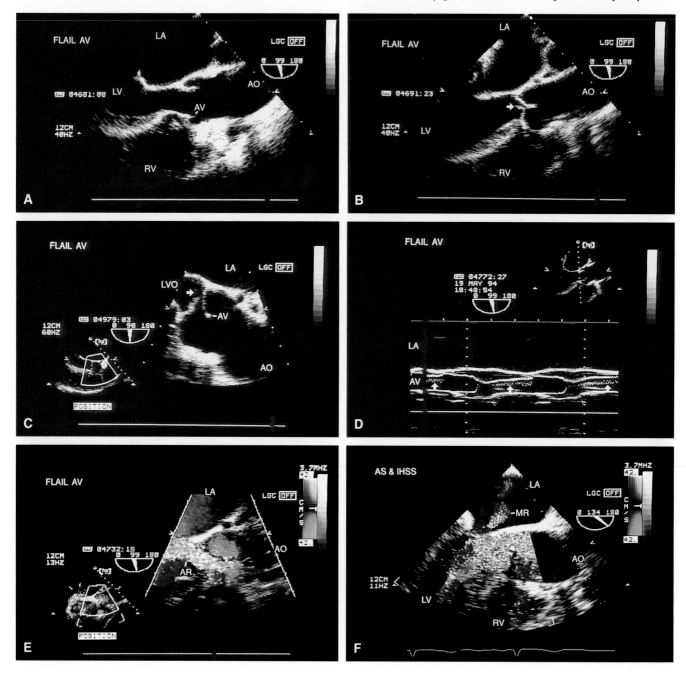

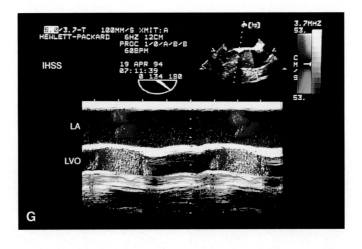

Figure 3.16. **Eversion of the aortic valve.** The distal portion of the left coronary cusp in this patient shows eversion causing noncoaptation with the right coronary cusp, which is only minimally everted.

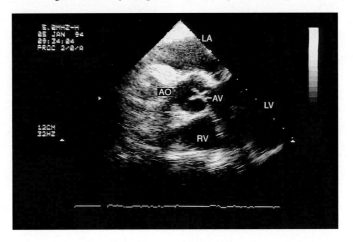

Figure 3.17. **Flail aortic valve in systemic lupus erythematosus. A.** Prominent prolapse of the right coronary cusp (arrow) into the LVOT during diastole and noncoaptation of the valve leaflets. **B.** The long-axis view of the aortic valve demonstrates an eccentric jet of severe aortic regurgitation (AR) directed toward the mitral valve. Note the prominent flow acceleration (FA), which also suggests severe regurgitation. **C.** Excised aortic valve. There is destruction of the right coronary cusp near the commissure (bottom left). No vegetations are seen. **D.** Gross specimen from another patient shows lupus valvulitis of both mitral and aortic valves. (**A-C** reproduced with permission from Mehta R, Agrawal G, Nanda NC, et al. Flail aortic valve in systemic lupus erythematosus. Echocardiography 1996;13:431–434.)

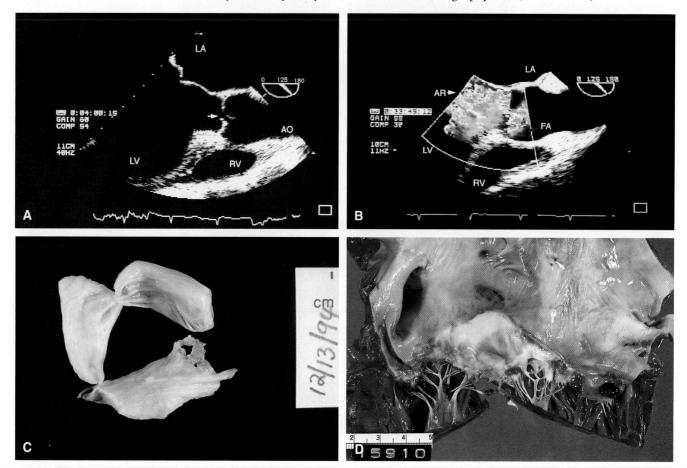

Figure 3.18. **Aortic valve vegetation. A-C.** A large vegetation (arrow) moving into the LVOT in diastole and back into the aortic root in systole.

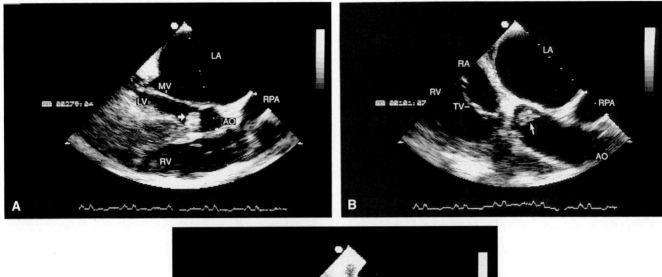

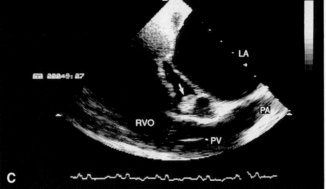

Figure 3.19. **Aortic valve vegetation. A-C.** A large vegetation (V) is shown prolapsing into the outflow tract with severe aortic regurgitation (AR). **D.** Pulsed Doppler of the distal ascending aorta demonstrates prominent pandiastolic backflow (AR) resulting from significant aortic regurgitation.

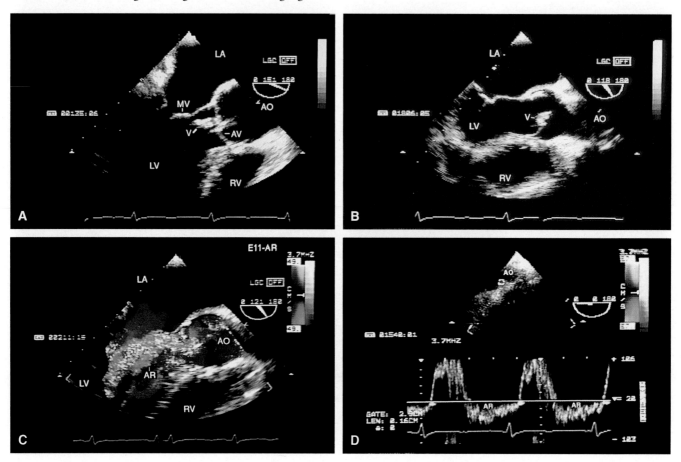

Figure 3.20. **Aortic valve vegetation. A.** A large vegetation (V) involving the aortic valve leaflets. **B.** Gross specimen shows aortic valve vegetations.

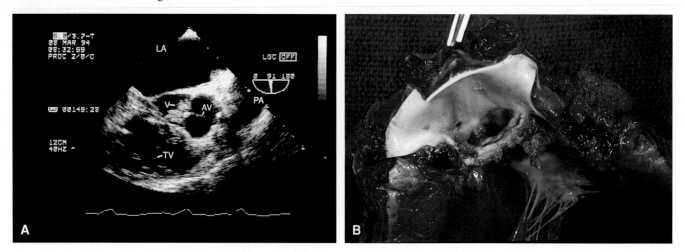

Figure 3.21. **Aortic valve vegetation with abscess formation.** The localized bounded echolucent area **(A,B)** is a large abscess communicating with the LVOT (arrow in **C**) and protruding into the left atrium. *V*, aortic valve vegetation. **D.** Torrential aortic regurgitation. **E.** Associated moderate mitral regurgitation resulting from annular dilatation. The mitral valve was not infected. **F.** Diastolic noncoaptation of infected aortic valve leaflets in another patient. **G.** Fistulous communication with the RA and RV (arrows) in the same patient seen in **F.**

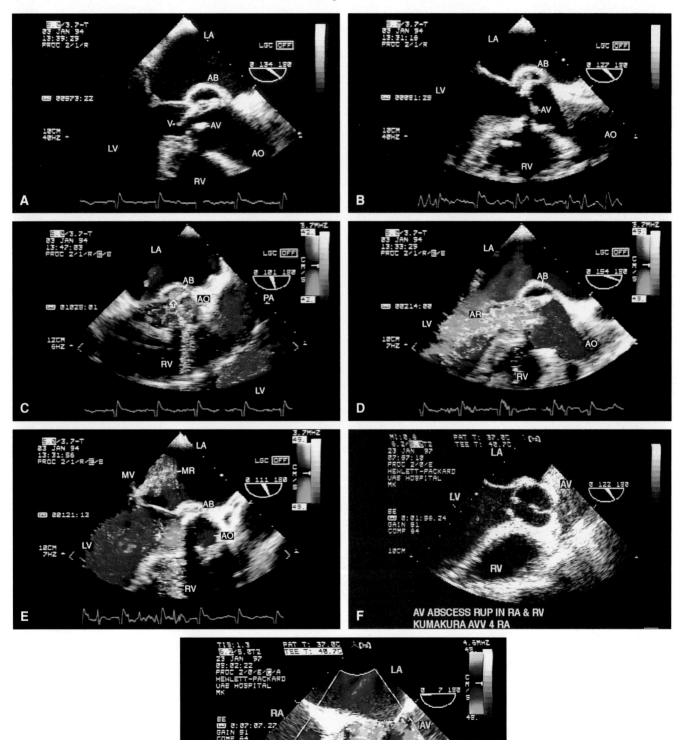

Figure 3.22. **Aortic valve abscess.** Abscess cavity (arrows) at the mitral–aortic junction **(A-C)** extending into the right atrium (arrowheads in **E** and **F**). Color-flow examination **(C,D)** shows the abscess cavity communicating with the LVOT (arrow in **D**).

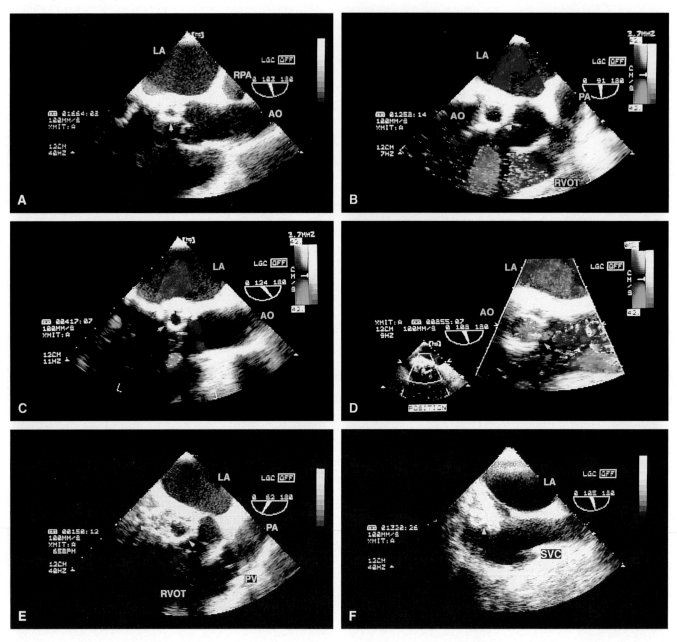

Figure 3.23.   **Aortic and mitral valve vegetations.** Vegetations involving both the aortic (open arrow) and the mitral (closed arrow) valves are shown.

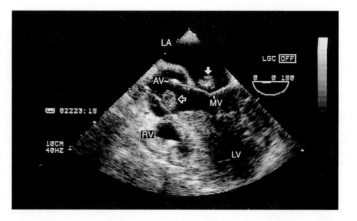

Figure 3.24. **Aortic and mitral vegetations. A-G.** Prominent vegetations (V, arrows) involving both mitral and aortic valves are shown. This demonstrates that infection of one valve can lead to infection of the contiguous valve. Note the presence of a vegetation at the mitral–aortic junction (closed arrow in **D**).

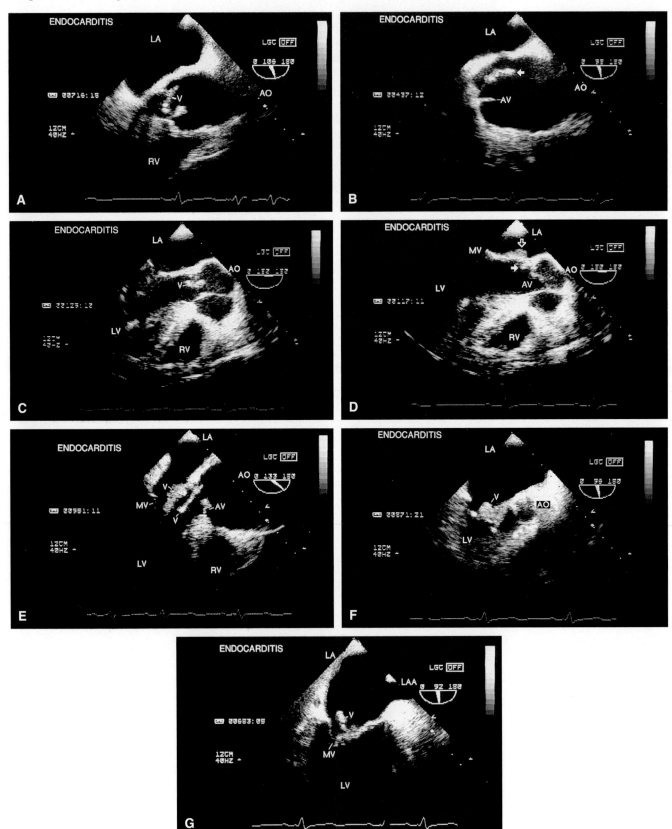

Figure 3.25.   **Aortic and mitral vegetations. A-C.** Another patient with mitral and aortic vegetations (V, arrow).

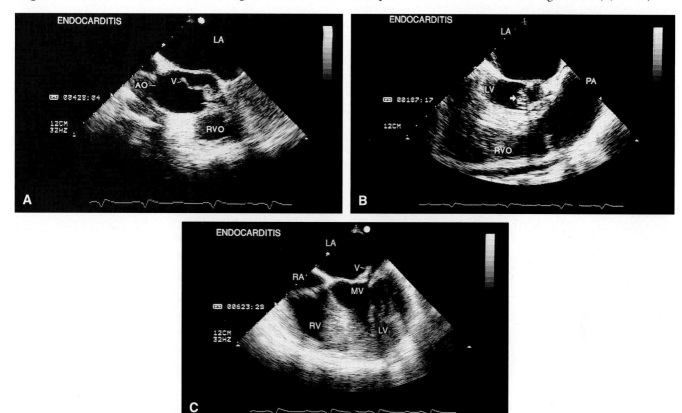

Figure 3.26. **Ascending aortic aneurysm.** The aneurysm measured 6 cm on echo and at surgery. **A.** Noncoaptation of the aortic valve leaflets (arrow) resulting from distortion by the aneurysm. **B.** Resulting severe aortic regurgitation with flow acceleration (FA). Note that the junction of the LVOT with the aortic root is not enlarged. **C,D.** Systolic frames.

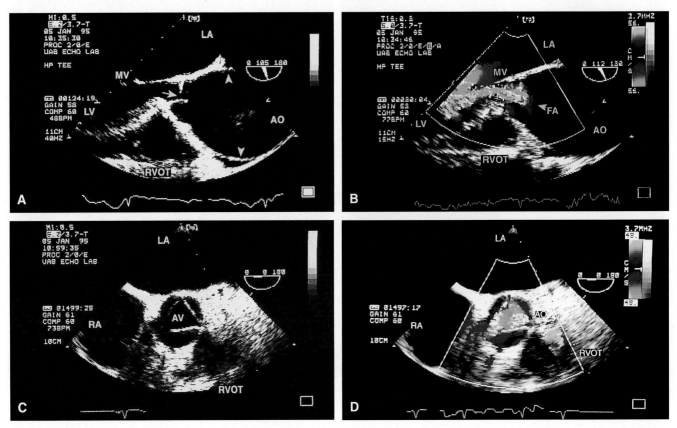

Figure 3.27. **Ascending aortic aneurysm.** Same patient seen in Figure 3.26, showing diastolic noncoaptation of the aortic valve leaflets (arrowheads in **A**) resulting in aortic regurgitation (red arrow in **B**).

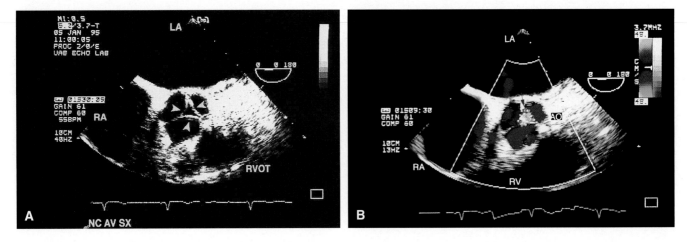

Figure 3.28. Ascending aortic aneurysm. **A-D**. Another example of a huge aneurysm with severe aortic regurgitation. **D** shows the aneurysm viewed in short axis with measurement of the anteroposterior (AP) and transverse (TR) diameters.[5]

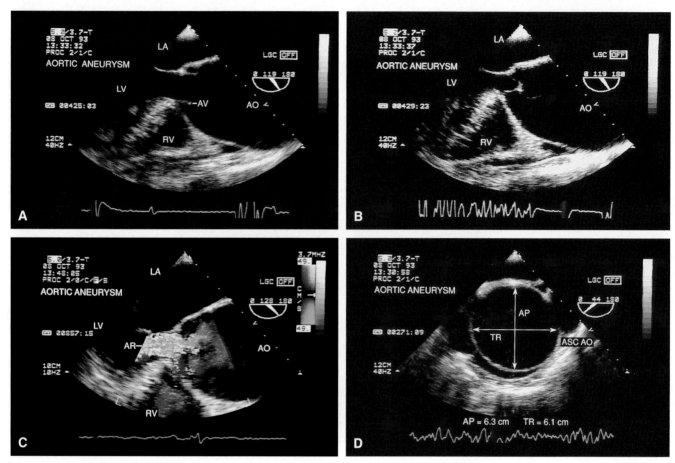

Figure 3.29. Ascending aortic aneurysm. **A.** The aneurysm of the ascending aorta in the short axis view measures 5.1 cm in the anteroposterior (A) diameter and 5.3 cm in the transverse (B) diameter. **B.** The descending aorta is normal in size.

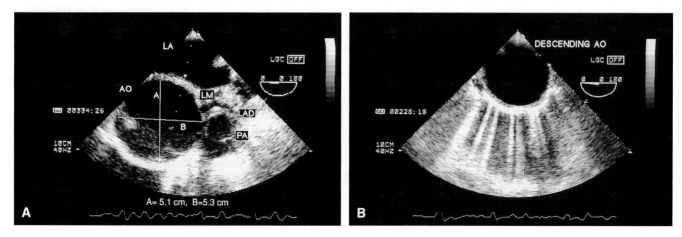

Figure 3.30. Aortic arch aneurysm. A-C. A large aneurysm with a thrombus (TH). *C,* aneurysm cavity.

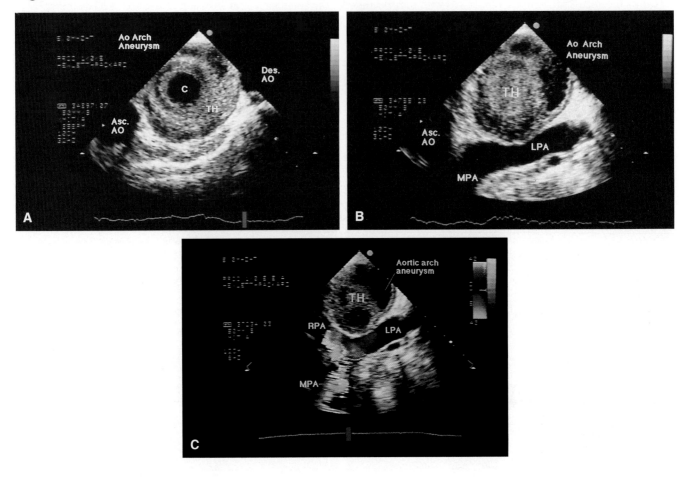

Figure 3.31. Descending aortic aneurysm. A,B. Two examples of descending thoracic aortic aneurysm (DTA) with thrombus (TH). An associated left pleural effusion (EFF) is present in **A.**

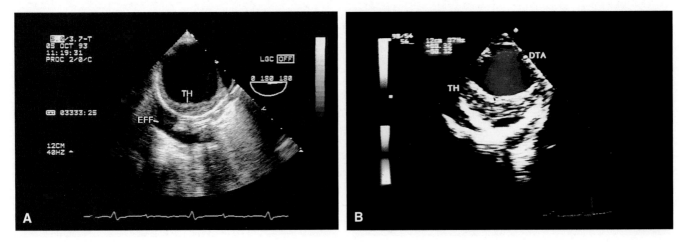

Figure 3.32. **Aortic dissection. A.** The dissection flap is clearly seen in the ascending aorta, close to but not involving the aortic valve leaflets. **B.** In another patient, the flap (F, arrowhead) is seen impinging on the aortic leaflets and interfering with their motion. **C,D.** Prolapse of a dissection flap (red arrow) into the LVOT and the resulting severe aortic regurgitation (AR) are shown in a different patient. **E.** Short-axis view shows a flap in the vicinity of the origin of the left main coronary artery (LMCA) but not involving it. **F,G.** On the other hand, in two other patients, the dissection flap can be seen extending into the lumen of the LMCA in **F** and into the right coronary artery (RCA) in **G**. **H,I.** Short-axis views at the level of the ascending aorta show a communication (C) between the true (TL) and false (FL) lumens as well as a thrombus (TH) in the false lumen. **J-L.** Long-axis views of the ascending aorta show prominent flow signals in both the true and false lumens. Note the absence of flow signals in the false lumen following surgery in **L** (right panel). **M-P.** Short-axis and long-axis views of the descending thoracic aorta show dissection. **Q,R.** Communications (C) between the true or perfusing (PL) and the false or nonperfusing (NPL) lumens. Note the presence of two communications in **R. S,T.** Pulse Doppler demonstrates to-and-fro flow between the perfusing and nonperfusing lumens. **U.** Spontaneous contrast in the NPL in the descending aorta consistent with low flow state. **V.** Thrombus formation. *CX*, left circumflex artery; *LAD*, left anterior descending coronary artery; *LPV*, left pulmonary vein. (**B, D, F-H, L-N,** and **R** reproduced with permission from Ballal R, Nanda NC, Gatewood R, et al. Usefulness of transesophageal echocardiography in assessment of aortic dissection. Circulation 1991;84:1903–1914. **C** reproduced with permission from Nanda NC et al. Transesophageal Echocardiography. American Heart Association Council on Clinical Cardiology Newsletter 1990; Summer: 3-22.)

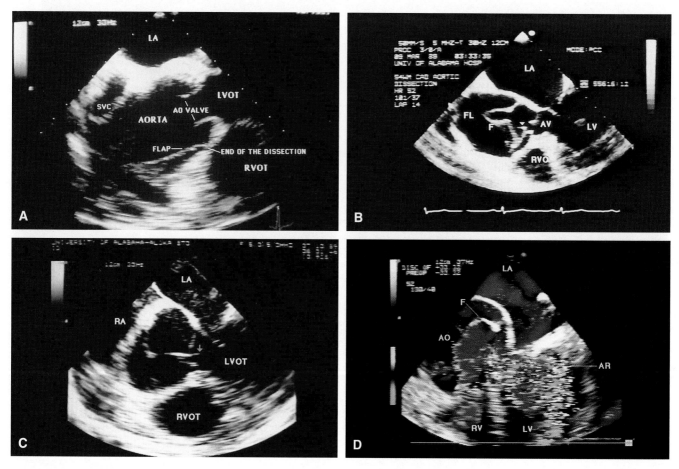

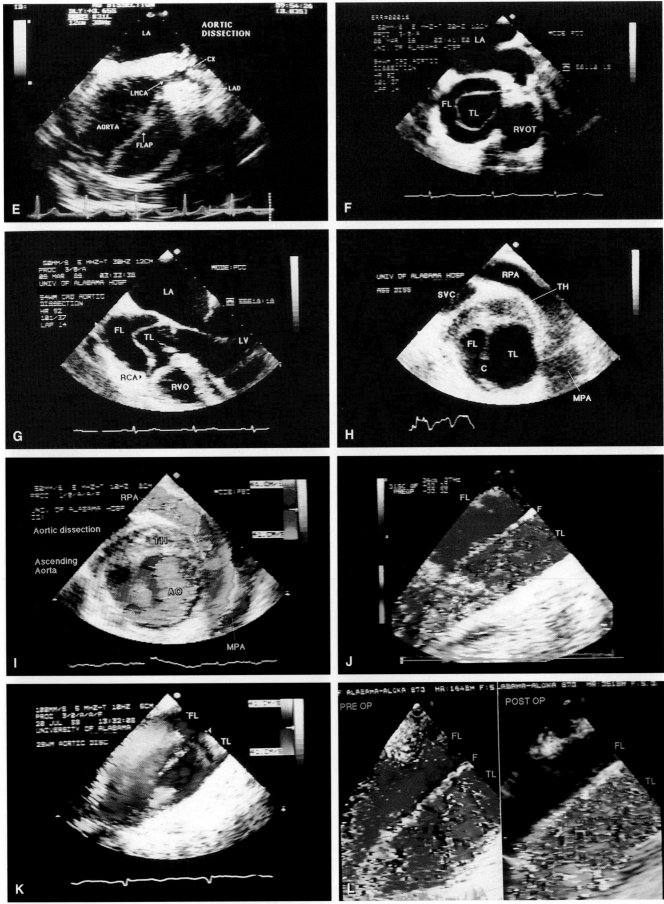

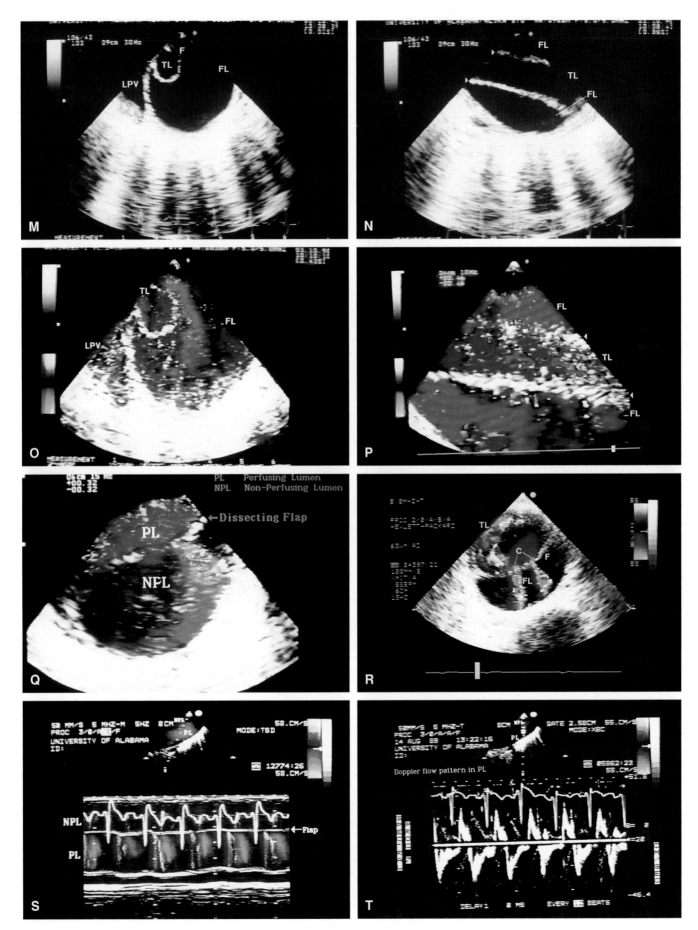

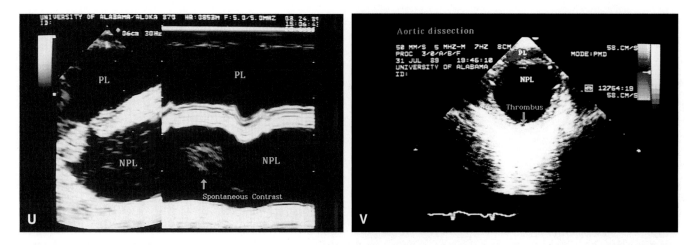

Figure 3.33. **Aortic dissection**. **A.** Long-axis view of the ascending aorta shows a thin linear echo (arrowheads) in the aortic lumen located very close to the anterior aortic wall, mimicking intimal thickening. This echo was immobile. **B.** Color Doppler examination, in the short-axis view, shows no flow signals in the false lumen (FL). This is an example of intramural dissection. There is no communication with the aortic lumen. (Reproduced with permission from Mehta R, Nanda NC, Roychoudhury D, et al. Atypical aortic dissection diagnosed by transesophageal echocardiography. Echocardiography 1994;11:261–263.)

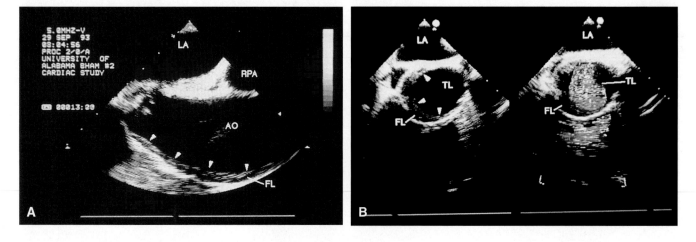

Figure 3.34. **Left sinus of Valsalva dissection**. **A,B.** Longitudinal plane examination of the aortic root. **A** depicts a sac-like dissection cavity (D) with a narrow neck (black arrow) connecting to the left sinus of Valsalva. **B** shows color Doppler flow signals entering the dissection cavity (D) as well as mosaic colored signals filling the whole of the left ventricular outflow tract in diastole, indicative of severe aortic regurgitation (AR). The left main coronary artery (LM) is not enlarged. **C-F.** Transverse plane examination of the aortic root. **C.** Systolic frame shows all three cusps of the aortic valve as well as the dissection cavity (D). **D.** Diastolic frame shows the dissection cavity (D) filled with color-flow signals as well as mosaic signals of aortic regurgitation. **E,F.** The hematoma (H) lining the dissection cavity near the origin of the anterior mitral leaflet (MV). (Reproduced with permission from Maxted W, Sanyal R, Nanda NC, et al. Transesophageal echocardiographic detection of sinus of Valsalva dissection. Echocardiography 1995;12:99–102.)

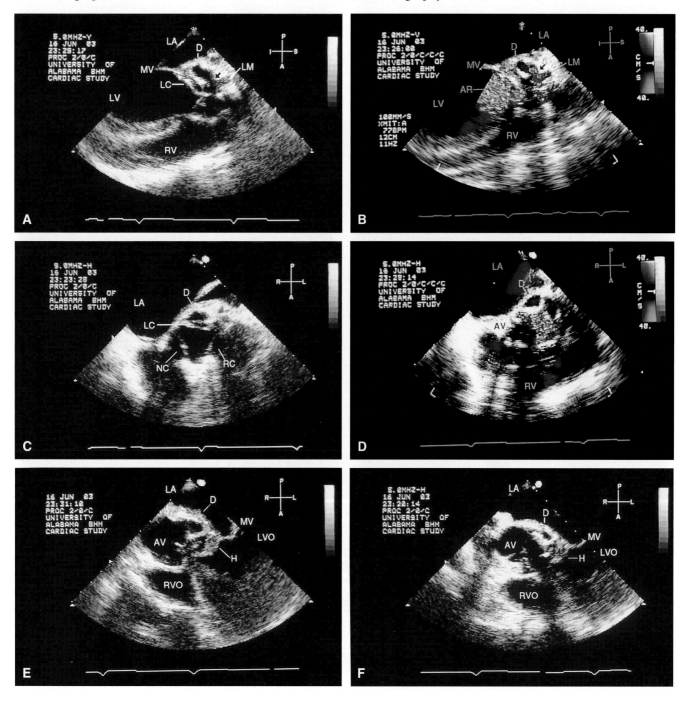

Figure 3.35. **Proximal right coronary artery dissection extending into the aortic root. A.** Coronary angiogram shows dissection (arrows) of the right coronary artery (RCA). **B.** Left ventriculogram shows the contrast dye (arrows) outside the lumen of the ascending aorta (AO). **C.** The aortic (AO) short-axis view demonstrates a dissection flap (solid arrow) in the lumen of the right coronary artery (RCA) as well as in the adjacent portion of the aortic root (open arrow). **D,E.** Longitudinal plane examination shows the dissection flap (open arrow, F) in the region of the right coronary sinus of the aortic root, viewed in oblique long-axis view. (Reproduced with permission from Varma V, Nanda NC, Soto B, et al. Transesophageal echocardiographic demonstration of proximal right coronary artery dissection extending into the aortic root. Am Heart J 1992;124:1055–1057.)

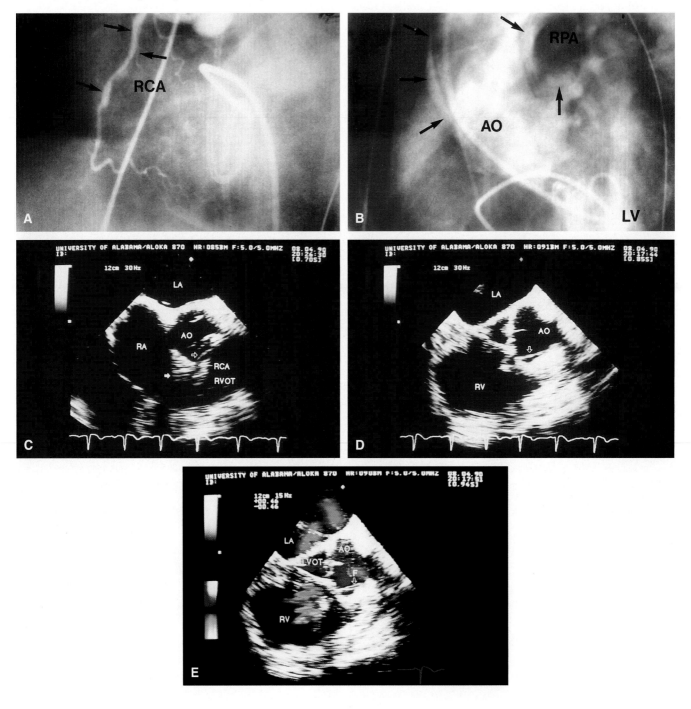

Figure 3.36. **Aortic dissection.** **A-D.** The dissection flap (F, arrow), together with associated severe aortic regurgitation (AR), is well visualized. **E.** The dissection flap (arrow) can be clearly distinguished from the aortic valve leaflets (arrowheads). **F.** The dissection flap (F, arrow) appears to involve the origin of the left main coronary artery (LM). **G,H.** A thrombus (TH) is seen in the false lumen. **I-L.** Dissection extending to involve the descending thoracic aorta. Communications between the true (TL) and false lumens (FL) are visualized in **I** and **L.** This patient underwent resuspension of the aortic valve and resection of the ascending aorta with placement of a Hemashield interposition graft.

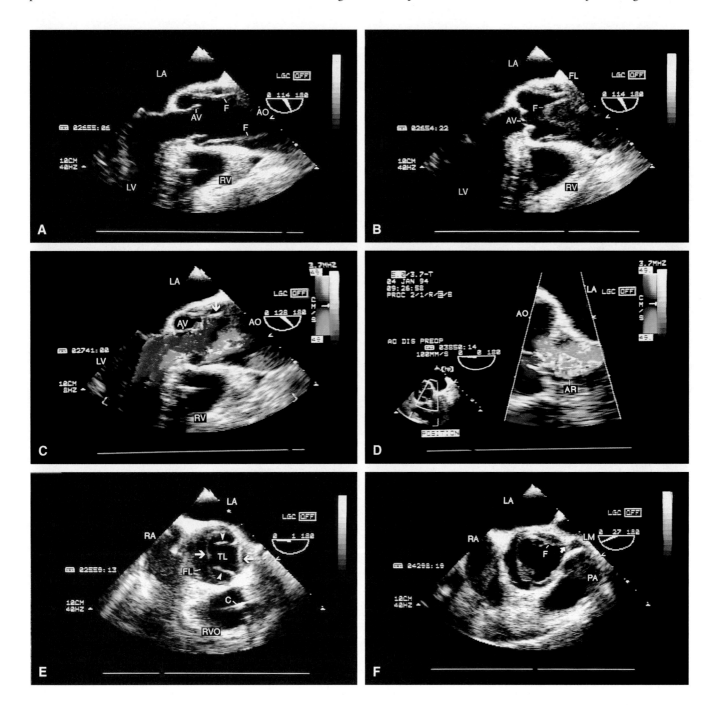

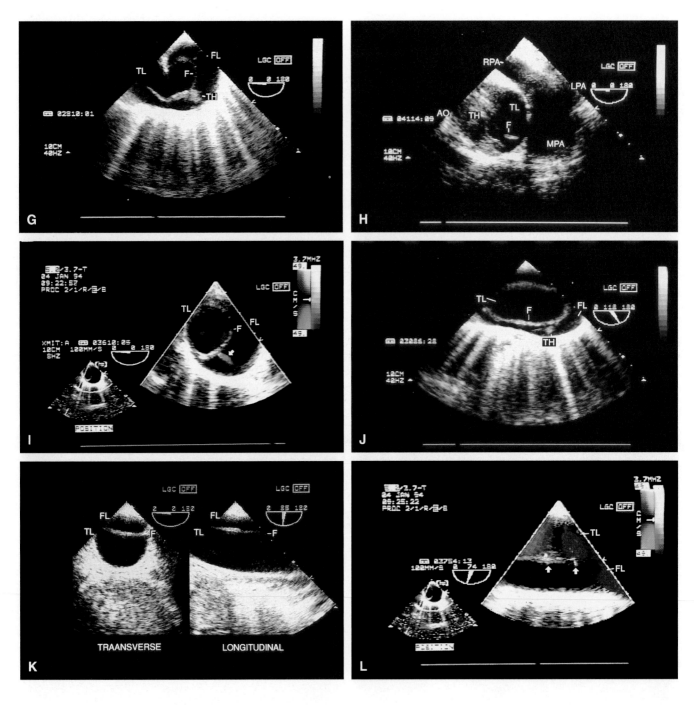

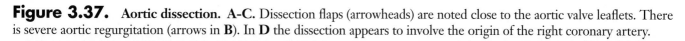

Figure 3.37. **Aortic dissection.** **A-C.** Dissection flaps (arrowheads) are noted close to the aortic valve leaflets. There is severe aortic regurgitation (arrows in **B**). In **D** the dissection appears to involve the origin of the right coronary artery.

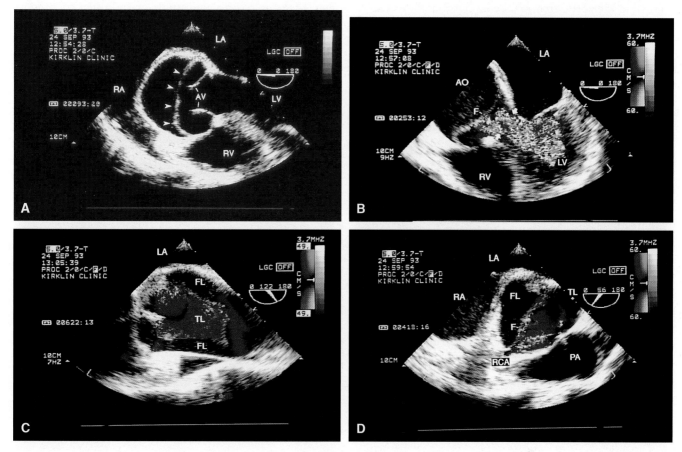

Figure 3.38. **Aortic dissection. A,B.** Because of the aortic valve–like motion of the dissection flap, this patient was initially labeled as having a double aortic valve. **C.** One large communication between the true (TL) and false lumens (FL) is noted in the aortic arch. **D.** Reduplication of the dissection flap (F). **E.** Two communications (arrowheads) are present in the descending aorta. **F.** Thrombus (TH) formation and another communication (arrowhead) are noted more distally in the descending aorta. **G.** Flow signals confined only to the true lumen in the descending aorta imaged in long axis.

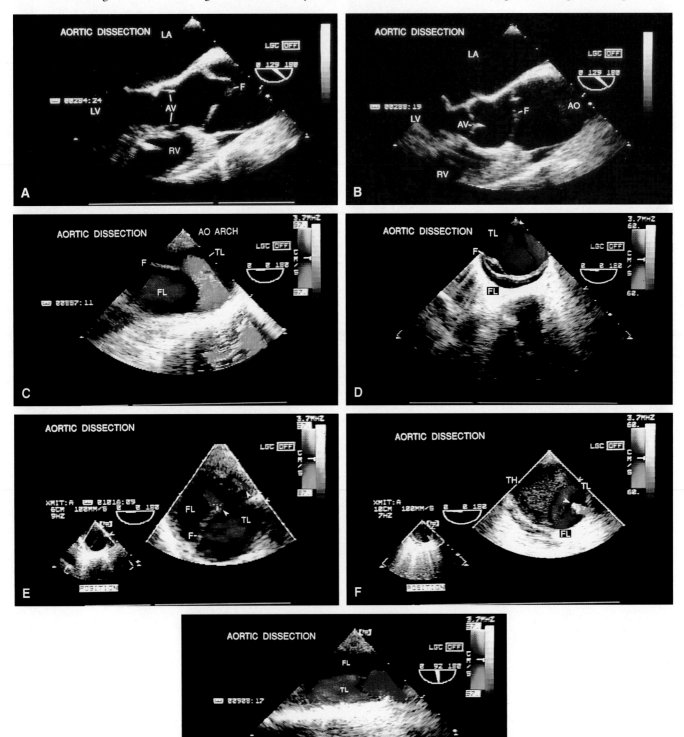

Figure 3.39.   **Aortic dissection. A-J.** The dissection flap (FL,F) appears to extend up to the origins of the right (RCA) and left main (LM) coronary arteries. Reduplication of the dissection flap is well seen in **D. G-J** shows extension of the dissection into the descending thoracic aorta imaged in long-axis and short-axis views. Collapse of the true lumen in diastole and expansion in systole, as shown in the short-axis view in **G,** result in a characteristic "help" sign when the descending aorta is viewed in real-time motion.

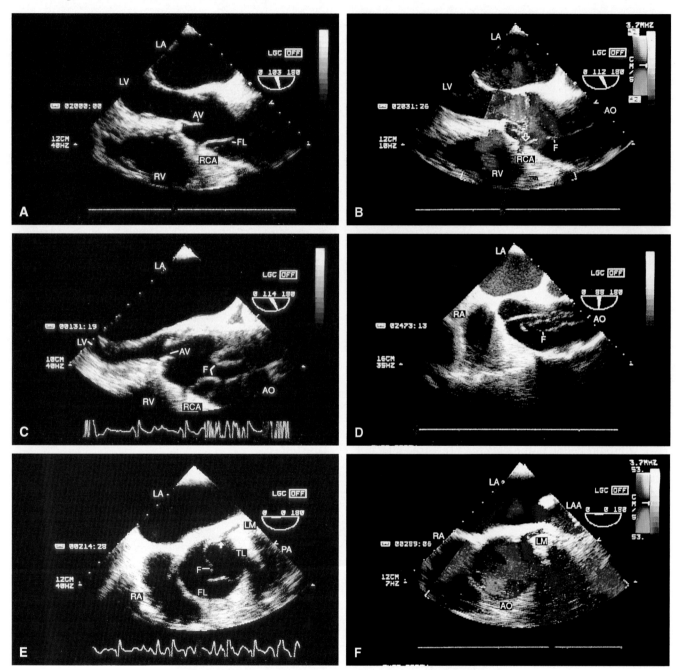

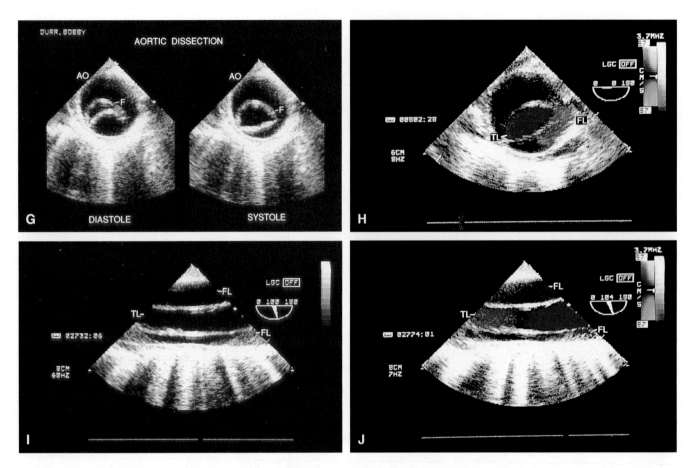

Figure 3.40. **Aortic dissection.** A prominent atherosclerotic plaque (arrowhead) in the true lumen could have predisposed to dissection in this patient. TL = true lumen; FL = false lumen.

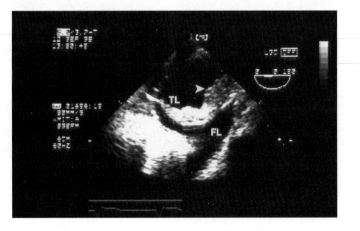

Figure 3.41. **Aortic dissection. A-C.** The dissection flap (F) is noted in the aortic root and ascending aorta (ASC AO), and there is severe AR. Because there was no involvement of the descending thoracic aorta, this dissection was classified as DeBakey type II.

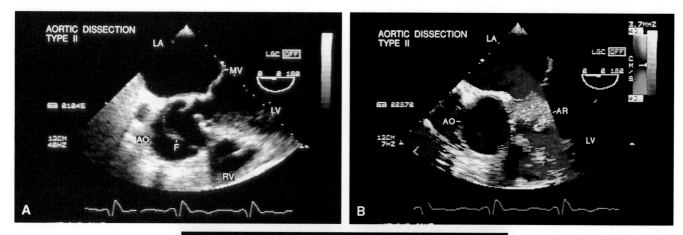

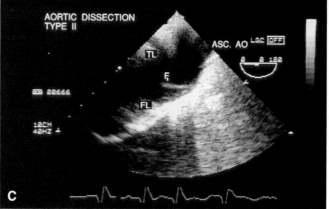

Figure 3.42. **Aortic dissection. A-C.** The dissection in this patient involves only the descending thoracic aorta, which is imaged in long and short axis (DeBakey type Ill or Stanford type B dissection). There is associated left pleural effusion (PLE). *F,* dissection flap; *FL,* false lumen; *L,* lung echoes; *TL,* true lumen.

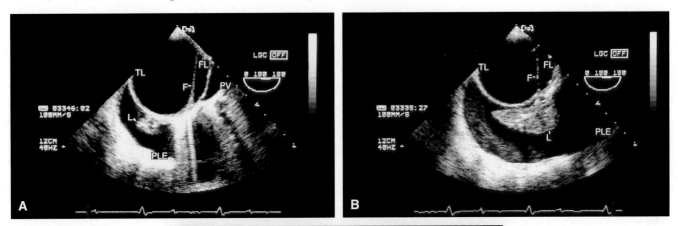

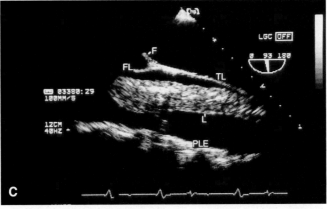

Figure 3.43.   **Aortic dissection. A,B.** Compression of the true lumen. The ascending aortic (AA, ASC AO) true lumen (TL) appears in this patient to be compressed (arrow in **B**) by the thrombosed (T, TH) false lumen (FL). *F*, dissection flap. **C,D.** Rupture into the mediastinum (another patient). The arrow in **C** points to the site of a contained rupture in the ascending aorta with the development of false aneurysm and hematoma (H) in the mediastinum. The hematoma extends around the pulmonary arteries and the left atrium (**D).** Contrast echoes are seen in the main and right pulmonary arteries; these resulted from an intravenous injection of normal saline. (Reproduced with permission from Ballal R, Nanda NC, Gatewood R, et al. Usefulness of transesophageal echocardiography in assessment of aortic dissection. Circulation 1991;84:1903–1914).

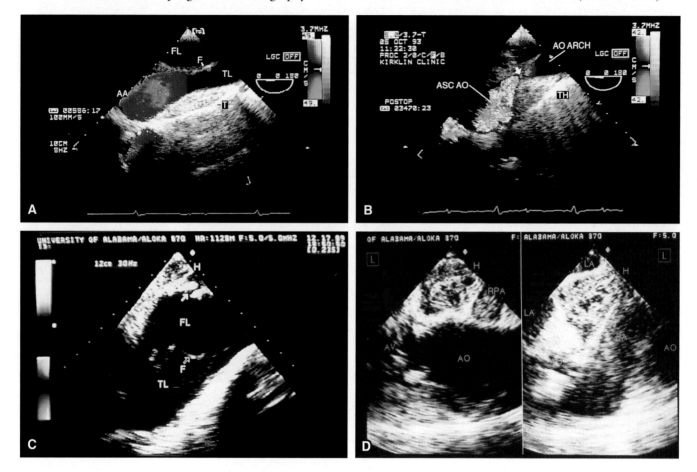

Figure 3.44. **Aortic dissection.** Rupture into the right ventricle. **A–D.** In addition to the typical dissection flap (F, DIFP) in the aortic root, an abnormal linear echo is seen in the right ventricle. **E,F.** Color Doppler demonstrates turbulent flow (arrows) in the right ventricle originating in the region of the linear echo, consistent with dissection rupture into the right ventricle. **G,H.** Communication (arrows) between the aorta and right ventricle is demonstrated. PAN, PANY, pseudoaneurysm.

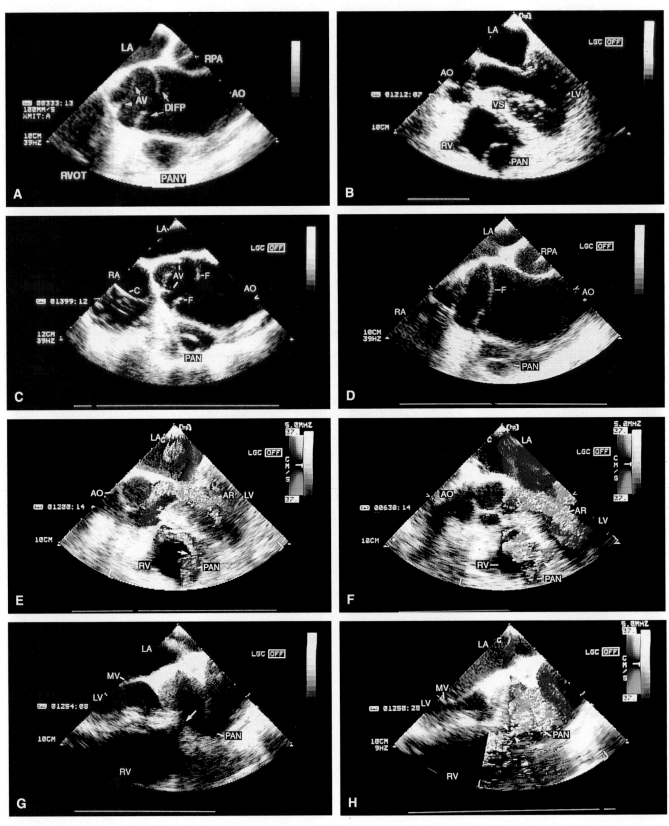

Figure 3.45. **Aortic dissection.** The side lobe (SL) artifact from a prosthetic aortic valve (P) can be distinguished from the dissection flap by its arc-like appearance and its extension to nonaortic structures such as the left atrium. *FL*, false lumen; *TH*, thrombus in false lumen; *TL*, true lumen.

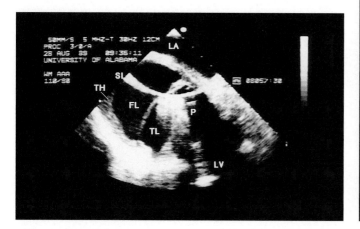

Figure 3.46. **Aortic dissection.** Graft replacement of the proximal aorta following aortic dissection. In this transgastric view the graft can be identified by its serrated appearance.

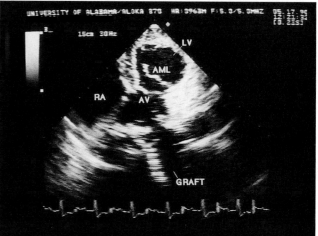

Figure 3.47. **Aortic dissection**. **A,B.** Graft to left main coronary artery. Transverse plane examination. Short-axis view of ascending aorta (AO) in the post-cardiopulmonary bypass period demonstrates a Cabrol graft (G) and its attachment to the left main coronary artery (LMCA). Closely packed, short linear echoes in the graft wall represent corrugations in the Dacron graft. (Reproduced with permission from Ballal R, Nanda NC, Gatewood R, et al. Usefulness of transesophageal echocardiography in assessment of aortic dissection. Circulation 1991;84:1903–1914).

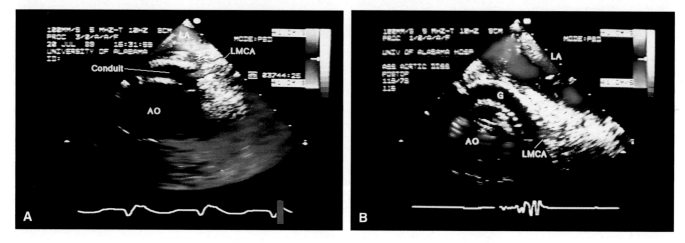

Figure 3.48. **Aortic dissection.** Intraluminal tube graft dehiscence. **A-H.** The large space between the graft (G) and the native aortic aneurysm walls (arrows in **A**) indicates graft dehiscence, which is definitively identified by the presence of flow signals moving from the graft into the space (arrows in **C,G**). Graft dehiscence is also suggested by discontinuity of the graft wall (arrow in **E**). Thus, the graft dehiscence in this patient occurred in its proximal attachment to the aortic aneurysm. **D** shows severe aortic regurgitation and a dissection flap (F) beyond the graft. **F** shows a portion of the dehisced graft (arrowhead) protruding into the native lumen. *LM,* left main coronary artery.

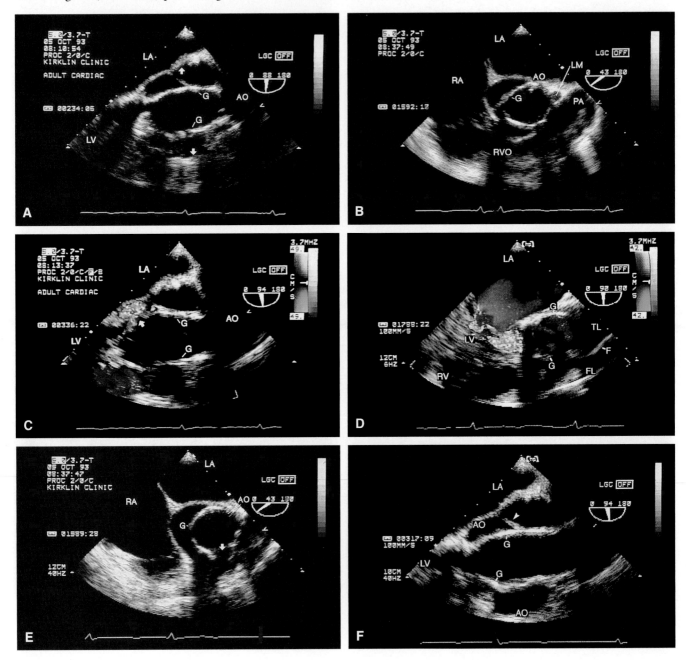

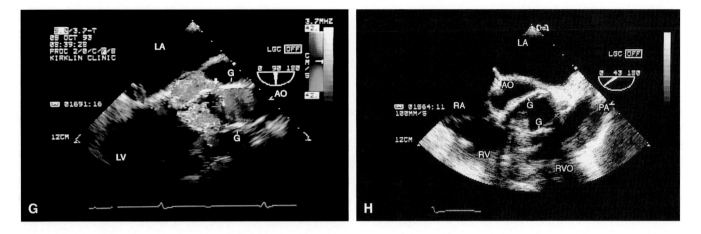

G
H

Figure 3.49. **Aortic dissection**. Intraluminal graft dehiscence at coronary anastomoses and pseudoaneurysm rupture into right atrium. **A-C.** Multiplane images at plane angles of 144°, 153°, and 51° demonstrate the aortic tube graft (G). Color Doppler flow imaging shows prominent signals within the tube graft, as well as in the aortic wrap-around/ aortic pseudoaneurysm (open arrow) in **B** and **C**. Localized kinking of the graft is also noted posteriorly in **A** (closed arrow). **D-I.** Two discrete areas of graft dehiscence with flow signals moving from the graft into the aortic pseudoaneurysm (AO) are noted in the regions of right (RCA, open arrow) and left main (LM, closed arrow) coronary anastomoses, visualized at various plane angulations. Ostia and proximal portions of both coronary arteries are patent and show good flow signals. **J,K.** Mosaic-colored signals (arrow) indicative of turbulent flow are noted in the right atrial appendage (RAA). (Reproduced with permission from Roychoudhury D, Nanda NC, Kim KS, et al. Transesophageal echocardiographic diagnosis of aortic graft dehiscence at coronary anastomoses and pseudoaneurysm rupture into right atrium. Echocardiography 1995;12:495–499.)

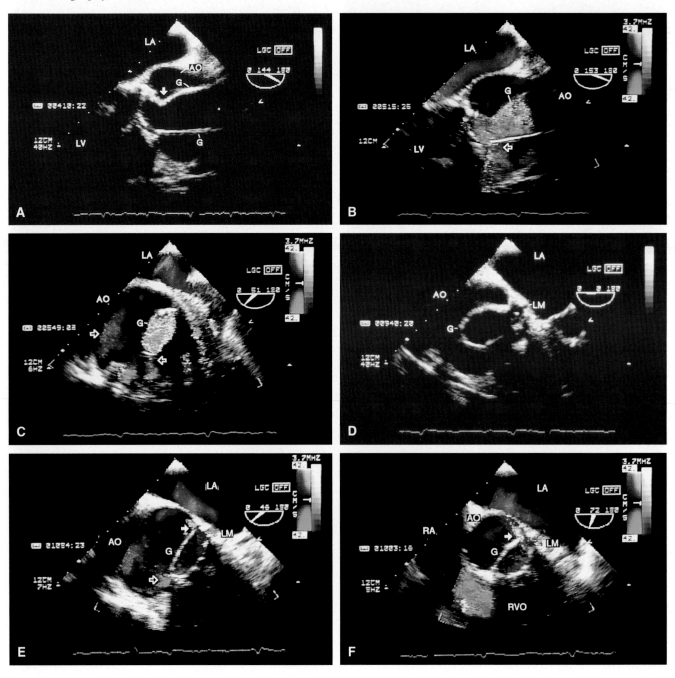

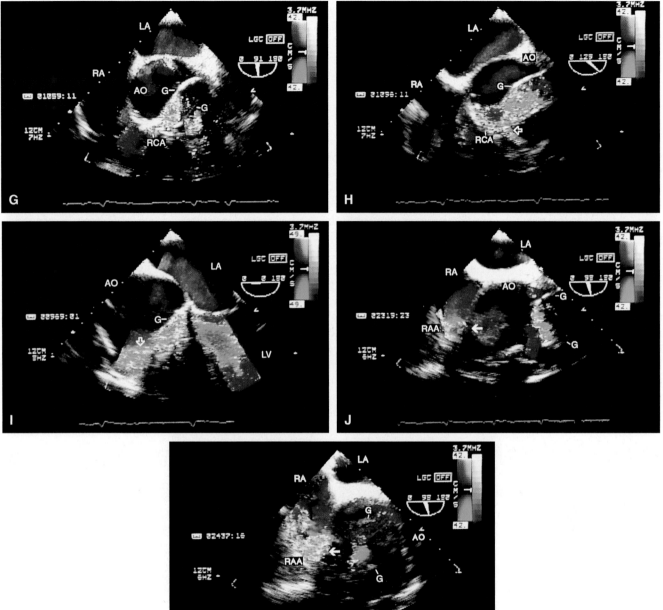

Figure 3.50. **Aortic dissection.** Graft dehiscence. **A-C.** Both the transverse (T) and longitudinal (L) planes demonstrate a large area (8 mm in maximum size) of posterior aortic (AO) graft (G) dehiscence (solid arrow) at the level of the aortic annulus. Prominent flow signals are noted moving in and out of the pseudoaneurysm (open arrow) during the cardiac cycle. The dehisced left main coronary artery (LMCA) arises from the pseudoaneurysm. **D,E.** Color M-mode and pulsed Doppler interrogation of the ascending aorta (AO) demonstrate prominent retrograde flow signals (arrow) during diastole, indicative of significant aortic regurgitation. **F.** Longitudinal (L) plane examination demonstrates a 5-mm dehiscence (closed arrow) in the posterior graft (G) at the level of the aortic annulus. In both longitudinal **(F)** and transverse plane views **(G,H)** flow signals are noted in the pseudoaneurysm (open arrow) posteriorly but not anterior to the graft, most likely caused by attenuation of flow signal intensity by the graft walls. **I,J.** Transverse (T) plane examination shows a large clot (C) in the pseudoaneurysm (open arrow) compressing (solid black arrow) the aortic graft (G) as well as flow signals moving through a localized area of the graft wall posteriorly into the pseudoaneurysm, consistent with dehiscence (solid yellow arrow). The site of dehiscence is located approximately 1.8 cm cephalad from the aortic annulus. **K.** Transverse (T) plane examination shows prolapse (arrow) of the noncoronary cusp of the aortic valve as well as flow signals filling approximately half of the proximal left ventricular outflow tract, consistent with moderately severe aortic regurgitation (AR). **L.** Intact attachment of the graft (G) with the distal ascending aorta (A). **M,N.** Longitudinal (L) plane examination shows dehiscence (solid arrow) of the aortic graft (G) approximately 2 cm above the annulus with flow signals moving in and out of the localized pseudoaneurysm (open arrow) during the cardiac cycle. The left main coronary artery (LMCA) is dehisced and arises from the pseudoaneurysm. **O.** The distal portion of the aortic graft (G) viewed in short axis during transverse (T) plane examination demonstrates a large space (arrow) anteriorly filled with flow signals, consistent with distal graft dehiscence. **P.** Longitudinal (L) plane examination shows mosaic flow signals completely filling the proximal left ventricular outflow tract in diastole, indicative of severe aortic regurgitation. In addition, flow signals are noted moving from the region of the aortic prosthesis (P) into the right ventricle (RV), denoting the presence of an aortic–right ventricular fistula (solid arrow). Pulsed Doppler interrogation of the fistula reveals continuous flow throughout the cardiac cycle (open arrow). **A-E, F-H, I-L,** and **M-P** are four different patients. (Reproduced with permission from Ballal RJ, Gatewood RP, Nanda NC, et al. Usefulness of transesophageal echocardiography in the assessment of aortic graft dehiscence. Am J Cardiol 1997;80:372–376.)

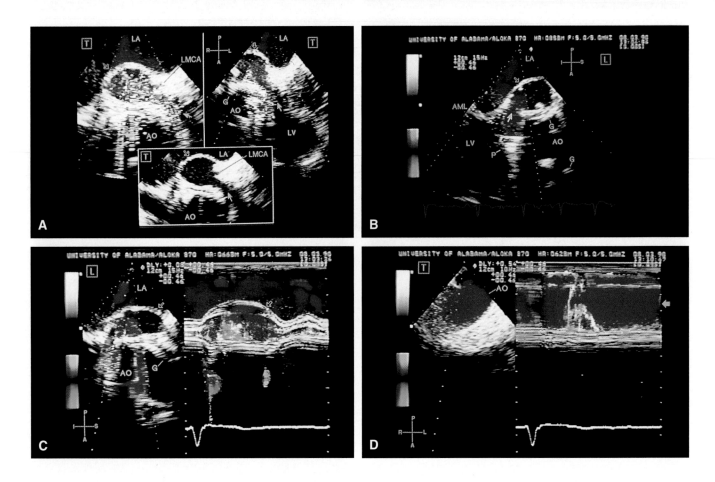

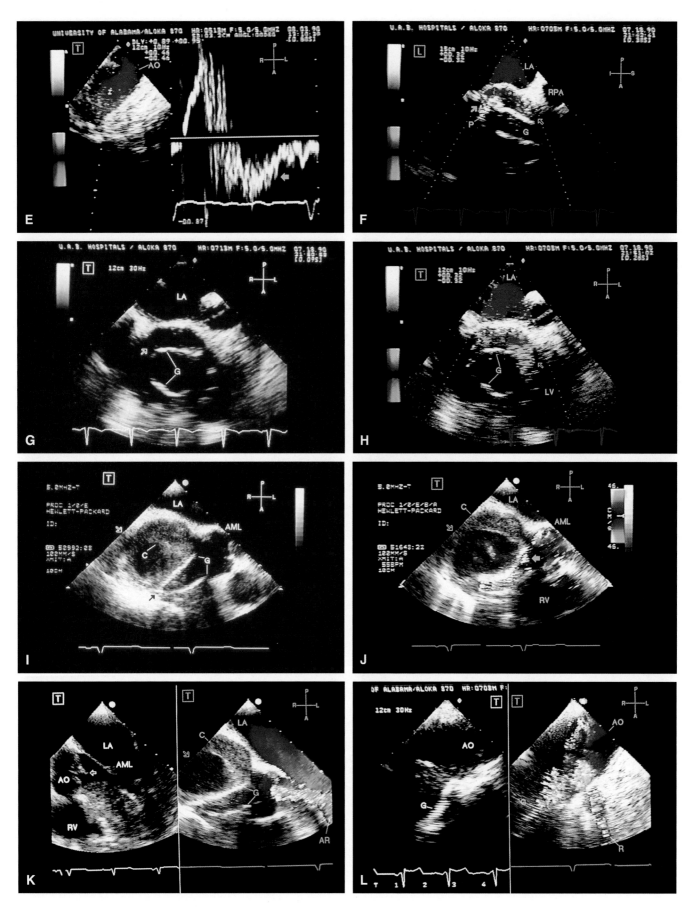

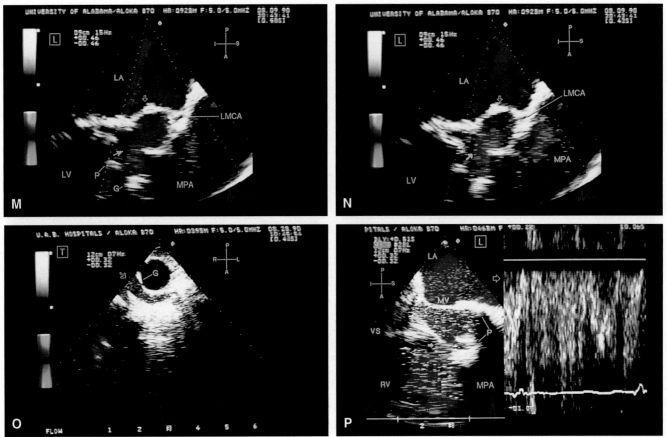

Figure 3.51. **Aortic dissection.** A patient with Marfan's syndrome who had previous graft repair of descending thoracic aortic dissection is shown. **A,B.** The junction of the graft (G) with the native descending aorta (DA) is well visualized. Note also the presence of the dissection flap (F) in the descending aorta beyond the graft junction and the communication (arrow) between the true lumen (TL) and the false lumen (FL). In addition, a hematoma (H) is visualized posteriorly between the aorta and the esophagus, indicative of a contained rupture, for which this patient underwent reoperation. **C,D.** Communication (arrow) between the true and false lumens imaged in short axis. **E.** Reduplication of the dissection flap. **F.** A linear, mobile echo (arrowhead) in the false lumen that could represent a fibrin plug, which helped contain the rupture, preventing exsanguination. The arrow points to the dissection flap (F). The patient also underwent aortic valve replacement because of severe aortic regurgitation (arrowhead in **H**) resulting from dilatation of the aortic root (AO) and sinuses (arrowheads in **G**). There was no evidence of dissection in the ascending aorta or the arch.

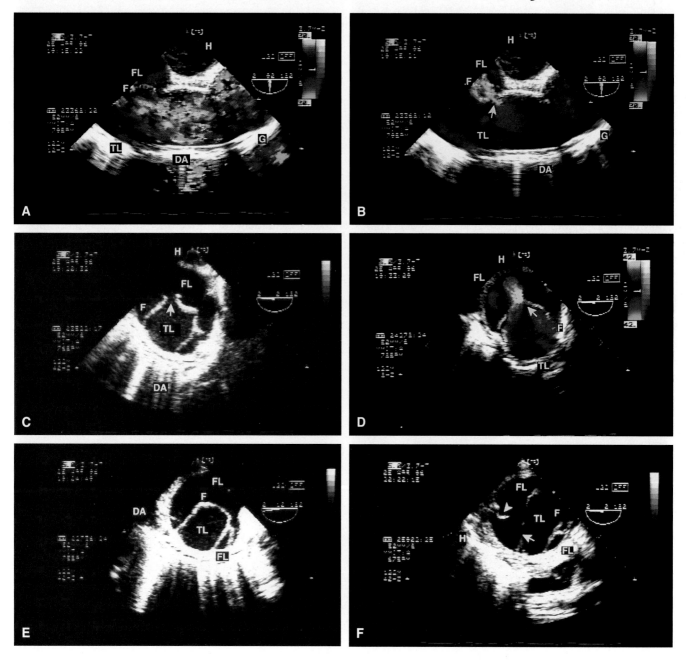

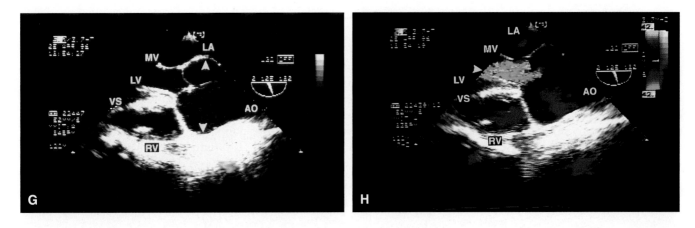

Figure 3.52. **Aortic dissection.** Graft replacement of abdominal aortic aneurysm. **A.** Transverse plane imaging of the descending thoracic aorta demonstrates a communication (arrow) in the dissection flap with prominent flow signals moving from the true lumen (TL) into the false lumen (FL) in systole (left) and from the false lumen into the true lumen in diastole (right). **B,C.** Transgastric views. **B.** *Left panel:* Longitudinal plane imaging demonstrates intact anastomosis (arrows) between the lower abdominal aorta (AO) and the graft (G). *Right panel:* Transverse plane imaging views the graft in short axis. **C.** Schematic representation. In this patient who underwent graft replacement of abdominal aortic aneurysm, transesophageal echocardiography was requested in the immediate postoperative period because of clinical suspicion of graft suture dehiscence. It was not possible to do a surface abdominal ultrasound study because of the dressings covering a fresh abdominal incision. The subsequent clinical course of the patient supported the transesophageal echocardiographic finding that the graft was intact. *IN,* intestines; *LRV,* left renal vein; *ST,* stomach. (Reproduced with permission from Chouinard M, Pinheiro L, Nanda NC, et al. Transgastric ultrasonography: a new approach for imaging the abdominal structures and vessels. Echocardiography 1991;8:397–403.)

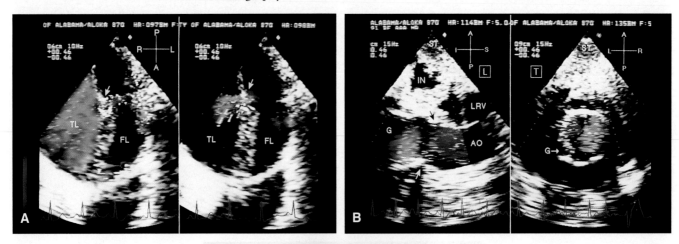

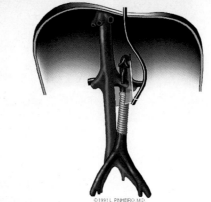

Figure 3.53. **Aortic atherosclerosis. A,B.** The descending aorta (DA), imaged in transverse (T) plane, shows multiple mobile linear echoes (arrows) representing atherosclerotic plaques protruding from the aortic wall into the lumen. **C,D.** Multiple toes with necrotic areas from peripheral systemic embolization, which developed following cardiac catheterization. **E.** Microscopic section of the punch biopsy taken from the sole of the left foot demonstrates clefts within the lumen of a vessel, which represent cholesterol crystals dissolved with histologic processing. (Reproduced with permission from Koppang J, Nanda NC, Coghlan C, Sanyal R. Histologically confirmed cholesterol atheroemboli with identification of the source by transesophageal echocardiography. Echocardiography 1992;9:379–383.)

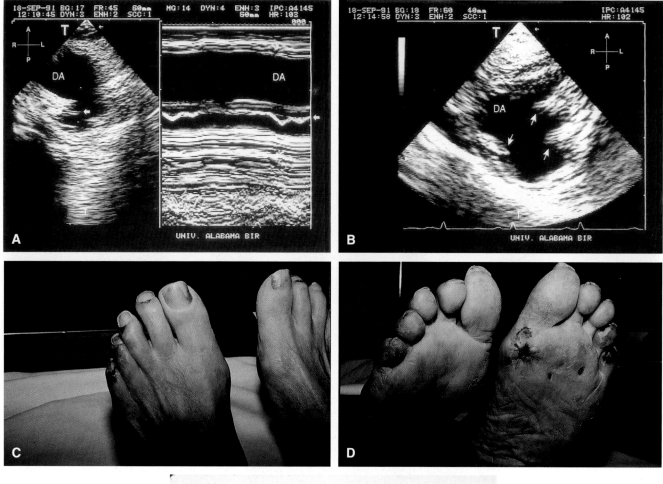

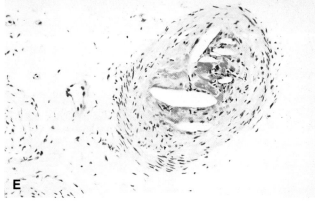

Figure 3.54. **Aortic atherosclerosis. A-E.** The arrows point to multiple, prominent mobile atherosclerotic plaques in the ascending aorta.

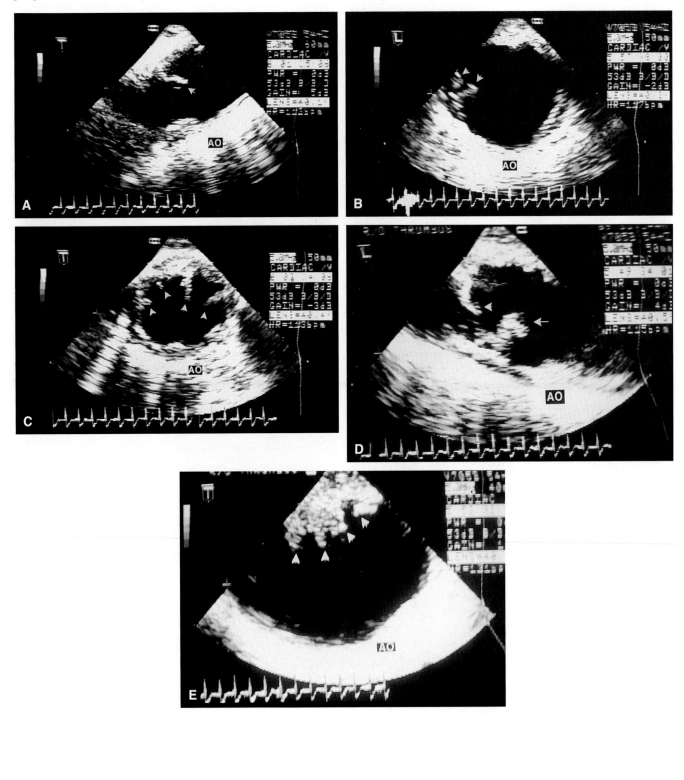

Figure 3.55. **Aortic atherosclerosis.** **A.** Three different types of atherosclerotic plaques are seen in the aortic arch: a linear plaque (upper solid arrow); a thick, rounded immobile plaque (lower solid arrow); and uniform intimal atherosclerotic thickening (lower open arrow). **B,C.** M-mode studies demonstrate plaque (PL) mobility.

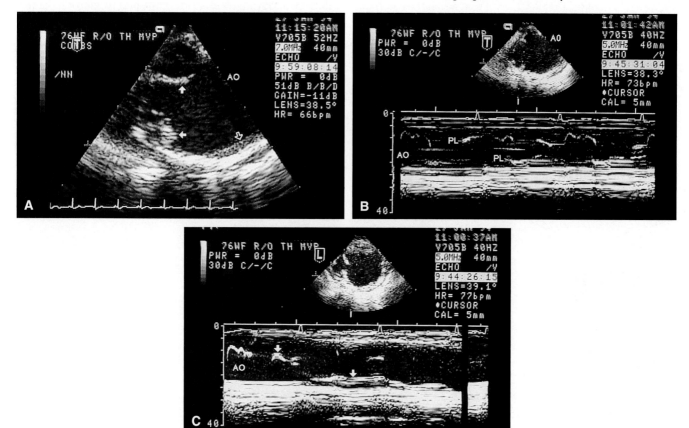

Figure 3.56. **Aortic atherosclerosis. A.** Multiple mobile and immobile plaques (arrows) are shown in the aortic arch. **B.** In another patient a shallow plaque ulceration (arrow) and a much deeper ulceration (arrowhead), which is more clearly identified because of flow signals in it, are seen. **C,D.** Other plaque ulcerations in the aortic arch in this patient are identified by color Doppler. **E-H.** Flow signals (arrows) outline deep penetrating ulcerations in the atherosclerotic plaques in the same patient shown in **A.**

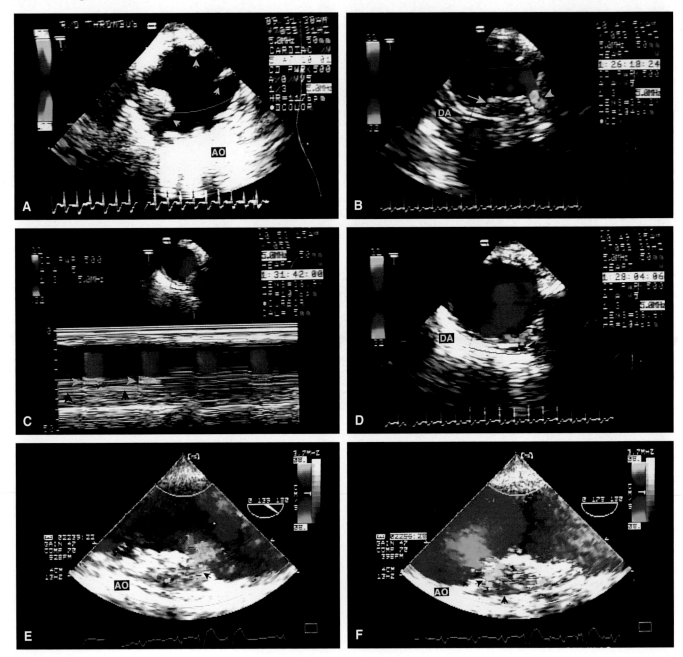

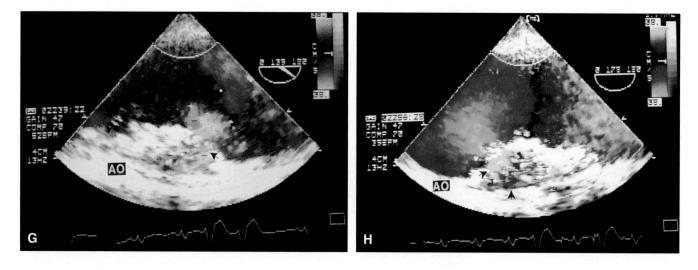

Figure 3.57. **Aortic atherosclerosis. A.** Uniform atherosclerotic intimal thickening (arrowheads) in the ascending aorta (AA) and arch (ACH). **B.** Shadowing (arrowheads) produced by a heavily calcified plaque (CA) present in the proximal ascending aorta in the same patient. **C.** A hematoma (H) is also present anteriorly behind the ascending aorta and arch. This patient had a contained aortic rupture, the presumed cause being atherosclerosis.

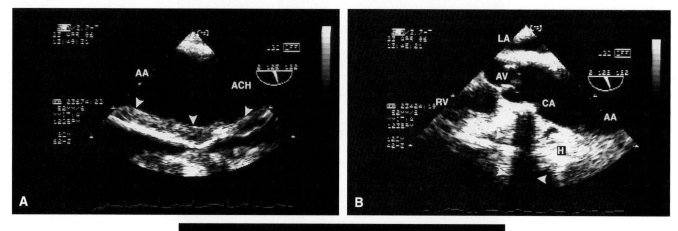

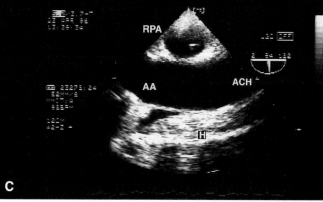

Figure 3.58. **Aortic atherosclerosis.** Descending aorta. **A-C.** Prominent atherosclerotic plaques (arrows) in the descending aorta (DA, DES AO) in two different patients.

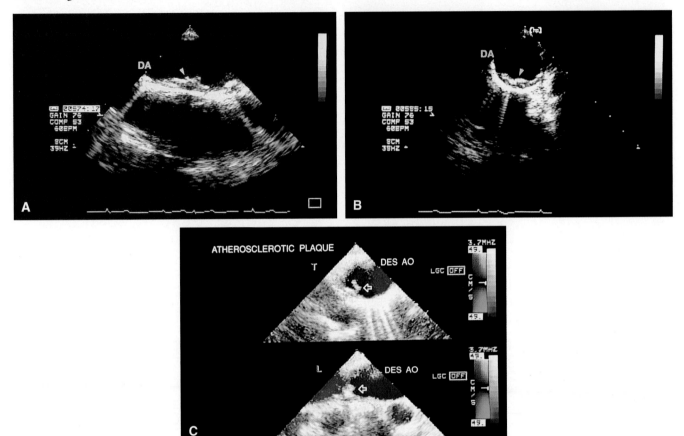

SUGGESTED READINGS

Appelbe AF, Olson S, Biby L, et al. Left brachiocephalic vein mimicking an aortic dissection on transesophageal echocardiography. Echocardiography 1993;10:67–69.

Armstrong WF, Bach DS, Carey L, et al. Spectrum of acute dissection of the ascending aorta: A transesophageal echocardiographic study. J Am Soc Echocardiogr 1996;9:646–656.

Ballal R, Gatewood R, Nanda NC, et al. Transesophageal echocardiography in the assessment of aortic graft dehiscence. Am J Cardiol 1997; 80:372-376.

Ballal R, Nanda NC, Gatewood R, et al. Usefulness of transesophageal echocardiography in assessment of aortic dissection. Circulation 1991; 84:1903–1914.

Borner N, Erbel R, Braun B, et al. Diagnosis of aortic dissection by transesophageal echocardiography. Am J Cardiol 1984;54:1157–1158.

Chan KL. Usefulness of transesophageal echocardiography in the diagnosis of conditions mimicking aortic dissection. Am Heart J 1991;122:495–504.

Chouinard M, Pinheiro L, Nanda NC, Sanyal R. Transgastric ultrasonography: A new approach for imaging the abdominal structures and vessels. Echocardiography 1991;8:397–403.

Cooke JP, Kazmier FJ, Orszulak TA. The penetrating aortic ulcer: pathologic manifestations, diagnosis, and management. Mayo Clin Proc 1988;63:718–725.

Cormier B, Iung B, Porte JM, et al. Value of multiplane transesophageal echocardiography in determining aortic valve area in aortic stenosis. Am J Cardiol 1996;77:882–885.

Erbel R, Borner N, Steller D, et al. Detection of aortic dissection by transesophageal echocardiography. Br Heart J 1987;58:45–51.

Erbel R, Oelert H, Meyer J, et al. Effect of medical and surgical therapy on aortic dissection evaluated by transesophageal echocardiography. Circulation 1993;88:1604–1615.

Espinola-Zavaleta N, Vargas-Barron J, Romero-Cardenas A, et al. Transesophageal echocardiographic diagnosis of periaortic abscess extending into interatrial septum. Echocardiography 1995;12:387–389.

Falcon-Eicher S, Eicher JC, Morvan Y, et al. False aneurysm of the aortic root and right ventricular outflow obstruction: an unusual complication of surgically treated infective endocarditis. Echocardiography 1996;13:75–79.

Fan P, Nanda NC, Gate RP Jr, et al. Transesophageal color Doppler evaluation of obstructive lesions using the new Quasar technology. Ultrasound Med Biol 1995;21:1021–1028.

Goldstein SA, Lindsay J. Thoracic aortic aneurysms: role of echocardiography. Echocardiography 1996;13:213–232.

Hashimoto S, Kumada T, Osakada G, et al. Assessment of transesophageal Doppler echocardiography in dissecting aortic aneurysm. J Am Coll Cardiol 1989;14:1253–1262.

Heinle SK, Kisslo J. The clinical utility of transesophageal echocardiography in patients with left-sided infective endocarditis. Am J Cardiac Imaging 1995;9:199–202.

Hofmann T, Kasper W, Meinertz T, et al. Determination of aortic valve orifice area in aortic valve stenosis by two-dimensional transesophageal echocardiography. Am J Cardiol 1987;59:330–335.

Karalis DG, Bansal RC, Hauck AJ, et al. Transesophageal echocardiographic recognition of subaortic complications in aortic valve endocarditis: clinical and surgical implications. Circulation 1992;86: 353–362.

Karalis DG, Chandrasekaran K, Victor MF, et al. Recognition and embolic potential of intraaortic atherosclerotic debris. J Am Coll Cardiol 1991;17:73.

Katz ES, Tunick PA, Rusinek H, et al. Protruding aortic atheromas predict stroke in elderly patients undergoing cardiopulmonary bypass: experience with intraoperative transesophageal echocardiography. J Am Coll Cardiol 1992;20:70–77.

Kim KS, Maxted W, Nanda NC, et al. Comparison of multiplane and biplane transesophageal echocardiography in the assessment of aortic stenosis. Am J Cardiol 1997;79:436–441.

Koppang J, Nanda NC, Coghlan C, Sanyal R. Histologically confirmed cholesterol atheroemboli with identification of the source by transesophageal echocardiography. Echocardiography 1992;9:379–383.

Kristensen SD, Ivarsen HR, Egeblad H. Rupture of aortic dissection during attempted transesophageal echocardiography. Echocardiography 1996;13:405–406.

Kronzon I, Tunick PA. Transesophageal echocardiography in thoracic aortic atherosclerosis. Echocardiography 1996;13:233–245.

Leung DY, Cranney GB, Hopkins AP, Walsh WF. Role of transesophageal echocardiography in the diagnosis and management of aortic root abscess. Br Heart J 1994;72:175–181.

Maxted W, Sanyal R, Nanda NC, et al. Transesophageal echocardiographic detection of sinus of Valsalva dissection. Echocardiography 1995;12:99–102.

Mehta R, Nanda NC, Roychoudhury D, et al. Atypical aortic dissection diagnosed by transesophageal echocardiography. Echocardiography 1994;11:261–263.

Mehta R, Agrawal G, Nanda NC, et al. Flail aortic valve in systemic lupus erythematosus. Echocardiography 1996;13:431–434.

Meyerowitz CB, Jacobs LE, Kotler MN, et al. Assessment of aortic regurgitation by transesophageal echocardiography: Correlation with angiographic determination. Echocardiography 1993;10:269–278.

Movsowitz C, Jacobs LE, Eisenberg S, et al. Discrete subaortic valvular stenosis: the clinical utility and limitations of transesophageal echocardiography. Echocardiography 1993;10:485–487.

Nienaber CA, Kodolitsch Y, Nicholas V, et al. The diagnosis of thoracic aortic dissection by noninvasive imaging procedures. N Engl J Med 1993;328:1–9.

Nishino M, Tanouchi J, Tanaka K, et al. Transesophageal echocardiographic diagnosis of thoracic aortic dissection with the completely thrombosed false lumen: differentiation from true aortic aneurysm with mural thrombus. J Am Soc Echocardiogr 1996;9:79–85.

Obeid A. Aortic dissection in progress diagnosed by transthoracic echocardiography. Echocardiography 1996;13:81–84.

Owen AN, Simon P, Moidl R, et al. Measurement of aortic flow velocity during transesophageal echocardiography in the transgastric five-chamber view. J Am Soc Echocardiogr 1995;8:874–878.

Ribakove GH, Katz ES, Galloway AC, et al. Surgical implications of transesophageal echocardiography to grade the atheromatous aortic arch. Ann Thorac Surg 1992;53:758–761.

Rosenzweig BP, Goldstein S, Sherrid M, et al. Aortic dissection with flap prolapse into the left ventricle. Am J Cardiol 1996;77:214–216.

Roudaut R, Chevalier JM, Barbeau P, et al. Mobility of the intimal flap and thrombus formation in aortic dissection: a transesophageal echocardiographic study. Echocardiography 1993;10:279–288.

Roychoudhury D, Nanda NC, Kim K, et al. Transesophageal echocardiographic diagnosis of aortic graft dehiscence at coronary anastomoses and pseudoaneurysm rupture into right atrium. Echocardiography 1995;12:495–499.

Schneider M, Mugge A, Daniel W. Imaging modalities in the diagnosis of acute aortic dissection. Echocardiography 1996;13:207–212.

Stoddard MF, Hammons RT, Longaker RA. Doppler transesophageal echocardiographic determination of aortic valve area in adults with aortic stenosis. Am Heart J 1996;132:337–342.

Stoddard MF, Arce J, Liddell NE, et al. Two-dimensional transesophageal echocardiographic determination of aortic valve area in adults with aortic stenosis. Am Heart J 1991;122:1415–1422.

Taams MA, Gussenhoven WJ, Bos E, Roelandt J. Saccular aneurysm of the transverse thoracic aorta detected by transesophageal echocardiography. Chest 1988;93:436–437.

Taams MA, Gussenhoven WJ, Schippers LA, et al. The value of transesophageal echocardiography for diagnosis of thoracic aorta pathology. Eur Heart J 1988;9:1308–1316.

Tardif JC, Miller DS, Pandian NG, et al. Effects of variations in flow on aortic valve area in aortic stenosis based on in vivo planimetry of aortic valve area by multiplane transesophageal echocardiography. Am J Cardiol 1995;76:193–198.

Tingleff J, Egeblad H, Gotzsche CO, et al. Perivalvular cavities in endocarditis: abscesses versus pseudoaneurysms? A transesophageal Doppler echocardiographic study in 118 patients with endocarditis. Am Heart J 1995;130:93–100.

Tribouilloy C, Shen WF, Peltier M, et al. Quantitation of aortic valve area in aortic stenosis with multiplane transesophageal echocardiography: comparison with monoplane transesophageal approach. Am Heart J 1994;128:526–532.

Tunick PA, Kronzon I. Protruding atheromas in the thoracic aorta: a newly recognized source of cerebral and systemic embolization. Echocardiography 1993;10:419–428.

Tunick PA, Kronzon I. Protruding atherosclerotic plaque in the aortic arch of patients with systemic embolization: A new finding seen by transesophageal echocardiography. Am Heart J 1990;120: 658–661.

Tunick PA, Kronzon I. Transesophageal echocardiography in embolic disease. Cardiol 1991;July:72.

Varma V, Nanda NC, Soto B, et al. Transesophageal echocardiographic demonstration of proximal right coronary artery dissection extending into the aortic root. Am Heart J 1992;123:1055–1057.

Wann S, Jaff M, Dorros G, Sampson C. Intramural hematoma of the aorta caused by a penetrating atheromatous ulcer. Clin Cardiol 1996; 19:438–439.

Wells KE, Alexander JJ, Piotrowski JJ, Finkelhor RS. Massive aortic thrombus detected by transesophageal echocardiography as a cause of peripheral emboli in young patients. Am Heart J 1996;132:882–883.

Tricuspid and
Pulmonary Valves

4

The tricuspid valve is well imaged on transesophageal echocardiography. The septal and anterior leaflets are seen in the transverse plane (four-chamber and right ventricular inflow views), and the anterior and posterior leaflets are imaged in the longitudinal plane. Tricuspid stenosis is unusual in the absence of mitral stenosis. Even small pressure gradients across a tricuspid valve may indicate significant stenosis.

Tricuspid regurgitation is far more common than stenosis. The most common cause of moderate or severe tricuspid regurgitation is right heart dilatation. Mild tricuspid regurgitation is commonly seen in normal healthy individuals and, therefore, often is not pathological. The absolute jet area is used to semiquantitate the severity of tricuspid regurgitation; therefore, it is important to image the tricuspid valve in multiple planes to find the maximum jet area. In the absence of an angiographic "gold standard," the criteria used for assessing the severity of mitral regurgitation also are used to grade the severity of tricuspid regurgitation. Mild tricuspid regurgitation is considered to be present when the maximum jet area is <4 cm^2, moderate when the jet area is 4 to 8 cm^2, and severe when the jet is >8 cm^2. Proximal flow acceleration is also an important marker of significant regurgitation.

Tricuspid prolapse most often accompanies mitral prolapse but can occur in its absence. The most specific pattern of prolapse occurs when one or more of the redundant leaflets shows a distinct bulge into the right atrium during systole. Prolapse may result in the entire spectrum of regurgitation, from mild to severe, and the regurgitant jet may be eccentric. In some patients, myxomatous degeneration may result in prominent thickening of a prolapsing tricuspid valve.

Pulmonary stenotic lesions are primarily the realm of congenital heart disease. However, mild pulmonary regurgitation often is noted in healthy individuals, and therefore may be considered "normal" or "physiologic." More severe degrees of pulmonary regurgitation result from pulmonary hypertension or right heart/pulmonary artery dilatation from other causes. In the absence of an angiographic "gold standard," the criteria used for assessment of the severity of aortic regurgitation have also been applied for grading the severity of pulmonary regurgitation. A ratio of jet width at its origin from the pulmonary valve to the right ventricular outflow tract diameter, taken at the same point, of 38% or less is considered mild or moderate pulmonary regurgitation, 39% to 74% is moderately severe, and 75% or more indicates severe regurgitation. The distance the pulmonary regurgitation jet travels in the right ventricular outflow tract also has been found useful in assessing its severity, especially in the presence of infundibular stenosis, which narrows the outflow tract. In our experience, a regurgitation jet reaching to within 1 cm of the tricuspid valve always denotes severe pulmonary regurgitation. It is particularly important not to rely on the presence of turbulent flow to identify tricuspid or pulmonary regurgitation since the regurgitant flow signals may be laminar and totally devoid of aliasing and variance when the right atrial or pulmonary artery diastolic pressures are high. In some such instances, torrential pulmonary and tricuspid regurgitation have been completely missed. The pulmonary valve may show redundancy, thickening, and prolapse resulting from myxomatous degeneration, and the resulting regurgitation may be eccentric. Pulmonary valve prolapse often is associated with prolapse of other valves. Both tricuspid and pulmonary valves may show evidence of infection, especially in drug addicts.

Figure 4.1.   **Tricuspid regurgitation**. **A.** A small jet of mild tricuspid regurgitation (TR). This is often seen in normal individuals. **B.** The regurgitant jet (arrow) is larger and represents moderate TR. Note the presence of flow acceleration on the ventricular aspect of the tricuspid valve. **C** through **G** show much larger jets, indicative of severe TR. Prominent flow acceleration is present in **C**. **D.** A relatively small zone of flow acceleration (arrow) is seen, even though the patient has torrential TR, almost completely filling the massively dilated right atrium (RA). Marked turbulence of the TR jet is seen in **E** and in the color M-mode (arrows, **F**). **G.** Transgastric view demonstrates severe TR. (**D** reproduced with permission from Rosenthal SM, Nanda NC. Assessment of valvular regurgitation by transesophageal echocardiography. J Invasive Cardiol 1992;4:366–372.)

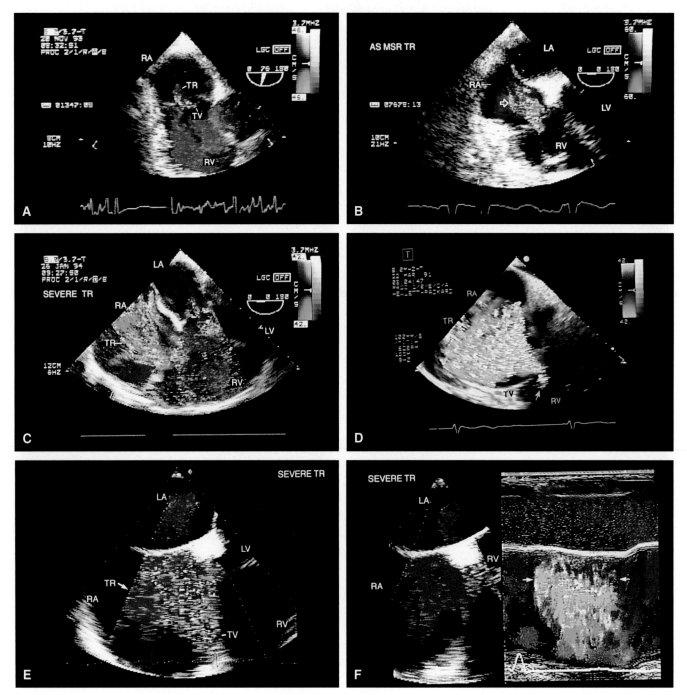

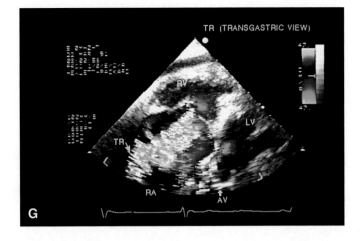

Figure 4.2. **Tricuspid valve prolapse.** **A.** Prolapse of both anterior (arrow) and septal leaflets of the tricuspid valve. **B.** Another patient with tricuspid valve prolapse. A medially located eccentric TR jet originating from the septal leaflet and extending into the inferior vena cava (IVC) and coronary sinus (CS) is seen. **C.** Four-chamber view of another patient with tricuspid valve (TV) prolapse (arrow). Note that the mitral valve (MV) is thickened but does not prolapse. **D–H.** Another patient with prolapse (arrow) of the septal leaflet of the TV with an eccentric TR jet directed along the RA free wall. Note the presence of flow acceleration on the ventricular side of the TV. Examination in the longitudinal plane shows two jets of TR in **G** and all three leaflets of the TV in **H.** *A*, anterior leaflet; *P*, posterior leaflet; *S*, septal leaflet. **I–O.** Another patient with TV prolapse. Marked prolapse of the TV with thickening (arrowheads) consistent with myxomatous degeneration is noted. In some views (**J, M, N,** and **O**) the marked thickening and redundancy produce the appearance of a mass. *ATV,* anterior tricuspid leaflet. (**I–O** are courtesy of Dr. Alan Schwadron, Montgomery, AL.)

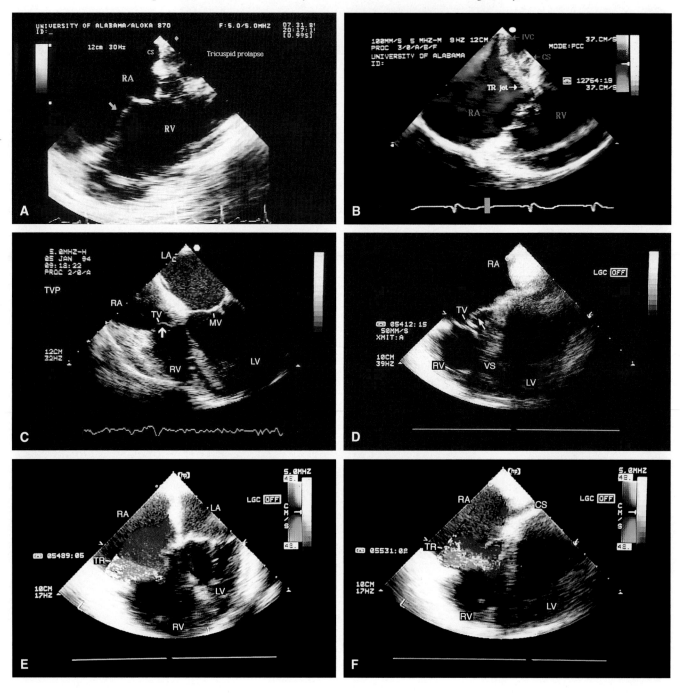

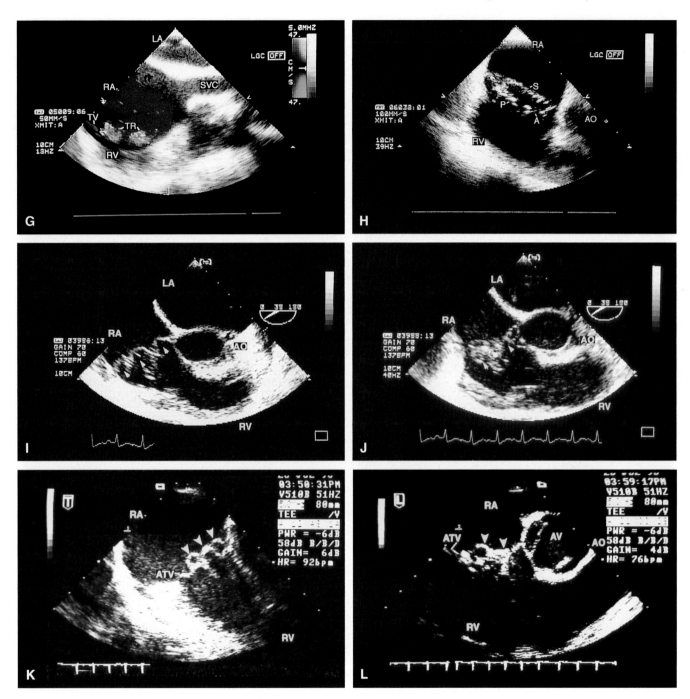

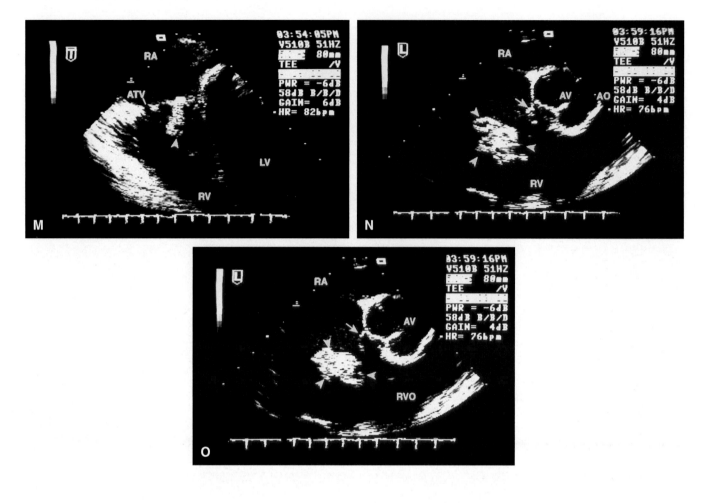

Figure 4.3. **Tricuspid regurgitation**. **A.** Two jets of TR are noted extending into the RA adjacent to the coronary sinus. **B.** Another patient with a TR jet impacting the atrial septum. **C–E.** A patient with both TR (arrows in **C–E**) and MR (upper arrow in **C**) impacting the atrial septum, mimicking atrial septal (AS) defect. Careful angulation of the multiplane probe helps to exclude the presence of an atrial septal defect.

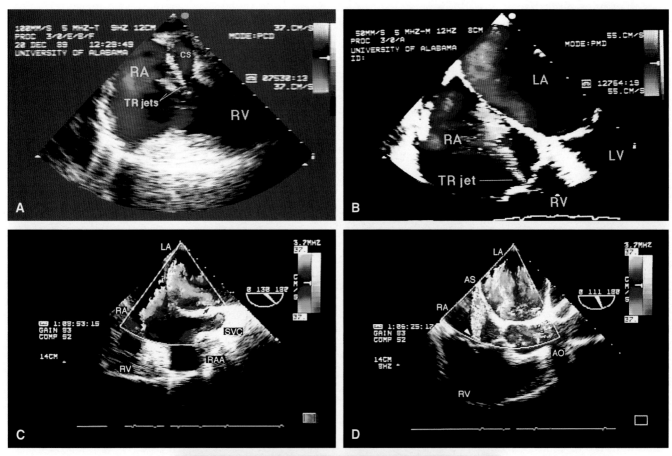

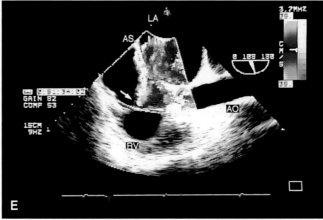

Figure 4.4. Tricuspid regurgitation. **A.** The anterior leaflet (arrow) and the septal leaflet (arrowhead), which demonstrate a localized prolapse. **B.** Note noncoaptation (arrow) of the anterior and septal leaflets of the TV in this patient with severe TR and massively dilated RA. **C,D.** Prominent flow acceleration and severe TR (arrows). The arrowhead in **D** shows associated mild MR. **E.** TR appears less severe, but the presence of large flow acceleration (arrow) suggests that the regurgitation is indeed severe. **F.** The patient shown in **E** underwent porcine replacement of the TV (arrows). **G.** Another patient with an eccentric TR jet (arrows), which initially moves along the septal leaflet and then is in contact with the atrial septum.

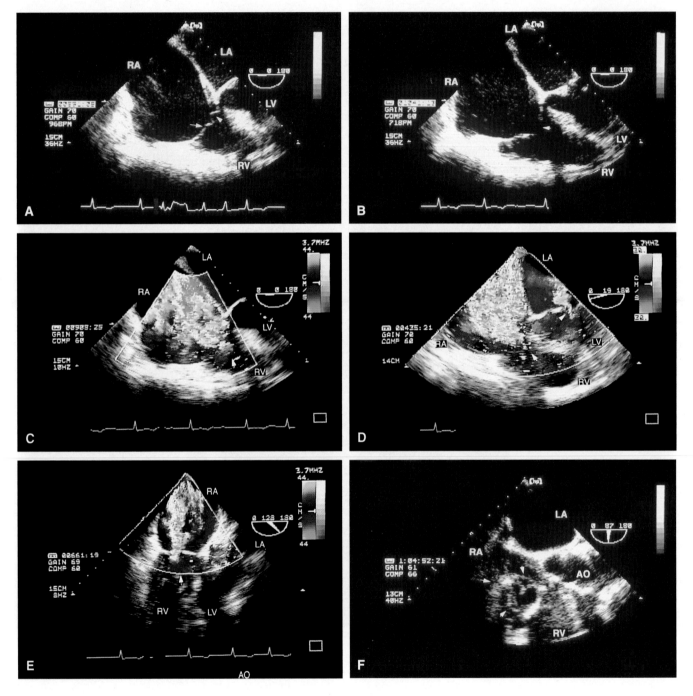

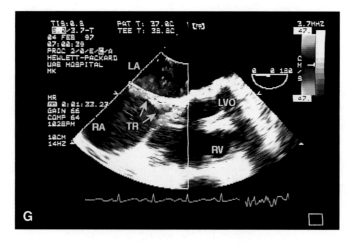

Figure 4.5. Tricuspid valve endocarditis. **A,B.** Multiplane examination shows a large vegetation (arrow) attached to the anterior (A) tricuspid leaflet. The posterior (P) tricuspid leaflet is not involved. (Reproduced with permission from Maxted W, Nanda NC, Kim KS, et al. Transesophageal echocardiographic identification and validation of individual tricuspid valve leaflets. Echocardiography 1994;11:585–590.)

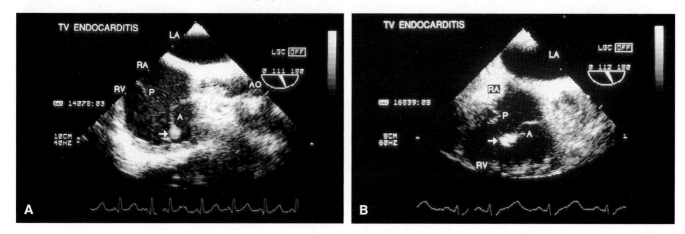

Figure 4.6. Pulmonic regurgitation. **A.** A very small jet of mild PR. **B.** The PR jet occupies almost the entire extent of the proximal RVOT, indicating severe regurgitation. This patient previously had patch repair of a ventricular septal defect.

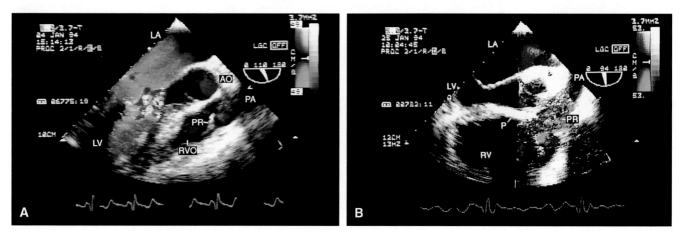

Figure 4.7. **Pulmonary valve prolapse. A,B**. Prolapse of the left and anterior cusps of the pulmonary valve (PV). **C,D**. All three leaflets of the pulmonary valve are seen in short axis. *A,* anterior; *L,* left; *P,* posterior. **E–H**. Associated eccentric jets of PR (arrowheads).

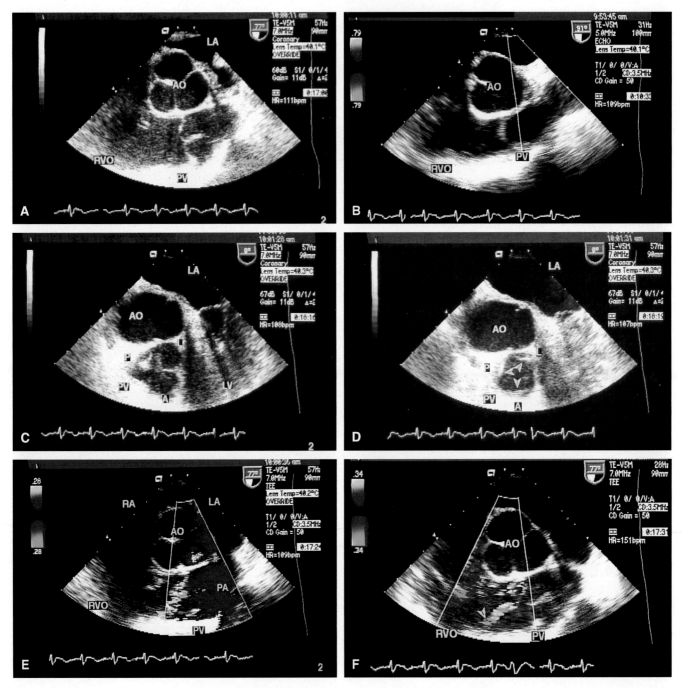

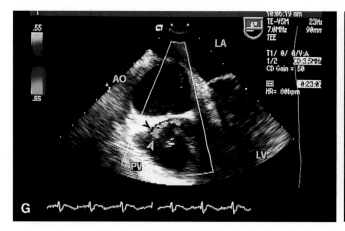

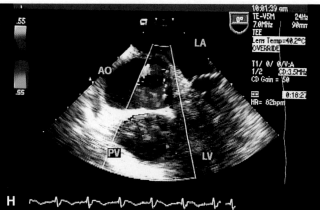

SUGGESTED READINGS

Cook JW. Accurate adjustment of de Vega tricuspid annuloplasty using transesophageal echocardiography. Ann Thorac Surg 1994;58:570–572.

Guarneri E, Tunick PA, Kennedy JT, et al. Horizontal plane transesophageal echocardiography may be false negative for large tricuspid vegetations. Echocardiography 1994;11:35–37.

Hancock HL, D'Cruz IA. Doppler-phonocardiographic findings in tricuspid valve prolapse. Echocardiography 1993;10:265–267.

Hutchison SJ, Rosin BL, Curry S, et al. Transesophageal echocardiographic assessment of lesions of the right ventricular outflow tract and pulmonic valve. Echocardiography 1996;13:21–34.

Kai H, Koyanagi S, Hirooka Y, et al. Right-to-left shunt across atrial septal defect related to tricuspid regurgitation: assessment by transesophageal Doppler echocardiography. Am Heart J 1994;127:578–584.

Karatasakis G, Karamintziou R, Taylor KM. Transthoracic and transesophageal echocardiographic diagnosis of a De Vega tricuspid annuloplasty rupture. J Am Soc Echocardiogr 1994;7:321–323.

Maxted W, Nanda NC, Kim KS, et al. Transesophageal echocardiographic identification and validation of individual tricuspid valve leaflets. Echocardiography 1994;11:585–590.

Meijburg HWJ, Bisser CA. Pulmonary venous flow as assessed by Doppler echocardiography: potential clinical applications. Echocardiography 1995;12:425–440.

Rollefson WA, Winslow TM, Adams CW, et al. Traumatic dehiscence of a tricuspid annuloplasty ring: diagnosis by transesophageal echocardiography. Am Heart J 1994;127:708–710.

Rosenthal SM, Nanda NC. Assessment of valvular regurgitation by transesophageal echocardiography. J Invasive Cardiol 1992;4:366–372.

Van TB, Halldorsson A, Baucum RW, et al. Retrieval of a distal right pulmonary artery vegetative embolus under transesophageal echocardiographic guidance. Echocardiography 1993;10:489–495.

Prosthetic Valves
and Rings

5

Prosthetic valves may be made from metal and other material or may be biologic grafts (i.e., heterografts, homografts, or autografts). Mechanical grafts last longer than bioprostheses but require long-term anticoagulation. The great potential advantage of the bioprostheses is that anticoagulation is required only early after placement unless indicated for other reasons, such as the presence of atrial fibrillation. Porcine heterografts are the most commonly used; they cannot be implanted in children, however, because of the relatively rapid calcification that occurs. Homografts (i.e., human valves) and autografts (i.e., grafts from the same individual—as in placement of the pulmonary valve in the aortic position) may be less prone to calcification. The Ross procedure is a recently developed surgical approach in which the patient's pulmonary valve is placed in the aortic position and a homograft is placed in the pulmonary position. The lower pressure gradient across the homograft in the pulmonary position may make it less subject to calcification. An important role of transesophageal echocardiography is measuring the size of the annulus to be certain that appropriately sized homografts are available and, in the case of the Ross procedure, to be certain that the pulmonary valve is the right size for placement in the aortic position.

The most commonly used mechanical valve is the St. Jude valve. Newer valves such as the Carbomedics (Sulzer Carbomedics Inc., Austin, TX) and Medtronic-Hall (Meditronics, Inc., Minneapolis, MN) valves are preferred by some surgeons, and their use is increasing. The echocardiographer must also be familiar with other valves, such as the Bjork-Shiley and Starr-Edwards valves, because large numbers of these implants are still functioning.

Problems that can occur with all valves include paravalvular leaks, infection, and thrombus. Bioprosthetic valves also may calcify and degenerate.

Because all mechanical and bioprosthetic valves are inherently somewhat stenotic, a region of flow acceleration often can be seen proximal to the valve during flow across the valve. Because of the presence of localized areas of high-velocity flow, the Doppler study may overestimate the gradient across the prosthetic valve. A baseline study performed at the time of surgery can be helpful so that changes in pressure gradients can be followed over time. It is important to investigate the motion of the occluder or leaflets when assessing stenosis. Immediately after the termination of cardiopulmonary bypass, the flow may be in-

adequate to open one of the leaflets of the mechanical prosthetic valve. This is a normal finding that resolves over time as cardiac output increases. For valves in the mitral position, a flat EF slope in association with a high velocity on conventional Doppler study suggests obstruction.

Valve prostheses may normally have a small amount of regurgitation. In the case of the St. Jude and CarboMedics valves, up to three small regurgitant jets are seen. These correspond to the two leaflets and to a central jet. Compared with pathologic regurgitant jets, these normal jets tend to be more laminar and narrow. In mitral prostheses the jets may, however, extend well back into the left atrium. In assessing the severity of the prosthetic mitral regurgitation, it is important to interrogate the pulmonary veins near their entry into the left atrium with conventional Doppler to search for systolic backflow, which is a reliable marker for severe regurgitation. The size of the proximal flow acceleration should be assessed as well. Finally, the area of the jet is important (<4 cm^2, mild regurgitation; 4 to 8 cm^2, moderate regurgitation; >8 cm^2, severe regurgitation), although jet area may be misleading if an eccentric jet is present. Multiple planes should be interrogated to find the plane in which the regurgitant jet has the largest area. The presence of spontaneous contrast in the left atrium suggests that any mitral regurgitation is not severe. In the case of aortic prostheses, the aortic regurgitant jet may be seen best by the transthoracic approach because there is acoustic shadowing of the jet on the transesophageal examination, caused by the metallic components and posterior calcification. For prostheses in the aortic position, the severity of the regurgitation is assessed by determining the ratio of jet width at its origin to left ventricular outflow tract diameter, also measured at the origin of the jet ($<38\%$, mild; 39% to 75%, moderate; $>75\%$, severe).

Paravalvular leaks may be important causes of regurgitation. These leaks may be caused by valve suture dehiscence and can be seen to originate beyond the extent of the prosthetic elements. The location of proximal flow acceleration outside the confines of the prosthesis also may help to determine that the leak is paravalvular.

Thrombi can lead to emboli or to obstruction or may interfere with the function of a valve and cause significant regurgitation. Thrombi may be present in the left atrium or left atrial appendage and may be well seen on the transesophageal study. Because the left atrial appendage may be partially or completely removed at the time of surgery, inability to image it should not be taken as evidence that there is a clot obscuring the appendage. Left ventricular function is better preserved if the papillary muscles are not completely removed; remnants of the papillary muscle and chordae left in place by the surgeon may be mistaken for a mobile clot. For this reason, a baseline transesophageal study is of great use for comparison.

The transesophageal and transthoracic examinations are complementary in patients with a mitral valve replacement. Transesophageal study is far more effective than is transthoracic examination in assessing the left atrium for the presence and severity of mitral regurgitation in patients with valves in the mitral position. On the transthoracic study, acoustic shadowing of the left atrium by the valve is present. Conversely, substantial acoustic shadowing and reverberation that degrade the transesophageal image of the left ventricle are present on transesophageal study but not on transthoracic examination.

Certain structures are well examined by transesophageal echocardiography. The short-axis view of a prosthetic valve permits a complete view of the valve suture line. Stents are well seen, and, in the case of mitral prostheses, may physically narrow the left ventricular outflow tract or may impinge on the left ventricular free wall or ventricular septum, producing arrhythmias or conduction system abnormalities. Bioprosthetic mitral cusp rupture resulting from degeneration or infection may be manifested as linear echoes protruding into the left atrium, with or without fluttering. Left atrial perforation or dissection may be seen. Abscesses may be visualized. They may be large and filled with pus. The presence of flow signals in the abscess cavity demonstrates that there is communication with an adjoining vessel or cavity. Abscesses may form fistulas to other structures. Following aortic valve replacement, systolic anterior motion of the mitral valve may be unmasked, and significant left ventricular outflow tract obstruction may develop in the presence of coexisting hypertrophic cardiomyopathy. Rarely, a left ventricular outflow tract gradient may be caused by an abscess narrowing the outflow tract. Pannus may cause obstruction and may be difficult to distinguish from clot. If the obstructing echo density is mobile, however, thrombus is more likely. Bioprosthetic valves may suffer cusp degeneration or calcification, which may produce obstruction. Linear echoes protruding into the left ventricular outflow tract are characteristic of prolapse caused by bioprosthetic aortic valve degeneration. Similar echoes also may be caused by infection.

Transesophageal echocardiography is also useful in the assessment of mitral annuloplasty rings, which are placed to reduce the severity of mitral regurgitation. Residual mitral regurgitation, as well as ring thrombus, obstruction, and dehiscence, are well demonstrated. Systolic anterior motion of the anterior mitral leaflet with left ventricular outflow tract obstruction also may occur after ring placement and can be diagnosed by echocardiography. In patients undergoing aortic valvuloplasty, the site of aortic valve repair and the severity of residual aortic regurgitation also are well assessed by transesophageal echocardiography.

Figure 5.1.   **St. Jude mitral prosthesis: normal.** The mitral prosthesis (MP) is seen in the closed **(A)** and open **(B)** positions. **A.** Prosthetic reverberations or artifacts (arrows) that clutter the LV. **B.** The two leaflets (1 and 2) of the prosthesis in the open position together with the reverberations. **C.** Aliased diastolic inflow into the left ventricle (LV) is seen with a small region of flow acceleration. **D–G.** Two to three small jets of mitral regurgitation (MR; arrows) are shown. These are normal findings. Usually, these jets are narrow and do not show significant turbulence but may extend deep into theleft atrium (LA). **G** illustrates the norm (not pansystolic). **H.** Small linear echoes are normally seen on both the atrial and ventricular aspects of the prosthesis and represent suture material. **I,J.** Immediately postsurgery, while the patient is still on partial bypass, one leaflet of the prosthesis (P) may intermittently fail to open. This should not be mistaken for dysfunction. When cardiac output improves, normal opening of both leaflets occurs consistently.

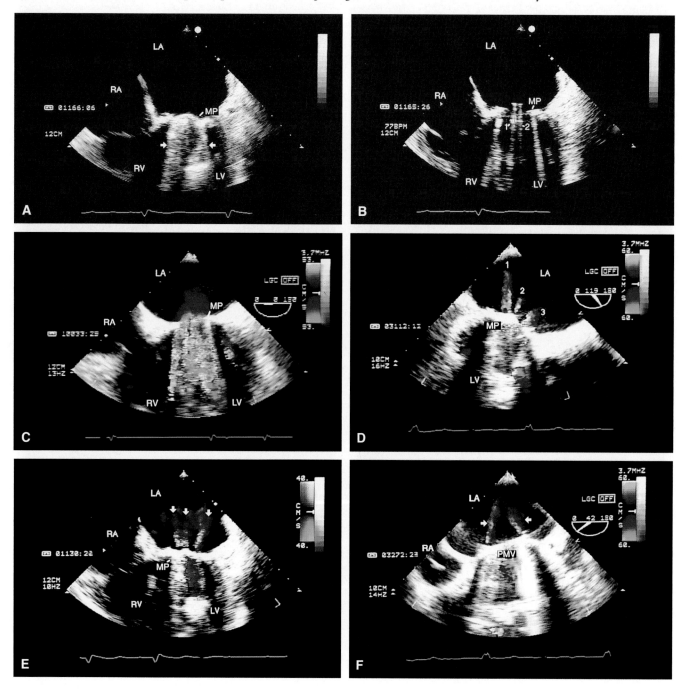

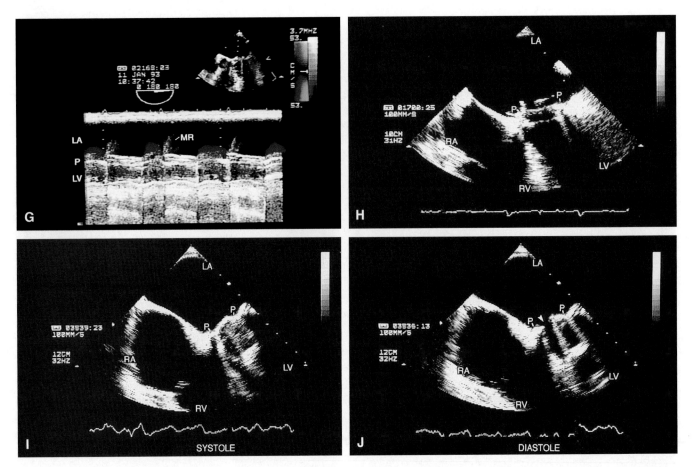

Figure 5.2. **St. Jude mitral prosthesis: thrombus. A–F.** Localized echo densities consistent with thrombus (T) are noted on the St. Jude prosthesis (P) in two different patients (**A,B** and **C–F**). In both patients, thrombus prevented opening of one of the leaflets of the prosthesis. **F.** Continuous wave Doppler shows a flat velocity profile in early diastole (arrows) as well as a high peak velocity of 152 cm/sec consistent with obstruction. **G** and **H** (one patient) and **I** (another patient) show two other patients with thrombosed (TH,T) St. Jude mitral prostheses. The echo densities representing thrombus are seen on the atrial side of the prosthesis. Thrombi are less dense than the metallic components of the prosthesis and are different from prosthetic reverberations, which are anteriorly directed, more prominent, and larger linear echoes. In addition, reverberations are not seen on the atrial aspect of the prosthesis.

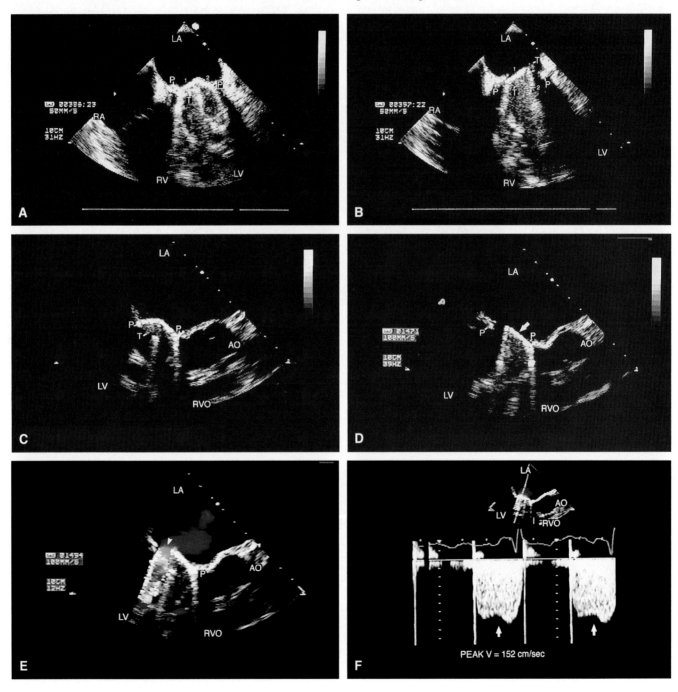

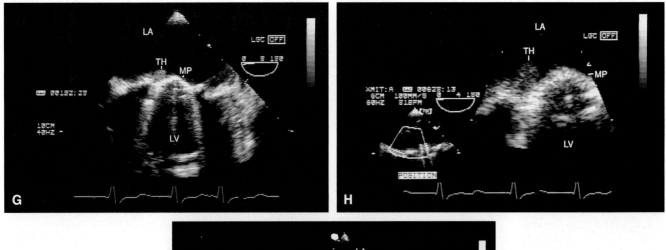

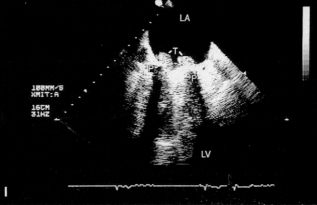

Figure 5.3. **St. Jude mitral prosthesis: paravalvular regurgitation. A.** A large eccentric jet (arrowheads) coursing medially along the atrial septum is seen originating beyond the edges of the prosthetic elements (P). **B.** The paraprosthetic leak (arrowheads) is located laterally. There is also a large zone of flow acceleration (FA), which is clearly located outside the confines of the prosthetic valve (P). **C.** The dehisced area (arrow) is clearly seen, and a wide jet of paravalvular regurgitation (oblique arrow) can be seen coursing through it **(D)**. The vertical arrows point to two small jets of normal valvular regurgitation through the St. Jude prosthesis. **E,F.** Another patient with dehiscence of sutures and pansystolic paravalvular regurgitation. **G,H.** Another patient with suture dehiscence (arrow in **G**) and severe eccentric MR (arrowheads), with a large flow acceleration on the ventricular aspect of this St. Jude prosthesis. **I.** There is eccentric periprosthetic MR (white arrows) as well as eccentric TR (yellow arrows) moving along the atrial septum. Two small normal jets of MR also are seen originating from the St. Jude prosthesis.

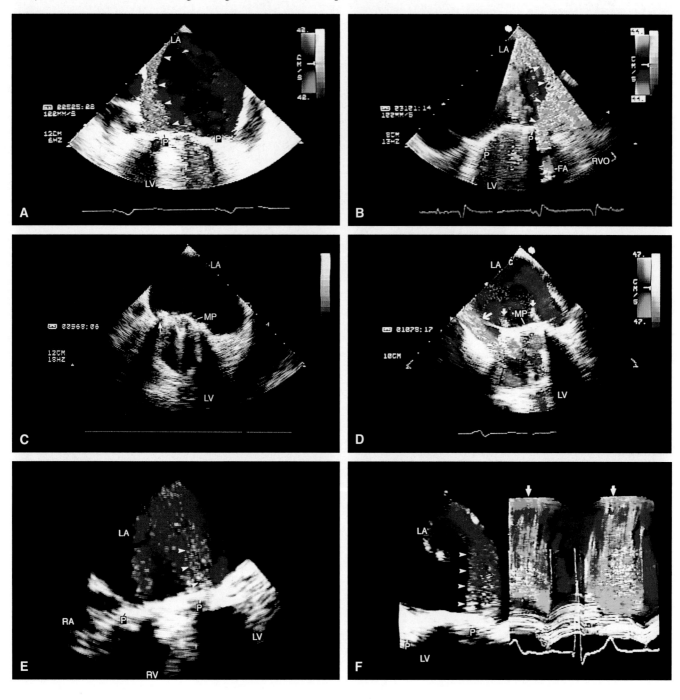

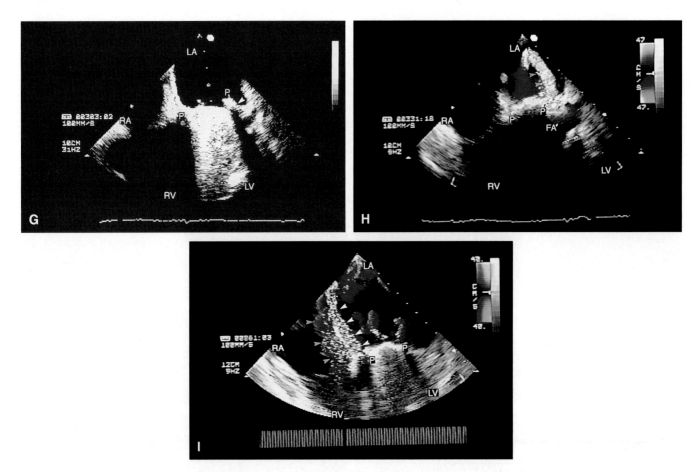

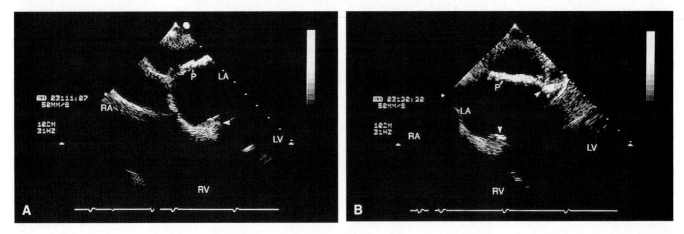

Figure 5.4. **A,B. St. Jude mitral prosthesis: ectopic position.** In this patient, the St. Jude prosthesis (P) is attached to the wall of the left atrium (upper arrowhead in **B**) rather than to the valve ring (lower arrowheads).

Figure 5.5. **CarboMedics mitral prosthesis: normal**. **A–C.** Schematics of the CarboMedics mitral prosthesis. In **A**, the CarboMedics aortic prosthesis also is shown. **C.** The mechanism of normally occurring MR through the hinge points (courtesy of Sulzer CarboMedics Inc., Austin, TX). **D.** The prosthesis is seen in the four-chamber view, demonstrating multiple reverberations (1, 2, 3, 4) partially obscuring the LV and RV cavities. **E.** Both leaflets of the prosthesis and the suture ring (arrow) are viewed in short axis. **F.** Individual sutures (arrowheads) are seen on the atrial aspect of the prosthetic valve. **G.** Diastolic flow acceleration (arrowhead) on the atrial aspect of the prosthesis. The LV inflow jet is large. **H,I.** Two small jets of normal prosthetic valvular regurgitation (arrowheads). *R*, prosthetic reverberations.

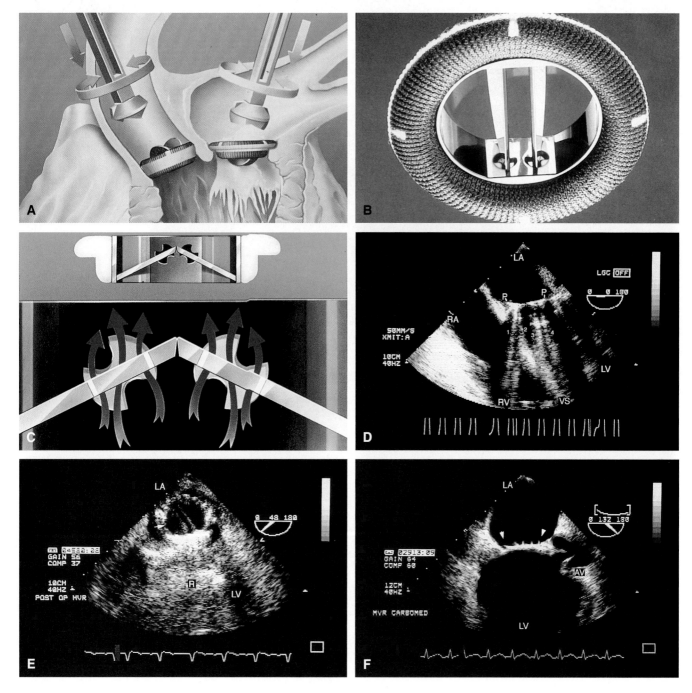

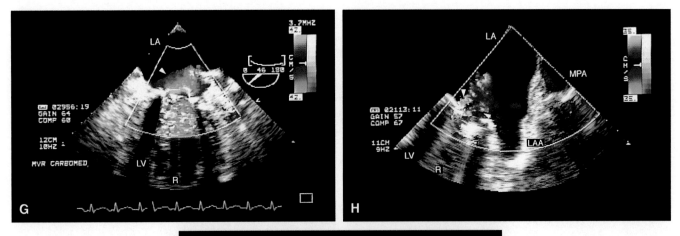

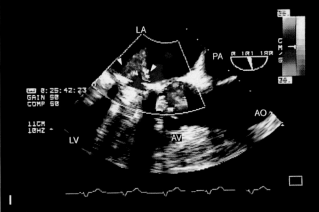

Figure 5.6. **A–E. CarboMedics mitral prosthesis: dehiscence of LA wall. A.** A small linear echo (vertical arrow) at the site of the paravalvular defect (horizontal arrow) consistent with suture material. **B.** Color Doppler examination shows a large paravalvular regurgitant jet originating at the site of the paravalvular defect (arrow) shown in **A.** **C.** An abnormal 1-cm linear echo (arrow) protrudes into the left atrium at the mid-interatrial septal level. **D,E.** Multiplane views at 105 and 111 degrees demonstrate a cavitary defect (arrows) involving the left atrial wall at the mid-interatrial septal level, indicative of dehiscence, which explains the presence of the linear echo in the left atrium seen in **C. F–H. CarboMedics mitral prosthesis: LA pseudoaneurysm. F.** A large pseudoaneurysm (AN; arrow) that developed following prosthetic replacement (MP, arrowhead) of the mitral valve. **G,H.** Color Doppler examination shows flow signals (arrowhead in **H**) moving from the LV into the aneurysm cavity. (**A** through **E** reproduced with permission from Howard J, Agrawal G, Nanda NC. Transesophageal echocardiographic diagnosis of left atrial wall dehiscence. Echocardiography 1997;14:299–302.)

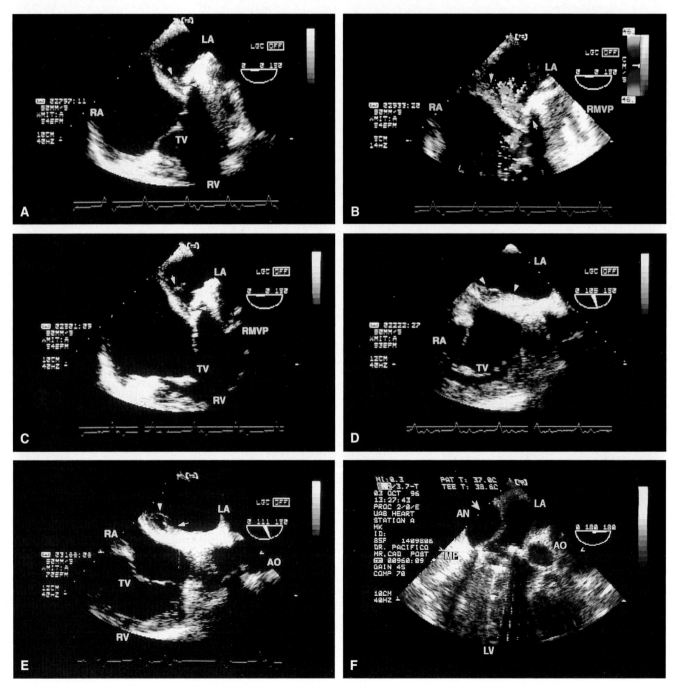

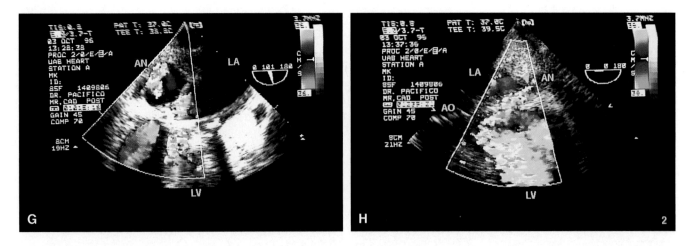

Figure 5.7. Bjork-Shiley mitral prosthesis: thrombus/pannus. **A.** A small echo density consistent with thrombus (T) is seen within the ring of the prosthesis (P). **B.** Its presence is confirmed by the flat diastolic velocity profile (arrows) and a high peak pressure gradient (16 mm Hg) across the prosthesis, consistent with obstruction. **C–K.** Another patient with a thrombosed Bjork-Shiley mitral prosthesis. Note the spontaneous contrast (SC) echoes in the LA in **C, G,** and **J. I.** A thrombus (TH) is well seen on the atrial aspect of the prosthesis (PMV) imaged with a probe in the esophagus, whereas the thrombus on the ventricular aspect is best visualized during transgastric examination **(I).** Another thrombus (TH) is present in LAA **(G).** Color Doppler–directed continuous wave Doppler reveals a very flat diastolic velocity profile with a very high peak velocity of 305 cm/sec, indicative of very severe flow obstruction. **K.** The arrowhead in **J** shows prominent flow acceleration on the atrial aspect of the prosthesis. *R,* prosthetic ring. **L.** Another patient with a Bjork-Shiley prosthesis. In this patient, the echo density on the ventricular aspect of the prosthesis (P) was found at surgery to be a pannus (PAN) rather than a thrombus. Spontaneous echo contrast (SEC) was present in LA. **M.** Gross specimen of a thrombosed mitral prosthetic valve.

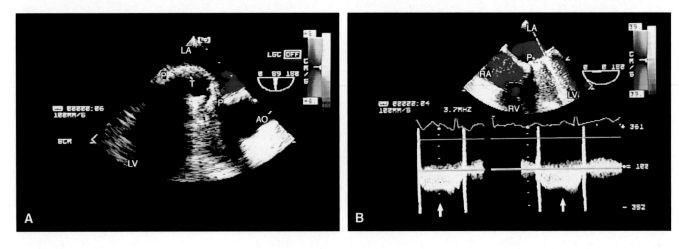

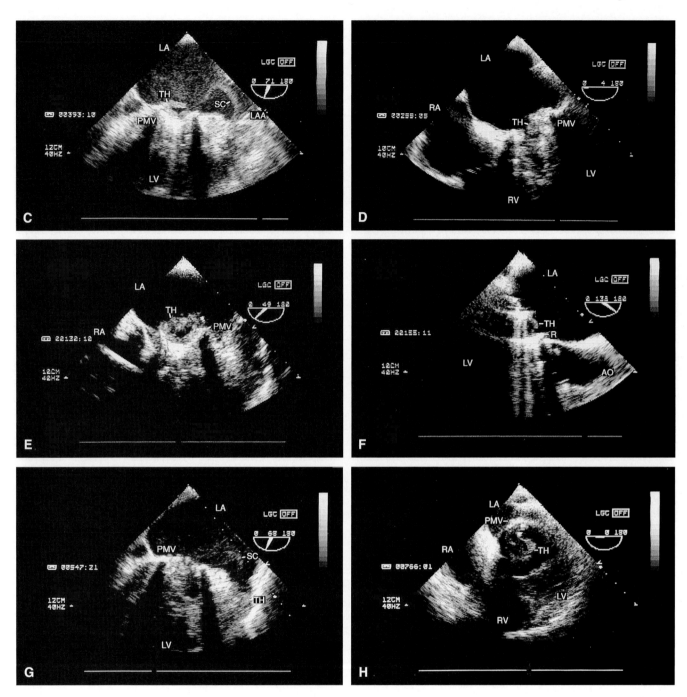

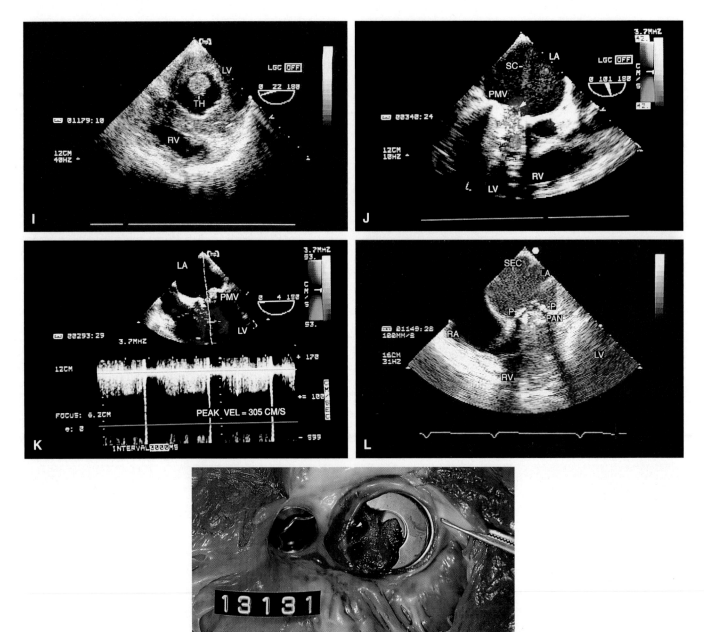

Figure 5.8. **Bjork-Shiley mitral prosthesis: suture dehiscence**. The arrow in **A** shows a large area of dehiscence with severe paraprosthetic (P) MR (arrow in **B**).

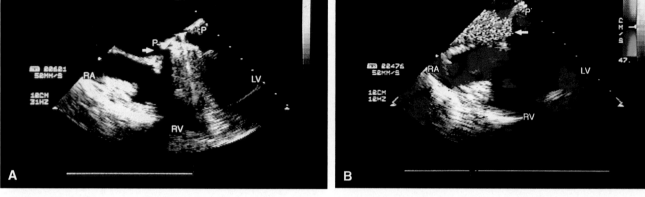

Figure 5.9. **Cooley-Cutter mitral prosthesis: stenosis. A.** Prosthetic reverberations (arrow). **B.** A questionable thrombus (arrow). **C,D.** Prominent flow acceleration (FA) is present on the atrial aspect of the prosthesis (MP,P). **E.** A high velocity of 176 cm/sec was measured across the prosthesis by continuous wave Doppler (arrows). **F.** Associated mild MR.

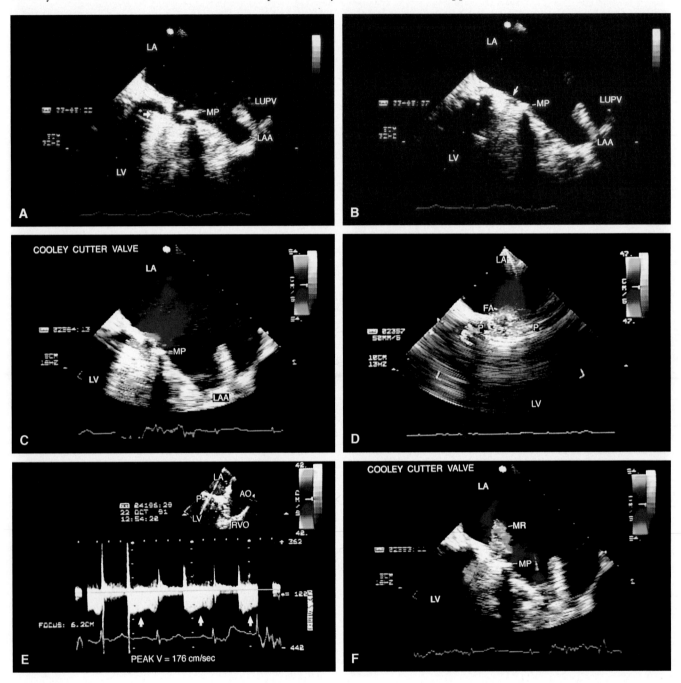

Figure 5.10.   **Starr-Edwards prosthesis: normal. A.** The rounded poppet (arrows) is seen in the open position in diastole and in the closed position in systole. **B.** Transgastric view shows the three prosthetic struts (arrows) together with the resulting reverberations imaged in short axis. **C.** Gross specimen shows Starr-Edwards prostheses in the aortic and mitral positions.

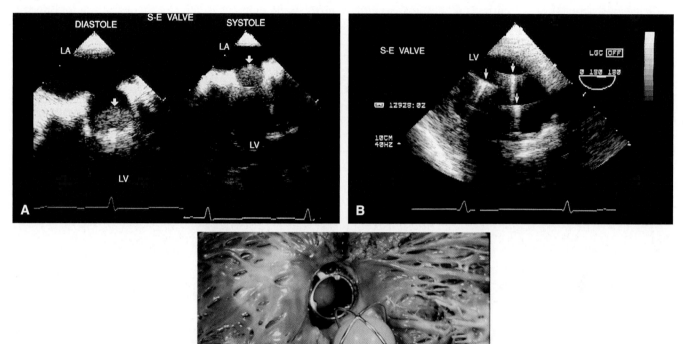

Figure 5.11. **Starr-Edwards mitral prosthesis: dehiscence.** The poppet, or ball (**B**), is seen in the closed (**A**) and open (**B**) positions. Note the reverberations from the ball partially obscuring the LV in **B**. **C,D.** Eccentric, severe paravalvular mitral regurgitation (arrowheads) originating beyond the prosthetic (P) elements is shown. **E.** Color M-mode examination demonstrates systolic backflow (arrowheads) in the left upper pulmonary vein (LUPV), confirming the presence of severe MR. C,C, mitral ring. **F.** Gross specimen shows suture dehiscence and clot involving a Starr-Edwards prosthesis.

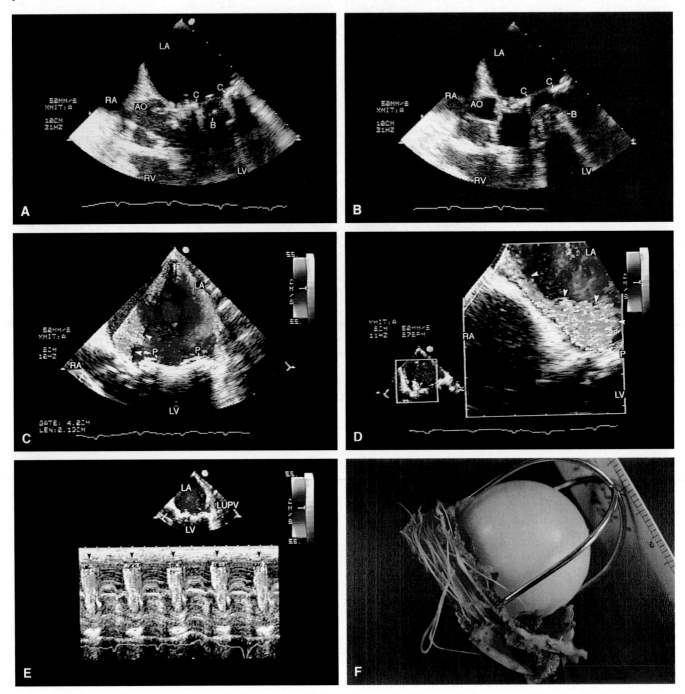

Figure 5.12. **Mitral annuloplasty rings. A.** *R* points to the Carpentier ring in the mitral position. There is no obstruction to mitral flow. **B.** Gross specimen of Carpentier ring. **C, D.** Duran ring in the mitral position (arrows in **C**). **D.** Color Doppler examination shows prominent flow acceleration and aliased flow resulting from narrowing of the mitral orifice by the ring.

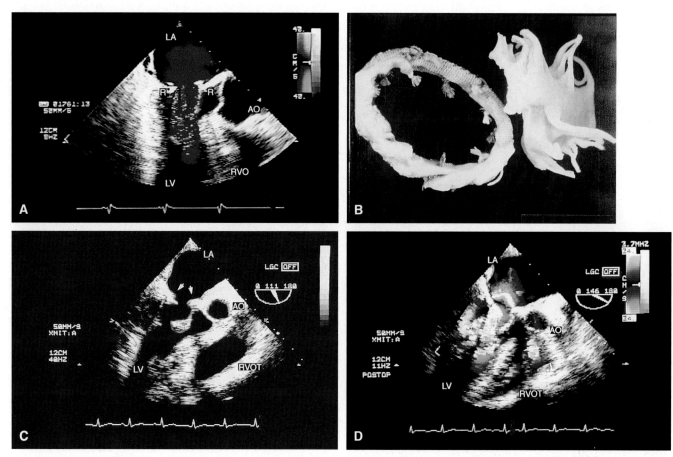

Figure 5.13. **Mitral annuloplasty ring. A.** *R* demonstrates an annuloplasty ring in the mitral position. *S*, sutures. **B.** Color Doppler examination shows aliased inflow signals and prominent diastolic flow acceleration (arrow) produced by narrowing of the mitral orifice by the ring. **C.** Pulsed Doppler examination of the left upper pulmonary vein shows a smaller S wave than D wave, consistent with moderate mitral regurgitation preoperatively. After ring placement, the S wave is equal to the D wave, suggesting a reduction in mitral regurgitation (in **D**). **E.** Another patient in whom the annulus size was reduced to 2.64 cm after placement of an annuloplasty ring for severe MR.

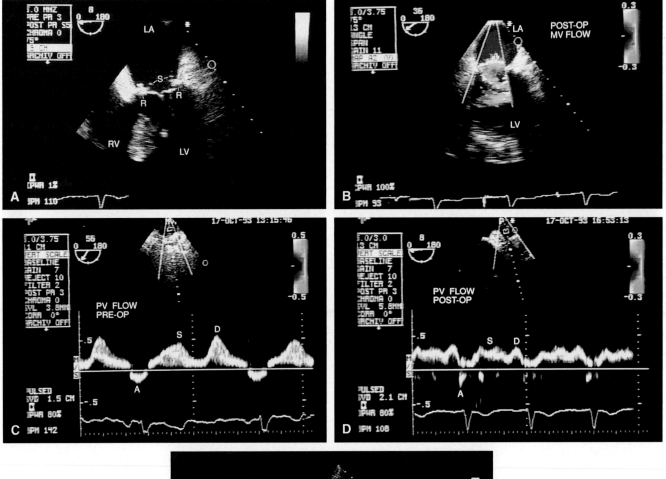

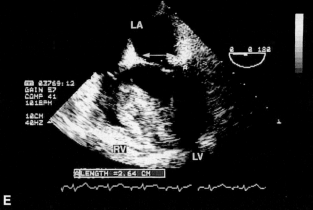

Figure 5.14. **Mitral annuloplasty ring.** The ring (R) is seen in diastole in **A** and in systole in **B**. **C**. Color Doppler examination shows moderate residual mitral regurgitation in this patient, who had severe MR before ring placement. **D**. A systolic frame shows ring (R) echoes in another patient following mitral annuloplasty.

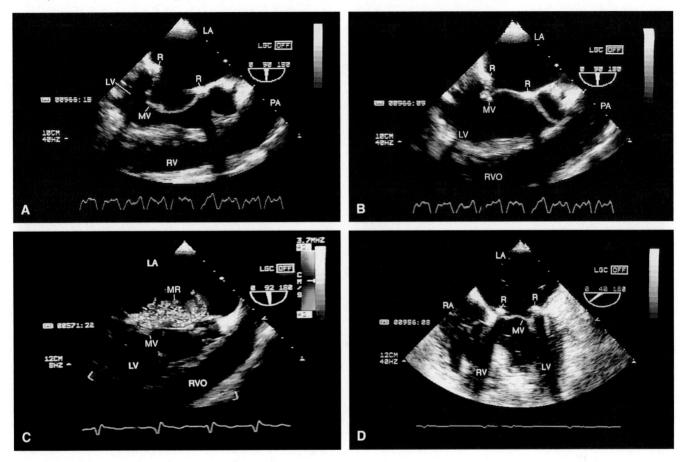

Figure 5.15. **Mitral annuloplasty ring: ruptured chordae. A.** Ruptured chordae (arrowheads) prolapsing into the LA in systole. *R*, mitral annuloplasty ring. **B,C.** Color Doppler examination demonstrates severe eccentric MR (arrowheads) through the ring with prominent systolic backflow (SBF) in the LUPV **(D).**

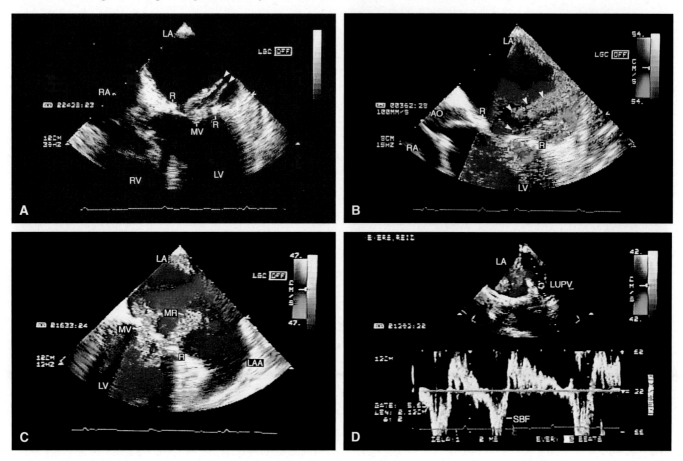

Figure 5.16.   **Mitral annuloplasty ring: obstruction. A,B.** Prominent diastolic flow acceleration (arrow) and a narrow inflow jet resulted from obstruction produced by a Duran ring in this patient.

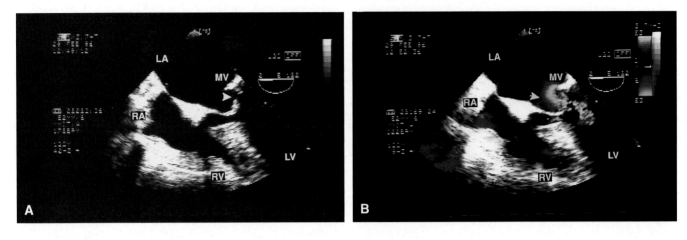

Figure 5.17.   **Mitral annuloplasty ring: thrombus/dehiscence. A.** A thrombus (arrow) involving the ventricular aspect of a Duran ring. There is severe mitral valve prolapse. **B–D.** Another patient with a flail Duran ring (R) and thrombus formation (arrow in **D**). In **B** the flail ring is shown in systole in the left atrium. **C.** Another systolic frame, showing the ring now prolapsing into the ventricle. In this patient, the Duran ring had dehisced and was attached only by a single remaining suture. (Reproduced with permission from Osman K, Willman B, Nanda NC, et al. Transesophageal echocardiographic findings of a dehisced duran mitral annuloplasty ring. Echocardiography 1995;12:441–446.)

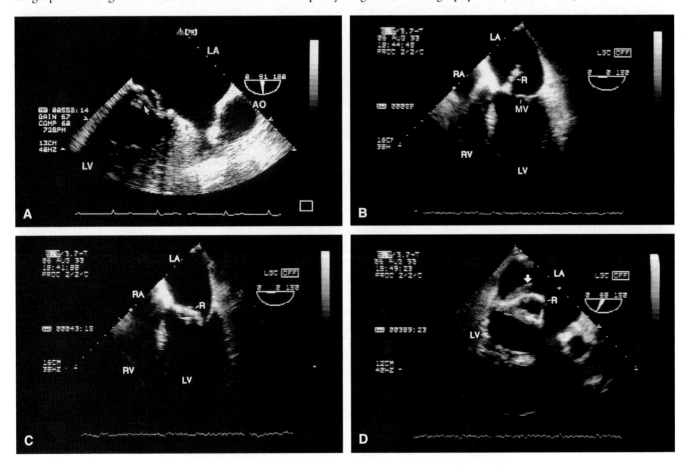

Figure 5.18. **Porcine mitral prosthesis: normal.** The porcine prosthesis is shown in the closed position (**A,B;** arrow in **B**) in systole and in the open position (arrow in **C**) in diastole. **D.** The porcine prosthesis imaged in short axis. **E.** Mitral prosthetic (P) inflow with a localized area of flow acceleration on the atrial side of the valve. **F.** A systolic frame demonstrates absence of regurgitation through the prosthesis (MP). **G.** *ST*, prosthetic stents in LV; *S*, sutures on the atrial side.

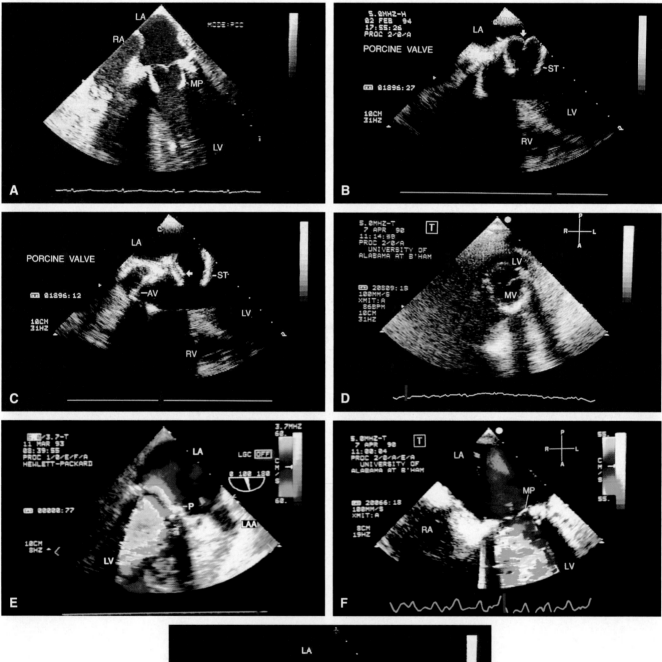

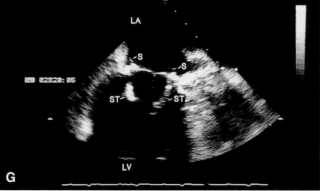

Figure 5.19. **Porcine mitral prosthesis: stenosis and regurgitation. A.** A large diastolic flow acceleration (arrowheads) on the atrial side of the prosthesis (P), suggesting the presence of obstruction. **B.** Thickening and calcification of the prosthesis resulting from degeneration. **C.** A decreased slope of the diastolic velocity profile with a measured mitral valve area (MVA) of 0.9 cm² measured by the pressure half-time technique, indicating significant obstruction. **D.** Associated severe valvular MR (arrowheads). Images **B** through **D** are from the same patient.

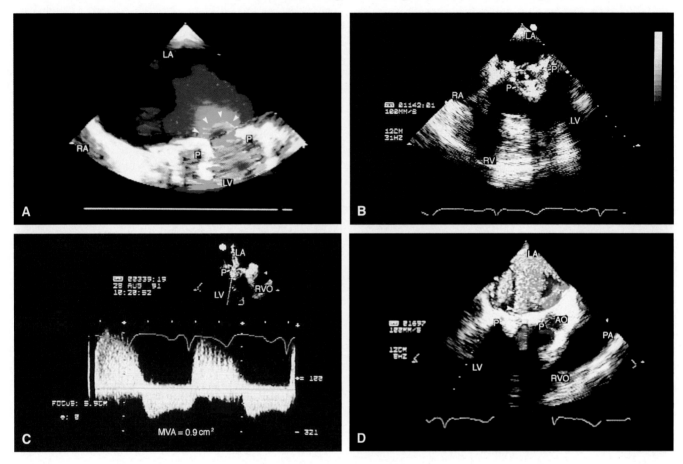

Figure 5.20. Porcine mitral prosthesis: spontaneous contrast and thrombus in LA. **A.** M-mode study shows spontaneous contrast (arrows). **B,C.** A large thrombus (TH) in the LAA. The prosthetic leaflets are only mildly thickened (**B**). **D.** Extensive thrombus formation (TH) in the left atrium in another patient with an obstructed porcine mitral prosthesis. (**C** reproduced with permission from Mahan EF III, Nanda NC. Transesophageal echocardiography. In: Rackley CE, ed. Challenges in Cardiology I. Mt. Kisco, NY: Futura, 1991:85–101.)

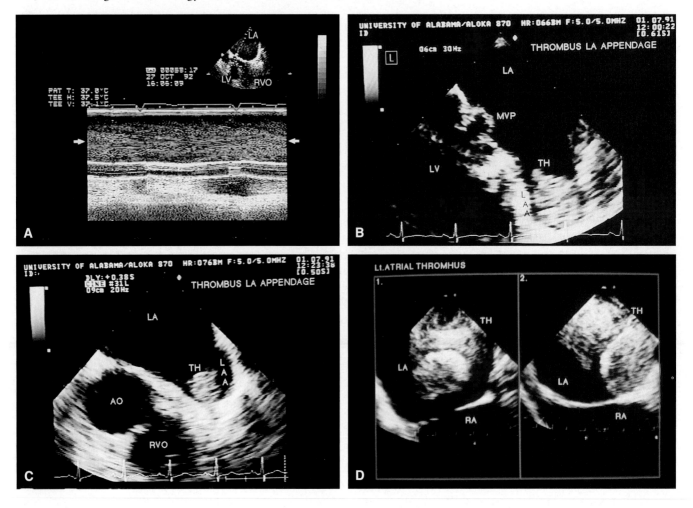

Figure 5.21. Porcine mitral prosthesis: paravalvular regurgitation. **A.** A laterally located area of prosthetic (MP) dehiscence (arrow). **B–D.** An eccentric jet of MR (arrowheads) originating in the area of prosthetic (P) dehiscence. **E.** Color M-mode demonstrates systolic backflow (arrows) in the LUPV, indicative of severe MR. After repair, the dehisced area is no longer seen **(F)**, and there is absence of systolic backflow in LUPV **(G).**

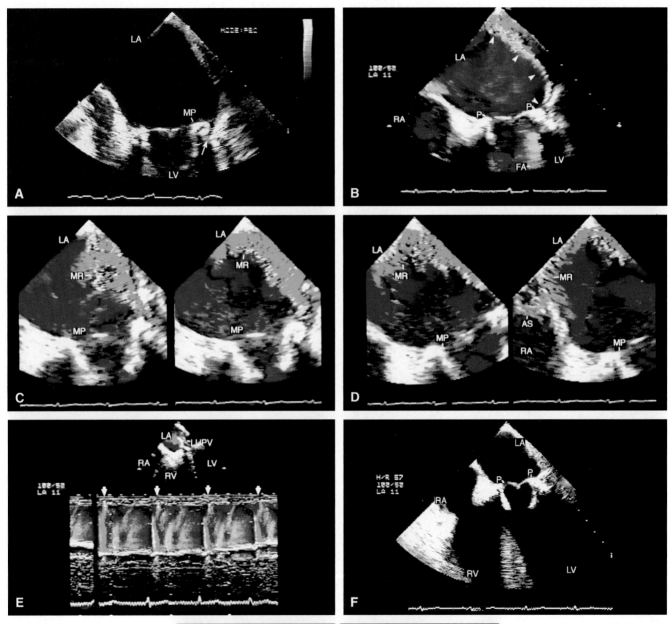

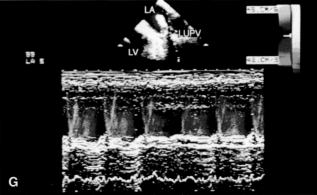

Figure 5.22. **Porcine mitral prosthesis: paravalvular and valvular regurgitation. A**. Thickened prosthetic (P) leaflets (arrowhead) and a large area of lateral dehiscence (arrow). **B**. Valvular and paravalvular MR (arrowheads). **C**. Prominent systolic backflow (arrows) is noted in the LUPV. **D–F**. Another patient with thickened prosthetic (MVR) leaflets and prominent diastolic flow acceleration as well as lateral paravalvular regurgitation (arrows). The MR jet is narrow as a result of the Coanda effect, caused by the jet impinging against the LA lateral wall. Systolic backflow was present in the LUPV, however, indicative of severe MR. This was confirmed by angiography.

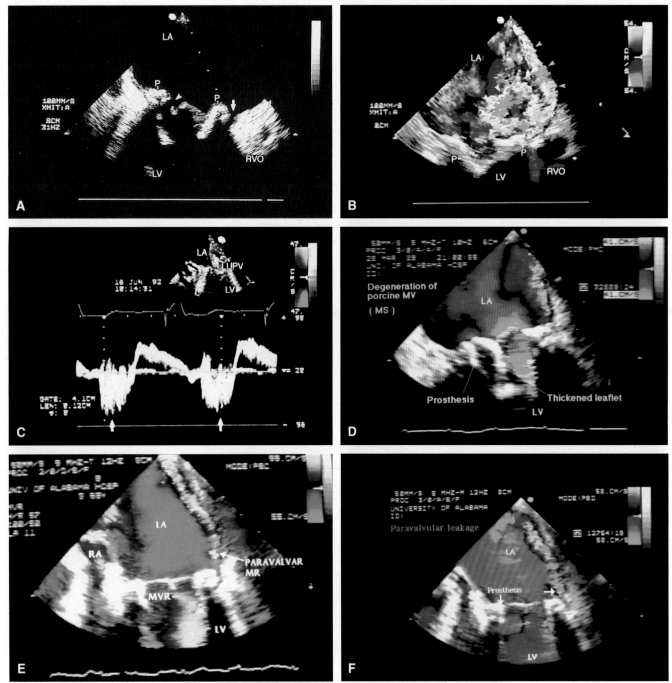

Figure 5.23. **Mitral prosthesis: valvular regurgitation. A–C.** *S* represents the valve stents, and the arrow in **B** points to a suture. Color Doppler examination demonstrates three jets of MR **(E)** associated with two areas (arrows) of prominent flow acceleration on the ventricular side of the prosthesis in **D. F.** Systolic backflow in LAA indicates severe MR. Although MR was pansystolic in this patient, the systolic backflow occurred only in mid- and late systole, because it takes some time for the MR jet to travel to LAA from the prosthesis. **G.** Postoperative study shows abscence of severe MR and two jets (arrows) of mild, normal mitral prosthetic (MP) regurgitation.

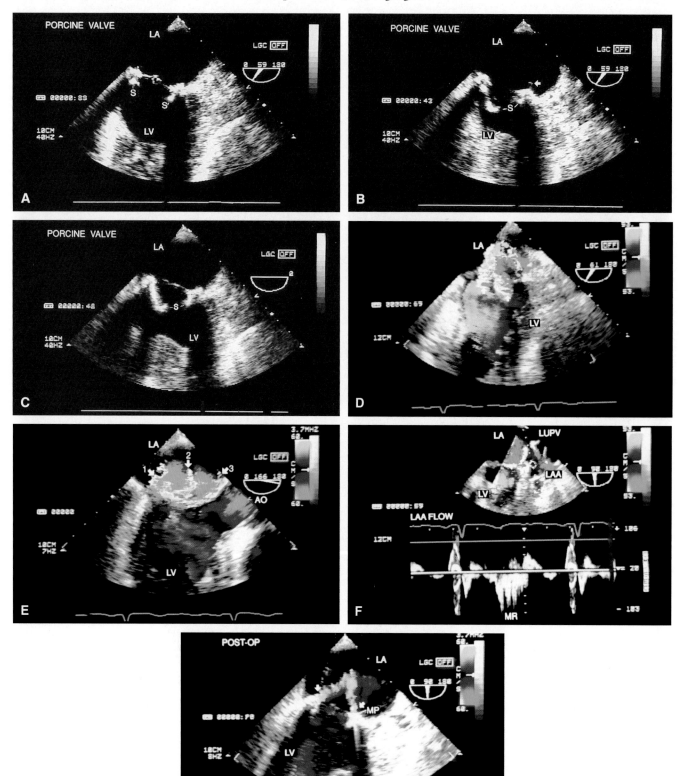

Figure 5.24. **Porcine mitral prosthesis: degeneration. A.** Heavily calcified mitral prosthetic (MP) leaflets (arrow). *S*, prosthetic stents (shown in **A** and **B**). **C,D.** The calcified leaflets (arrows) as well as the prosthetic ring (R) are viewed in short axis.

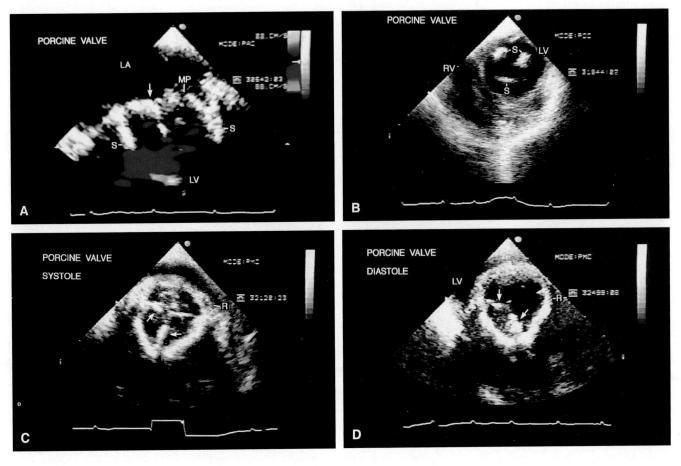

Figure 5.25.   Porcine mitral prosthesis: cusp rupture. **A.** Marked bowing (arrow) of the prosthetic (P) leaflets into the left atrium caused by prolapse. There is no evidence of cusp rupture. **B–F.** Rupture of the cusps (arrowheads) is seen. Note prominent linear protrusion of the ruptured leaflets into LA. **F.** Coarse systolic flutter of a ruptured cusp (arrowhead). **G.** Torrential MR together with a large area of flow acceleration (FA) on the ventricular aspect of the prosthesis. **B** and **C** are from one patient; **D** through **G** are from another patient. **H,I.** Another patient with porcine cusp prolapse and rupture (arrowhead in **H**), with severe MR (arrowheads) and prominent flow acceleration (FA) in **I.** **J–L.** Rupture of thickened porcine mitral cusps (arrowheads in **J,K**) with severe, eccentric MR (arrowheads in **L**) through the prosthesis (P). **M.** Another patient with porcine (P) cusp rupture with severe MR (arrows) shown in both color two-dimensional and M-mode images (arrows). **N.** The arrow points to severe valvular MR from cusp rupture; arrowheads show associated severe paravalvular MR. **O,P.** Gross specimens show porcine prosthetic cusp rupture.

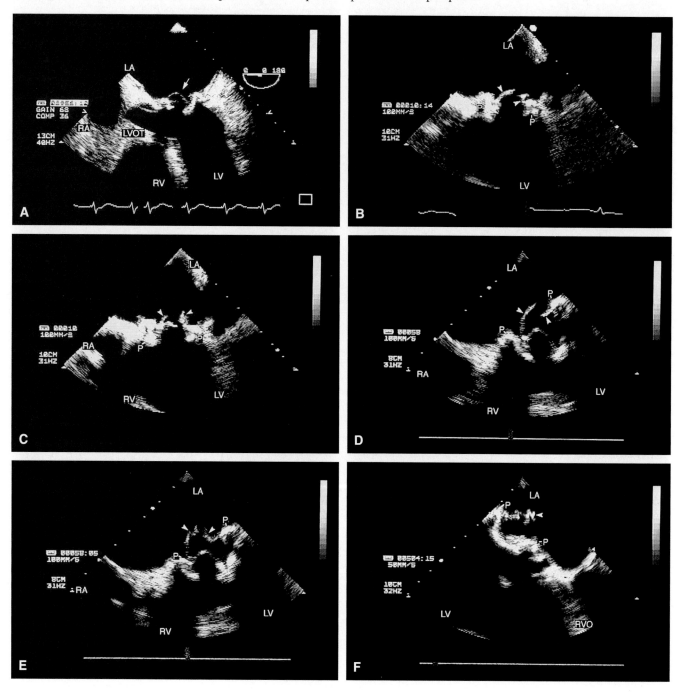

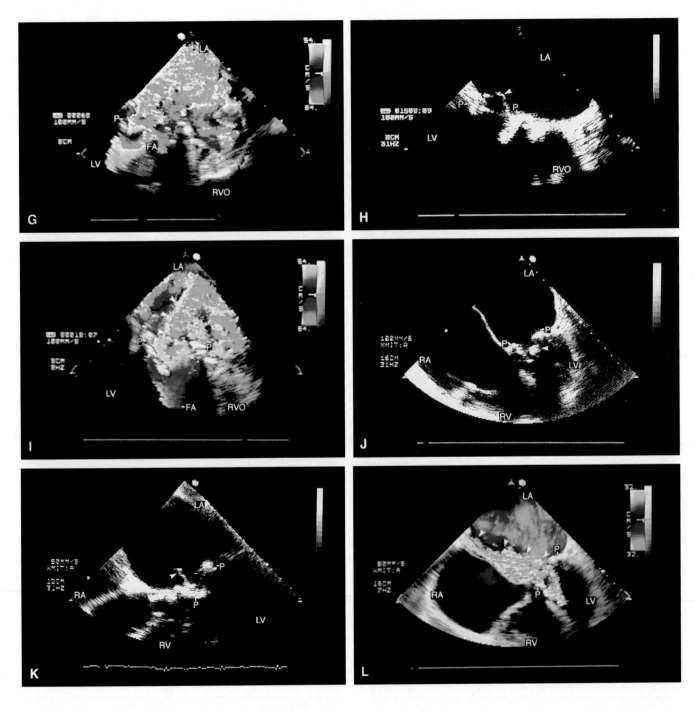

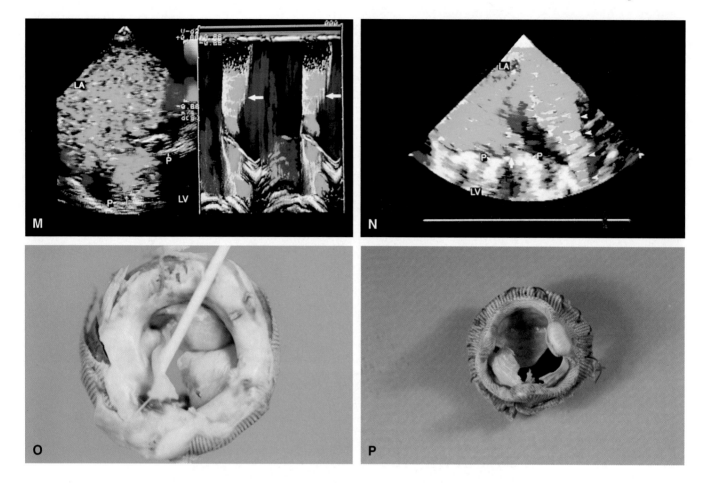

Figure 5.26. **Porcine mitral prosthesis: LA pseudoaneurysm**. Apical two-chamber view (longitudinal plane examination). **A.** A narrow, 2-mm wide channel (arrow) is seen extending from the left atrium into a 1.3-cm pseudoaneurysm cavity (circled). **B.** A diastolic frame shows color flow signals moving from the pseudoaneurysm into the left atrium during diastole (arrow). **C.** Pulsed Doppler interrogation shows to-and-fro motion of blood flow signals, which move into the pseudoaneurysm in systole and out of it into LA during diastole. *MP*, mitral prosthesis. (Reproduced with permission from Ballal R, Nanda NC, Sanyal R. Intraoperative transesophageal echocardiographic diagnosis of left atrial pseudoaneurysm. Am Heart J 1992;123:217–218.)

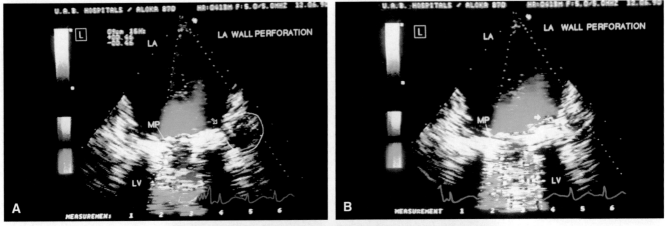

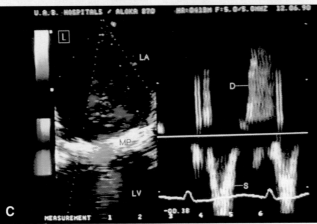

Figure 5.27.   **Porcine mitral prosthesis: regurgitation. A.** Color Doppler–guided pulsed Doppler interrogation of LUPV demonstrates prominent systolic backflow (arrow), indicative of severe MR. Because LUPV is dilated, there is systolic swirling of blood flow, with forward flow (red) seen medially and backflow (blue) more laterally. Color guidance is important for placing the pulsed Doppler sample volume in the blue and not in the red flow signals to demonstrate systolic backflow diagnostic of severe MR. **B.** Reduced S wave (arrows) suggests moderate mitral regurgitation in another patient. There is no systolic backflow.

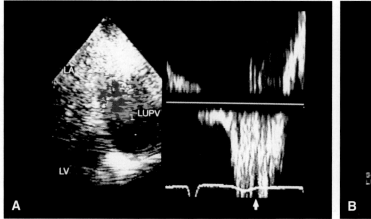
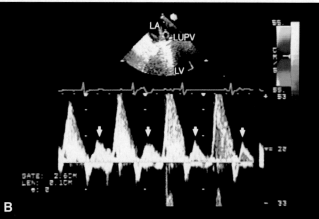

Figure 5.28. St. Jude aortic prosthesis: normal. **A.** Prosthetic aortic valve (PAV) leaflets (arrowhead) and suture ring (arrow), imaged in short axis. **B.** *R* marks the suture ring, also imaged in short axis but without the leaflets. **C,D.** M-mode tracings demonstrate normal motion of the prosthesis (AV). **E.** An arc-like prosthetic side lobe artifact (R). G is the intraluminal tube graft in the aorta (AO).

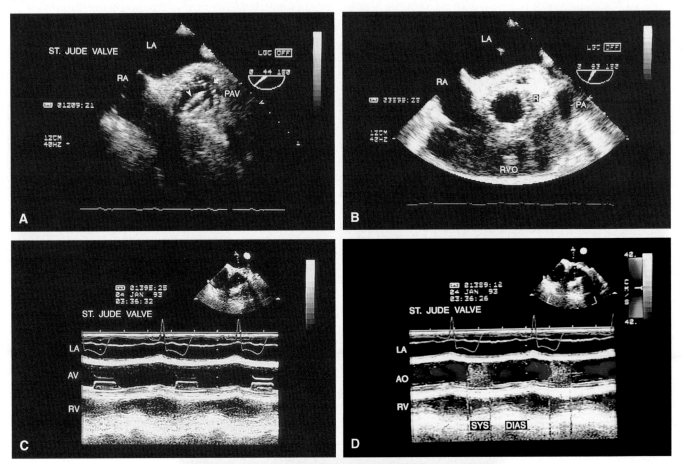

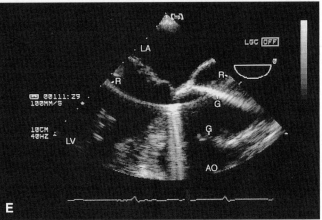

Figure 5.29. **A–E. St Jude aortic prosthesis: paravalvular leak. A.** Prosthetic (P) ring dehiscence (arrow). **B,E.** Color-flow Doppler demonstrates paravalvular AR (arrows) moving through the dehisced area into the LVOT. **C.** A large flow acceleration (FA) and significant AR.

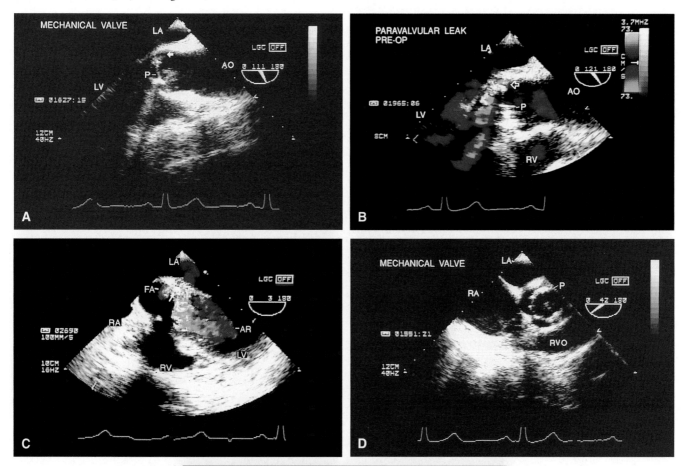

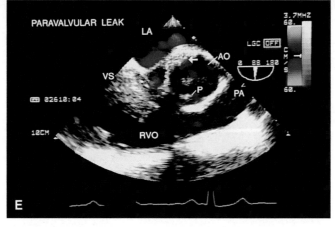

Figure 5.30. **CarboMedics aortic prosthesis: normal. A.** The prosthesis in the closed position in diastole (arrowhead). **B.** Both leaflets in the open position (arrow) in systole. **C.** The leaflets (arrowhead) are open in systole. The suture ring is also seen in **C** and in **D** and **E** (arrow). **F,G.** Two jets of normal mild AR (arrows) that are eccentrically located.

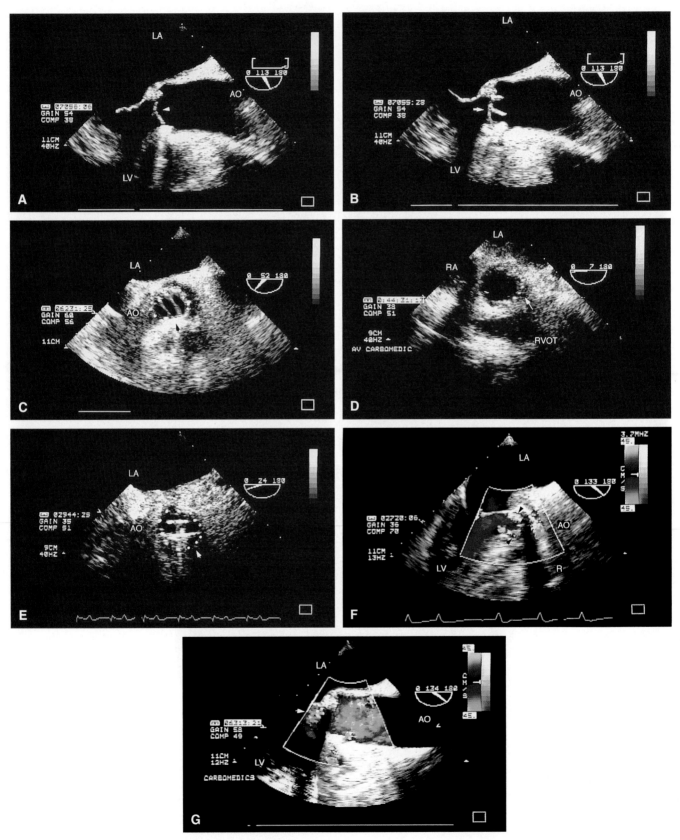

Figure 5.31. **CarboMedics aortic prosthesis: paravalvular regurgitation. A,B.** The AR jet occupies essentially the entire LVOT proximally, indicative of severe regurgitation. In both **A** and **B** the most proximal portion of the AR jet is not imaged because of acoustic shadowing (S) caused by the metallic prosthesis (P), calcification, or both.

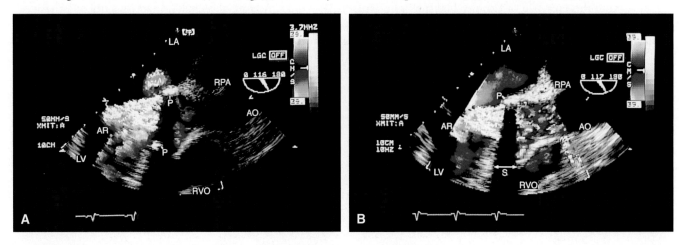

Figure 5.32. Bjork-Shiley aortic prosthesis: thrombus/dehiscence/abscess. **A,B.** A large thrombus (T) involving the aortic prosthesis (P). **C.** Another patient with a thrombus on the aortic prosthesis (AP) and severe associated AR. Diastolic MR caused by severe AR is also noted. **D.** Paravalvular AR caused by dehiscence of prosthetic (P) sutures (arrow). Note the presence of two arc-like side lobe artifacts (R). **E–H.** A large abscess (A) involving the prosthesis (P) posteriorly together with severe AR (arrowheads in **G**). **I–K.** Another patient with an abscess cavity (AB) located on the posterior aspect of the prosthesis (PAV) and communicating with the LVOT **(K).** **L.** A patient with an infected Bjork-Shiley prosthesis with associated perforation at the base of the anterior mitral leaflet. The arrowheads demonstrate the MR jet moving through the perforation. The large flow acceleration (FA) suggests the presence of severe MR, even though the jet through the perforation appears small. Note a second tiny MR jet arising from the coaptation point. (Reproduced with permission from Mahan EF III, Nanda NC. Transesophageal echocardiography. In: Rackley CE, ed. Challenges in Cardiology I. Mt. Kisco, NY: Futura, 1991:85–101.)

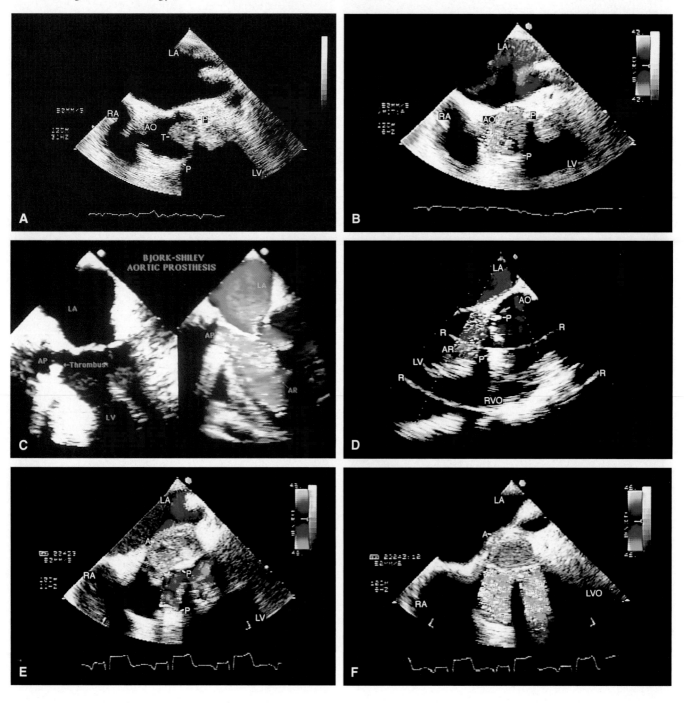

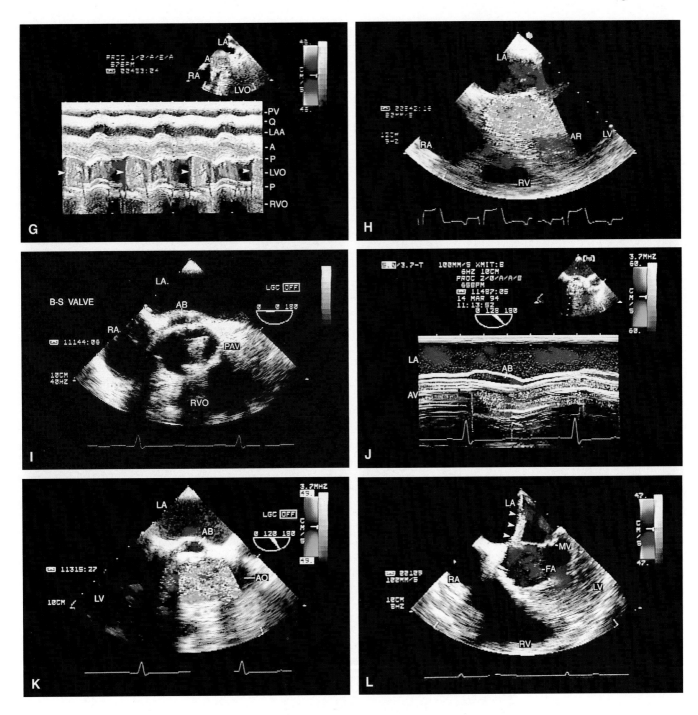

Figure 5.33. **Starr-Edwards aortic prosthesis: normal.** The arrows in **A** and **C** point to the three struts of the prosthesis. *LM*, left main coronary artery. **B.** Labels *1* and *2* point to reverberations from the strut that partially obscure the RV. **B–D.** The acoustic shadowing produced by the poppet (ball, **B**) is well seen (arrow in **D**). **E.** Gross specimen of a normal Starr-Edwards prosthesis in the aortic position.

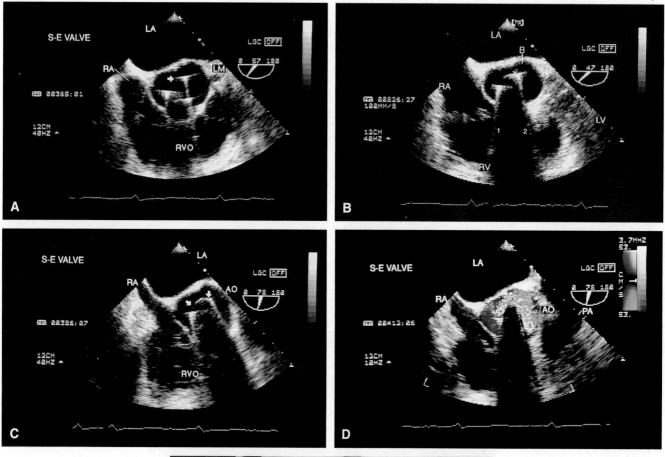

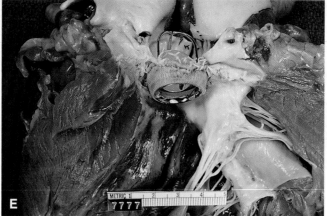

Figure 5.34. **Starr-Edwards prosthesis: paravalvular regurgitation. A.** Note the presence of acoustic shadowing (S) in the systolic frame. **B.** An eccentric jet of paravalvular prosthetic (P) AR. **C.** Another patient with severe paravalvular AR (arrowhead) from a Starr-Edwards prosthesis that was placed 32 years earlier. **D.** Following replacement with another mechanical prosthesis a small fistulous communication is noted into the LA (arrowhead).

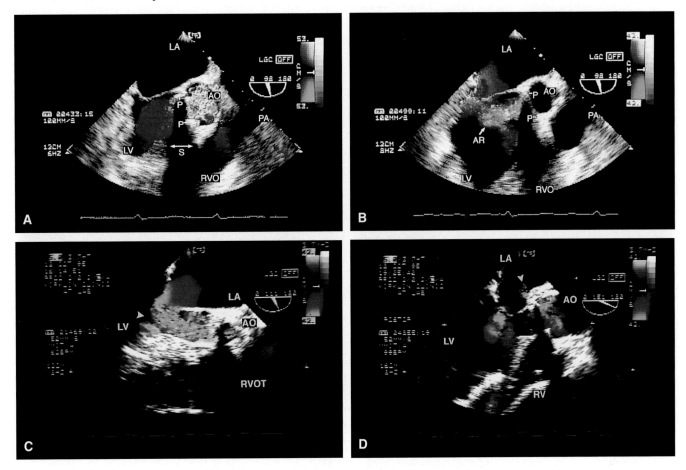

Figure 5.35. Medtronic-Hall prosthesis: abscess/paravalvular leak. **A.** A large abscess cavity (A) is noted in the area of the prosthesis. *R*, a prominent reverberation artifact. **B.** Eccentric paravalvular AR (arrow), with prominent flow acceleration on the aortic side of the valve. **C.** Severe aortic regurgitation (arrowheads) with some proximal acoustic shadowing is noted. **D–G.** Another patient with multiple abscesses (A) involving the prosthesis (P). An abscess (A) encroaches on the anterior mitral leaflet **(E)**. **G.** Color Doppler examination shows flow signals within the abscess cavity, indicating communication with the aorta or left ventricle. This patient underwent homograft replacement of the infected Medtronic-Hall prosthesis. **H.** A small hematoma (H) is noted posterior to the prosthesis (P) in the postoperative study.

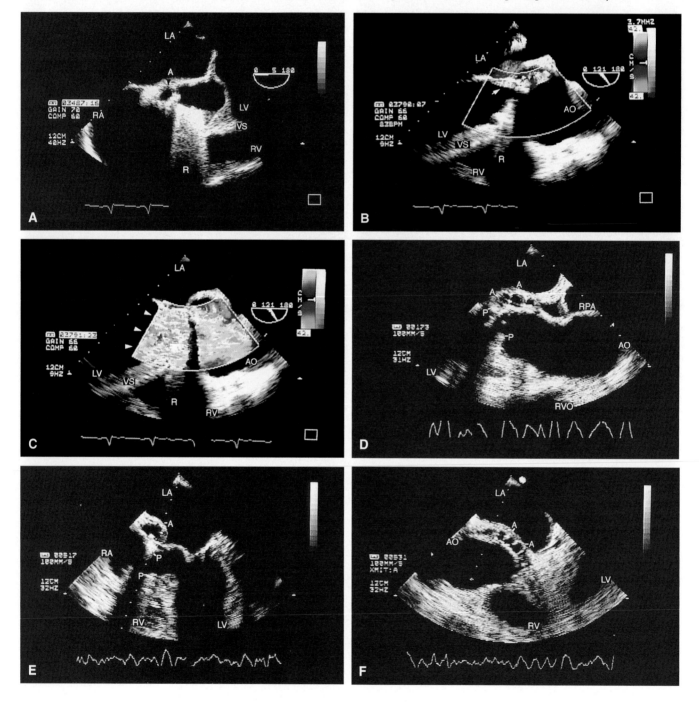

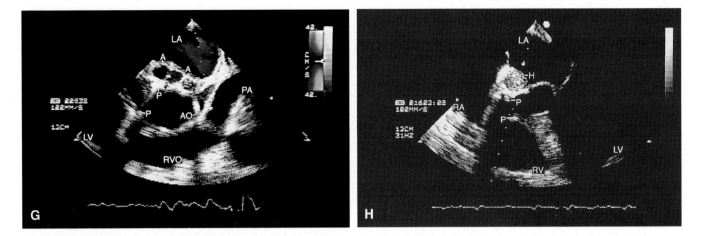

Figure 5.36. Medtronic-Hall prosthesis: abscess/aortopulmonary fistula. **A–E.** The modified four-chamber and five-chamber views demonstrate a portion of the aortic prosthesis (arrow) protruding into the LVOT. The anterior leaflet of the mitral valve shows two perforations, one at the base (1) and the other in the midportion (2). Mitral regurgitation jets are seen moving into the left atrium through these perforations (MR-1, MR-2) and also from the coaptation area of the mitral leaflets (MR-3). **B.** The diastolic frame shows the prosthesis in contact with the body of the anterior mitral leaflet in the area of the perforation. **E.** Both valvular (V) and paravalvular (P) aortic regurgitation (AR) are noted. **F,G.** Modified aortic short-axis views demonstrate the fistulous connection between the aortic root (A) and the main pulmonary artery (PA) through an abscess cavity (A3). Two other abscess cavities (A1, A2) are also noted. **H,I.** Abscess cavity A2 is well demonstrated. **J,K.** The relationship of the abscess cavity A1 to the superior vena cava (SVC) during transverse (**J**) and longitudinal (**K**) plane examinations is demonstrated. **L–N.** Longitudinal plane examination shows the abscess cavity A3. Its communication with the main pulmonary artery (PA) is seen in **N.** (Reproduced with permission from Chen CH, Nanda NC, Fan PH, et al. Transesophageal echocardiographic diagnosis of aortopulmonary fistula. Echocardiography 1993;10:85–90.)

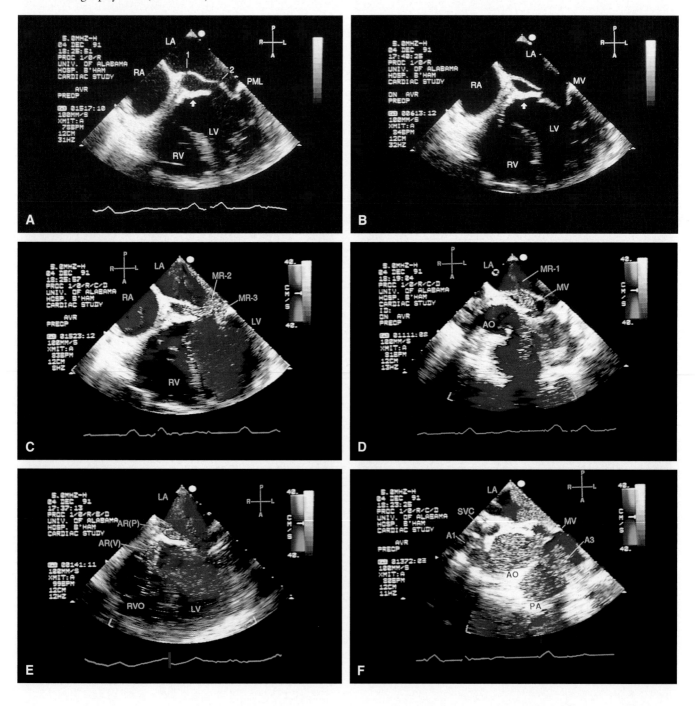

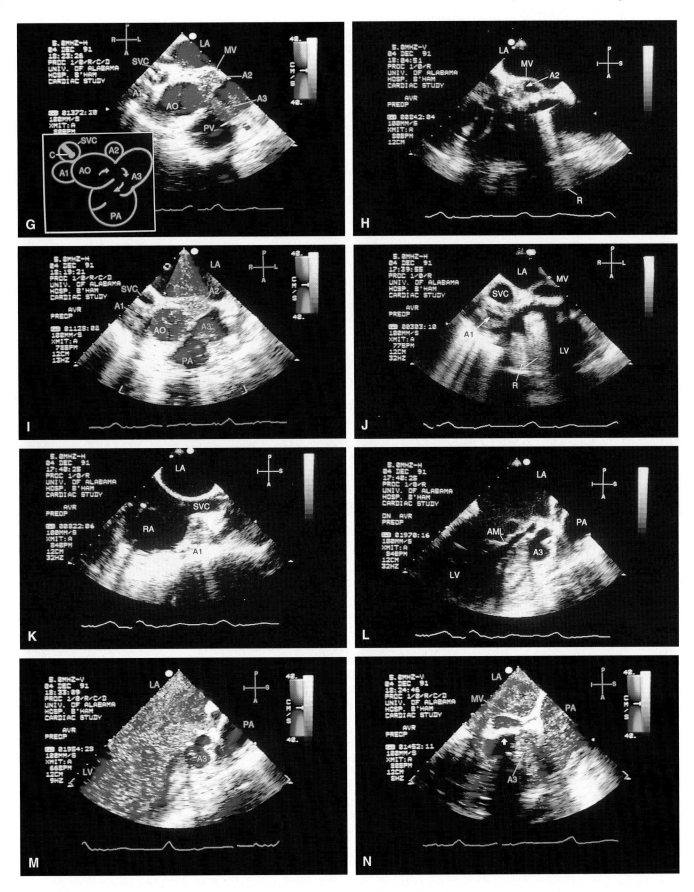

Figure 5.37. **A–H. Porcine aortic prosthesis: normal.** The leaflets (**A**, arrowheads in **C–E** and **G**, arrow in **F**) and the stents (ST, arrows in **E** and **G**) of the prosthesis (P) are well seen. Because the metallic stents are highly echogenic, they may obscure the thin leaflets. It may be necessary to use multiple transducer angulations to see the leaflets as completely as possible. **F.** M-mode tracing of the prosthesis (AP) shows it in the open and closed position (arrows). **H.** Gross specimen of a normal porcine prosthesis in the aortic position.

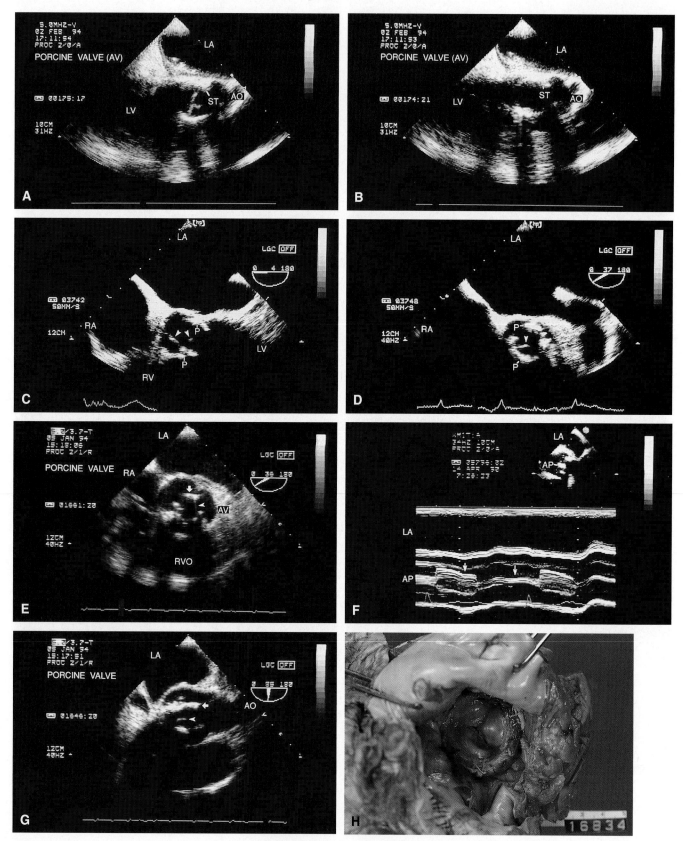

Figure 5.38. Porcine aortic prosthesis: degeneration/prolapse/valvular regurgitation. **A.** A thickened, stenotic prosthesis (P) with marked restriction of the opening (arrowhead) in systole. **B–E.** Another patient with thickened prosthetic leaflets (arrows in **B,C**) prolapsing into the LVOT. **D.** The proximal portion of the AR jet (arrows) is not imaged because of acoustic shadowing produced by the calcified prosthesis. **E.** Severe AR (arrow) is seen in this patient. **F.** Another patient with very mild thickening and degeneration of the porcine prosthesis (PAV). **G.** More severe thickening and degeneration of the prosthesis (P) than that seen in **F**. **H,I.** Another patient with a degenerated porcine aortic prosthesis (PAV). The arrow in **H** points to a linear echo protruding from the prosthesis in diastole. This finding is common in the setting of degeneration. **J–L.** A different patient with a heavily calcified prosthesis (P) that prolapses into the LVOT (arrows). Associated severe AR is shown in **L**. **M,N.** Linear echoes (arrows) that prolapse into the LVOT in a patient with a thickened, degenerated heterograft prosthesis (P). **O.** Prolapse (arrowhead) of a heterograft prosthesis (P) in a patient who has an aortic (AO) aneurysm. **P.** Mild thickening and degeneration of a heterograft prosthesis (P) in another patient with aortic root aneurysm and dissection. *F*, dissection flap; *FL*, false lumen. **Q,R.** Gross specimens with calcification and thickening on the ventricular **(Q)** and aortic **(R)** aspects of a heterograft prosthesis.

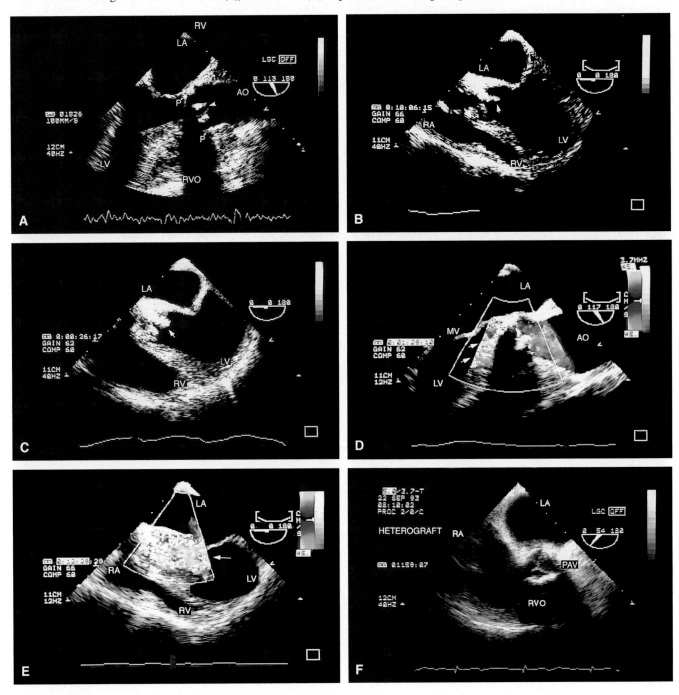

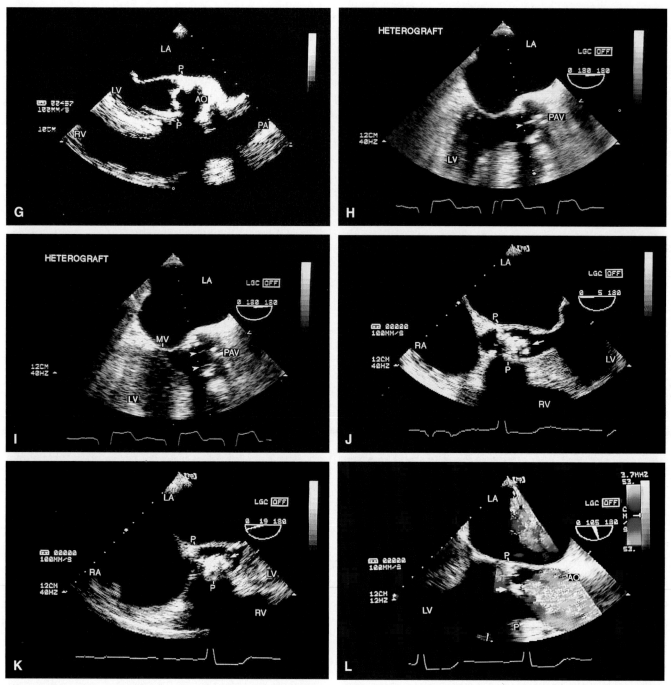

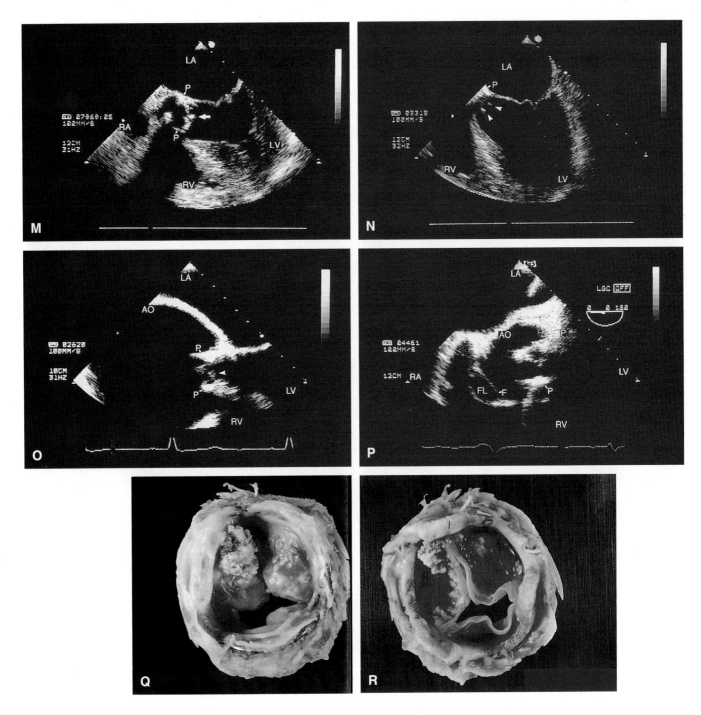

Figure 5.39. Porcine aortic prosthesis: valvular and paravalvular regurgitation. **A.** Prolapse (arrowhead) of a thickened and degenerated prosthesis (P). **B–D.** AR flow signals are shown moving into the LVOT posteriorly from beyond the confines of the prosthesis, indicative of a paravalvular leak. **C.** Associated valvular regurgitation originating from within the confines of the aortic prosthesis. An anterior paraprosthetic leak also is demonstrated (white arrow). The black arrows in **B** and **C** show the site of the posterior paravalvar leak. **E.** Another patient with heterograft prosthesis (P) cusp prolapse demonstrating severe AR.

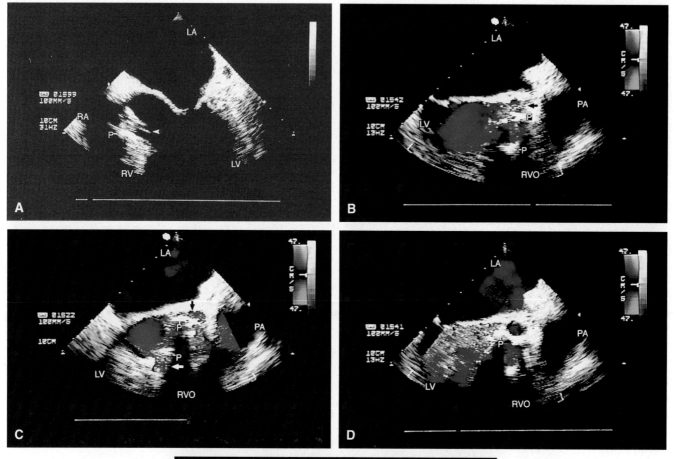

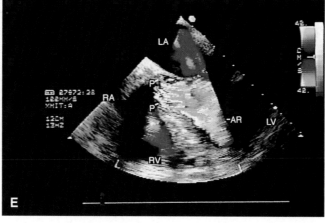

Figure 5.40.   **Porcine aortic prosthesis: cusp rupture.** The arrowheads in **A** and **B** show a ruptured cusp prolapsing into the LVOT, with severe AR shown in **C** through **E** (arrowheads in **D**, arrows in **E**). Diastolic MR (arrowheads) from severe AR is noted in **C**. **F** is a gross specimen of a thickened and calcified porcine aortic valve with cusp rupture (circled).

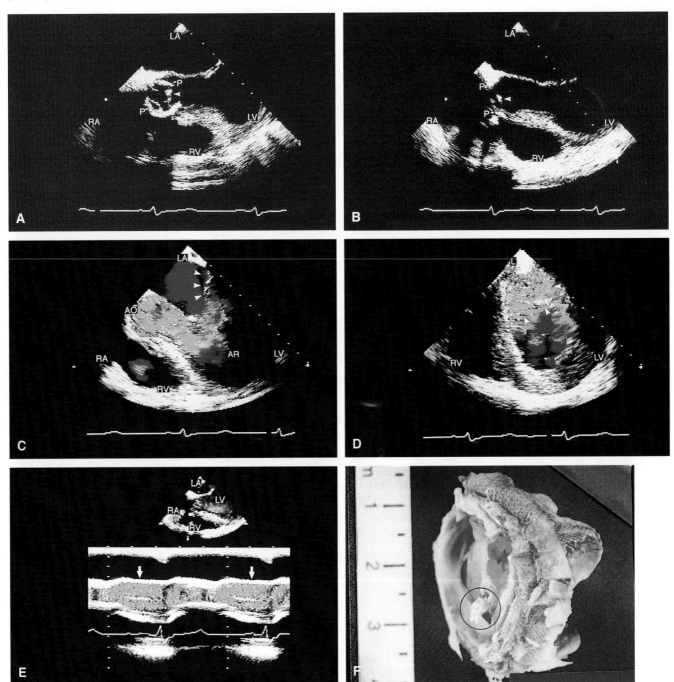

Figure 5.41. **Porcine aortic prosthesis: tear of right coronary cusp.** The arrowhead in **A** shows a torn right coronary cusp of the porcine prosthesis P prolapsing into the LVOT with severe AR **(B)**.

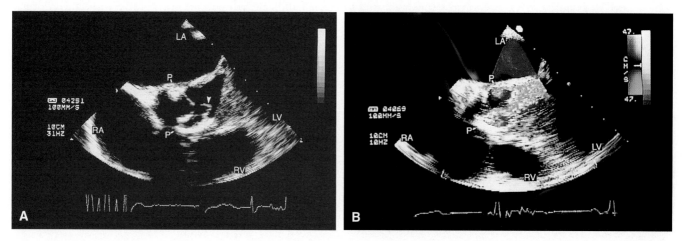

Figure 5.42. **Porcine aortic prosthesis: paravalvular regurgitation. A.** The arrow points to a mildly thickened porcine aortic valve (PAV). **B.** Eccentric paravalvular AR (arrow) originating in the vicinity of the posterior prosthetic stent (S). There is no valvular regurgitation.

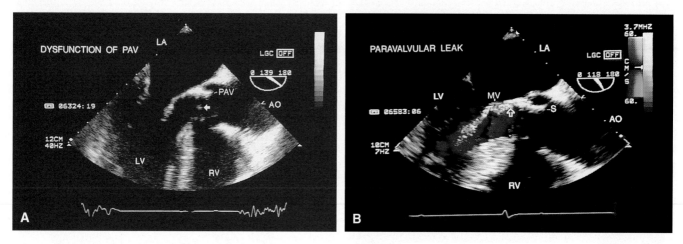

Figure 5.43. **Porcine aortic prosthesis: abscess/fistula. A,B.** A large abscess cavity is noted posteriorly communicating with the LVOT. *P*, prosthesis. **C–I.** Another patient with a large abscess cavity (A,AB, arrow in **G**) located on the posterior aspect of the prosthesis (P,AP). **H,I.** Color Doppler studies in the same patient show the abscess cavity communicating with the LVOT in diastole (**H**) and systole (**I**). **J–L.** Another patient with a heterograft who has a rounded abscess cavity, best seen in **K** (arrow), protruding into the LA and close to the aortic-mitral junction. **J.** The prosthetic leaflets (closed arrow) and the stents (open arrows) do not appear to be abnormally thick. **L.** Color Doppler examination shows the presence of significant AR. **M,N.** Another patient with an infected porcine prosthesis showing a fistula into the RV (arrows).

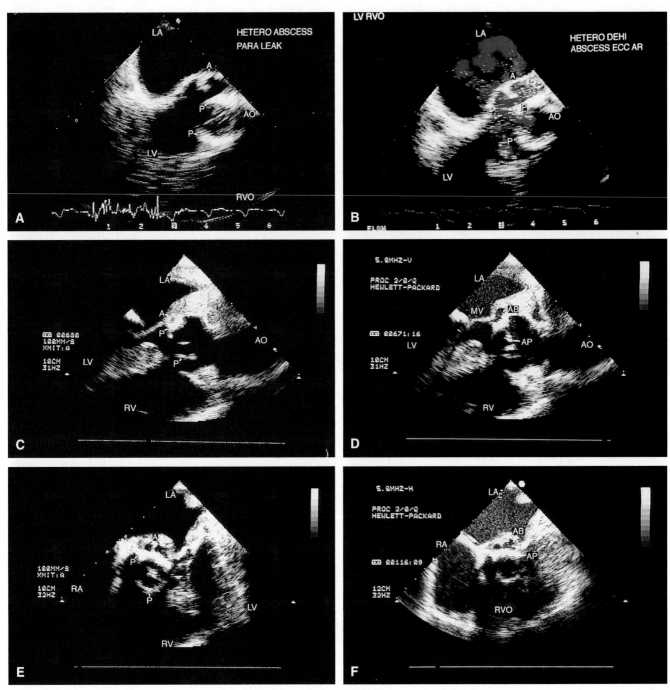

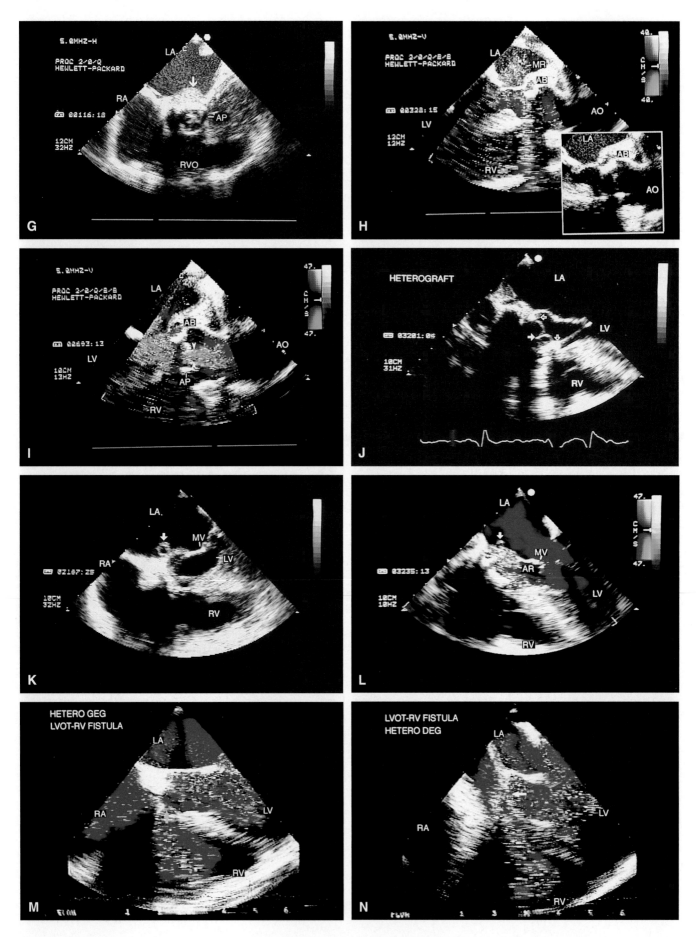

Figure 5.44.   Ionescu-Shiley porcine prosthesis: prolapse/abscess/regurgitation. The arrow in **A** shows prolapse of a cusp into the LVOT with associated severe prosthetic (P) AR **(B).** This patient was found to have cusp rupture at surgery. **C–H.** Another patient with the same type of prosthetic (P) valve showing prolapse and abscess formation. The arrowhead in **C** shows cusp prolapse into the LVOT. An abscess (A) cavity is seen on the posterior and lateral aspects of the prosthesis **(C,D). E,F.** Color Doppler examination shows the abscess cavity (arrow in **F**) communicating with the LVOT. **G,H.** Diastolic MR (arrowheads) resulting from severe AR (arrows) is seen.

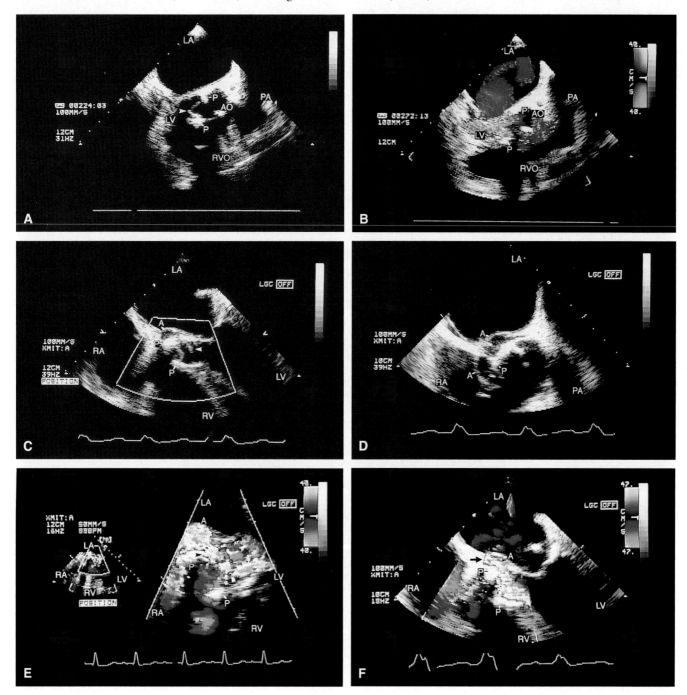

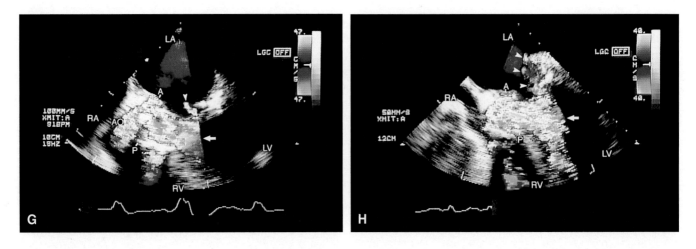

Figure 5.45. **Porcine aortic prosthesis: hypertrophic cardiomyopathy.** In this patient, systolic anterior motion (SAM) of the mitral valve developed after porcine aortic valve replacement for aortic stenosis, which had masked coexisting hypertrophic cardiomyopathy. Note that the LVOT is narrowed to less than 20 mm in this patient.

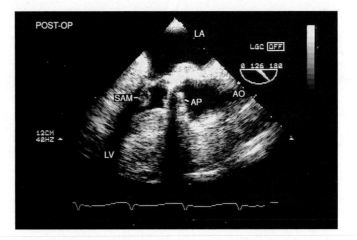

Figure 5.46. Homograft aortic prosthesis: degeneration/stenosis/prolapse/regurgitation/infection. **A.** Thickening and calcification of the prothesis (P) with marked restriction of opening during systole is indicative of stenosis. **B.** Color Doppler shows a very narrow jet (arrowheads) originating from the prosthesis in systole, also indicative of obstruction. **C–F.** Another patient with prosthetic (P) cusp prolapse (arrow in **C**), with severe eccentric AR and prominent flow acceleration (FA in **D,E**) on the aortic side. The AR jet is directed posteriorly and abuts against the anterior mitral leaflet. This valve was replaced with a St. Jude prosthesis (P) **(F)**. Labels *1* and *2* indicate normal small prosthetic AR jets. Jet 1 originates anteriorly but is directed posteriorly (red). Conversely, jet 2 originates posteriorly but is directed anteriorly (blue). *H*, a small hematoma. **G,H.** Another patient with prosthetic (P) cusp prolapse (arrow) resulting in diastolic noncoaptation with the right coronary leaflet and producing severe AR **(H). I.** A patient with homograft prosthetic degeneration and severe AR (arrowheads). **J.** Color Doppler study of another patient with a homograft aortic prosthesis (P) showing severe AR (arrows). Note that the jet shows largely laminar flow with only a small amount of turbulence (variance) because of the nonperpendicular orientation of the ultrasonic beam relative to the direction of blood flow. **K–N.** A patient with homograft endocarditis. **K.** Marked diastolic prolapse (arrows) of the thickened prosthetic leaflets (P) with noncoaptation. A large vegetation (V) is seen prolapsing into the LVOT in diastole in **L** and into the aortic root in systole in **M. N.** Color Doppler examination shows severe AR and minimal PR. **O–V.** Another patient with endocarditis involving a homograft prosthesis (P). The arrows in **O, P,** and **R** show prosthetic dehiscence and a large pseudoaneurysm posteriorly. **Q–V.** A fistula (F, arrows) from the aortic root into the RV and an abscess cavity (AB in **S** and **T**) are seen. **V.** Color Doppler–guided continuous wave Doppler shows flow through the fistula throughout the cardiac cycle.

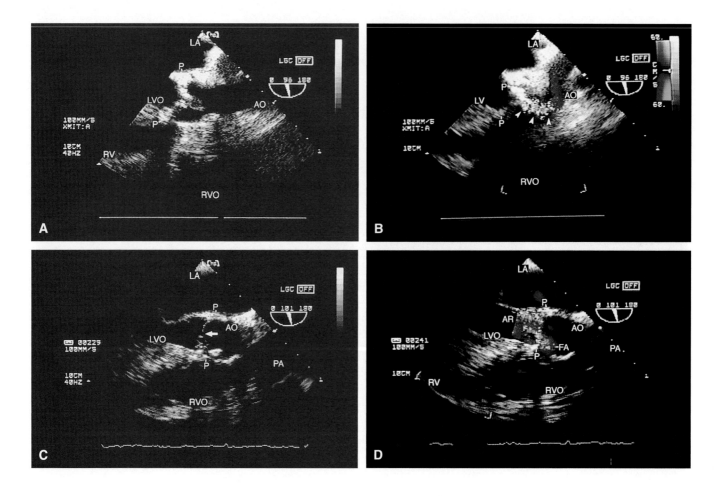

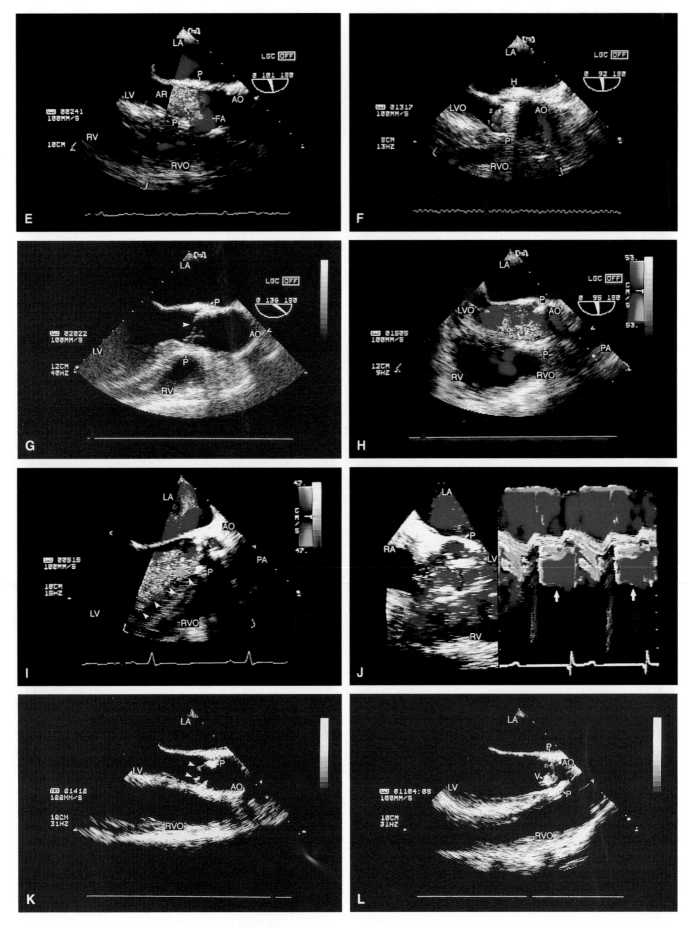

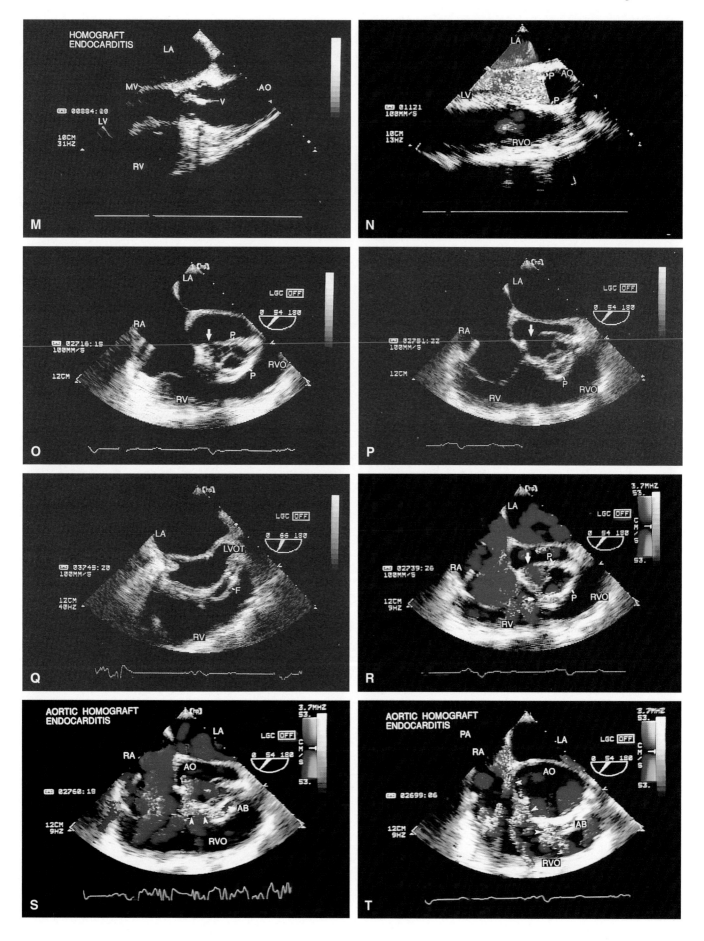

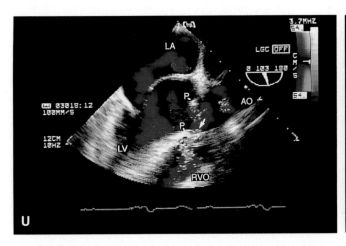

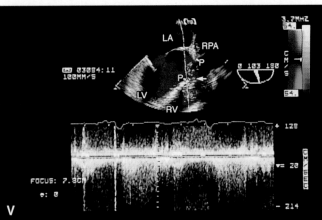

Figure 5.47.   **Homograft aortic prosthesis: endocarditis. A–C.** Abscess cavities (arrows) communicating with the aortic root. The prosthetic leaflets are thickened. **D,E.** Color Doppler examination demonstrates flow signals (arrow in **D**) in the abscess (AB) cavity. **F.** Fistula (arrow) from the aorta to the right ventricle. **G,H.** Severe AR (arrows) is demonstrated.

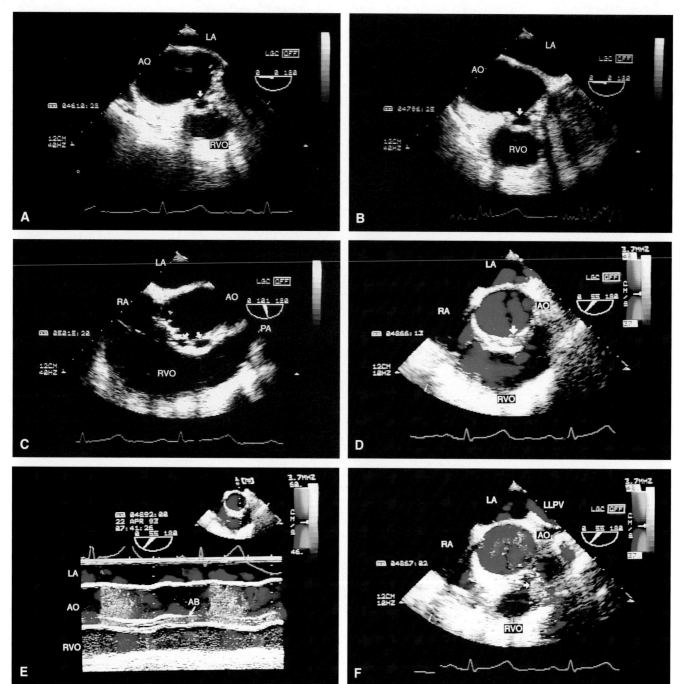

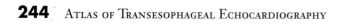

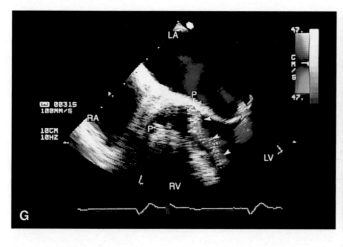

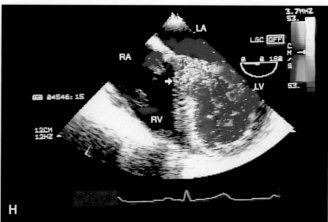

Figure 5.48.   **Homograft aortic prosthesis: subaortic obstruction produced by abscess.** Longitudinal **(A)** and transverse **(B)** plane examinations showed abscess cavity (arrows) and narrowing of LVOT more clearly than did transthoracic study. The abscess cavity communicates with LVOT posteriorly; anteriorly, it appears closed. Homograft aortic valve (AV) leaflets are only mildly thickened. **C.** *Left panel:* a systolic frame shows aliasing and narrowing of the flow channel in LVOT, indicative of subaortic obstruction (longitudinal plane examination). *Right panel:* a diastolic frame shows color Doppler flow signals occupying less than 25% of the proximal left ventricular outflow tract, consistent with mild AR (transverse plane examination). (Reproduced with permission from Sanyal RS, Roychoudhury D, Nanda NC, et al. Transthoracic and transesophageal echocardiographic diagnosis of severe subaortic obstruction produced by an abscess cavity. Am Heart J 1994;128:1252–1255.)

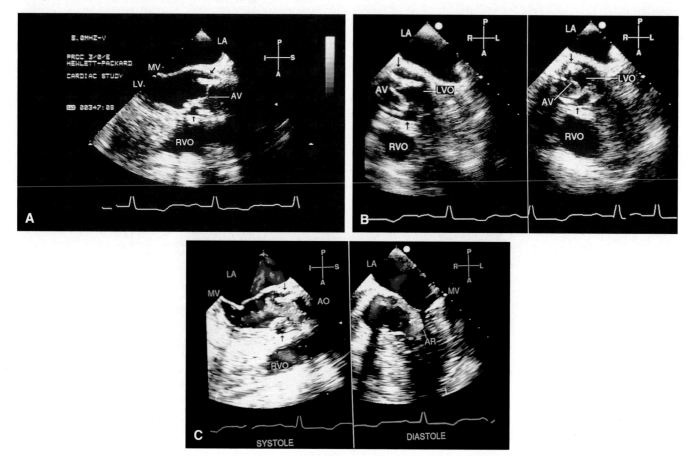

Figure 5.49. Pulmonary autograft in the aortic position with homograft replacement of the pulmonary valve (Ross operation): prolapse/valvular and paravalvular regurgitation. **A.** Prolapse (arrowhead) of the prosthesis (P) placed in the aortic position. **B,C.** Severe posteriorly directed eccentric regurgitation (arrows). **D–F.** Another patient with prolapse of the autograft. The arrow in **D** shows noncoaptation caused by severe prolapse of the noncoronary cusp (NCC). Resulting severe AR (arrow) with prominent flow acceleration is seen in **E.** The arrow in **F** points to redundancy and noncoaptation of the prosthetic leaflets viewed in short axis. **G.** Another patient with an autograft who has a hole (upper arrow) in the right coronary cusp. The homograft pulmonary valve (lower arrow) in this patient is mildly thickened. **H.** Another patient with a pulmonary autograft in the aortic position with suture dehiscence and a posterior paravalvular leak.

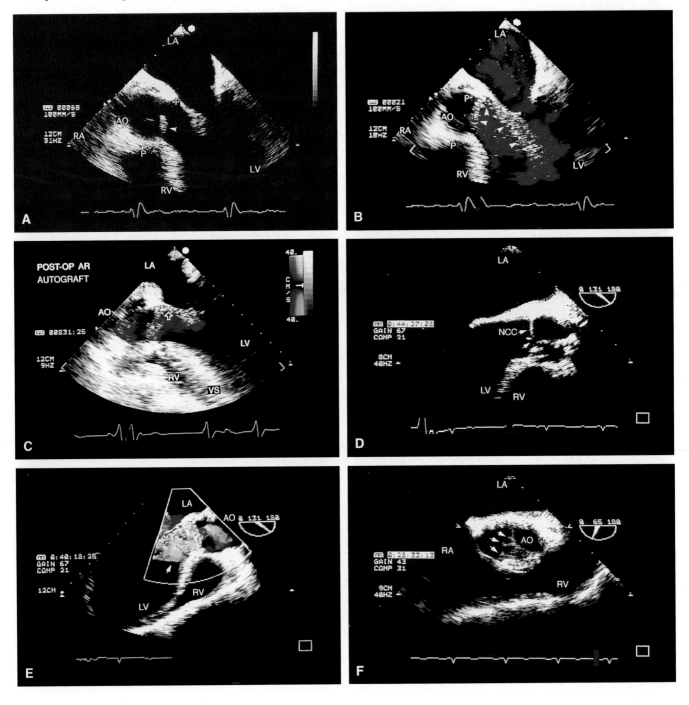

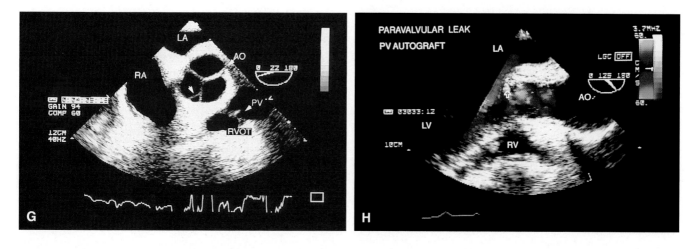

Figure 5.50. **Aortic valve annuloplasty.** This patient presented with severe prolapse and noncoaptation (arrow in **A**) of the aortic valve leaflets, resulting in severe AR (arrowheads in **B**). Following aortic valve annuloplasty, AR is reduced and now is only mild (arrow in **C**).

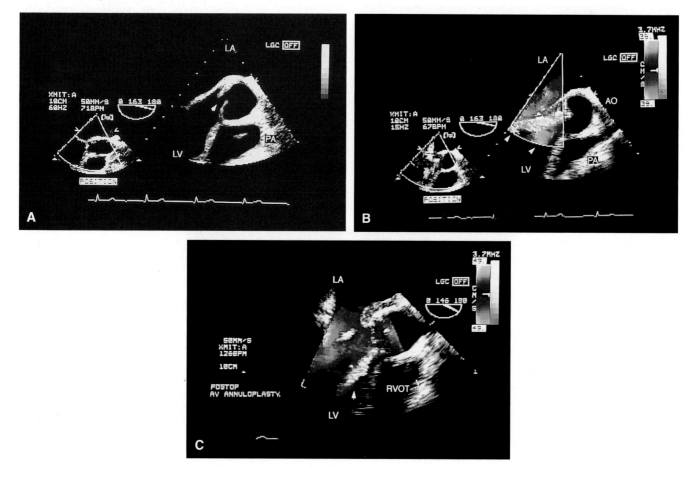

Figure 5.51.   **Tricuspid valve prosthesis and ring. A.** A pannus (arrow) involving a metallic tricuspid prosthesis valve (TVP). **B.** Mild TR (arrow) in the same patient. *S,* acoustic shadowing caused by the prosthesis. **C.** Turbulent inflow into the RV (arrow) is seen in the diastolic frame. This metallic prosthesis was replaced by a CarboMedics prosthesis. **D,E.** Another patient with a normal porcine tricuspid prosthesis (P). **F.** A Carpentier annuloplasty ring (R) in the tricuspid position in another patient.

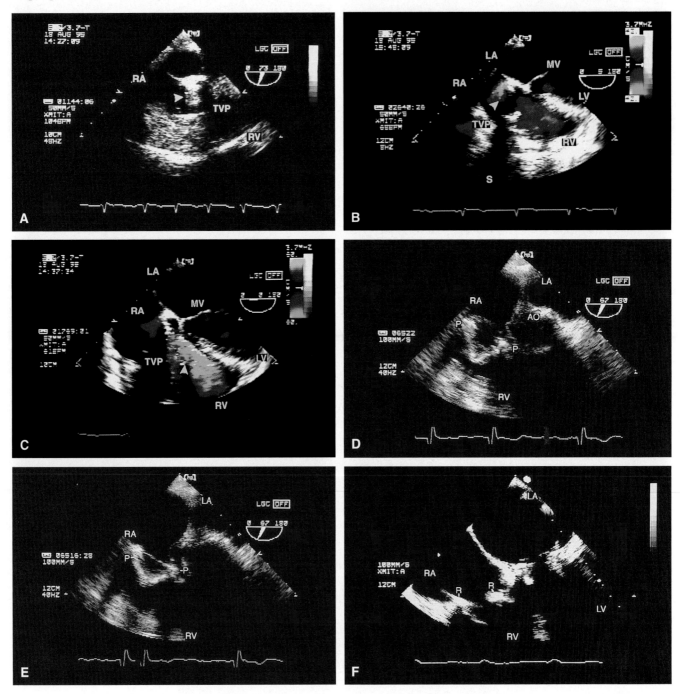

Figure 5.52.   **Pulmonary valve prosthesis.** A prosthesis (PP) is shown in the pulmonary position in this patient, who also had repair of a ventricular septal defect (arrows in **A,E**). **B.** Turbulent flow (arrow) in the pulmonary artery in systole. The peak velocity by continuous wave Doppler measured 2.48 m/sec **(C),** which is within normal limits for a prosthetic valve. **D.** Associated severe PR is shown. **E.** This patient also had moderate AR.

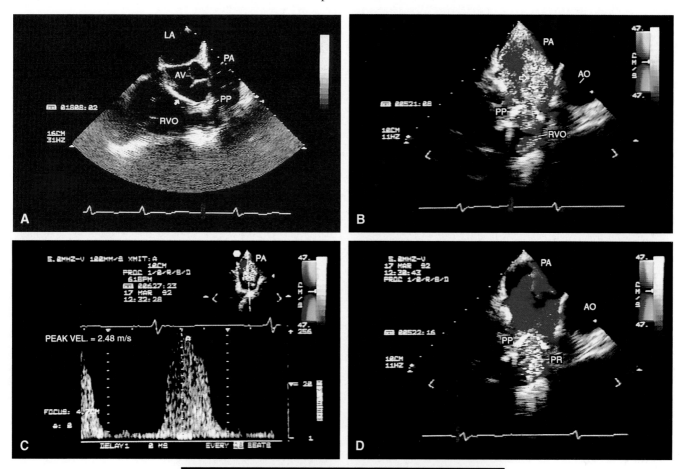

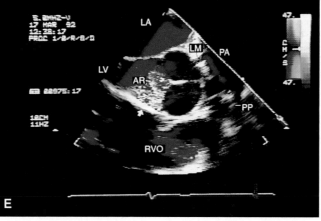

SUGGESTED READINGS

Alam M, Rosman HS, Sun I. Transesophageal echocardiographic evaluation of St. Jude medical and bioprosthetic valve endocarditis. Am Heart J 1992;123:236–239.

Andrade A, Vargas-Baron J, Romero-Cardenas A, et al. Transthoracic and transesophageal echocardiographic study of pulmonary autograft valve in aortic position. Echocardiography 1994;11:221–226.

Azari DM, DiNardo JA. The role of transesophageal echocardiography during the Ross procedure. J Cardiothorac Vasc Anesth 1995;9:558–561.

Ballal R, Nanda NC, Sanyal R. Intraoperative transesophageal echocardiographic diagnosis of left atrial pseudoaneurysm. Am Heart J 1992;123:217–218.

Cape EG, Nanda NC, Yoganathan AP. Quantification of regurgitant flow through bileaflet heart valve prostheses: theoretical and in vitro studies. Ultrasound Med Biol 1993;19:461–468.

Chen CH, Nanda NC, Fan PH, et al. Transesophagealechocardiographic diagnosis of aortopulmonary fistula. Echocardiography 1993;10:85–90.

Daniel LB, Grigg LE, Weisel RD, Rakowski H. Comparison of transthoracic and transesophageal assessment of prosthetic valve dysfunction. Echocardiography 1990;7:83–95.

Faletra F, De Chiara F, Corno R, et al. Additional diagnostic value of multiplane echocardiography over biplane imaging in assessment of mitral prosthetic valves. Heart 1996;75:609–613.

Flachskampf FA, Hoffmann R, Franke A, et al. Does multiplane transesophageal echocardiography improve the assessment of prosthetic valve regurgitation? J Am Soc Echocardiogr 1995;8:70–78.

Freedberg RS, Goodkin GM, Perez JL, et al. Valve strands are strongly associated with systemic embolization: a transesophageal echocardiographic study. J Am Coll Cardiol 1995;26:1709–1712.

Freeman WK, Schaff HV, Khandheria BK, et al. Intraoperative evaluation of mitral valve regurgitation and repair by transesophageal echocardiography: incidence and significance of systolic anterior motion. J Am Coll Cardiol 1992;20:599–609.

Garcia MJ, Vandervoort P, Stewart WJ, et al. Mechanisms of hemolysis with mitral prosthetic regurgitation. Study using transesophageal echocardiography and fluid dynamic simulation. J Am Coll Cardiol 1996;27:399–406.

Hixson CS, Smith MD, Mattson MD, et al. Comparison of transesophageal color flow Doppler imaging of normal mitral regurgitant jets in St. Jude Medical and Medtronic Hall cardiac prostheses. J Am Soc Echocardiogr 1992;5:57–62.

Howard J, Agrawal G, Nanda NC. Transesophageal echocardiographic diagnosis of left atrial wall dehiscence. Echocardiography 1997;14:299-302.

Jaggers J, Chetham PM, Kinnard TL, Fullerton DA. Intraoperative prosthetic valve dysfunction: detection by transesophageal echocardiography. Ann Thorac Surg 1995;59:755–757.

Jebara VA, Mihaileanu S, Acar C, et al. Left ventricular outflow tract obstruction after mitral valve repair. Results of the sliding leaflet technique. Circulation 1993;88:1130–1134.

Khandheria BK, Seward JB, Oh JK, et al. Value and limitations of transesophageal echocardiography in assessment of mitral valve prostheses. Circulation 1991;83:1956–1968.

Khandheria BK. Transesophageal echocardiography in the evaluation of prosthetic valves. Am J Cardiac Imaging 1995;9:106–114.

Labbe L, Roudaut R, Lorient-Roudaut MF, et al. Relationship between intravascular hemolysis and bright sparkling echoes detected by TEE in the vicinity of mechanical mitral prosthesis. Echocardiography 1996;13:381–386.

Lange HW, Olson JD, Pederson WR, et al. Transesophageal color Doppler echocardiography of the normal St. Jude medical mitral valve prosthesis. Am Heart J 1991;122:489–494.

Lee TM, Chou NK, Su SF, et al. Left atrial spontaneous echo contrast in asymptomatic patients with a mechanical valve prosthesis. Ann Thoracic Surg 1996;62:1790–1795.

Mahan EF III, Nanda NC. Transesophageal echocardiography. In: Rackley CE, ed. Challenges in Cardiology I. Mt. Kisco, NY: Futura, 1991:85–101.

Mohr-Kahaly S, Kupferwasser I, Erbel R, et al. Regurgitant flow in apparently normal valve prostheses: improved detection and semiquantitative analysis by transesophageal two-dimensional color-coded Doppler echocardiography. J Am Soc Echocardiogr 1990;3:187–195.

Nagueh SF, Bozkurt B, Li GA, et al. Progressive dehiscence and dynamic compression of an aortic root homograft— detection and characterization by transesophageal echocardiography. Am Heart J 1996;132:1070–1073.

Nellessen U, Schnittger I, Appleton CP, et al. Transesophageal two-dimensional echocardiography and color Doppler flow velocity mapping in the evaluation of cardiac valve prostheses. Circulation 1988;78:848–855.

Orsinelli DA, Pasierski TJ, Pearson AC. Spontaneously appearing microbubbles associated with prosthetic cardiac valves detected by transesophageal echocardiography. Am Heart J 1994;128:990–996.

Orsinelli DA, Pearson AC. Detection of prosthetic valve strands by transesophageal echocardiography: clinical significance in patients with suspected cardiac source of embolism. J Am Coll Cardiol 1995;26:1713–1718.

Osman K, Willman B, Nanda NC, et al. Transesophageal echocardiographic findings of a dehisced Duran mitral annuloplasty ring. Echocardiography 1995;12:441–446.

Pederson WR, Walker M, Olson JD, et al. Value of transesophageal echocardiography as an adjunct to transthoracic echocardiography in evaluation of native and prosthetic valve endocarditis. Chest 1991;100:351–360.

Robert F, Roudaut R, Pepin C, et al. Significance of "strands" on mitral mechanical prostheses during late follow-up after surgery. Echocardiography 1996;13:265–270.

Sanyal RS, Roychoudhury D, Nanda NC, et al. Transthoracic and transesophageal echocardiographic diagnosis of severe subaortic obstruction produced by an abscess cavity. Am Heart J 1994;128:1252–1255.

Stoddard MF, Dawkins PR, Longaker RA. Mobile strands are frequently attached to the St. Jude Medical mitral valve prosthesis as assessed by two-dimensional transesophageal echocardiography. Am Heart J 1992;124:671–674.

Taams MA, Gussenhoven EJ, Cahalan MK, et al. Transesophageal Doppler color flow imaging in the detection of native and Bjork-Shiley mitral valve regurgitation. J Am Coll Cardiol 1989;13:95–99.

van den Brink RBA, Visser CA, Basart DCG, et al. Comparison of transthoracic and transesophageal color Doppler flow imaging in patients with mechanical prostheses in the mitral valve position. Am J Cardiol 1989;63:1471–1474.

Vered Z, Mossinson D, Pelege E, et al. Echocardiographic assessment of prosthetic valve endocarditis. Eur Heart J 1995;16(Suppl B):63–67.

Weinert L, Karp R, Vignon P, et al. Feasibility of aortic diameter measurement by multiplane transesophageal echocardiography for preoperative selection and preparation of homograft aortic valves. J Thorac Cardiovasc Surg 1996;112:954–961.

Ischemic Heart Disease

6

Careful transesophageal imaging can reveal a great deal of information about the anatomy of the coronary tree. The presence of stenosis is indicated by compromise of the lumen. To be certain that what is being imaged is truly a stenosis rather than an artifact produced by an oblique section through the vessel, it is necessary to be able to see normal lumen on either side of the obstruction. Poststenotic dilatation may be present; it suggests a severe stenosis. Other markers of severe stenosis are an elevated pressure gradient across the stenosis by conventional Doppler and the presence of turbulence in the region of the stenosis on color-flow Doppler. The use of echocardiographic contrast may enhance flow visualization. Additional segments of the coronary vessels may be visualized and stenosis identified in these segments following contrast injection. The left main and proximal segments of the left anterior descending, left circumflex, and right coronary artery, together with some of their branches, can be visualized by transesophageal echocardiography. With newer color Doppler equipment, smaller epicardial and intramyocardial vessels (e.g., septal perforators) also can be seen.

Wall motion abnormalities also are well visualized by transesophageal echocardiography, especially using the transgastric approach. Mitral regurgitation in ischemic heart disease can be recognized and its severity assessed. Mitral annular dilatation and dilatation of the left atrium and left ventricle imply long-standing, significant mitral regurgitation. When the head of the papillary muscle is ruptured, it often can be imaged prolapsing into the left atrium. In up to 30% of patients, however, the ruptured head may not prolapse into the left atrium. In these cases the diagnosis is made by noting chaotic movement of the ruptured head in the left ventricle. Meticulous examination is important in these cases.

The term *pseudoaneurysm* refers to a rupture of the ventricle that is walled off by clot before the patient experiences fatal tamponade. These lesions have a narrow neck (which distinguishes them from true aneurysms) that leads to a walled-off cavity. Pseudoaneurysms are inherently unstable in that they have a propensity to rupture. They should be resected even if discovered late after a myocardial infarction in an otherwise stable patient.

Other mechanical complications that can result from ischemic heart disease include ventricular septal rupture, which is easily seen on color-flow Doppler. Posterior ventricular septal defects often are best visualized using the transgastric approach.

Figure 6.1.   **Coronary lesions. A-G. Left main disease. A.** A linear atherosclerotic plaque that produced a 33% stenosis of the left main lumen (LM). *A*, width of nonstenotic lumen; *B*, width of stenosed lumen. **B.** An eccentric, highly reflectile atherosclerotic plaque (upper arrow) that produced more than 80% stenosis of the left main coronary artery (LMCA). The presence of normal-sized lumen beyond the stenosed area increases the diagnostic confidence, because it excludes the possibility of artificial narrowing produced by an oblique section through the coronary vessel. **C.** Another view of the coronary artery shown in **B**, demonstrating the atherosclerotic plaque (arrow) as well as bifurcation of the left main coronary artery (LMCA) into the left circumflex (LCX) and left anterior descending (LAD) arteries. **D,E.** A patient with left main ostial stenosis. **D.** A very narrow color-flow jet (arrow) in the ostium with distal widening. **E.** Doppler interrogation demonstrates high-velocity (1.13 m/sec) diastolic (DS) flow, further confirming the presence of ostial stenosis. A lower velocity antegrade systolic flow (SF) also is noted. The ostial velocity in this patient is underestimated because of the nonperpendicular orientation of the ultrasound beam relative to the blood flow direction. *SV*, Doppler sample volume. **F,G.** Another patient with severe mid-left main stenosis with turbulent flow seen beyond the lesion. Pulsed Doppler interrogation reveals a high diastolic velocity. **H-J. Left anterior descending (LAD) stenosis.** The upper vertical arrows in **H** point to two atherosclerotic plaques, one located at the ostium and the other more distally, producing severe stenosis. Note the presence of a normal LAD lumen beyond the second lesion. **I.** Another patient in whom significant proximal LAD stenosis was identified because of flow acceleration and aliasing (arrow). **J.** Another patient in whom a localized flow acceleration and aliasing (red arrow) identified discrete stenosis at the origin of the LAD. **K,L. Left circumflex stenosis.** Discrete severe stenosis (arrow), about 1 cm from its origin, with post-stenotic dilatation in the circumflex (LCX) coronary artery. **M,N. Right coronary artery stenosis.** Two discrete areas of severe stenosis (arrows), one at the ostium and the other a little more distal, involving the right coronary artery (RCA). **O-Q. Contrast echocardiography in assessing coronary stenosis. O.** *Left panel*: Color flow signals are seen filling the left main coronary artery and the proximal LAD completely following IV injection of 3 g of Levovist (an echo contrast agent). *Right panel*: Before injection hardly any flow signals are apparent. **P.** *Left panel*: linear flow signals (arrows) are demonstrated in the LAD (without demonstrating the walls) following IV injection of Levovist. *Right panel*: This LAD segment could not be demonstrated without contrast injection. **Q.** *Left panel*: IV injection of Levovist not only demonstrated flow signals in the LAD but also showed an area of flow acceleration and aliasing corresponding to an area of severe stenosis in the proximal LAD on the coronary angiogram. *Right panel*: a smaller area of flow signals with a smaller flow acceleration persisting from a previous Levovist injection. Contrast enhancement is useful in demonstrating additional segments of the coronary arteries not visualized on routine examination and demonstrating stenoses in these segments. **R-V. Left anterior descending stenosis.** The arrowheads in **R** and **S** show narrowing and interruption of color flow signals in the LAD (2), indicative of severe stenosis. Color Doppler-guided pulsed Doppler examination **(T)** in this patient demonstrates a high diastolic velocity of 1 m/sec, also consistent with stenosis. *1*, left main coronary artery; *3*, left circumflex artery; *4*, left atrial branch. Aliased signals in another patient **(U)** suggest narrowing in the proximal LAD, which is supported by the presence of a high diastolic velocity of 1.3 m/sec obtained by pulsed Doppler examination **(V)**. The red flow signals next to the aliased area in **U** represent antegrade flow in the anterior interventricular vein, which accompanies the LAD. *LM*, left main coronary artery. **W-Y. Saphenous vein graft.** The arrows in **W-Y** demonstrate a saphenous vein graft (G) originating from the medial aspect of the ascending aorta (AO). (**C, D, H,** and **K** reproduced with permission from Samdarshi TE, Nanda NC, Gatewood RP Jr, et al. Usefulness and limitations of transesophageal echocardiography in the assessment of proximal coronary artery stenosis. J Am Coll Cardiol 1992;19:572-580.)

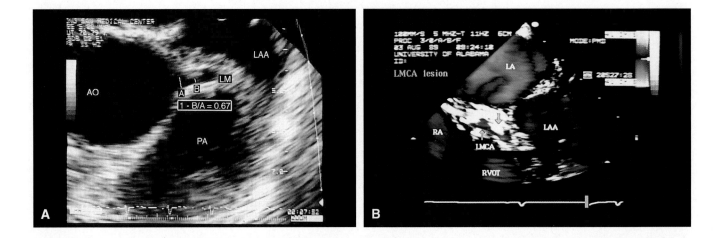

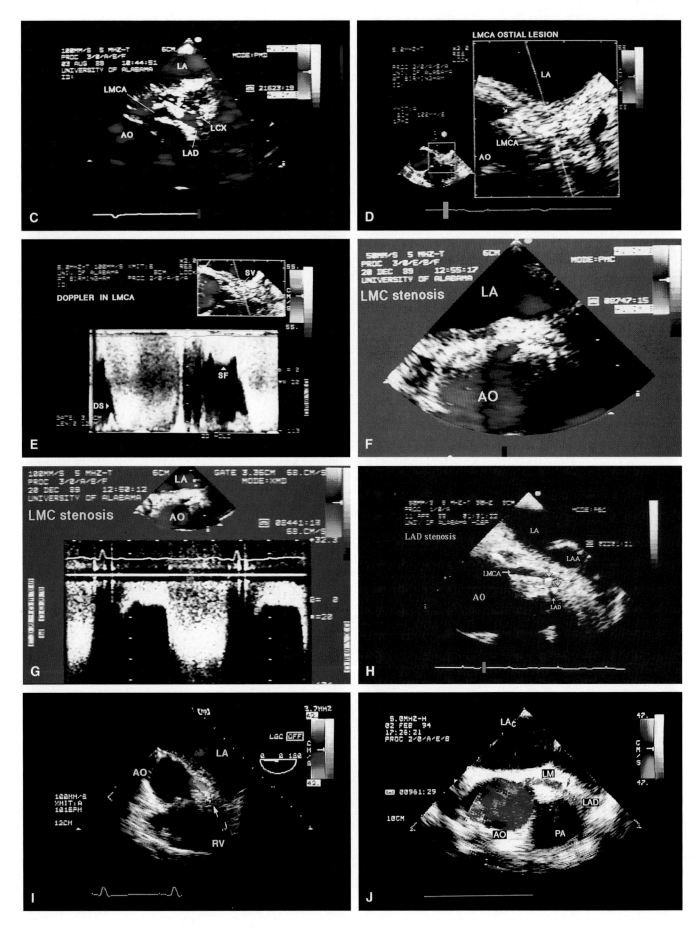

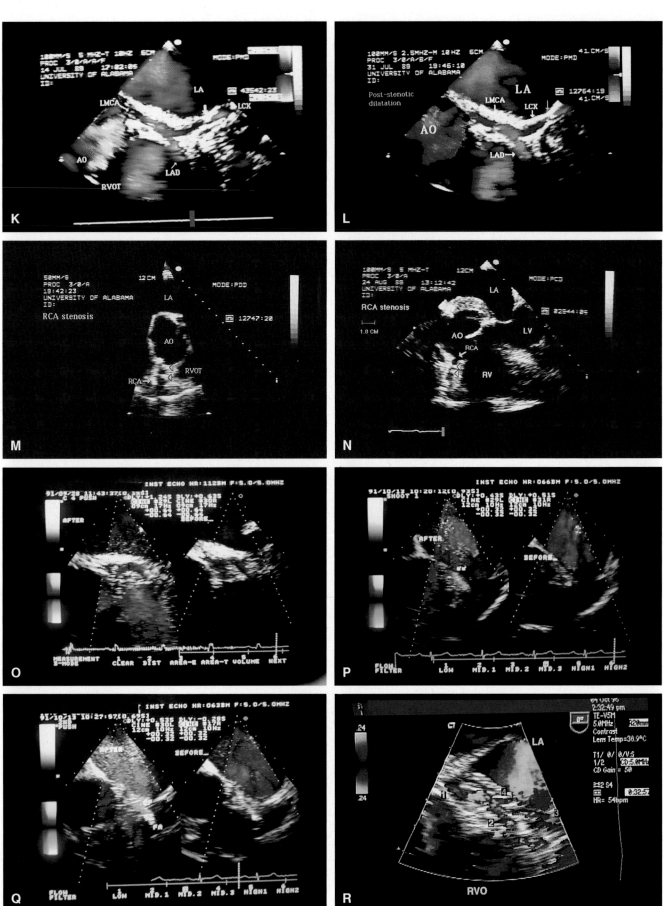

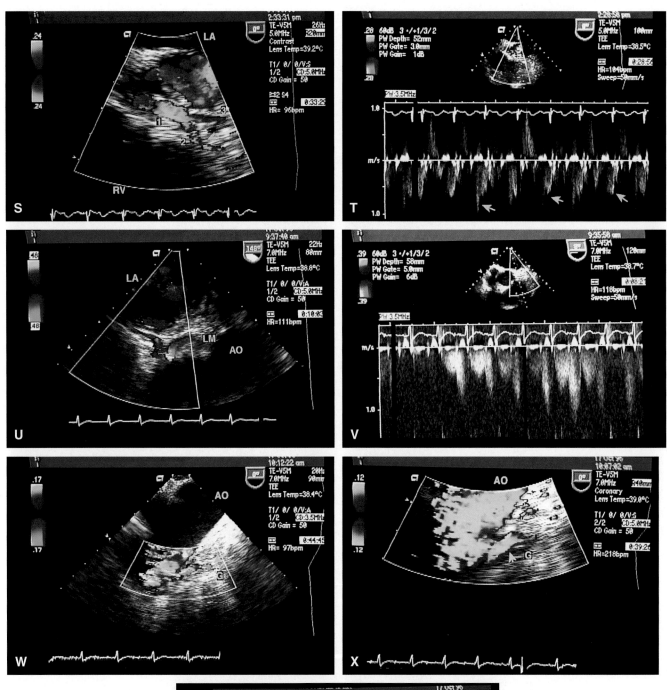

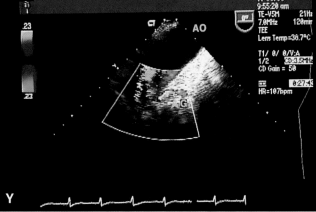

Figure 6.2. **Left ventricular dysfunction. A.** Marked hypokinesis of the anterior septum (arrowheads) is seen in this patient with ischemic heart disease. The inferior wall is also hypokinetic. **B.** M-mode image from the same patient shows hypokinesis of anterior (ANT) and inferior walls (POST). **C.** Color Doppler examination in this patient demonstrates two MR jets resulting from LV dysfunction. **D.** Another patient with moderate MR resulting from ischemic heart disease. **E,F.** Two other patients with mild (**E**) and severe (**F**) MR. Because the mitral valve leaflets appear to be structurally normal, the MR is presumed to be ischemic in origin. In both patients the LV as well as the mitral annulus were enlarged. **G.** Dyskinesis of the LV anterior free wall (black arrow) in this transgastric systolic frame in another patient. *IW*, LV inferior wall.

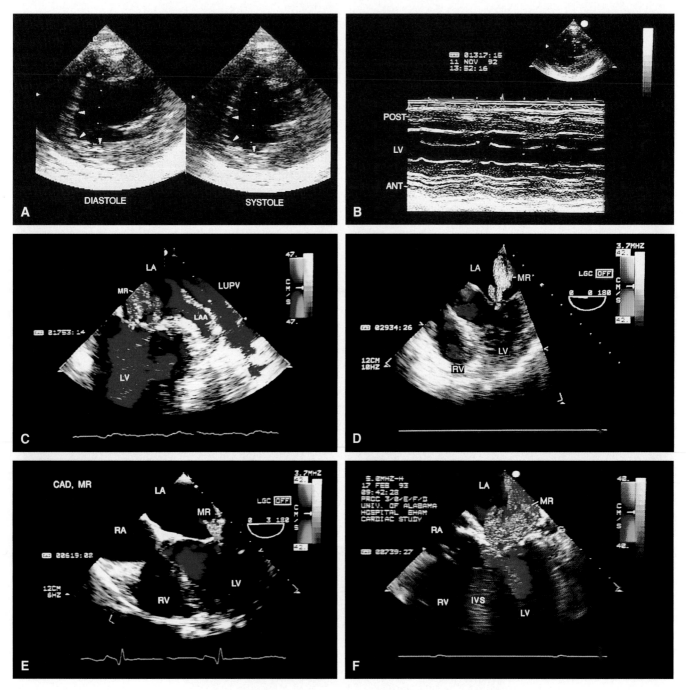

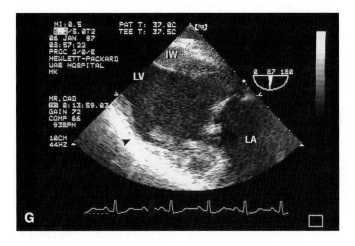

Figure 6.3.   **LV apical aneurysm. A.** A bright, fibrotic scar (arrowhead) in the aneurysmal apex. **B.** A huge LV apical aneurysm (arrowheads). **C.** Gross specimen of LV apical aneurysm caused by an acute myocardial infarction. **D-F.** Another patient with a large apical aneurysm containing a thrombus (arrowheads). **F.** Color Doppler examination shows the presence of associated MR. **G,H.** Gross specimens of LV aneurysm with mural thrombus. **I.** Aneurysmal proximal inferior wall (arrowheads) is seen in the two-chamber view. Note the myocardial thinning, which is well seen.

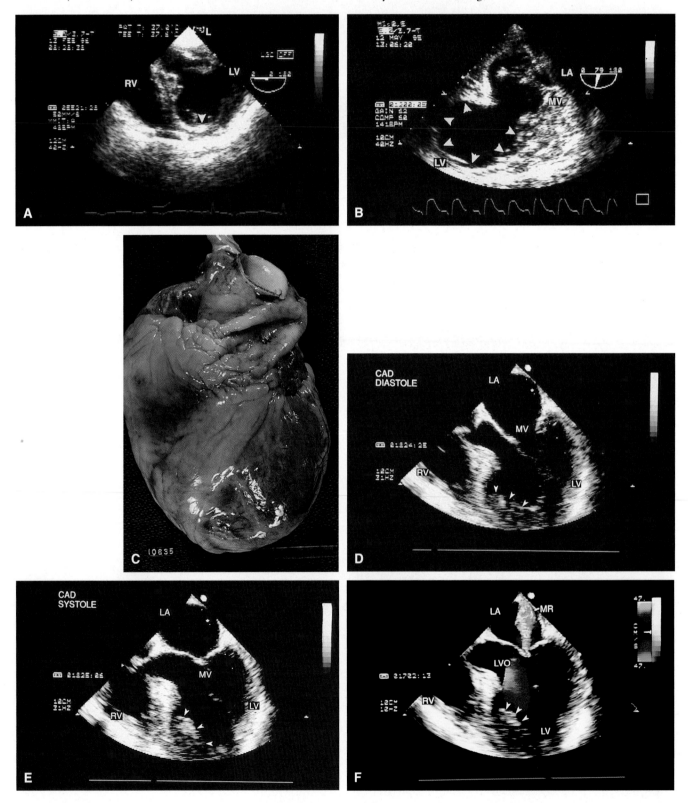

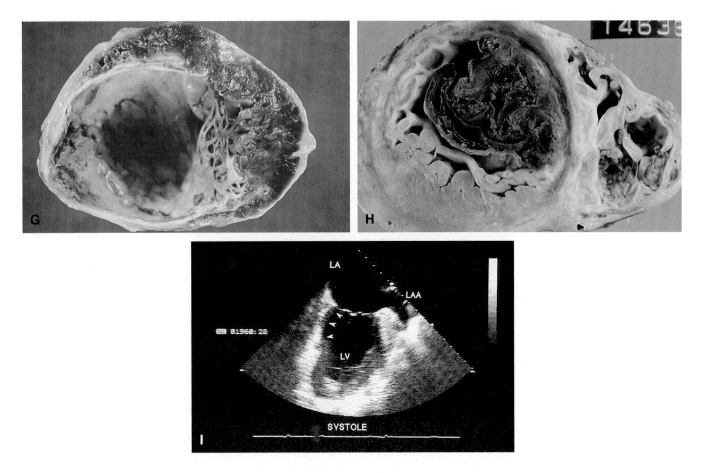

Figure 6.4. **LV pseudoaneurysm.** The arrows in **A** and **B** show the communication of the LV with a large pseudoaneurysm (PSA). In **B** and **C** the pseudoaneurysm appears to be larger than the LV cavity. **D.** Color Doppler examination reveals flow signals moving from the LV into the PSA through the relatively narrow neck (arrowheads). Pseudoaneurysms are differentiated from true aneurysms by their narrow necks-in pseudoaneurysms the neck or mouth is smaller than the aneurysm cavity, whereas in true aneurysms the mouth or neck is much larger, often as large as or larger than the cavity.

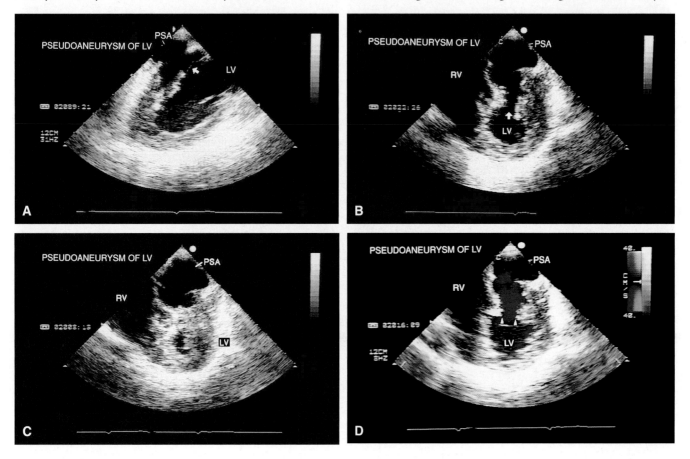

Figure 6.5. Contained slit-like cardiac rupture following acute myocardial infarction. **A-E.** Transgastric views **(A,B)** show a large and narrow color jet (arrow) within the LV posterior wall. **B** also shows color flow signals partially filling the pseudoaneurysm cavity (PAN). In **C**, the color Doppler was turned off, revealing an echo-free space (arrow), which corresponded to the site of the color jet seen in **A**; however, it could not otherwise be distinguished from an artifactual echo "dropout." Associated moderate MR is noted in **D**. **E.** Postoperative image shows absence of color flow signals within the myocardial wall. **F.** Gross specimen from another patient shows a contained LV rupture. **(A-E** reproduced with permission from Rao A, Garimella S, Nanda NC, Chung SM. Transesophageal color Doppler echocardiographic diagnosis of cardiac rupture following acute myocardial infarction. Echocardiography 1996;13:309-312.)

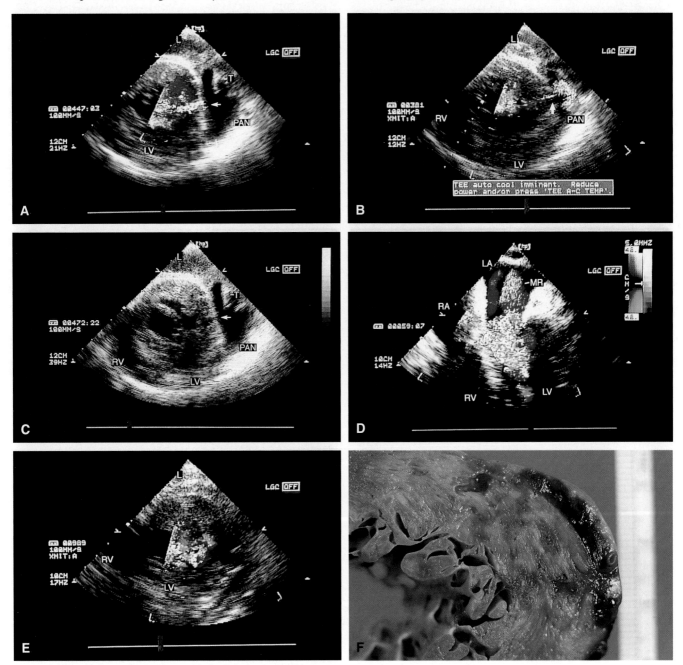

Figure 6.6. **Ventricular septal rupture. A-C.** Ventricular septal rupture (R) with an apical aneurysm (AN). **D,E.** Color Doppler examination shows shunting of flow across the ruptured interventricular septum into RV (arrows). **F.** Gross specimen from another patient shows a probe passing through a ruptured ventricular septum.

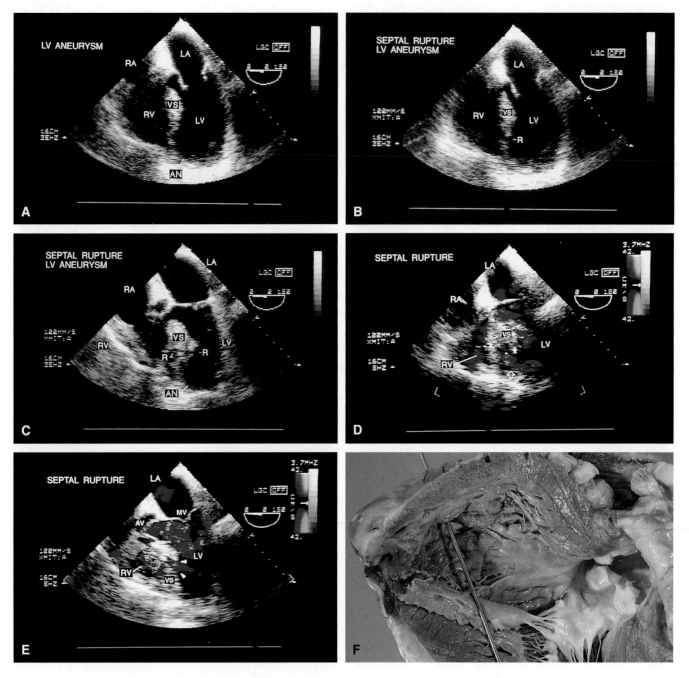

Figure 6.7. Ventricular septal rupture after acute anterior myocardial infarction. **A.** Apical five-chamber view. Flow signals are seen moving from the LV into the RV through the large apical defect (arrows). **B.** The patch (solid arrow) used to close the defect. **C.** Transgastric views (transverse plane imaging) from the same patient show marked enlargement and widening of the ventricular septum (VS), with large areas of echolucency consistent with dissection (horizontal open arrows in **C**). Color Doppler imaging shows prominent color flow signals (maximal width 10 mm) moving from the LV into the VS (vertical open arrow in **C**) and occupying the large echolucent areas seen on the non-color Doppler image. The prominent area of localized relatively high-velocity signals (flow acceleration) noted in the LV measured 9 mm at the site of the defect. No corresponding defect at the same level is seen on the right ventricular aspect, but two smaller sites of rupture, both 5 mm in size, are noted on the right side further posteriorly (solid arrows in **C**). These are associated with smaller areas of flow acceleration (1.5 to 2 mm). These defects are not delineated on the two-dimensional image, but are visualized only during color Doppler examination. Thus, the patient has four defects in the VS, one very large and located in the apical region, and the other three much smaller and located more posteriorly. None of the findings noted in **C** were demonstrated by transthoracic echocardiography. *VSD*, ventricular septal defect. (Reproduced with permission from Ballal RS, Sanyal RS, Nanda NC, Mahan EF III. Usefulness of transesophageal echocardiography in the diagnosis of ventricular septal rupture secondary to acute myocardial infarction. Am J Cardiol 1993;71:367-370.)

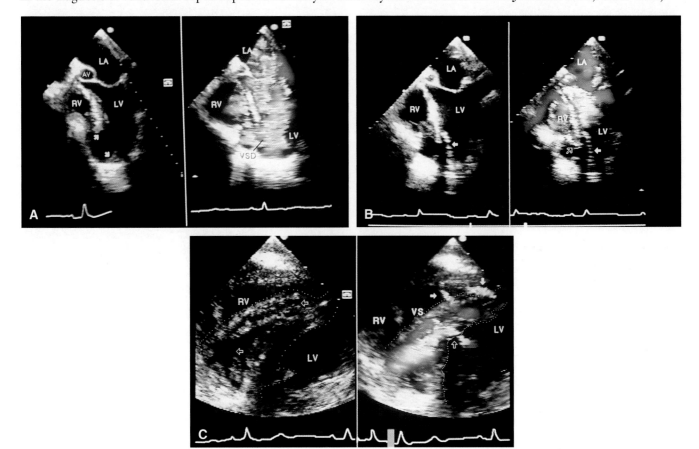

Figure 6.8. **Ventricular septal rupture after acute inferior myocardial infarction.** Transgastric views. **A.** Transverse plane imaging demonstrates mosaic color signals indicative of turbulent blood flow moving from the LV through the posterior ventricular septum (P) into the RV. The arrow indicates a localized area of increased velocity with aliasing (flow acceleration) on the left ventricular side of the defect. Note that the defect is not identified on the non-color Doppler two-dimensional image. *Top A,* ascitic fluid; *bottom A,* anterior ventricular septum. **B,C.** Longitudinal plane imaging demonstrates mosaic signals moving from the LV into the RV through the inferior portion of the ventricular septum during systole (left panel in **B** and **C**). The diastolic frame (right panel in **B**) reveals right-to-left shunt (red flow signals) through a large area of ventricular septal defect (VSD, arrow heads). With use of both transverse and longitudinal plane imaging, the site of rupture was correctly identified in the inferior aspect of the posterior septum. *L,* liver; *C,* Swan-Ganz catheter. **D.** Color M-mode examination shows flow signals moving from the RV into the LV during diastole (open arrow). Mosaic-colored signals in the RV during systole are denoted by solid arrows. (Reproduced with permission from Ballal RS, Sanyal RS, Nanda NC, Mahan EF III. Usefulness of transesophageal echocardiography in the diagnosis of ventricular septal rupture secondary to acute myocardial infarction. Am J Cardiol 1993;71:367-370.)

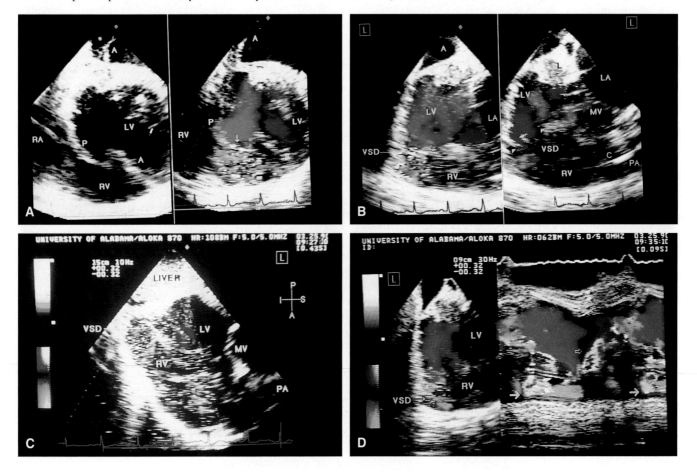

Figure 6.9. Ventricular septal rupture after acute inferior myocardial infarction. **A.** Four-chamber view shows an irregular defect that extends from the middle of the VS on the left side to the apical region on the right side (arrows). In addition, a large echo density (arrowhead) is seen attached to a TV leaflet or chord, which demonstrates marked prolapse into the RA. At surgery, the patient was found to have RV papillary muscle rupture in addition to VS rupture. **B.** Another four-chamber view from the same patient demonstrates localized widening (arrows) of the apical portion of the ventricular septum consistent with dissection. **C.** The same defect (solid arrow) viewed from the transgastric approach (transverse plane imaging). Color Doppler examination shows complete filling of the markedly enlarged right atrium with aliased flow signals during systole, indicative of severe tricuspid regurgitation (TR). Aliased flow signals also are seen moving from the LV into the RV through the defect. The open arrow points to the moderator band in the right ventricle (RV). *L*, liver; *PM*, posteromedial papillary muscle. (Reproduced with permission from Ballal RS, Sanyal RS, Nanda NC, Mahan EF III. Usefulness of transesophageal echocardiography in the diagnosis of ventricular septal rupture secondary to acute myocardial infarction. Am J Cardiol 1993;71:367-370.)

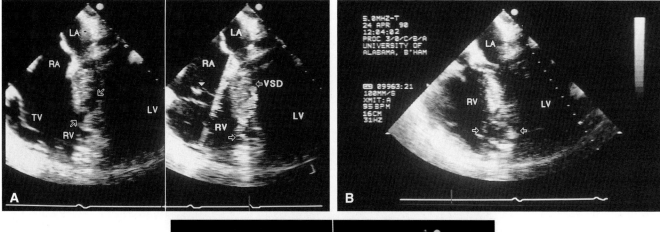

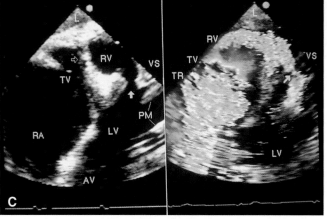

Figure 6.10. **LV papillary muscle rupture. A,B.** Classic findings of prolapse (arrows) of the ruptured papillary muscle head into the LA in two patients. **A.** The ruptured head involved the anterior papillary muscle. **B.** In this case it involved the posterior muscle. (Reproduced with permission from Moursi MH, Bhatnagar SK, Vilacosta I, San Roman JA, Espinal MA, Nanda NC. Transesophageal echocardiographic assessment of papillary muscle rupture. Circulation 1996;94:1003-1009.)

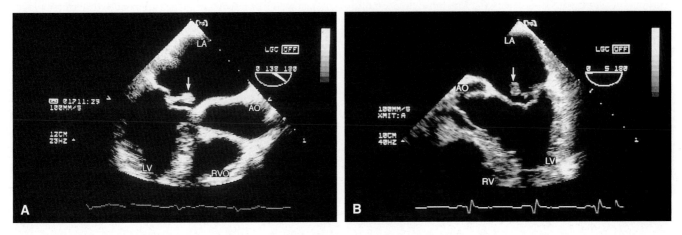

Figure 6.11. LV papillary muscle rupture. **A–C** and **D–G** represent transgastric views in two different patients, both of whom demonstrated erratic motion of the ruptured papillary muscle head (arrows) in the LV. The ruptured head, which involved the posterior papillary muscle in both patients, did not prolapse into the LA in either case. (Reproduced with permission from Moursi MH, Bhatnagar SK, Vilacosta I, San Roman JA, Espinal MA, Nanda NC. Transesophageal echocardiographic assessment of papillary muscle rupture. Circulation 1996;94:1003-1009.)

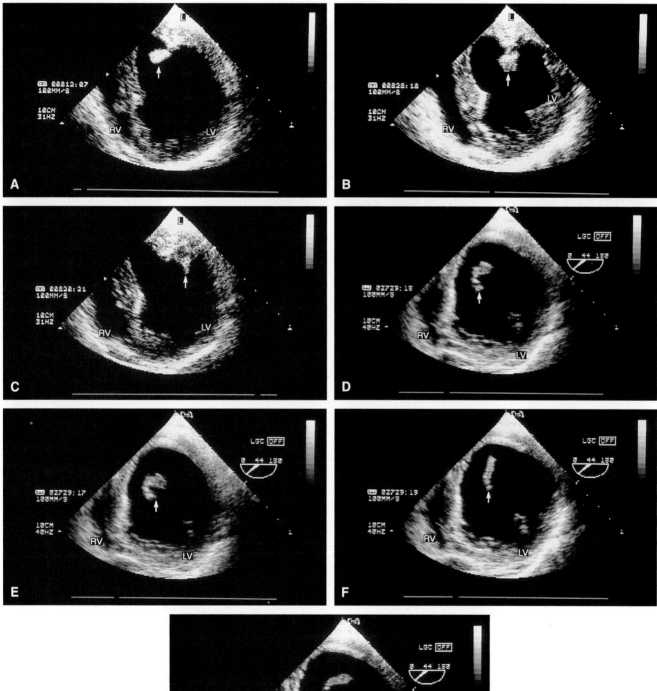

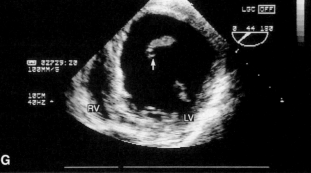

Figure 6.12. **LV papillary muscle rupture. A.** Five-chamber view shows a flail anterior mitral leaflet (arrowhead) prolapsing into the LA, but the ruptured papillary muscle head (arrow) remains in the LV just beneath the posterior leaflet. **B.** Transgastric view demonstrates the anterior position of the ruptured head (arrow), which involved the anterior papillary muscle. (Reproduced with permission from Moursi MH, Bhatnagar SK, Vilacosta I, San Roman JA, Espinal MA, Nanda NC: Transesophageal echocardiographic assessment of papillary muscle rupture. Circulation 1996;94:1003-1009.)

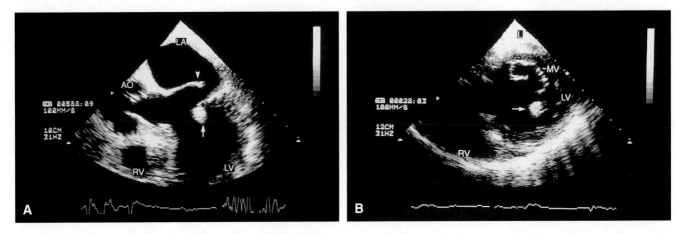

Figure 6.13. **LV papillary muscle rupture. A-C.** The ruptured posterior papillary muscle head (arrows) moving back and forth between LV and LA.

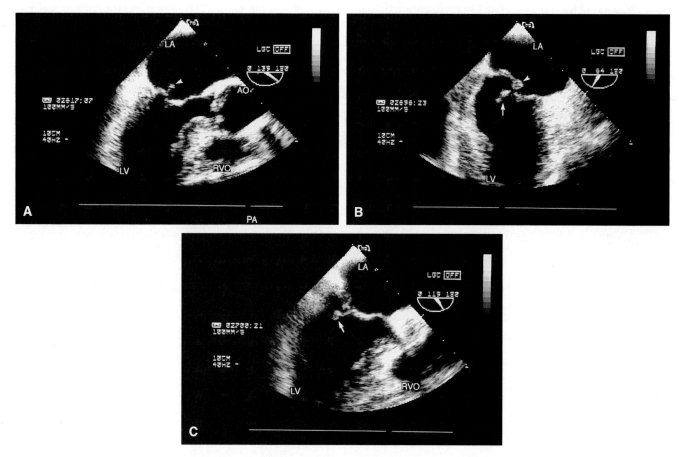

Figure 6.14. **LV papillary muscle rupture.** Color M-mode examination in another patient with papillary muscle rupture shows systolic backflow (arrows) extending deep into the right upper pulmonary vein (RUPV), indicative of torrential MR.

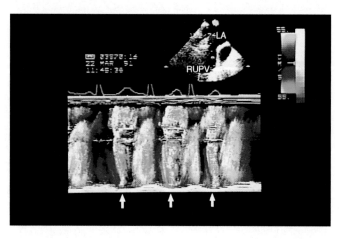

Figure 6.15. **LV papillary muscle rupture. A,B.** The ruptured papillary muscle head is not visualized in LA, and the findings resemble chordae (CH) rupture (arrow in **B**). **C-G.** Careful examination, however, clearly shows the ruptured papillary muscle head (arrow) moving back and forth between the LV and the LA. **D.** The site of rupture of the papillary muscle (PM) is clear; the shape of the ruptured head (arrow) matches that of the papillary muscle (PM) still attached to the LV wall. **F,G.** Chordae (arrowheads) in the LV. **H,I.** Color Doppler examination shows an unimpressive small eccentric MR jet. However, the zone of flow acceleration (arrowheads in **H**) is large, and color Doppler-guided pulsed Doppler examination **(J)** shows prominent aliased systolic backflow (SBF) in the LUPV, indicative of severe MR. Note the presence of associated mild TR in **I**. *D,A*, diastolic and atrial systolic waves in the pulmonary vein tracing.

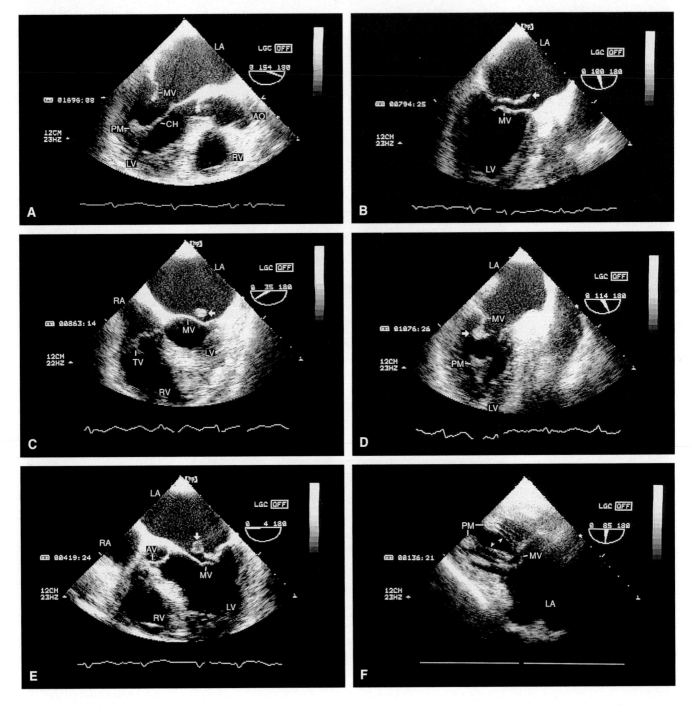

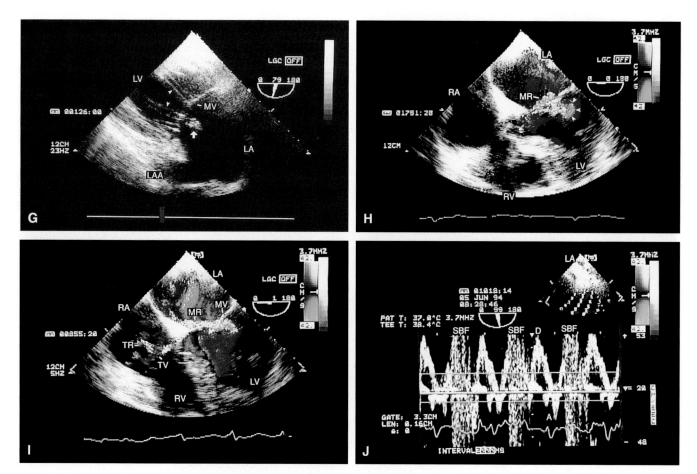

Figure 6.16. **LV papillary muscle rupture. A.** Diastolic frame. **B,C.** A small ruptured head (arrows) prolapsing into the LA.

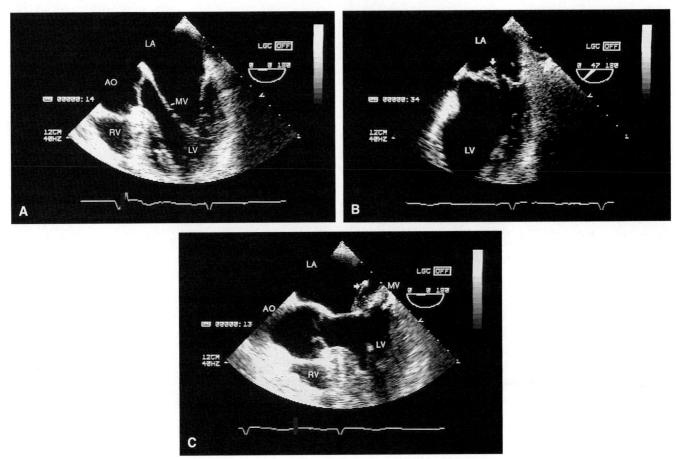

Figure 6.17. **LV papillary muscle rupture. A.** The ruptured head (arrow), which remains in LV in systole and does not prolapse into LA. In our experience, in approximately 30% of patients the ruptured head does not prolapse into the LA and the diagnosis is made by observing its chaotic motion in LV. **B.** Gross specimen from another patient shows a ruptured papillary muscle.

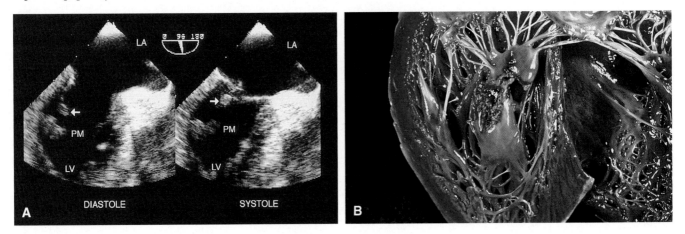

Figure 6.18. RV papillary muscle rupture. **A,B.** Transgastric views. **A.** The ruptured posterior right ventricular papillary muscle (M) is seen in the region of the posterior tricuspid leaflet (P) in systole. **B.** Anterior (A) and posterior (P) leaflets in the open position in diastole. **C.** The ruptured papillary muscle (M) in the RA. The arrow points to an associated ventricular septal rupture. **D.** Associated severe TR. *S*, septal tricuspid leaflet. (Reproduced with permission from Maxted W, Nanda NC, Kim KS, et al. Transesophageal echocardiographic identification and validation of individual tricuspid valve leaflets. Echocardiography 1994;11:585-591.)

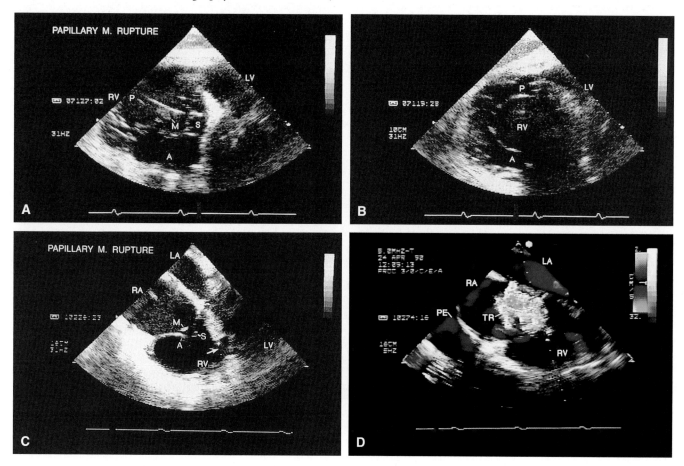

SUGGESTED READINGS

Abd El-Rahman SM, Khatri G, Nanda N, et al. Transesophageal three-dimensional echocardiographic assessment of normal and stenosed coronary arteries. Echocardiography 1996;13:503–510.

Agarwal KK, Gatewood RP, Nanda NC, Chopra KL. Improved transesophageal echocardiographic assessment of significant proximal narrowing of the left anterior descending and left circumflex coronary arteries using echo contrast enhancement. Am J Cardiol 1994;73:1131–1133.

Amuchastegui LM, Amuchastegui M, Moreyra E, Salomone O. Embolic accident following heparin therapy for a left ventricular clot diagnosed by TEE: a case report. Echocardiography 1994;11:197–200.

Ballal RS, Sanyal RS, Nanda NC, Mahan EF III. Usefulness of transesophageal echocardiography in the diagnosis of ventricular septal rupture secondary to acute myocardial infarction. Am J Cardiol 1993;71:367–370.

Caiati C, Aragona P, Iliceto S, Rizzon P. Improved Doppler detection of proximal left anterior descending coronary artery stenosis after intravenous injection of a lung-crossing contrast agent: a transesophageal Doppler echocardiographic study. J Am Coll Cardiol 1996;27:1413–1421.

D'Cruz IA, Hayes M, Killam HAW. Echocardiographic features of large posterobasal left ventricular aneurysms. Echocardiography 1996;13:65–70.

Fein SA, Vargas M. Transesophageal echocardiographic diagnosis of cardiac rupture. J Am Soc Echocardiogr 1991;4:415–416.

Koenig K, Kasper W, Hofmann T, Meinertz T, Just H. Transesophageal echocardiography for diagnosis of rupture of the ventricular septum or left ventricular papillary muscle during acute myocardial infarction. Am J Cardiol 1987;59:362.

Kozakova M, Palombo C, Benanti C, et al. Analysis of right ventricular kinesis by means of transesophageal echocardiography: present problems and perspectives. Echocardiography 1996;11:179–187.

Kozakova M, Palombo C, Zanchi M, et al. Increased sensitivity of flow detection in the left coronary artery by transesophageal echocardiography after intravenous administration of transpulmonary stable echocontrast agent. J Am Soc Echocardiogr 1994;7:327–336.

Kozakova M, Palombo C, Pittella G, Distante A. Transesophageal echocardiography in myocardial ischemia: a review. Echocardiography 1995;12:479–494.

Kozlowski CM, Dorogy ME. Transesophageal echocardiography and concurrent coronary angiography for the rapid assessment of papillary muscle rupture. Echocardiography 1994;11:47–49.

Maxted W, Nanda NC, Kim KS, et al. Transesophageal echocardiographic identification and validation of individual tricuspid valve leaflets. Echocardiography 1994;11:585–591.

Moursi MH, Bhatnagar SK, Vilacosta I, San Roman JA, Espinal MA, Nanda NC. Transesophageal echocardiographic assessment of papillary muscle rupture. Circulation 1996;94:1003–1009.

Obarski TP, Rogers PJ, Debaets DL, et al. Assessment of postinfarction ventricular septal ruptures by transesophageal Doppler echocardiography. J Am Soc Echocardiography 1995;8:728–734.

Patel AK, Miller FA, Khandheria BK, et al. Role of transesophageal echocardiography in the diagnosis of papillary muscle rupture secondary to myocardial infarction. Am Heart J 1989;118:1330–1333.

Rao A, Garimella S, Nanda NC, Chung SM. Transesophageal color Doppler echocardiographic diagnosis of cardiac rupture following acute myocardial infarction. Echocardiography 1996;13:309–312.

Saka K, Nakamura K, Hosoda S. Transesophageal echocardiographic findings of papillary muscle rupture. Am J Cardiol 1991;68:561–563.

Samdarshi TE, Nanda NC, Gatewood RP Jr, et al. Usefulness and limitations of transesophageal echocardiography in the assessment of proximal coronary artery stenosis. J Am Coll Cardiol 1992;19:572–580.

Sastry BKS, Krishna RN, Venkateshwar RG, et al. An unusual complication during a transesophageal echocardiographic procedure in a patient with left ventricular pseudoaneurysm. Echocardiography 1994;11:51–54.

Schrem SS, Tunick PA, Slater J, Kronzon I. Transesophageal echocardiography in the diagnosis of ostial left coronary artery stenosis. J Am Soc Echocardiogr 1990;3:367–373.

Sheikh KH, Bengtson JR, Rankin JS, et al. Intraoperative transesophageal Doppler color flow imaging used to guide patient selection and operative treatment of ischemic mitral regurgitation. Circulation 1991;85:594–604.

Stoddard MF, Dawkins PR, Longaker RA, et al. Transesophageal echocardiography in the detection of left ventricular pseudoaneurysm. Am Heart J 1993;125:534–539.

Stoddard MF, Keedy DL, Kupersmith J. Transesophageal echocardiographic diagnosis of papillary muscle rupture complicating acute myocardial infarction. Am Heart J 1990;120:690–692.

Topol EJ, Weiss JL, Guzman PA, et al. Immediate improvement of dysfunctional myocardial segments after coronary revascularization: detection by intraoperative transesophageal echocardiography. J Am Coll Cardiol 1984;4:1123–1134.

Yoshida K, Yoshikawa J, Hozumi T, et al. Detection of left main coronary artery stenosis by transesophageal color Doppler and two-dimensional echocardiography. Circulation 1990;81:1271–1276.

Zotz RJ, Dohmen G, Genth S, et al. Diagnosis of papillary muscle rupture after acute myocardial infarction by transthoracic and transesophageal echocardiography. Clin Cardiol 1993;16:665–670.

Cardiomyopathy

7

Hypertrophic cardiomyopathy (HCM) is characterized by inappropriate hypertrophy of the ventricle. Although asymmetric septal hypertrophy is the classical presentation, any wall or even the entire ventricle may be involved. Systolic anterior motion (SAM) of the mitral valve occurs and results in obstruction to outflow. The result is mitral regurgitation and a subvalvular gradient across the left ventricular outflow tract. The obstruction of the left ventricular outflow tract (LVOT) results in turbulent flow that is recognizable as such using color-flow Doppler. The velocity waveform obtained from conventional Doppler examination of the outflow tract shows a high peak velocity, reflecting the increased pressure gradient. Additionally, there is a slow upslope of the velocity waveform and a more rapid downslope. This differentiates it from fixed LVOT obstruction, in which the velocity waveform is symmetric.

Midsystolic notching of the aortic valve is another common finding. There often is evidence of reduced diastolic compliance of the left ventricle, resulting in an abnormally increased A-to-E ratio on conventional Doppler examination of mitral inflow. The surgical treatment of hypertrophic cardiomyopathy is myomectomy of the ventricular septum. This resection appears as a "scooped-out" area by echocardiography.

Dilated cardiomyopathy (DCM) is recognized by dilatation of the cardiac chambers and poor ventricular function. The sluggish flow that occurs in these patients may result in thrombus formation that is visible by echocardiography.

Ventricular assist devices have been used to support the left and right ventricles. Some examples of imaging of the conduits that are placed in these patients are shown in this chapter.

Figure 7.1. **Hypertrophic cardiomyopathy. A.** Prominent systolic anterior motion (SAM) (arrowhead) of the anterior mitral leaflet touching the ventricular septum (VS). **B.** SAM of both the anterior and posterior mitral leaflets with noncoaptation. The resulting eccentric mitral regurgitation (MR) jet (arrowheads) is demonstrated in **C. D,E.** M-mode studies demonstrate midsystolic preclosure of the aortic valve (AV; arrowhead in **D**) and coarse systolic fluttering (arrowheads in the second beat in **E**).

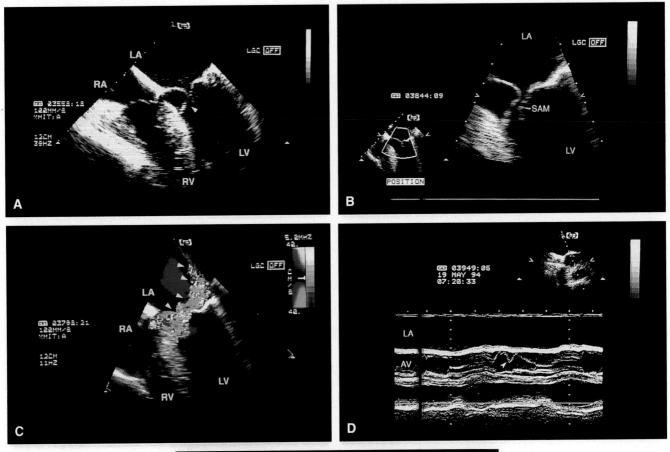

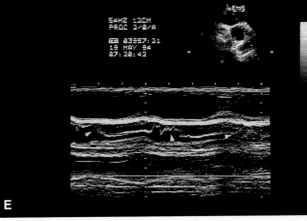

Figure 7.2. **Hypertrophic cardiomyopathy. A-I.** Serial frames demonstrate closing motion of the mitral leaflets and development of systolic anterior motion of both anterior and posterior leaflets.

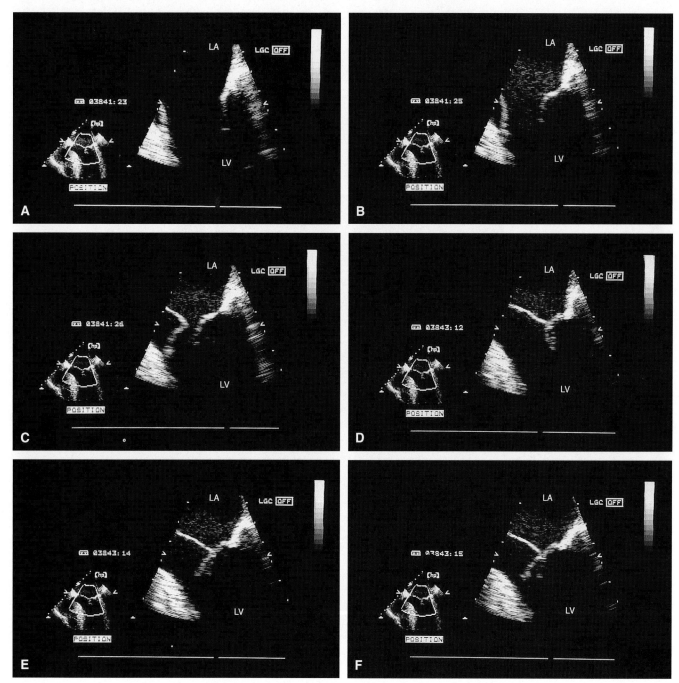

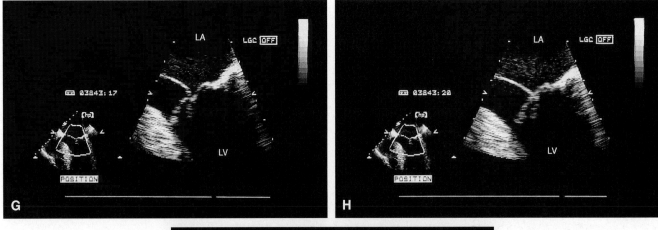

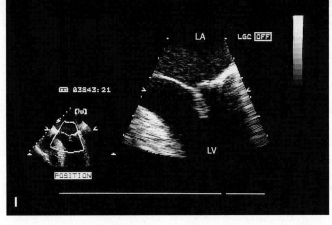

Figure 7.3. **Hypertrophic cardiomyopathy: mitral regurgitation.** Serial frames demonstrate changing severity of MR. **A.** MR appears to be severe. **B.** There is no MR, or only trace MR. **C-E.** The MR is eccentric. **F.** Mild MR. **G.** Aliased LV inflow is noted with the leaflets open in diastole.

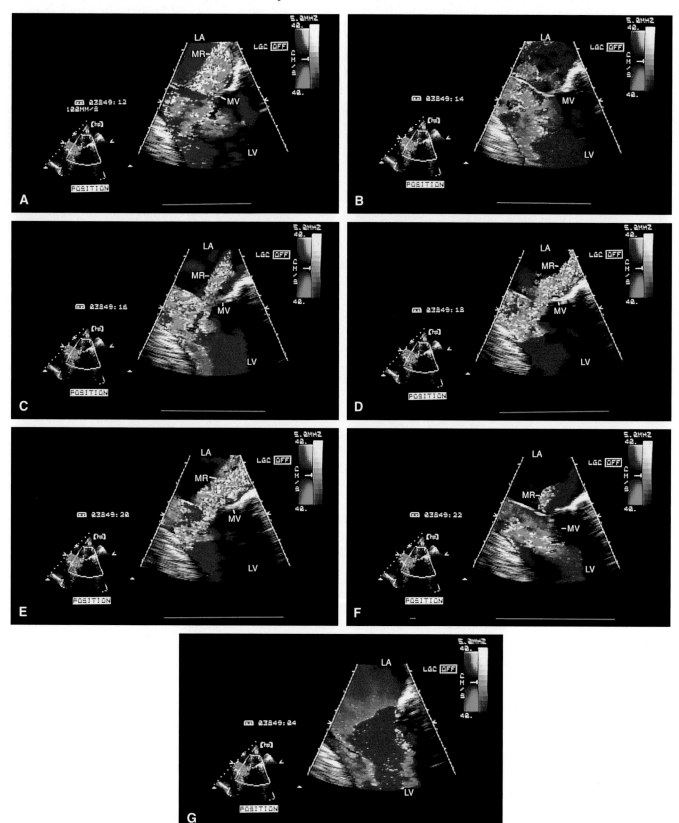

Figure 7.4. **Hypertrophic cardiomyopathy. A.** Prominent SAM of the anterior mitral leaflet touching the VS is seen. **B.** Prominent systolic turbulent flow in the narrowed LVOT as well as significant eccentric MR. **C.** A schematic shows asymmetric VS hypertrophy (ASH), narrow LVOT with turbulent flow, SAM of anterior mitral leaflet and MR.

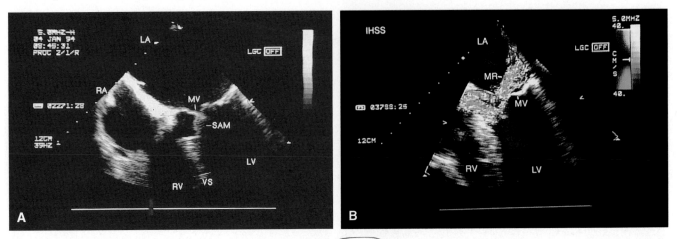

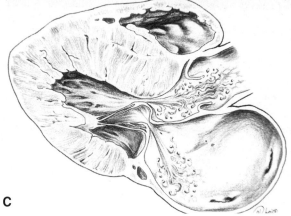

Figure 7.5. **Hypertrophic cardiomyopathy. A,B.** Turbulent systolic flow in the narrowed LVOT and eccentric MR jet. **C.** Color flow-directed continuous wave Doppler demonstrates a high velocity of 3 m/sec in the LVOT. The slope of the upstroke of the Doppler velocity waveform is less (slower) than the downslope, typical of hypertrophic cardiomyopathy.

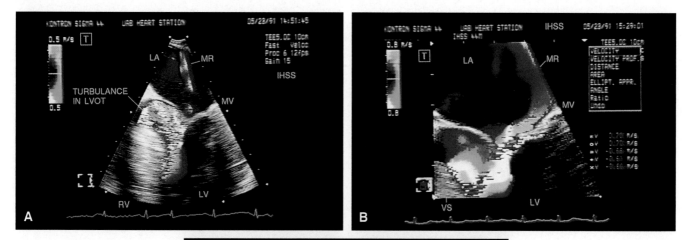

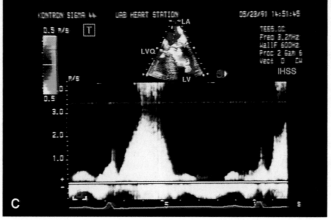

Figure 7.6. **Hypertrophic cardiomyopathy. A-C.** SAM of anterior mitral leaflet touching the VS, with turbulent systolic flow in LVOT and MR. This patient underwent a myectomy. **D.** The site of myectomy (scooped-out portion of the VS).

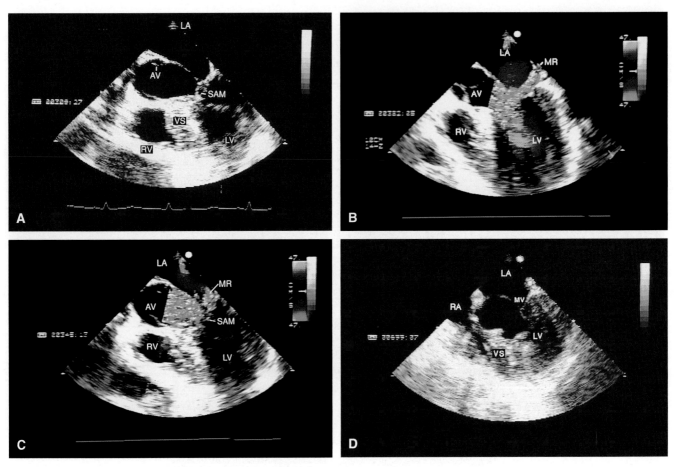

Figure 7.7. **Hypertrophic cardiomyopathy. A-C.** SAM of mitral valve, turbulent systolic flow in the LVOT, and a large MR jet with a large zone of flow acceleration as well as systolic backflow (SBF) in the LUPV indicative of severe MR. **D.** This patient also underwent myectomy; the arrow shows the scooped-out site. Note the presence of residual SAM.

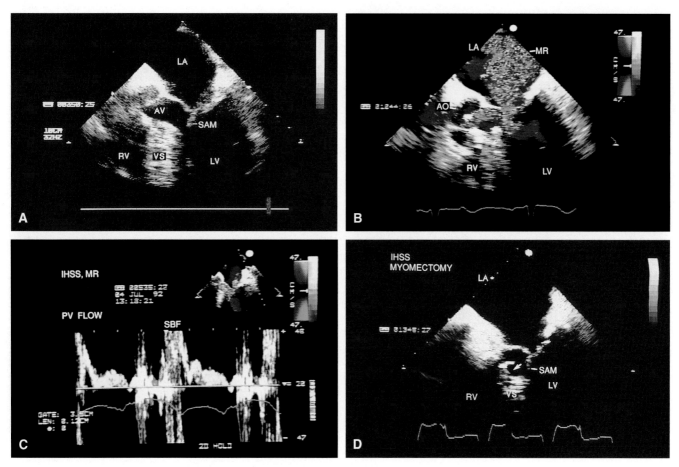

Figure 7.8. **Hypertrophic cardiomyopathy. A,B.** SAM of anterior MV leaflet is well seen. **C.** A transgastric view shows marked LVH. **D.** Turbulent systolic flow in LVOT and mild MR. **E.** Following myectomy, the LVOT has widened and the SAM has practically disappeared. The arrow shows the characteristic scooped-out appearance of the VS after myectomy.

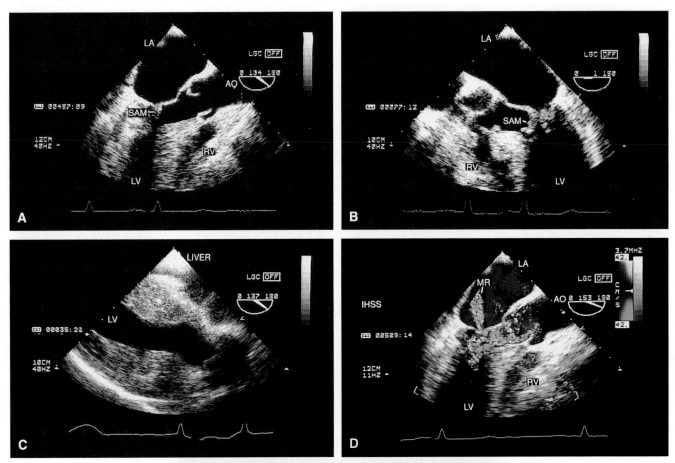

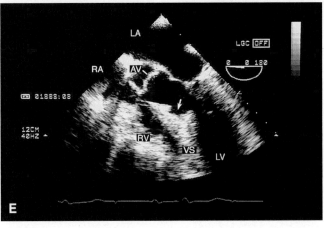

Figure 7.9. **Hypertrophic cardiomyopathy. A.** The scooped-out area (arrow) of myectomy following surgery. *Inset:* The preoperative image demonstrates mitral SAM (arrowheads) and a narrow LVOT. **B.** The left upper pulmonary vein (PV) and mitral inflow tracings from another patient with hypertrophic cardiomyopathy are shown. Note the presence of a small E and a large A wave on the mitral tracing and a large S wave, small D wave, and a prominent biphasic A wave on the pulmonary vein flow tracing. The increased duration of pulmonary vein A wave compared to the mitral A wave is indicative of increased LV end-diastolic pressure. **C-E.** Gross specimens from three other patients show hypertrophic cardiomyopathy. **D,E.** RV hypertrophy, often associated with this entity, is seen.

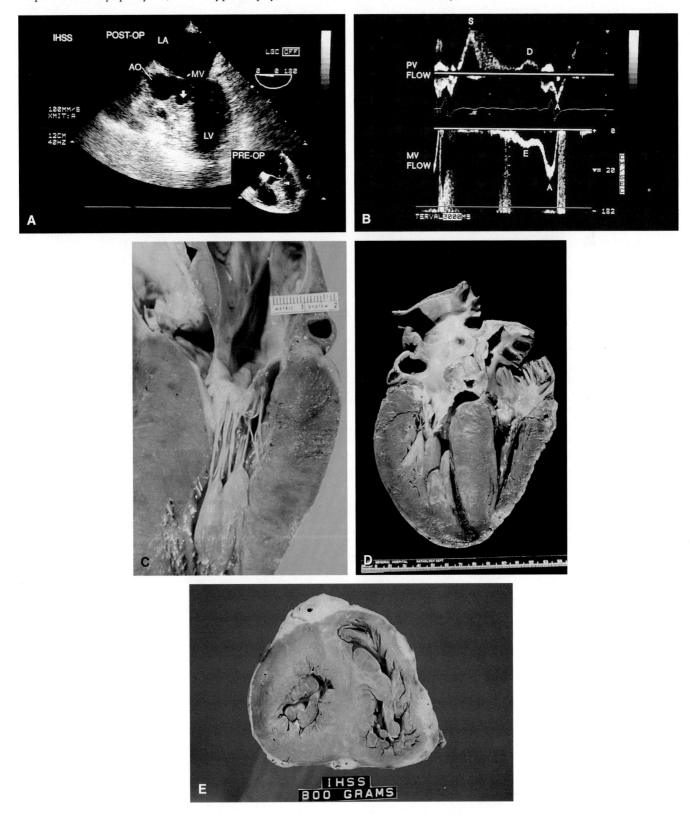

Figure 7.10. **Apical hypertrophic cardiomyopathy. A-C.** The arrow shows marked hypertrophy in the LV apical region. The proximal VS, seen well in **A**, is only mildly hypertophied. **D,E.** Postoperative images; the arrowheads show the area of muscle resection. **F.** A short-axis view of the LV shows marked hypertrophy of the LV free wall (open arrow) and mild hypertrophy of the VS (closed arrow) and inferior wall.

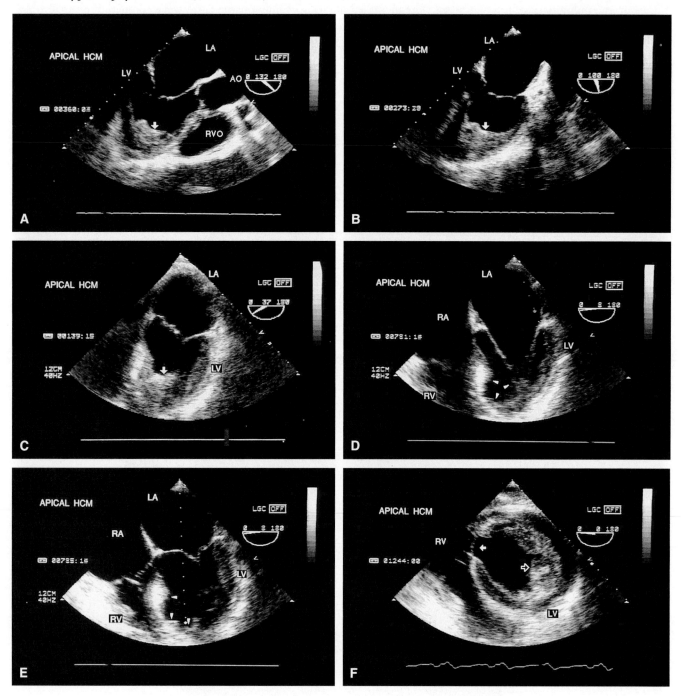

Figure 7.11. **Dilated cardiomyopathy.** Diastolic (**A**) and systolic (**B**) frames show poor LV function. **C.** Midsystolic notching of the AV is seen on M-mode examination, consistent with low cardiac output and significant MR. **D.** A thrombus in the LAA imaged from the transgastic approach. **E.** Diminished systolic S wave in the left upper pulmonary vein (PV) Doppler tracing is consistent with poor LV function and moderate MR. **F.** Dilated RA, RV, and coronary sinus (CS), also typical of dilated cardiomyopathy. **G.** Prominent trabeculation (arrowheads) in the RA free wall resulting from hypertrophy. These should not be confused with thrombi. **H.** RA free wall hypertrophy. **I.** Four-chamber view from a patient with dilated cardiomyopathy shows dilatation of all four cardiac chambers. **J.** Another patient with dilated cardiomyopathy demonstrating a thrombus (arrowhead) located in LV adjacent to the posterior mitral leaflet. **K,L.** Gross specimens show dilated LV and RV.

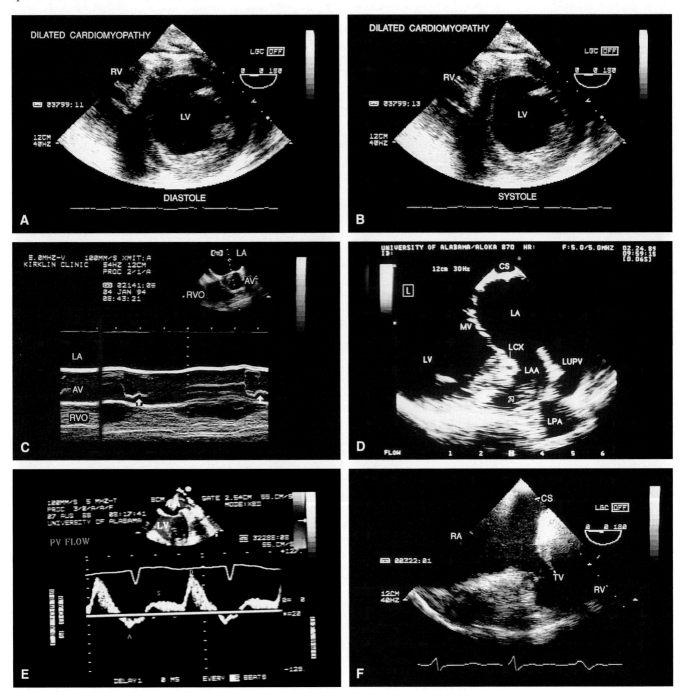

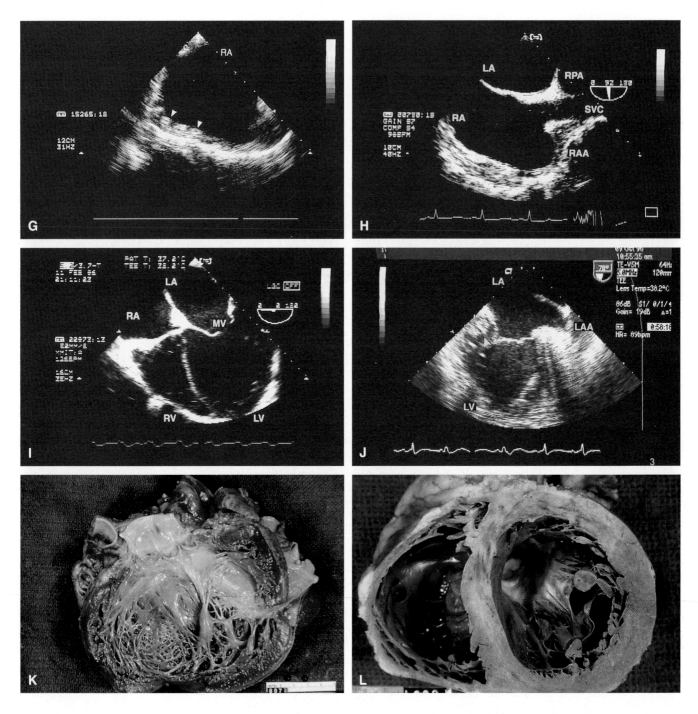

Figure 7.12. **Dilated cardiomyopathy: RV assist device. A,B.** An RV assist device (arrows) placed in this patient with dilated cardiomyopathy. The arrowheads demonstrate acoustic shadowing produced by the metallic device.

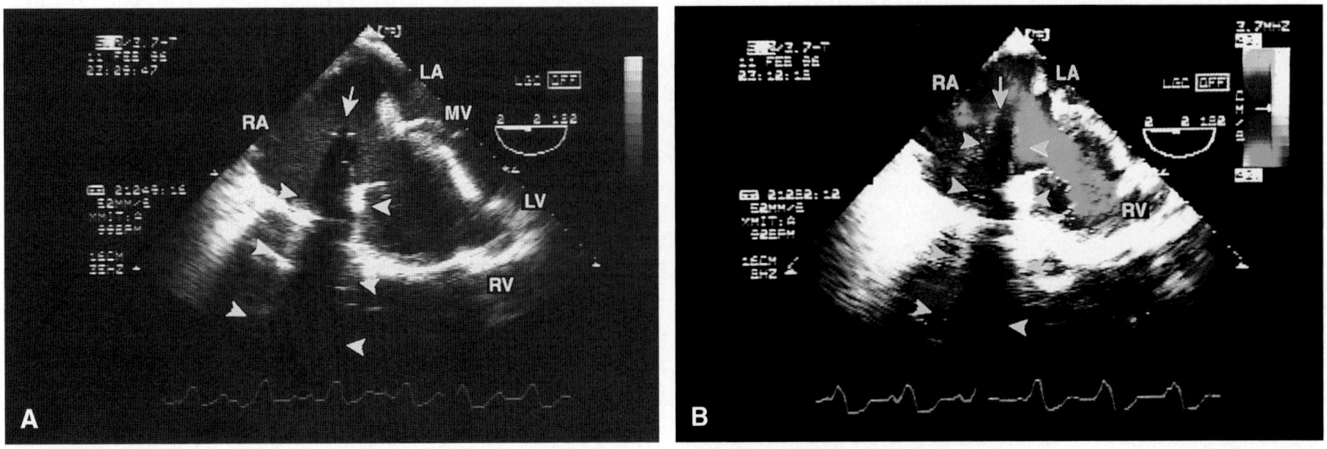

Figure 7.13. **Mechanical biventricular assist device.** The arrangement for a biventricular assist device, with the right-sided device pumping blood from the right atrium to the pulmonary artery and the left-sided device pumping blood from the left atrium to the aorta. (Reproduced with permission from Holman W. VAD Approved as a bridge to transplantation. UAB Insight 1989; Vol 1, No. 2.)

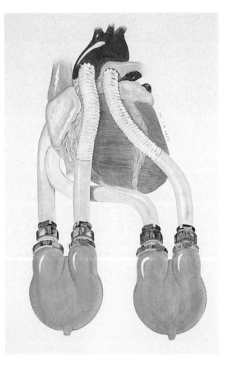

Figure 7.14. **Mechanical biventricular assist device. A.** Using biplane imaging, the Teflon conduit (arrows) is identified by the transverse serrations in its walls, and its attachment to the ascending aorta (AO) is well delineated. The main pulmonary artery (PA) is imaged posterior to the aorta. **B.** Mosaic-colored signals indicative of turbulent flow are noted moving through the conduit into the ascending aorta. Similar flow signals also are noted in the main pulmonary artery. **C.** Pulsed-Doppler interrogation of the conduit reveals prominent phasic flow signals. The electrocardiogram here and in **A** shows ventricular fibrillation. **D.** Using the standard single plane technique, the communication between the conduit and the aorta could not be delineated, even on extensive exploration of this region. **E.** Examination of the LV shows a large thrombus occupying the apical region. (Reproduced with permission from Parks J, Nanda NC, Bourge RC, et al. Transesophageal echocardiographic evaluation of mechanical biventricular assist device. Echocardiography 1990;7:561-566.)

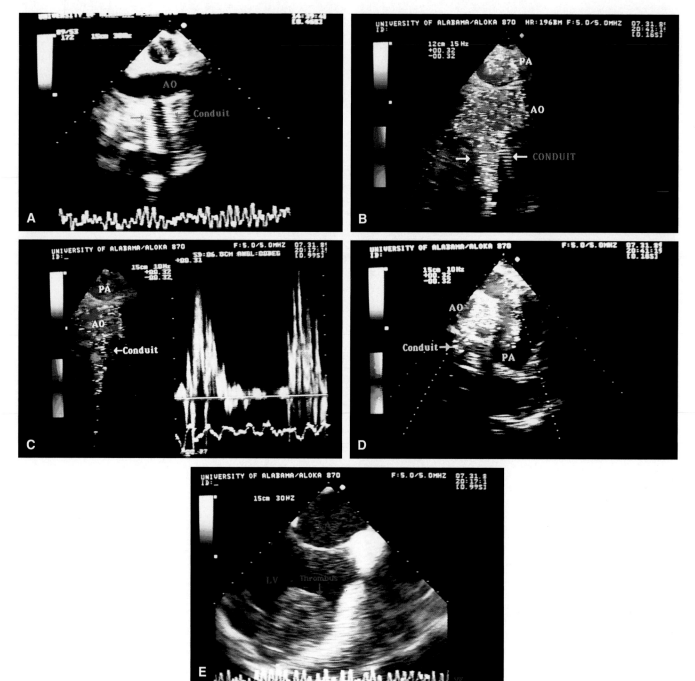

Figure 7.15. **Malpositioned Thoratec RV assist device. A.** The four-chamber view shows the Thoratec cannula (T) lodged in the LA. **B,C.** Color Doppler examination shows a prominent right-to-left atrial shunt (arrowhead). (Reproduced with permission from Snoddy BD, Nanda NC, Holman WL, et al. Usefulness of transesophageal echocardiography in diagnosing and guiding correct placement of a right ventricular assist device malpositioned in the left atrium. Echocardiography 1996;13:159-163.)

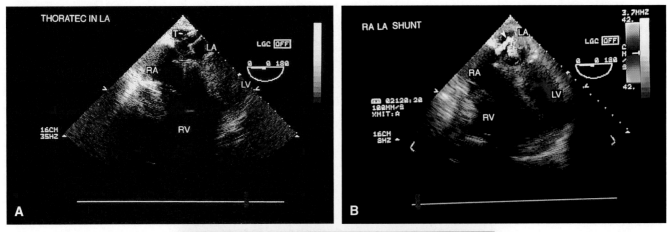

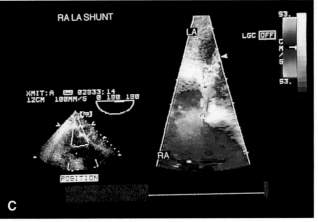

Figure 7.16. **Malpositioned RV assist device.** Same patient as in Fig. 7.15. **A,B.** As the cannula (T) was being withdrawn into the RA, a large left-to-right atrial shunt (arrowhead) developed. Note the distortion of the atrial septum in the fossa ovalis region. (Reproduced with permission from Snoddy BD, Nanda NC, Holman WL, et al. Usefulness of transesophageal echocardiography in diagnosing and guiding correct placement of a right ventricular assist device malpositioned in the left atrium. Echocardiography 1996;13:159-163.)

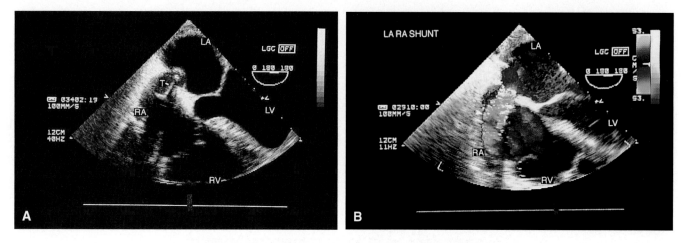

Figure 7.17. **Malpositioned RV assist device.** Same patient as in Figs. 7.15 and 7.16. **A,B.** When the cannula (T) was securely placed in the RA, the left-to-right atrial shunt (arrowhead) became very small. **C.** Four-chamber view demonstrates TR and MR and a small left-to-right atrial shunt (arrowhead). The cannula was in the RA. **D.** Descending thoracic aorta (AO) shows a dissection flap (F). *SC,* spinal canal; *VB,* vertebral body. (Reproduced with permission from Snoddy BD, Nanda NC, Holman WL, et al. Usefulness of transesophageal echocardiography in diagnosing and guiding correct placement of a right ventricular assist device malpositioned in the left atrium. Echocardiography 1996;13:159-163.)

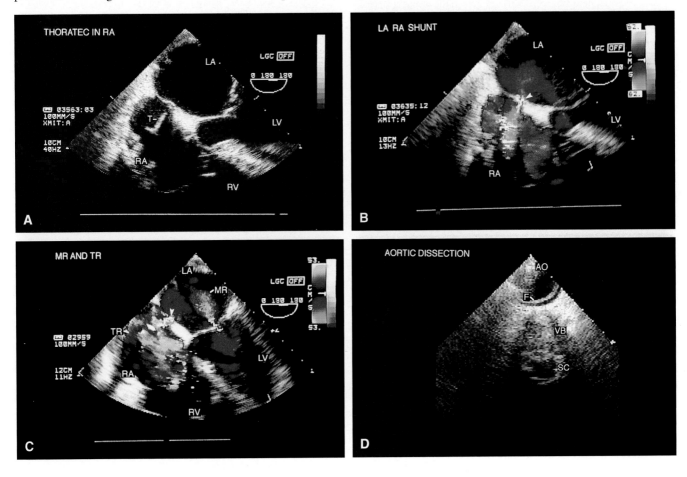

SUGGESTED READINGS

Baron A, Roychoudhury D, Kim KS, et al. Transesophageal echocardiographic findings of a patient with hypertrophic cardiomyopathy, mitral valve prolapse, and coronary artery disease: a case report. Echocardiography 1995;12:501-505.

Grigg LE, Wigle ED, Williams WG, et al. Transesophageal Doppler echocardiography in obstructive hypertrophic cardiomyopathy: clarification of pathophysiology and importance in intraoperative decision making. J Am Coll Cardiol 1992;20:42-52.

Ito T, Suwa M, Hirota Y, et al. Influence of left atrial function on Doppler transmitral and pulmonary venous flow patterns in dilated and hypertrophic cardiomyopathy: evaluation of left atrial appendage function by transesophageal echocardiography. Am Heart J 1996;131:122-130.

Lim YC, Doblar DD, Frenette L, et al. Intraoperative transesophageal echocardiography in orthotopic liver transplantation in a patient with hypertrophic cardiomyopathy. J Clin Anesth 1995;7:245-249.

Oki T, Fukuda N, Tabata T, et al. Transesophageal echocardiographic analysis of the systolic pattern of the anterior mitral leaflet in patients with flat chest: differentiation from mitral valve prolapse. Echocardiography 1995;12:351-358.

Oki T, Fukuda N, Iuchi A, et al. Transesophageal echocardiographic evaluation of mitral regurgitation in hypertrophic cardiomyopathy: contributions of eccentric left ventricular hypertrophy and related abnormalities of the mitral complex. J Am Soc Echocardiogr 1995;8:503-510.

Parks J, Nanda NC, Bourge RC, et al. Transesophageal echocardiographic evaluation of mechanical biventricular assist device. Echocardiography 1990;7:561-566.

Snoddy BD, Nanda NC, Holman WL, et al. Usefulness of transesophageal echocardiography in diagnosing and guiding correct placement of a right ventricular assist device malpositioned in the left atrium. Echocardiography 1996;13:159-163.

Stewart WJ, Schiavone WA, Salcedo EE, et al. Intraoperative Doppler echocardiography in hypertrophic cardiomyopathy: correlations with the obstructive gradient. J Am Coll Cardiol 1987;10:327-335.

Widimsky P, Ten Cate FJ, Vletter W, et al. Potential applications for transesophageal echocardiography in hypertrophic cardiomyopathies. J Am Soc Echocardiogr 1992;5:163-167.

Congenital Heart Disease

8

Part 1
OVERVIEW OF CONGENITAL HEART DISEASE

The excellent results obtained in infants and children using transthoracic echocardiography limit the need to use the transesophageal approach to elucidate the lesions of congenital heart disease. In some patients, however, it is not possible to perform adequate transthoracic studies, particularly in adults with congenital heart disease. Furthermore, transesophageal echocardiography is the only practical method for assessing operative results during the procedure.

The septum primum covers the septum secundum and closes the fossa ovalis. In about 25% of patients this coverage is not complete, and a flow may occur across the septum. This is particularly likely in the setting of elevated right-sided pressures, which can open the patent foramen and result in paradoxic embolus. The secundum defect occurs at the level of the fossa ovalis and is the most common of the atrial septal defects. These lesions often present as a single large defect but may be fenestrated or multiple. Defects smaller than 2 cm in diameter can be closed by transcatheter patch closure, but larger defects must be closed surgically. The size of the defect is easily assessed by transesophageal echocardiography, especially if the multiplane probe is used.

The ostium primum type of atrial septal defect (partial atrioventricular septal defect or partial atrioventricular canal defect) occurs at the base of the septum. It often is associated with a cleft in the anterior mitral valve leaflet, which is regurgitant as a result. In contrast, sinus venosus atrial septal defects occur in the superior part of the septum. Drainage of the right upper pulmonary vein into the right atrium is a commonly associated anomaly. The superior vena cava may override the defect. In adults, this defect may be difficult to visualize by transthoracic echocardiography. When an atrial septal defect is suspected based on other findings but is not found on transthoracic examination, transesophageal echocardiography is indicated.

Ventricular septal defects, especially small ones, often are visualized more effectively on transthoracic than on transesophageal echocardiography, because more planes are available from the transthoracic approach. Patent ductus arteriosus and other aortopulmonary communications,

both congenital and surgically created, can be visualized by transesophageal echocardiography.

Stenosis of the pulmonary veins usually is diagnosed early. It can be seen as narrowing of the vein, and Doppler examination demonstrates a high-velocity narrow jet with turbulence and spectral broadening. In adults, congenital stenosis must be differentiated from acquired narrowing produced by mediastinal lesions such as a tumor or sclerosing mediastinitis and pulmonary vein obstruction occurring after lung transplantation. In cor triatriatum, a membrane partitions the left atrium (or, rarely, the right atrium) into two chambers in such a way that the pulmonary veins are on one side of the membrane and the left atrial appendage is on the other side. Cor triatriatum is different from a supravalvar mitral membrane, which is located below and inferior to the left atrial appendage. These lesions may or may not result in obstruction to flow. Congenital mitral stenosis is a rare lesion, similar in presentation to mitral stenosis. The valve is thickened and domes in diastole. Associated abnormalities of the papillary muscle and chordae may be present.

Subvalvular aortic stenosis results from a fibromuscular membrane that has a location that is variable relative to the aortic valve. These membranes are most commonly attached to the base of the anterior mitral leaflet and to the ventricular septum. Subvalvular membranes appear as linear echoes in the left ventricular outflow tract. Turbulent flow and a high gradient may be present, and there is often associated aortic regurgitation. Early, as opposed to mid- or late, systolic closure of the aortic valve is commonly seen. It may involve only one cusp.

In congenital aortic stenosis the valve domes in systole. The short-axis view shows a typical "circle within a circle" appearance. Careful planimetry yields a good estimate of the valve area. Care must be taken to move the probe up and down the esophagus to visualize even the smallest flow-limiting orifice at the top of the domed valve. Color Doppler allows visualization of the width of the jet. A jet that is 7 mm or smaller suggests severe aortic stenosis in an adult. The jet width should be measured at its origin from the aortic valve. Color Doppler should be turned off during planimetry of the orifice because it tends to overestimate the area. It is, however, useful in identifying the aortic orifice in patients with heavily calcified valves that show no discernible opening movement in systole (i.e., fixed orifice). In these cases, the first appearance of turbulent flow signals in early systole helps identify the stenotic orifice, which can then be studied via planimetry with the color Doppler turned off. After valvotomy the jet size is larger, and the planimetered area is also greater. Because the transesophageal study can be performed intraoperatively, it is useful in guiding surgery. Supravalvular aortic stenosis is a rare lesion that may present as a discrete membrane or may be tubular. Coarctation of the aorta is best seen on transthoracic echocardiography but also may be evaluated by the transesophageal approach. The best results are obtained with a multiplane probe.

Membranes occur in the right atrium. Examples include eustachian valves and Chiari networks. Obstruction is rare but may occur. Right ventricular muscle bundles may be prominent and are associated with right ventricular hypertrophy. Rarely, the hypertrophy may be sufficient to cause obstruction in the body of the ventricle. A small ventricular septal defect may be associated, and it is suspected that the jet from the defect may, at least in some cases, stimulate hypertrophy. Infundibular stenosis may occur alone or in association with tetralogy of Fallot. The right ventricular outflow tract is best viewed in long axis using longitudinal plane examination.

In congenital pulmonary stenosis the valve domes in systole and also may be thickened. Stenosis in the proximal segments of the right or left pulmonary arteries can be visualized by transesophageal echocardiography; however, stenosis in distal segments or in the peripheral branches cannot be visualized using echocardiographic techniques.

The pathophysiologic features of complete atrioventricular canal defect (atrioventricular septal defect), including absence of the atrioventricular septum, deficiency of the adjacent atrial and inlet ventricular septum, a common atrioventricular annulus, and shunting from the left atrium into the right atrium and from the left ventricle into the right ventricle, are well seen using the transesophageal approach. The severity of atrioventricular valve regurgitation can also be evaluated.

In tricuspid atresia the tricuspid valve is absent and both atrial and ventricular septal defects are necessarily present to ensure patient survival. This lesion often is associated with a hypoplastic right ventricle. For the purpose of surgical planning, it is necessary to delineate the right ventricular outflow tract, the pulmonary valve, and the pulmonary artery. Surgical correction (i.e., the Fontan procedure) involves closure of the atrial septal defect, closure of any ventricular septal defect, and placement of a shunt from the right atrium to the pulmonary artery.

In transposition of the great vessels, the connection of the vessels to the ventricles can be seen and the relation of the pulmonary artery and the aorta can be delineated. Associated pulmonary valve stenosis can be seen, as can banding of the pulmonary artery. Coexisting atrial or ventricular septal defects and atrioventricular or semilunar valve regurgitation also can be assessed by transesophageal echocardiography. The adequacy of the Mustard procedure can be assessed immediately after operation. Intraatrial baffle leak or obstruction can be delineated. In congenitally corrected transposition of the great vessels, the discordant atrioventricular and ventriculoarterial connections, together with the presence and degree of Ebsteinization of the left-sided atrioventricular valve, can be assessed by transesophageal echocardiography.

Ebstein's anomaly is characterized by apparent displacement of one or more tricuspid valve leaflets into the right ventricle, resulting from a variable extent and degree of plastering of the leaflets to the contiguous ventricular septum or right ventricular wall. The degree of this displacement determines the size of the functional right ventricle. Transesophageal echocardiography is useful in assessing both these abnormalities and the severity of tricuspid regurgitation, which is often considerable. A patent foramen ovale or an atrial septal defect may be present, and may result in right-to-left shunting and cyanosis because of increased right atrial pressure. The anatomic features and the flow patterns of other complicated lesions, such as tetralogy of Fallot, double outlet right ventricle, and single ventricle also can be assessed via the transesophageal approach.

Abnormalities of the coronary arteries can be well seen. These include aneurysms, thrombi, and anomalous origins and course of the coronary arteries.

An important lesion is the sinus of Valsalva aneurysm. It may appear as a tubelike structure protruding into the right ventricle or the right atrium. Rupture may result in shunting into the right ventricle or the right atrium.

In the first part of this chapter of the book, the most common shunt lesions are illustrated first, then the obstructive lesions (both left-sided and right-sided), and, finally, the more complex congenital pathologies. The second and third parts of this chapter supplement the material shown in the first part and provide an enhanced understanding of the role of transesophageal echocardiography in the assessment of congenital cardiac lesions.

Figure 8.1.1. **Patent foramen ovale.** A defect in the midportion of the atrial septum that measures 1 cm or less is most likely a patent foramen ovale (PFO). **A.** Five-chamber view shows a small defect in the interatrial septum, consistent with a PFO. **B.** After a peripheral venous bolus of normal saline, contrast echoes are noted moving from the RA into the LA through the defect. The mildly thickened edges of the defect are outlined by the arrows. This patient presented with refractory hypoxemia from right-to-left shunting across a PFO secondary to increased RA pressure following acute inferior myocardial infarction with RV wall involvement. The RV inferior wall was akinetic on the transthoracic study. **C.** Another patient with a small defect (D), measuring about 1 cm, in the interatrial septum. **D–G.** Another patient with PFO. The black arrow in **D** shows bulging of the atrial septum (AS) into the LA, which occurred when the patient was asked to cough after receiving an intravenous injection of agitated normal saline. This resulted in the contrast echoes moving from the RA through the PFO into the left atrium (arrowheads in **D, F,** and **G**). Both cough and the Valsalva maneuver are useful in diagnosing a PFO because they transiently raise the RA pressure higher than that on the left, producing a right-to-left shunt. The lower arrowhead in **F** points to contrast echoes arriving in the aortic arch subsequent to their appearance in the LA. **H,I.** Right-to-left shunting (arrows) through a PFO demonstrated by color Doppler in another patient. Color Doppler examination usually is less sensitive than contrast echocardiography in detecting a PFO because the shunt flow velocity often is lower than the velocity threshold set for color Doppler. **J.** Left-to-right shunting (arrow) shown by color Doppler through a PFO in a patient with a large LA. Note the bulging of the atrial septum toward the RA. Contrast echocardiography was negative in this patient because coughing and the Valsalva maneuver failed to increase the RA pressure higher than the left, as evidenced by the absence of bulging of the atrial septum into the LA. **K.** A PFO (arrow) is well visualized on the two-dimensional image. **L,M.** Although the atrial septum appears intact in **L**, color Doppler examination clearly shows shunting into the RA. An area of flow acceleration is seen on the LA aspect of the atrial septum (AS). **N–P.** Another patient with a PFO. Right-to-left shunting is shown by both color Doppler (arrowheads in **N** and **O**) and peripheral venous saline contrast injection **(P).** **Q,R.** A different patient in whom minimal right-to-left shunting (arrowheads) through a PFO could be demonstrated by color Doppler. In these latter two patients, a recently introduced high-resolution color Doppler system was used. **S–V.** An elderly female with orthodeoxia in whom right-to-left shunting through a PFO was demonstrated by peripheral venous saline contrast injections (arrowheads in **S** and **T**). **U.** Shunting (arrow) also was demonstrated through the left upper pulmonary vein (LPV). Examination of the right lower and upper pulmonary veins did not show any contrast echoes. **V.** Contrast echoes (arrowheads) are seen in the SVC and PA but not in the RUPV following intravenous normal saline injection. Left pulmonary artery angiogram did not show any evidence of a pulmonary arteriovenous malformation or fistula. We believe the shunting into the LUPV is based on pulmonary capillary dilatation as a result of mild pulmonary fibrosis, which was found on her CT scan. (**A** and **B** reproduced with permission from Cox D, Taylor J, Nanda NC. Refractory hypoxemia in right ventricular infarction from right-to-left shunting via a patent foramen ovale: efficacy of contrast transesophageal echocardiography. Am J Med 1991;91:653–655. **S–V** reproduced with permission from Thakur AC, Nanda NC, Malhotra S, et al. Combined interatrial and intrapulmonary shunting in orthodeoxia detected by transesophageal echocardiography. Echocardiography January 1998 (in press.)

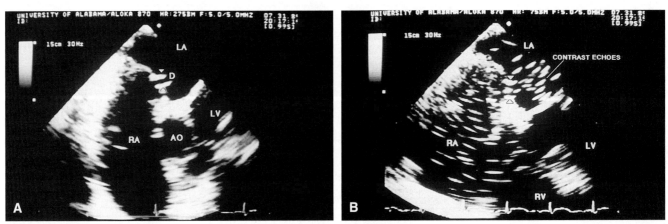

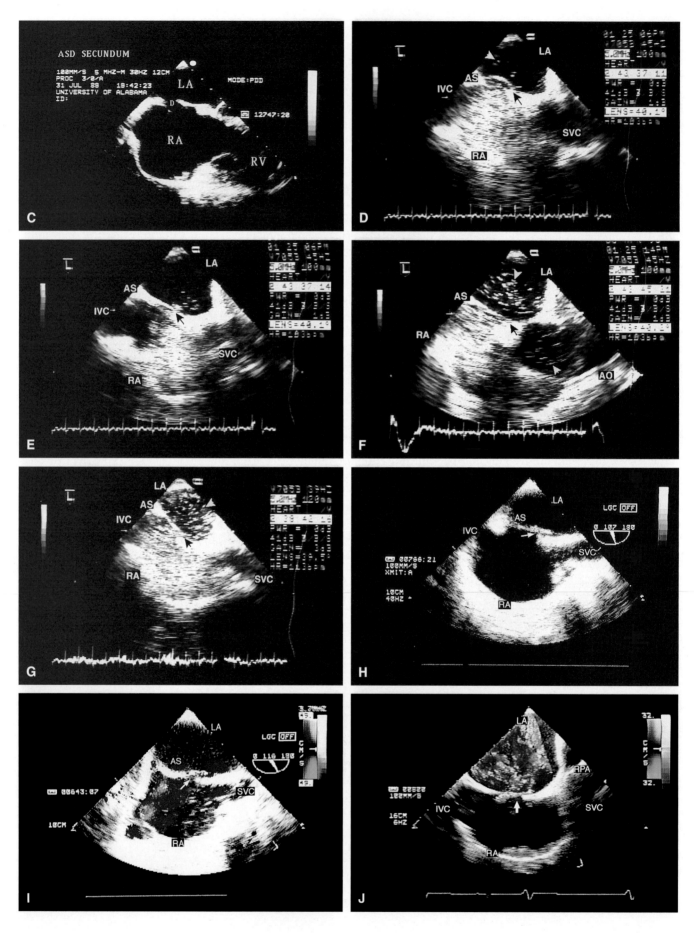

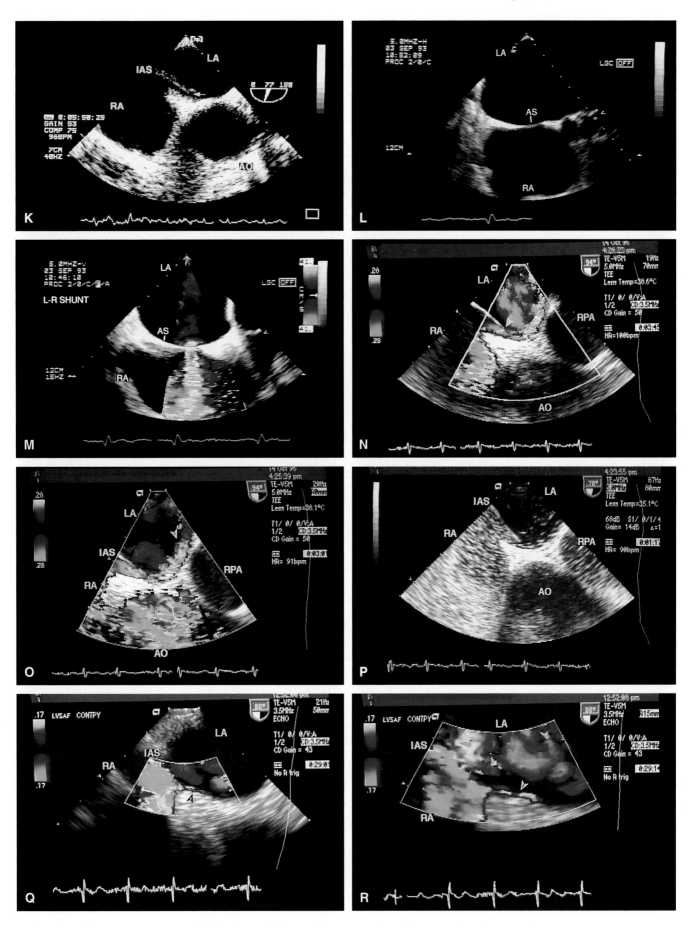

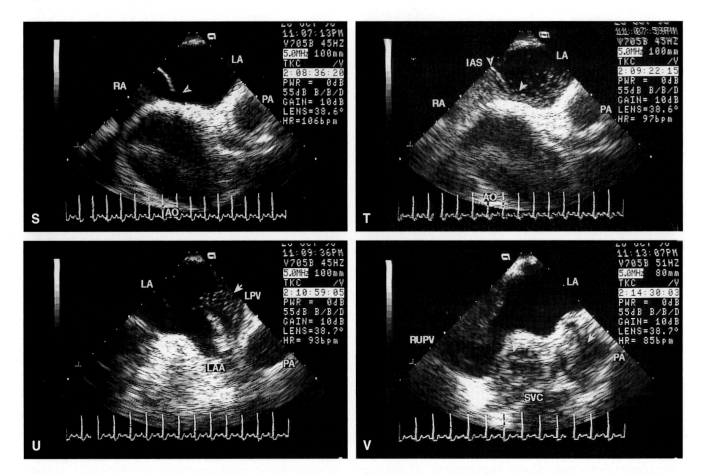

Figure 8.1.2. **Right-to-left shunting in hepatopulmonary syndrome. A,B.** Contrast echoes (arrowheads) appear in the left upper pulmonary vein (LUPV) following IV injection of normal saline. Contrast appeared in the pulmonary vein before appearing in the LA, which indicates that the shunt is at the level of the pulmonary vasculature. This patient has hepatopulmonary syndrome resulting from cirrhosis. In this syndrome, the pulmonary capillaries are dilated, allowing passage of contrast from the right to the left circulation.

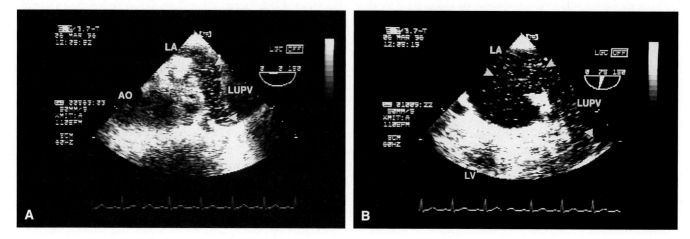

Figure 8.1.3. **Secundum atrial septal defect. A.** Gross specimen shows a large atrial secundum defect (ASD) in the fossa ovalis region. **B.** Schematic shows a secundum ASD. **C.** Arrowheads demonstrate a secundum ASD. Note the enlarged RA. *CT*, crista terminalis. **D,E.** Arrows show a large secundum ASD. Color flow signals are visualized moving from the LA into the RA through the ASD **(E)**. **F.** Secundum ASD in another patient. The defect measures 2.19 cm in the longitudinal plane (right panel) and 0.89 cm in the transverse plane (left panel), which illustrates that it is important to view the defect in multiple planes to assess its true size and extent. **G–J.** Large secundum defect in another patient. Color Doppler examination **(G)** shows a large defect (D) in the interatrial septum (IAS). Color M-mode **(H)** and pulsed Doppler **(I,J)** studies demonstrate the shunt to be left-to-right throughout the cardiac cycle except for a tiny right-to-left component during the isovolumic relaxation period (red signals in **H** and minimal flow signals above the baseline in **I** and **J**). Shunt volume in ASD can be estimated as follows: the maximal Doppler color-flow jet width (cm) at the defect site is taken as the diameter (D) of the defect, which is assumed to be circular. The area of the defect is then calculated using the formula $\pi D^2/4$. The mean velocity of the shunt flow (V) in cm/sec across the defect and the flow duration (T) in sec are next obtained by placing the pulsed Doppler sample volume (SV) at the defect site in the area of brightest or aliased color flow signals and parallel to the flow direction and then applying planimetry to the Doppler spectral trace so obtained over one cardiac cycle. The shunt volume (L/min) across the defect is calculated as a product of the area of the defect, mean velocity, flow duration and heart rate (beats/min) divided by 1000. The diameter of the defect in the patient shown in **G** through **J** was 2 cm, mean shunt flow velocity was 60 cm/sec, flow duration was 0.5 sec, and heart rate 95 beats/min. His shunt volume was calculated as follows: $(\pi D^2/4 \times V \times T \times HR/1000 = 3.14 \times (4/4) \times 60 \times 0.5 \times 95/1000 = 8.95$ L/min. **K,L.** A different patient with secundum atrial septal defect. An eccentric medially directed TR jet is seen moving into the LA through the defect **(K)**. **L.** The patch used to close the defect. **M,N.** Another adult patient with two large secundum-type defects seen by two-dimensional echocardiography **(M)**. Color Doppler study **(N)** demonstrates two large and one very small defect (numbered 1, 2, and 3). These findings were confirmed at surgery. (**G** and **J** reproduced with permission from Mehta RH, Helmcke F, Nanda NC, et al. Transesophageal Doppler color flow mapping assessment of atrial septal defect. J Am Coll Cardiol 1990;16:1010–1016.)

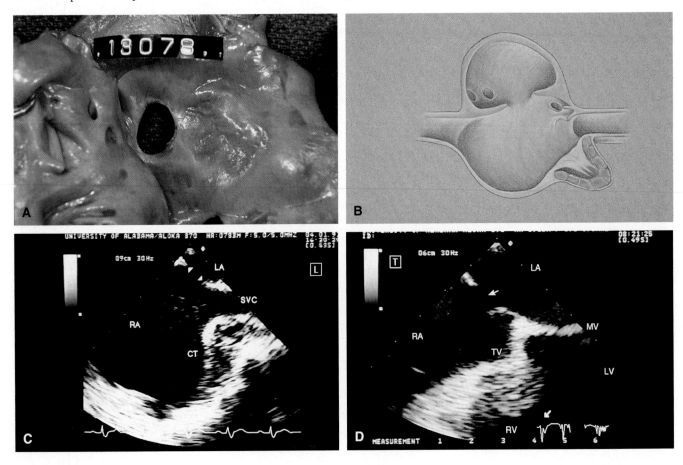

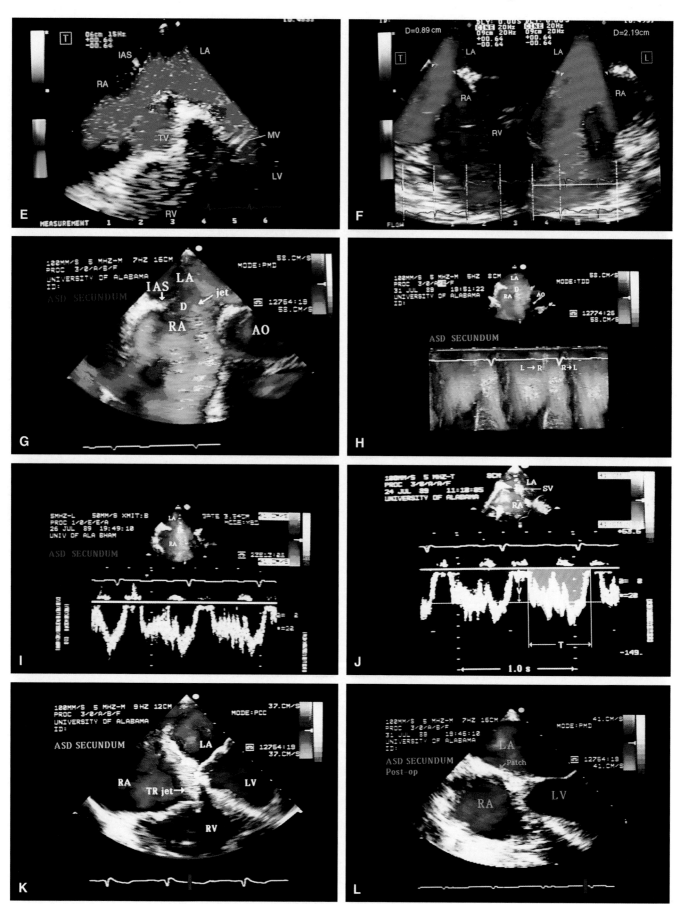

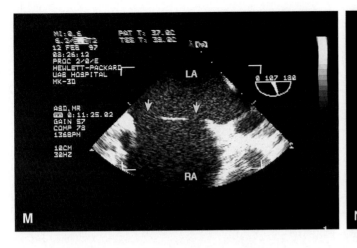

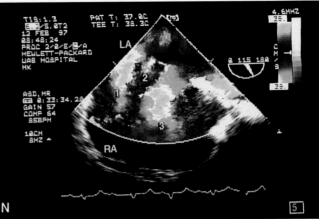

Figure 8.1.4. **Atrial septal aneurysm. A.** Biplane study shows the atrial septal aneurysm (AN) bulging into the RA during systole when examined in the longitudinal plane (right). In the transverse plane (left), the aneurysm appears as a circular structure in the short-axis view. **B.** Transverse plane imaging demonstrates the aneurysm in short axis as it bulges into the RA in systole and its relation to the RAA. **C,D.** Longitudinal plane examination demonstrates the aneurysm bulging into the LA during diastole. **E.** In this view, the transverse plane skims the surface of the aneurysm, resulting in an erroneous appearance of a mass lesion in the LA. **F.** M-mode examination shows the atrial septal aneurysm (arrow) bulging into the LA during diastole and into the RA during systole. The arrow in **G** and **H** shows another patient with an atrial septal aneurysm, which mimics a LA cyst in **H**. *P*, pericardial effusion; *RPA*, right pulmonary artery. (**A** through **F** reproduced with permission from Zboyovsky KL, Nanda NC, Jain H. Transesophageal echocardiographic identification of atrial septal aneurysm. Echocardiography 1991;8:435–437.)

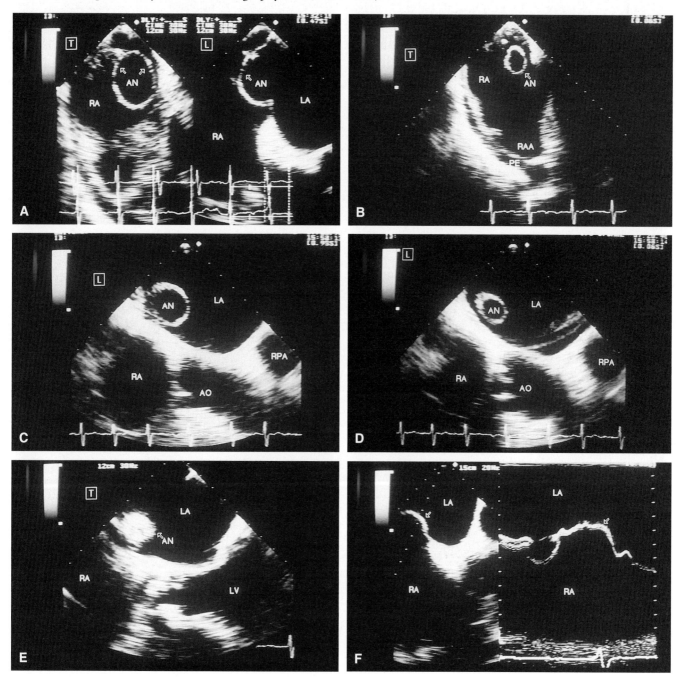

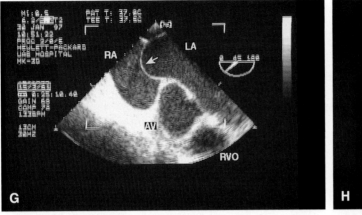

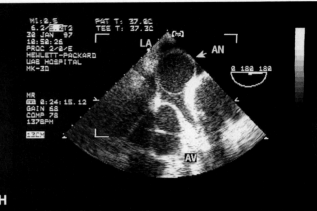

Figure 8.1.5. Partial atrioventricular septal (canal) defect. **A–C.** A large defect (D) is shown in the basal (inferior) portion of the atrial septum with no intact septum separating it from the attachment of the atrioventricular valves. **B.** Color Doppler examination demonstrates flow signals moving from the LA through the defect into the RA, then through the open TV into the RV. **C.** Color M-mode shows left-to-right shunting throughout the cardiac cycle except for a very small right-to-left component (dark red signals) occurring during the isovolumic relaxation period. **D–F.** Another patient with a partial atrioventricular canal defect. **D.** Left-to-right shunt (arrow) in the basal portion of the atrial septum. **E.** An associated PFO (arrow). **F.** Patch closure (arrow) of the defect. Note absence of shunting. **G.** Schematic demonstrates a large atrioventricular canal defect, an aneurysm of the membranous ventricular septum, and mitral regurgitant flow passing through the defect into the RA. **H–J.** Another patient with partial atrioventricular canal defect. In **H,** the arrow points to the defect and the arrowhead to prolapse of the anterior mitral leaflet. **I,J.** Color Doppler examination shows left-to-right shunting (arrowhead in **I**) through the defect. (**A** reproduced with permission from Mehta RH, Helmcke F, Nanda NC, et al. Transesophageal Doppler color flow mapping assessment of atrial septal defect. J Am Coll Cardiol 1990;16:1010–1016.)

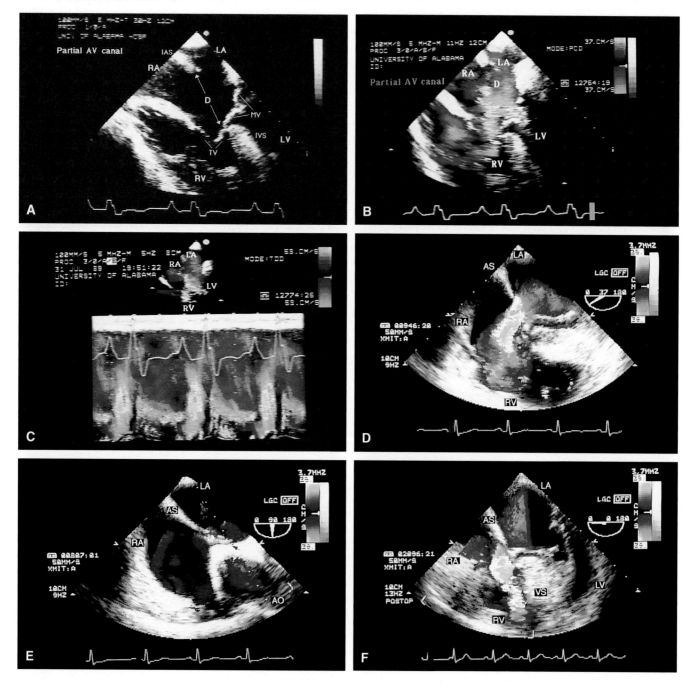

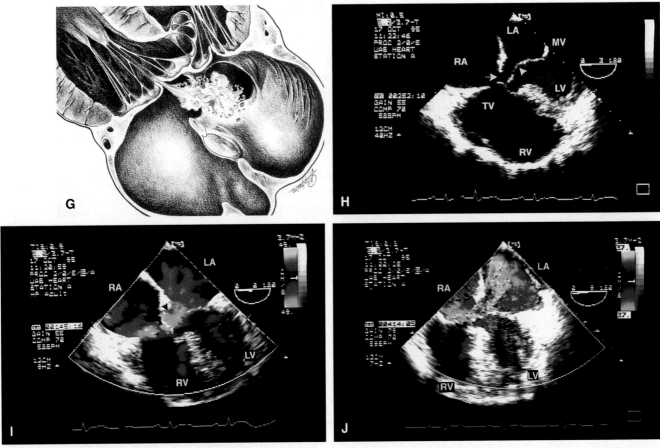

Figure 8.1.6. **Sinus venosus atrial septal defect. A.** Gross specimen shows a large sinus venosus atrial septal defect (ASD). **B–E.** A large defect is seen in the superior portion of the atrial septum, with flow signals (arrows) moving from the LA through the defect to the RA in **C** and from the RA to the LA in **D. E.** The SVC is seen straddling the atrial septum. Flow signals (arrow) are seen moving from the anomalous RUPV into the RA and then through the defect into the LA. **F,G.** Postoperative studies show the patch (upper arrow in **F**, arrow in **G**) used to close the defect.

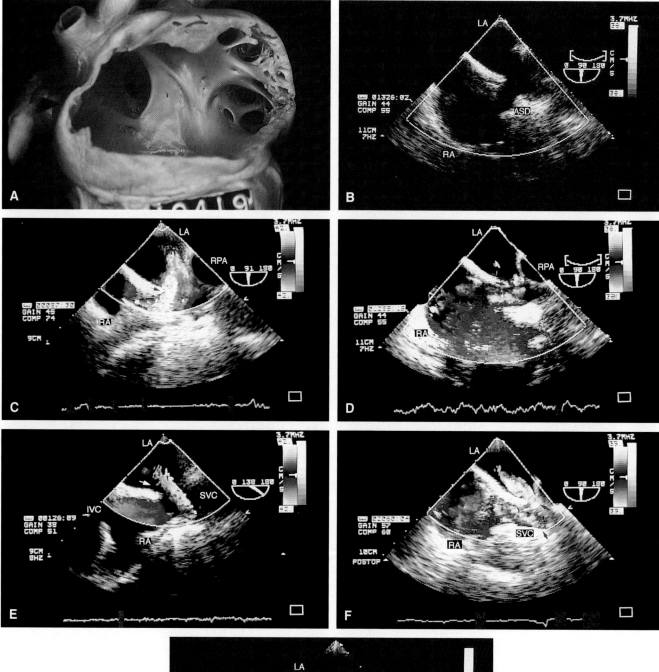

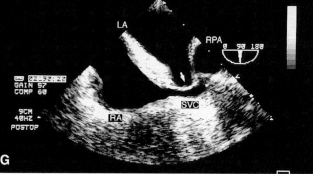

Figure 8.1.7.   **Sinus venosus atrial septal defect. A,B.** Examination at a plane angulation of 106° demonstrates the defect (D) in the superior portion of the atrial septum. The entrance of SVC into the RA is identified by the presence of the prominent crista terminalis (CT). **C.** Examination at a plane angulation of 76° fails to reveal the presence of the defect in the superior portion of the atrial septum. **D.** Color Doppler examination at a plane angulation of 126° shows the right superior pulmonary vein (RSPV) entering the SVC near its entrance into the RA. This was confirmed at surgery. **E,F.** An associated left superior vena cava (LSVC) is seen entering an enlarged coronary sinus (CS) in **F. G.** The patch (P) used to close the defect. (Reproduced with permission from Maxted W, Finch A, Nanda NC, et al. Multiplane transesophageal echocardiographic detection of sinus venosus atrial septal defect. Echocardiography 1995;12:139–143.)

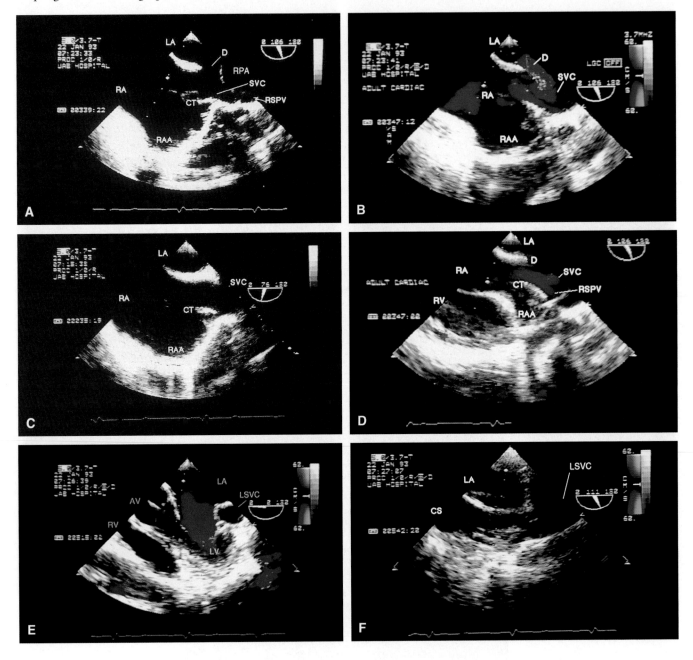

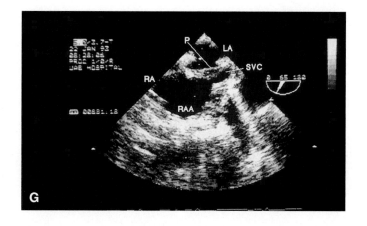

Figure 8.1.8. **Sinus venosus atrial septal defect. A,B.** Examination at a plane angulation of 97° demonstrates the defect (D) in the superior portion of the atrial septum. **C.** Color Doppler examination at a plane angulation of 17° shows the opening of the right superior pulmonary vein (RSPV) into the RA. (Reproduced with permission from Maxted W, Finch A, Nanda NC, et al. Multiplane transesophgeal echocardiographic detection of sinus venosus atrial septal defect. Echocardiography 1995;12:139–143.)

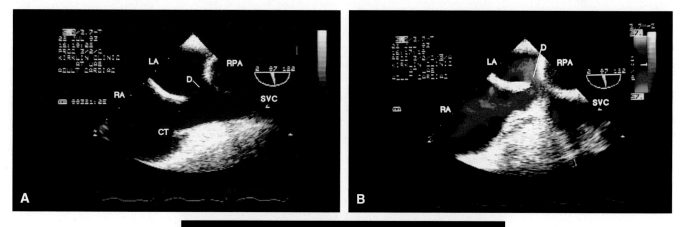

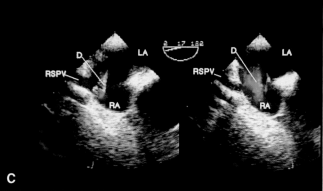

Figure 8.1.9. **Sinus venosus atrial septal defect. A.** A large defect (D) is seen in the transverse and longitudinal planes together with a left-to-right shunt. **B.** A large sinus venosus defect (D) with left-to-right shunting (blue signals) is shown in another patient. Flow signals (red) from an anomalous RUPV are seen moving into the RA and then through the defect into the LA. **C–F.** Another patient with a large sinus venosus defect (D) with left-to-right shunting (D). **E.** Flow signals (red) are seen moving from an anomalous RUPV into RA and then through the defect into LA. **F.** Postoperative study shows patch closure of the defect. RUPV flow signals are now seen entering the LA.

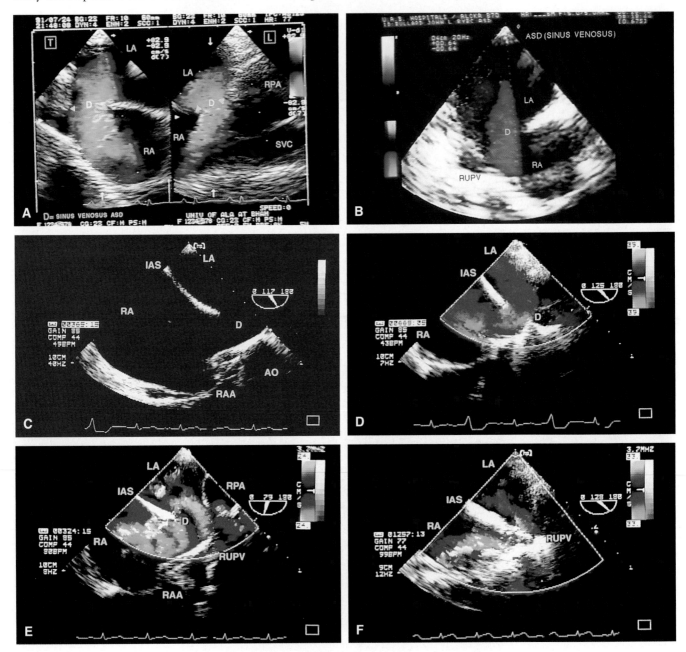

Figure 8.1.10. **Isolated anomalous LUPV drainage. A.** The left upper pulmonary vein (LPV) is imaged in its usual position. **B.** Instead of draining into the LA, the LPV opens into the RA underneath the atrial septum (arrow). **C.** Estimation of shunt flow volume in isolated partial anomalous pulmonary venous connection in another patient. The Doppler spectral trace (right) was obtained by placing the pulsed Doppler sample volume cursor parallel to the flow direction in a pulmonary vein (left; APV), located on the left side but not connected to the LA. The shunt flow volume (L/min) was calculated as a product of the cross-sectional area of the APV (obtained by the formula $\pi D^2/4$, with D equal to 0.98 cm, representing the lumen width at the site of pulsed Doppler interrogation), the mean flow velocity (38 cm/sec), the flow duration (T, 0.79 second), and the heart rate (84 beats/min), and dividing it by 1000. The shunt flow volume was calculated to be 1.90 L/min in this patient. (**C** reproduced with permission from Mehta RH, Jain SP, Nanda NC, et al. Isolated partial anomalous pulmonary venous connection: echocardiographic diagnosis and a new color Doppler method to assess shunt volume. Am Heart J 1991;122:870–873.)

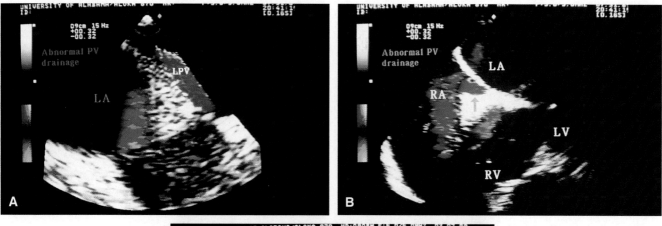

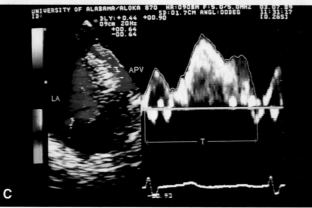

Figure 8.1.11.   Isolated right-sided anomalous pulmonary venous return into the RA. **A.** Simultaneous biplane (*T*, transverse plane; *L*, longitudinal plane) study shows red flow signals (V1) in the area normally occupied by the right superior pulmonary vein. Note that these flow signals do not extend into the LA as they normally should. **B–D.** Longitudinal plane examination. Prominent blue signals are noted in the RA in the vicinity of the right pulmonary artery (RPA) and originating just anterior to the interatrial septum (arrow), just across from where the right superior pulmonary vein signals should normally be seen entering the LA. These represent the RA entrance and course of the flow signals from the anomalous pulmonary vein (V1). **D.** Spatial waveform obtained by pulsed Doppler interrogation of V₁. (Reproduced with permission from Sanyal RS, Nanda NC, Snell D, et al. Transesophageal echocardiographic findings of complete unilateral anomalous pulmonary venous connection of right lung to right atrium. Echocardiography 1994;11:93–100.)

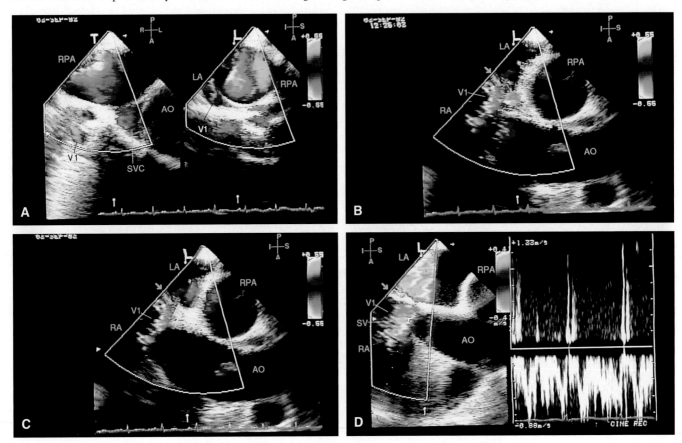

Figure 8.1.12. **Isolated right-sided anomalous pulmonary venous return into the RA.** Same patient as in Figure 8.1.11. **A–D.** Longitudinal planes. **A,B.** The extracardiac course and entrance of the second anomalous pulmonary vein (V2) into the RA are seen. **C,D.** The IVC is separately visualized and enters the RA more posteriorly. **E.** The left superior pulmonary vein (LSPV) enters the left atrium (LA) normally. (Reproduced with permission from Sanyal RS, Nanda NC, Snell D, et al. Transesophageal echocardiographic findings of complete unilateral anomalous pulmonary venous connection of right lung to right atrium. Echocardiography 1994;11:93–100).

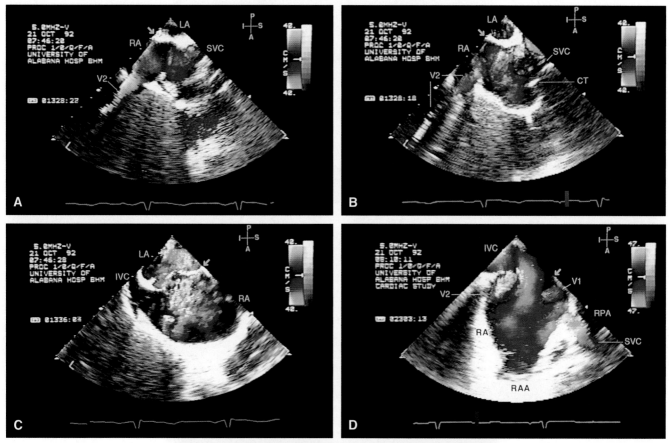

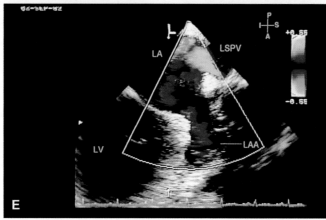

Figure 8.1.13. **Isolated right-sided anomalous venous return into RA.** Same patient as in Figure 8.1.11 and 8.1.12. Transverse plane. Following surgery, pulmonary vein flow signals from the right side (RPV) are seen entering the LA posterior to the surgically inserted patch (P). (Reproduced with permission from Sanyal RS, Nanda NC, Snell D, et al. Transesophageal echocardiographic findings of complete unilateral anomalous pulmonary venous connection of right lung to right atrium. Echocardiography 1994;11:93–100.)

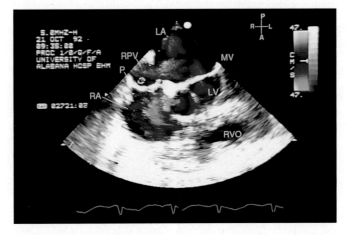

Figure 8.1.14. **Left-sided SVC. A–F.** The large rounded echo-free space lateral to the MV in **A** is the left-sided superior vena cava (LSVC). Longitudinal plane examination **(B,C)** demonstrates the LSVC imaged anterior to the left atrium **(B). C.** Following intravenous left arm injection of normal saline, contrast signals are seen in the LSVC. **D–G.** The LSVC imaged behind the aortic arch (ACH) in the same patient. **E–G.** Contrast signals (arrowheads) in the LSVC following intravenous left arm injection of normal saline. In suspected cases, contrast echocardiography is useful in confirming the diagnosis.

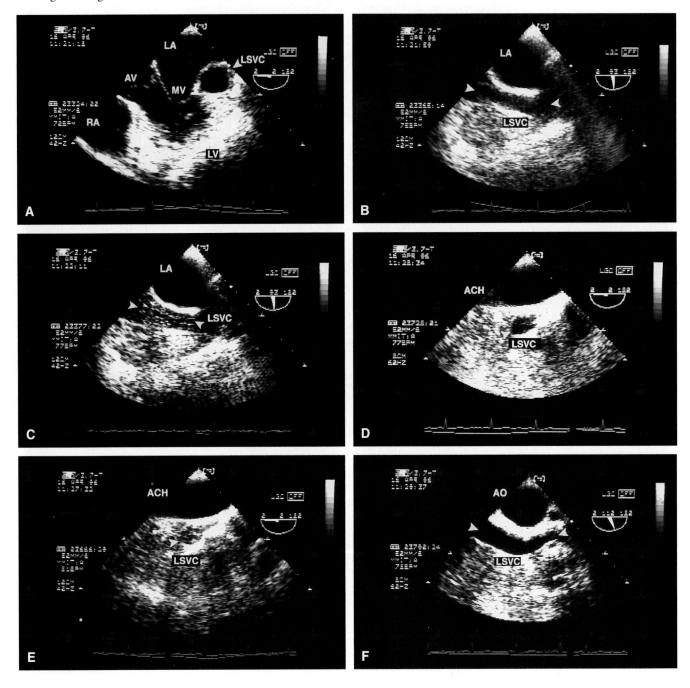

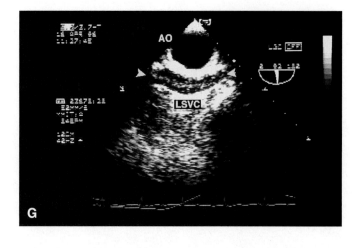

Figure 8.1.15. **Left-sided SVC**. Diagrammatic representation of left-sided superior vena cava (LSVC) draining into the coronary sinus (CS). *Left:* The more common course of the LSVC, anterior to the left pulmonary artery (LPA). *Right:* The much less common course of LSVC, posterior to the LPA. *LAZ*, left azygos vein; *LPV*, left-sided pulmonary veins; *RAZ*, right azygos vein; *RSVC*, right-sided superior vena cava. (Reproduced with permission from Nanda NC, Pinheiro L, Sanyal R, et al. Transesophageal echocardiographic examination of left-sided superior vena cava and azygos and hemiazygos veins. Echocardiography 1991;8:731–740.)

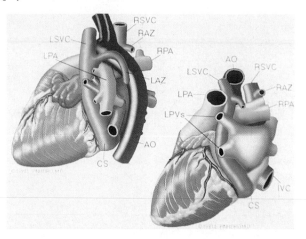

Figure 8.1.16. **Left-sided SVC draining into the coronary sinus.** A 47-year-old man with nephrotic syndrome and no other congenital cardiac abnormality. **A.** Transverse (T) imaging planes. The five-chamber (left) view shows enlargement of the coronary sinus (CS), resulting from drainage of the left-sided superior vena cava (LSVC), which is imaged in the aortic short-axis plane (right). **B.** Longitudinal (L) imaging planes. The two-chamber plane (left) views both the LSVC and the CS, but fails to show their continuity. Counterclockwise rotation of the transducer from this position shifts the plane to the left, resulting in a long-axis delineation of the LSVC and its entrance into the CS (right). **C.** The relationship of enlarged CS to left circumflex coronary artery (LCX) viewed in transverse and longitudinal planes. **D,E.** Composite illustrations shows the connection of the LSVC to the CS and their relationship to adjacent cardiac structures. The images used to generate each of these composites were taken from three different but adjacent transverse planes obtained by rotation with slight withdrawal of the probe when imaging the LSVC. **E, inset.** A spectral trace obtained from color Doppler–guided pulsed Doppler interrogation of the LSVC. **F,G.** Another set of composite illustrations, each acquired by combining two adjacent transverse plane images. These demonstrate the LSVC and left azygos vein (LAZ) and their relation to other cardiac structures. **H.** Longitudinal plane examination shows the relationship of the right SVC to the right pulmonary artery (RPA, left) and the relationship of the LSVC to the left pulmonary artery (LPA, right). The RSVC was imaged by clockwise rotation of the transducer so that the plane was shifted to the right (*1* in the inset), whereas the LSVC was imaged by counterclockwise rotation, which moved the plane to the left (*2* in the inset). **I.** Transverse plane examination demonstrates the LSVC located anterior to the LPA (left). The image on the right, obtained by slightly withdrawing the transducer, shows the entrance of the LAZ into the LSVC. Because the LAZ enters the LSVC in almost a perpendicular manner, the axes of the vessels are practically at right angles to each other. In this instance, the LAZ is imaged in long axis, whereas the LSVC is viewed in short axis. These images were obtained by withdrawing the transducer to acquire a standard transesophageal plane, which views the distal ascending aorta in short axis together with the main pulmonary artery bifurcation and then rotating the transducer counterclockwise to move the plane to the left. **J.** Transverse and longitudinal plane examination demonstrates the relation of the LAZ to the descending thoracic aorta (DA). These planes were obtained by advancing the transducer and rotating it counterclockwise (plane moves to the left) from the position used to obtain images shown in **I**. *PE*, pericardial effusion. (Reproduced with permission from Nanda NC, Pinheiro L, Sanyal R, et al. Transesophageal echocardiographic examination of left-sided superior vena cava and azygos and hemiazygos veins. Echocardiography 1991;8:731–740.)

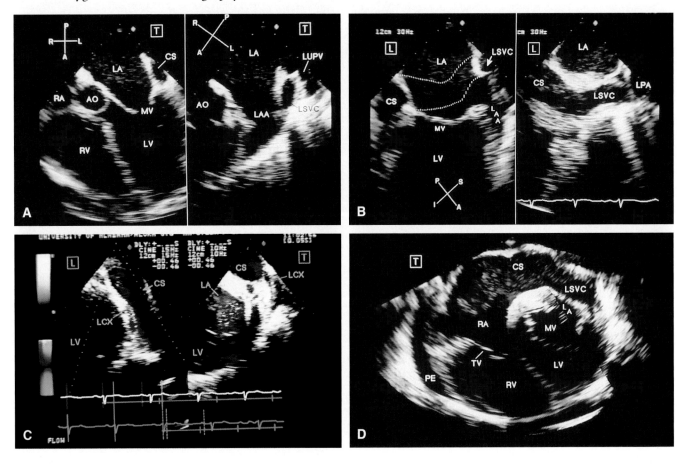

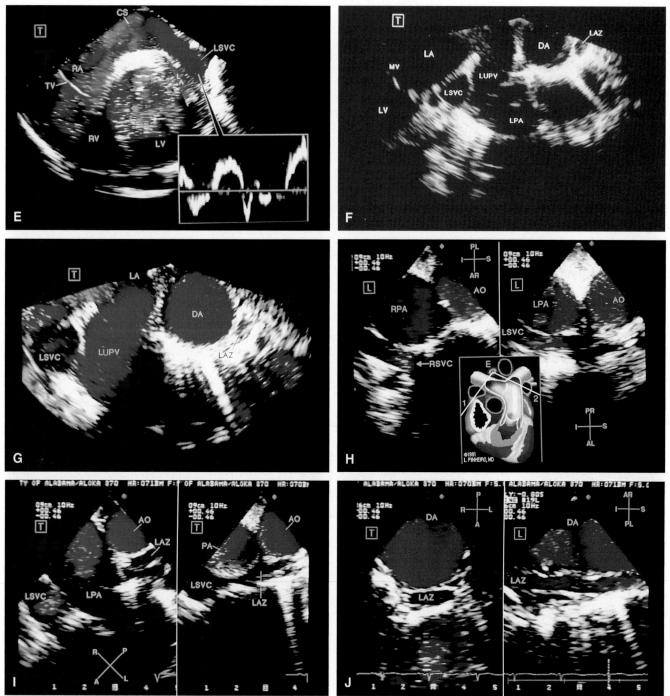

Figure 8.1.17. **Left-sided SVC draining into the coronary sinus**. A 40-year-old woman, status post-repair of an atrial septal defect, presented with systemic hypertension, left ventricular hypertrophy, and mitral regurgitation (MR). **A.** Four-chamber view shows a dilated coronary sinus (CS) resulting from the drainage of the left-sided superior vena cava (LSVC), noted at surgery for repair of atrial septal defect. Contrast injection into a left arm vein using normal saline demonstrates contrast echoes in the CS, RA, and RV. **B.** Transverse plane examination (left) at the level of the aortic root (AO) demonstrates the relationship of the LSVC to the LAA and left upper pulmonary vein (LUPV). Longitudinal plane examination (right) demonstrates the coexistence of a right-sided superior vena cava (RSVC). **C,D.** Composite illustrations prepared by combining two transverse plane images obtained by rotation of the transesophageal probe demonstrate an enlarged CS entering the RA. The inset in **D** represents a spectral trace obtained by color Doppler–guided pulsed Doppler interrogation of the CS. **E.** Longitudinal plane examination. The two-chamber view (left) shows marked enlargement of the CS. Note also the presence of MR in this systolic frame. Withdrawing the probe and rotating it counterclockwise (to shift the plane to the left) brings into view the entrance of the LSVC into the CS (right). **F.** The probe is withdrawn further to the level where the distal ascending aorta and the main pulmonary artery bifurcation are visualized. When the probe is rotated counterclockwise (to move the plane to the left), it demonstrates the LSVC (imaged in short axis) to be located posterior to the LPA and in the vicinity of the AO in this transverse plane examination (left), in contrast to Figure 8.1.11, where the LSVC was located anterior to the LPA. In the longitudinal plane examination (right), the LSVC is imaged in long axis. **G.** Withdrawing the probe and rotating it counterclockwise to image the proximal DA brings into view the LAZ, which is seen to enter LSVC in the transverse plane examination (left). Longitudinal plane examination (right, top) shows a posterior intercostal vein (ICV) joining the LAZ posterior to the DA, viewed in long axis. The spectral trace (right, bottom) was obtained by color Doppler–guided pulsed Doppler interrogation of the ICV. LAZ = left azygos vein. (Reproduced with permission from Nanda NC, Pinheiro L, Sanyal R, et al. Transesophageal echocardiographic examination of left-sided superior vena cava and azygos and hemiazygos veins. Echocardiography 1991;8:731–740.)

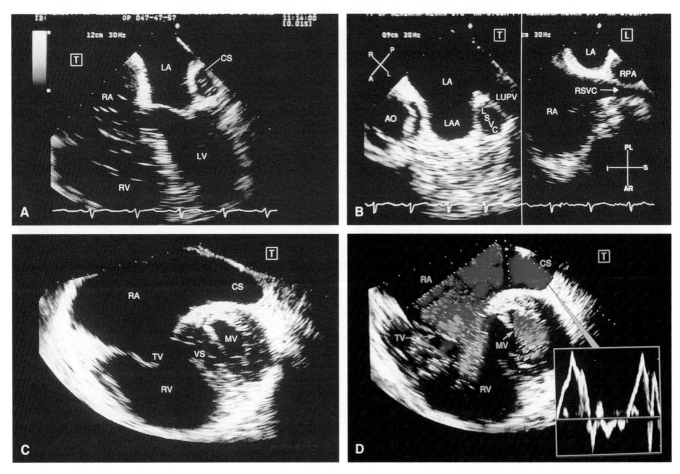

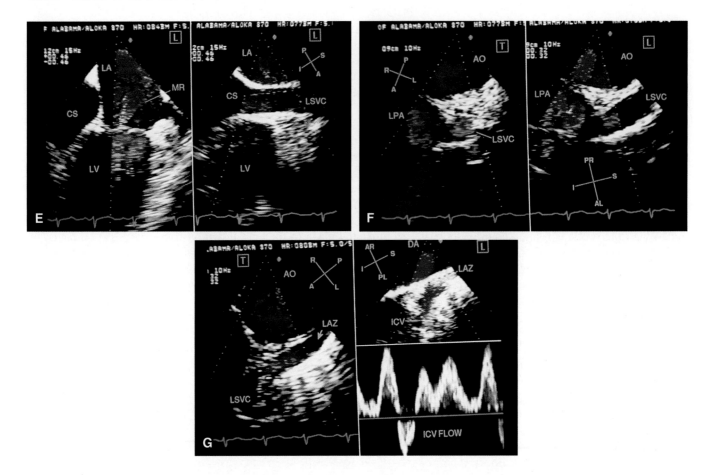

Figure 8.1.18. **Left-sided SVC entering the coronary sinus.** A 20-year-old man with tetralogy of Fallot and pulmonary atresia. In this patient, the IVC also drained into the coronary sinus (CS). The right superior vena cava (RSVC) drained normally into the RA. **A.** Transverse plane examination shows enlargement of the CS due to LSVC drainage (left). Longitudinal plane examination (right) shows the left azygos vein (LAZ) joining the LSVC. **B,C.** Composite illustrations, each prepared by placing together contiguous images obtained during transverse **(B)** and longitudinal **(C)** plane examinations. The IVC is clearly seen entering the CS. This finding and the presence of LSVC were confirmed angiographically. *HV,* hepatic vein. (Reproduced with permission from Nanda NC, Pinheiro L, Sanyal R, et al. Transesophageal echocardiographic examination of left-sided superior vena cava and azygos and hemiazygos veins. Echocardiography 1991;8:731–740.)

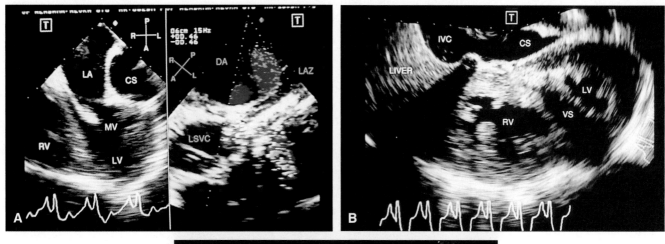

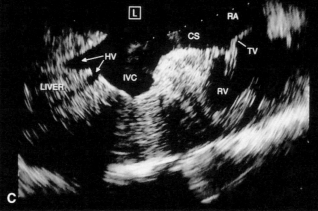

Figure 8.1.19. **Left-sided SVC. A,B.** Enlargement of the coronary sinus (CS) resulting from anomalous drainage of the left-sided SVC. **C.** Pulsed Doppler interrogation of the enlarged coronary sinus shows prominent flow signals throughout the cardiac cycle. *LPV*, left upper pulmonary vein.

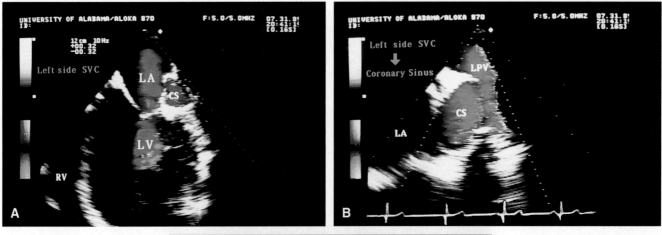

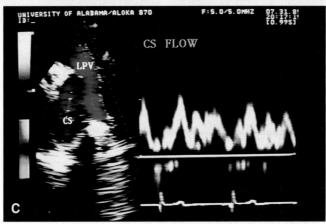

Figure 8.1.20. Left-sided SVC. **A,B.** Relationship of the left-sided superior vena cava (LSVC) to the LUPV and LA. **C.** Contrast signals (arrowheads) moving from the markedly enlarged coronary sinus (CS) into the RA following a left arm vein saline contrast injection. The coronary sinus is enlarged as a result of the increased (anomalous) flow. **D.** Pulsed Doppler interrogation of the LSVC imaged behind the aorta in the same patient shows continuous flow throughout the cardiac cycle (arrowheads).

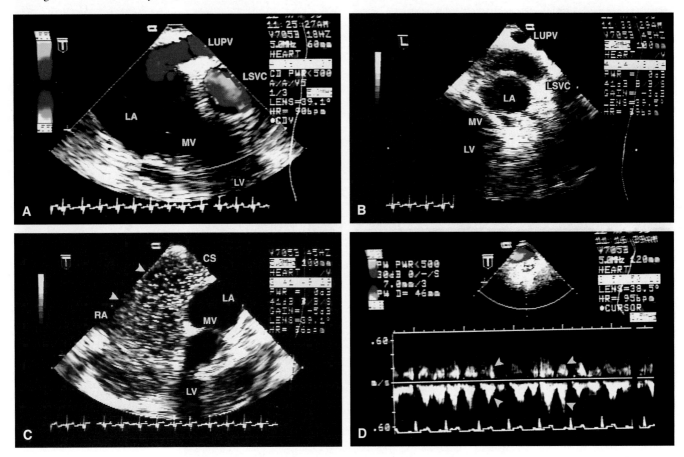

Figure 8.1.21. **Ventricular septal aneurysm. A,B.** An aneurysm (arrows) of the membranous septum bulging into the RV. **C,D.** Another patient with a trabecular ventricular septal aneurysm (arrows) associated with a defect. Flow signals are seen moving from LV to RV through the ventricular septal defect. **E.** Associated severe TR.

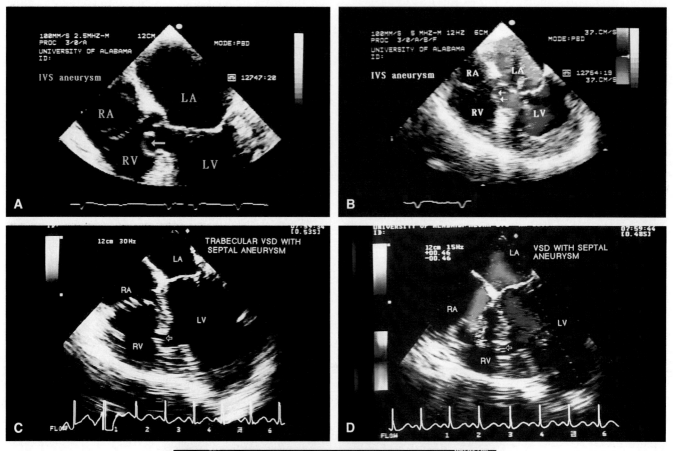

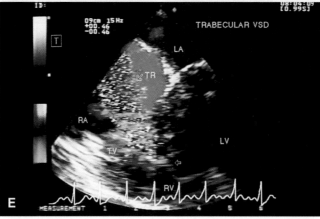

Figure 8.1.22. **Perimembranous ventricular septal defect.** The defect (D in **A** and the arrow in **B**) is demonstrated together with an aneurysm (AN) of the ventricular septum.

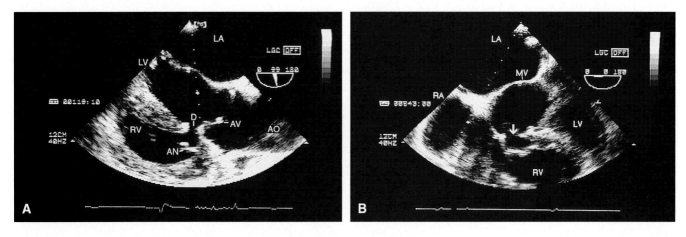

Figure 8.1.23. Trabecular ventricular septal defect. A large defect (D) is seen in the trabecular (muscular) portion of the ventricular septum (VS).

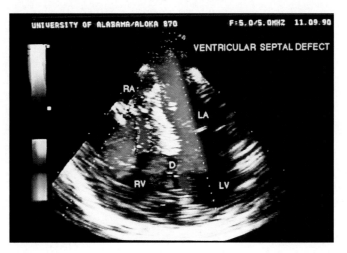

Figure 8.1.24. Perimembranous ventricular septal defect. **A–E.** A large defect (D) is seen just below the tricuspid and aortic valves with flow signals (arrow in **B**) moving through it into the RV. **C.** A large zone of flow acceleration (arrow) on the LV side of the defect. Color Doppler–guided continuous wave Doppler shows a high velocity of 5 m/sec. Using the Bernoulli equation, this translates into a pressure gradient of 100 mm Hg across the defect. Because this patient's systolic blood pressure was 125 mm Hg, the PA systolic pressure is estimated to be about 25 mm Hg. Thus, pulmonary hypertension is absent. **E.** A smaller second VSD (D2) is noted in addition to the large defect (D1) seen earlier. **F,G.** A perimembranous ventricular septal defect (arrowheads) with left-to-right shunting in another patient. **H,I.** Schematics show a perimembranous VSD.

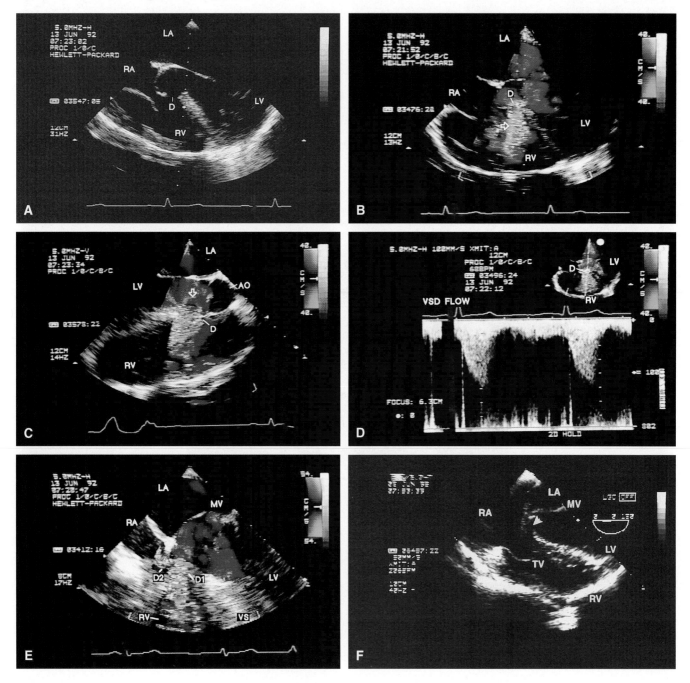

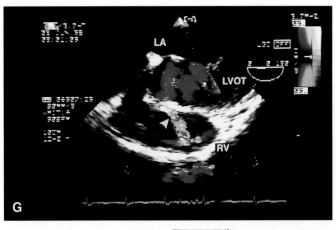

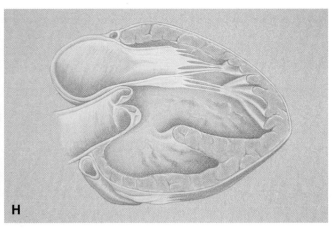

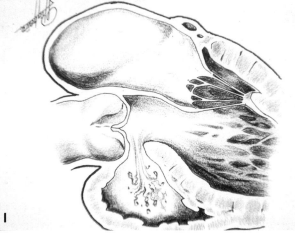

Figure 8.1.25. **Ventricular septal defect associated with atrial septal defect. A.** A large ventricular septal defect (open arrow) and an associated secundum atrial septal defect (closed arrow). **B,C.** Color Doppler examination. **B.** Flow signals moving from the LA to the RA (upper arrow) and from the LV to the RV (lower arrow). **C.** The ventricular septal defect is seen just underneath the TV, demonstrating its perimembranous location.

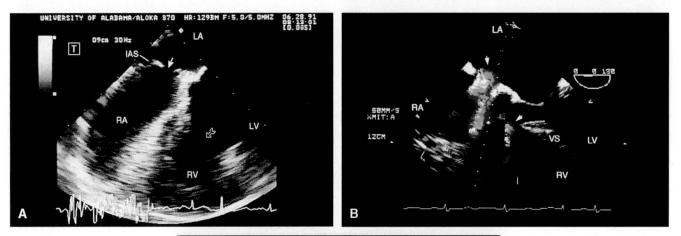

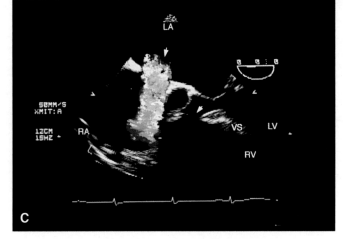

Figure 8.1.26. **Ventricular septal defect mimic**. A side-lobe artifact (arrows), which simulates the presence of a ventricular septal defect in all three patients shown here.

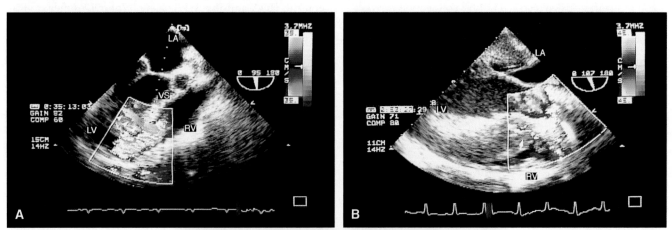

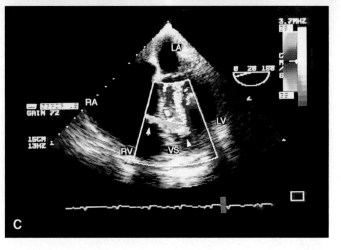

Figure 8.1.27. **Patent ductus arteriosus**. **A,B.** Turbulent flow (arrow) in the main pulmonary artery (MPA) produced by a patent ductus arteriosus (PDA) in this adult patient. **C.** Continuous wave Doppler examination shows flow throughout the cardiac cycle. **D.** The connection (arrow) between the PDA and the MPA. **E–G.** Color Doppler examination also delineates the PDA and its connection with the MPA. **H.** The relationship of the PDA with the MPA and the left pulmonary artery (LPA) is shown. **I.** Schematic shows a PDA. **J,K.** These views, obtained after surgery, show absence of turbulence in the MPA.

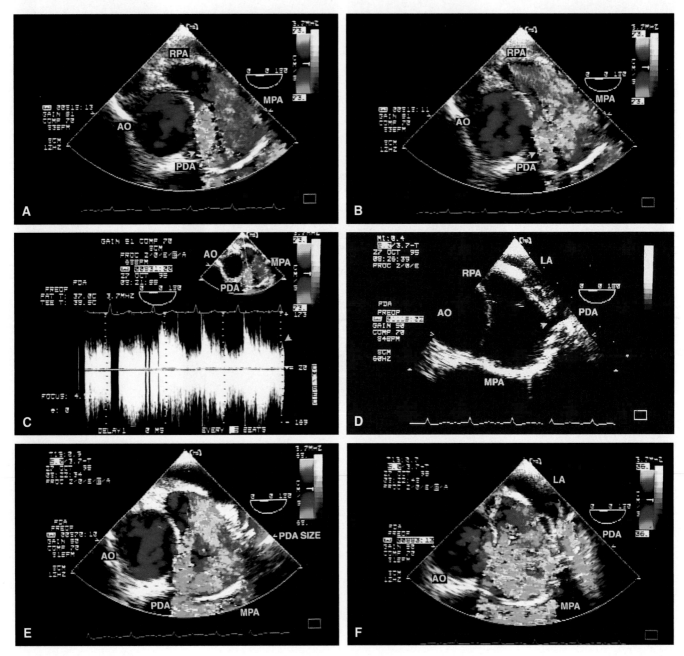

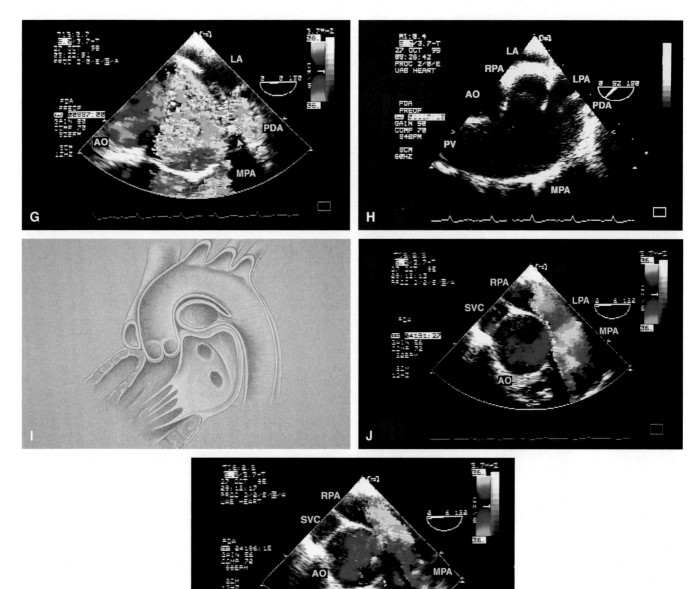

Figure 8.1.28. **Patent ductus arteriosus. A.** Color Doppler examination shows turbulent flow signals moving from the aorta (AO) into the pulmonary artery (PA) through the ductus (PDA). Color M-mode in **B** and pulsed Doppler in **C** show continuous flow throughout the cardiac cycle through the PDA. *DA*, descending aorta; *SV*, Doppler sample volume. **D.** Gross specimen shows a PDA.

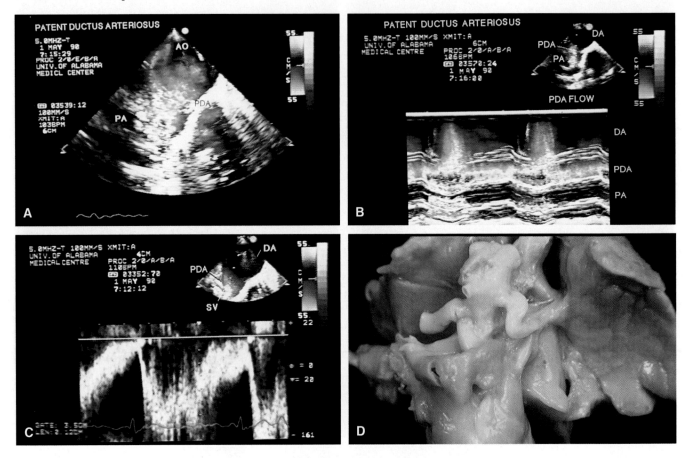

Figure 8.1.29. **Left pulmonary vein obstruction.** **A.** An extensive, thick linear echo indicative of a membrane (M) is seen interposed between dilated left-sided pulmonary veins (PV) and the LA in this 9-year-old boy. **B.** Color Doppler examination. Narrow jet (J) is visualized originating from a small area of discontinuity in the membrane and moving into the LA. The jet measured 2 mm at its origin, indicative of severe obstruction. **C.** High-pulse-repetition-frequency Doppler interrogation of the jet demonstrates a high peak velocity of 1.8 m/sec and continuous flow throughout the cardiac cycle with little phasic variation. Note also the presence of spectral broadening, indicative of turbulent flow. **D.** Postoperative study. After surgical repair there is marked increase in proximal jet width, to 7 mm; significant reduction in peak velocity, to 1.3 m/sec; and development of prominent phasic variations. Spectral broadening is still noted and indicates persistence of turbulent flow. **E.** Postoperative study shows pulmonary veins communicating with the LA through two relatively wide channels, one located posteriorly (upper closed arrows) in the usual location of the pulmonary vein—the LA junction, and the other more anteriorly (lower closed and open arrows), representing direct anastomosis of the left common pulmonary vein with the LAA. (Reproduced with permission from Samdarshi TE, Morrow R, Helmcke FR, Nanda NC, Bargeron LM Jr, Pacifico AD. Assessment of pulmonary vein stenosis by transesophageal echocardiography. Am Heart J 1991;122:1495–1498.)

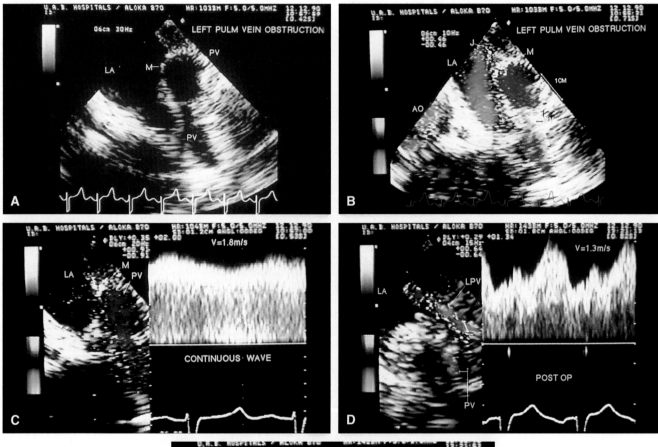

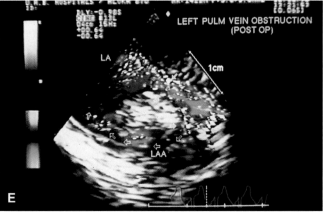

Figure 8.1.30. **Cor triatriatum. A.** Schematic shows a membrane separating the LA into two chambers, with pulmonary veins on one side and the LAA on the other. Notice the small orifice in the membrane causing obstruction to blood flow. **B–I.** An adult patient with a cor triatriatum membrane (arrowheads). In **F** through **H**, the membrane appears to be an extension of the "Q-tip" separating the LAA from the LUPV. In **E**, the membrane (arrowheads) appears to have a double attachment to the interatrial septum (IAS). **G,I.** Color Doppler examination shows laminar flow signals moving through the membrane, indicative of absence of obstruction. **J,K.** Another adult patient with cor triatriatum. **J.** A wide opening (1.4 cm; arrow) in the membrane is seen separating the LUPV from the LAA. **K.** Color Doppler study demonstrates some turbulence, but the peak velocity measured less than 1 m/sec, indicating absence of any significant obstruction to flow.

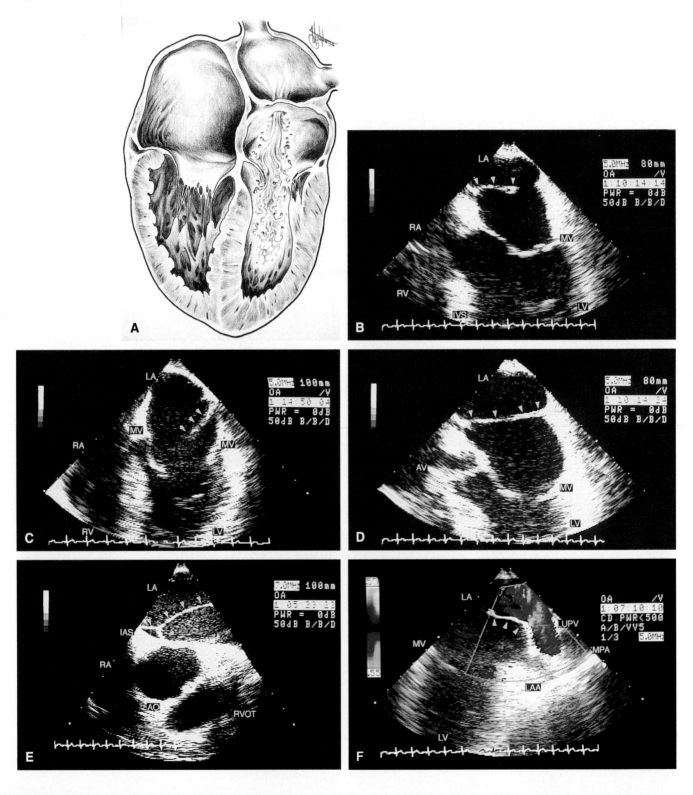

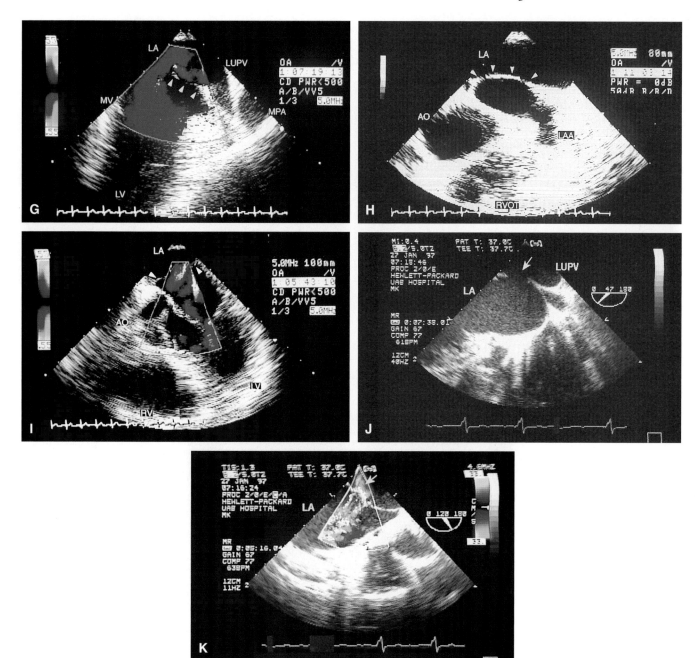

Figure 8.1.31. **Congenital mitral stenosis.** Diastolic frames demonstrate thickened mitral leaflets with a very small orifice and a narrow flow jet (arrow in **B**), indicative of severe stenosis. Note the unobstructed opening of the TV in **A**. This patient was known to have mitral stenosis since childhood.

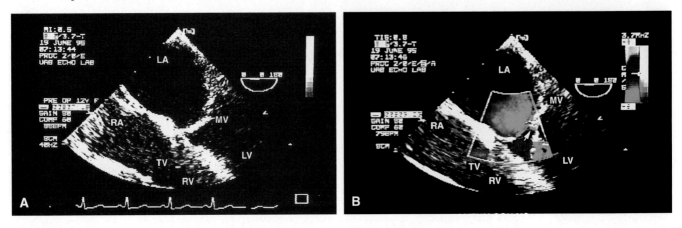

Figure 8.1.32. **Abnormal papillary muscle insertion.** The papillary muscle inserts directly into the anterior mitral leaflet. Note the absence of the chordae tendinae.

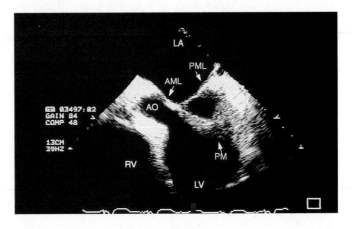

Figure 8.1.33. **Discrete subaortic membranous stenosis.** The arrows in **A, C,** and **D** and *MB* in **B** point to a prominent subaortic membrane. **E.** Two jets (arrowheads) of moderate AR. **F.** Postoperative study shows absence of the membrane in the LVOT.

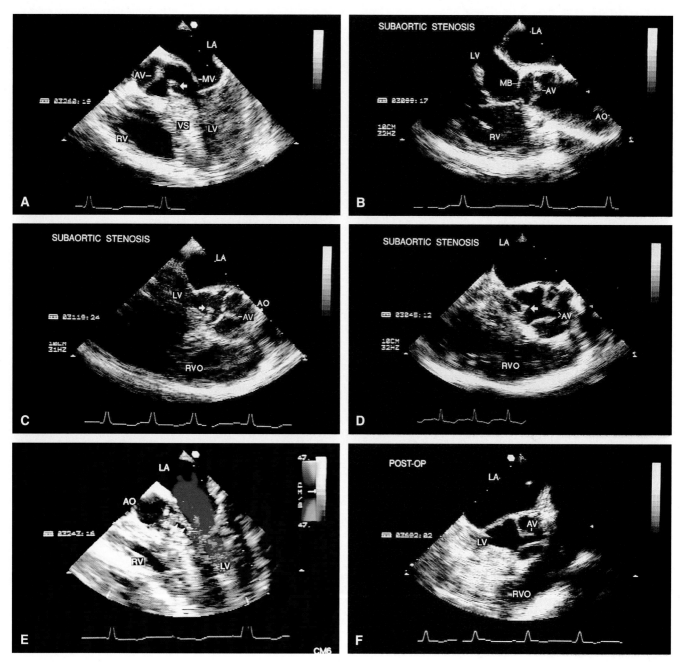

Figure 8.1.34. **Discrete subaortic membranous stenosis. A,B.** A discrete membrane (arrows) is shown attached to the base of an aortic cusp in **A** and to the anterior mitral leaflet in **B. C.** Flow acceleration and turbulence in the LVOT (arrowhead) produced by the membrane. **D.** Postoperative study shows widening of the LVOT and absence of the membrane.

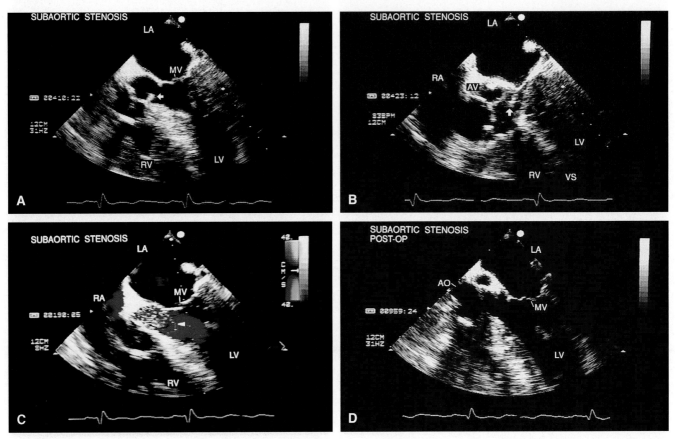

Figure 8.1.35. **Discrete subaortic membranous stenosis. A,B.** The membrane (M) is clearly separated from the AV cusps. **C.** Prominent early systolic preclosure of the AV (arrow) with coarse fluttering typical of this entity. **D.** The attachment of the membrane (M) to the base of the anterior mitral leaflet is well seen.

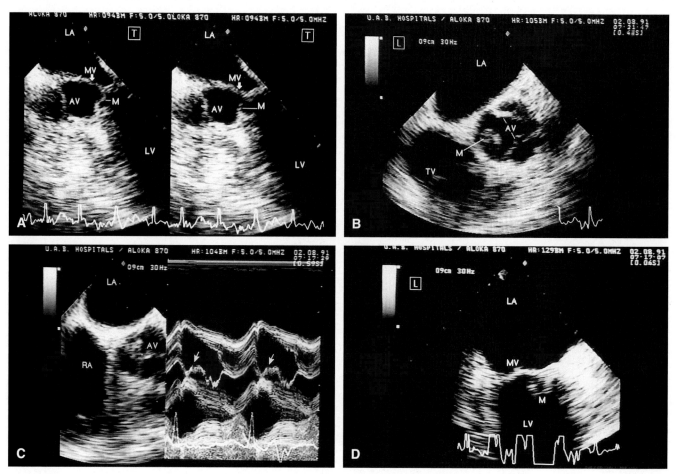

Figure 8.1.36. **Discrete subaortic membranous stenosis. A.** A narrow jet (arrow) in the LVOT results from obstruction produced by a subaortic membrane. **B.** Gross specimen of the subaortic membrane resected from the patient shown in **A.**

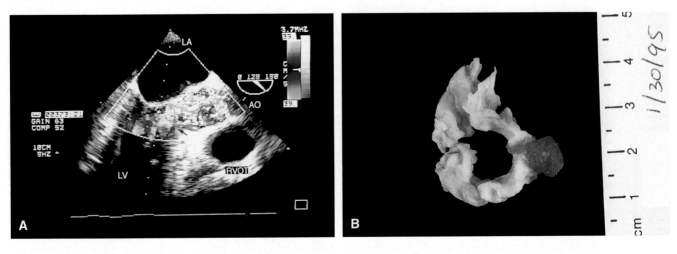

Figure 8.1.37. **Discrete subaortic membranous stenosis.** Modified Konno's operation. In this patient the LVOT was widened by surgically creating a ventricular septal defect and then closing it with a patch. **A.** During systole the patch bulges into the RV, widening the LVOT. **B.** Color Doppler examination shows minimal turbulence in the LVOT. Note the presence of associated mild MR in this patient.

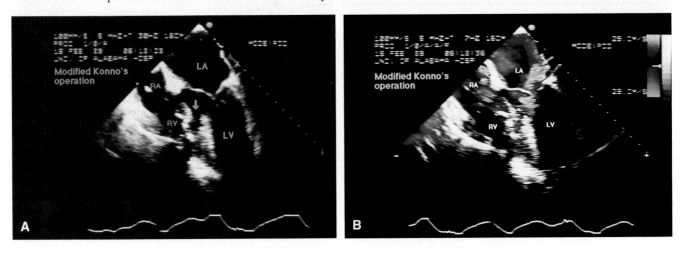

Figure 8.1.38. Bicuspid AV. **A.** A vertically oriented, redundant bicuspid AV in diastole. **B.** Another patient with a vertically oriented bicuspid valve with restricted opening, consistent with stenosis. **C.** Schematic corresponds to the echo image in **B**. **D,E.** Two other patients show an obliquely oriented bicuspid aortic valve (AOV in **E**) with a raphe (R in **E**) that extends from the anterior cusp to the aortic wall in both patients.

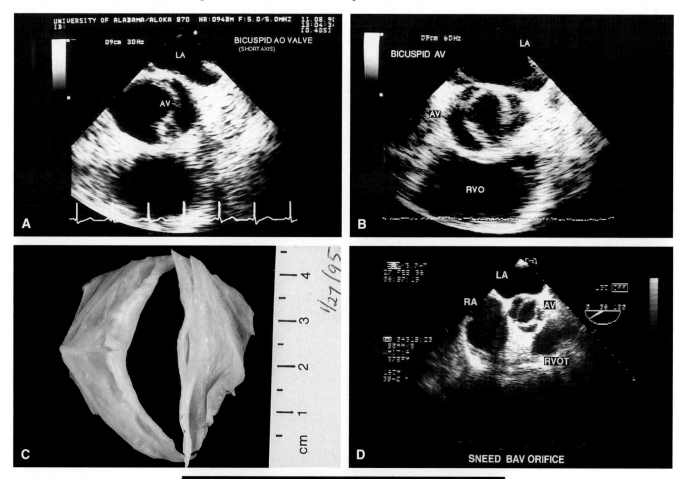

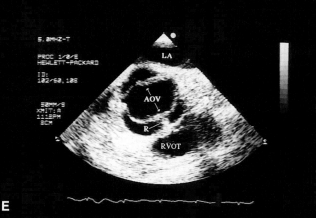

Figure 8.1.39. **Quadricuspid AV. A**. Diastolic frame in a 69-year-old woman clearly shows four aortic cusps with a large eccentrically located area of leaflet noncoaptation. **B**. Systolic frame shows the four cusps in the open position. **C**. Color Doppler examination in the five-chamber view (plane angle 0°) shows mosaic colored signals filling the proximal LVOT completely in diastole, indicative of severe AR. **D**. Color Doppler examination shows flow signals from the AR filling the area of cusp noncoaptation. **A, B**, and **D** were imaged at a plane angle of 44°. *1*, accessory cusp; *2*, left cusp; *3*, right cusp; *4*, noncoronary cusp. (Reproduced with permission from Patel JN, Osman K, Nanda NC, et al. Quadricuspid aortic valve diagnosed by multiplane transesophageal echocardiography. Echocardiography 1994;11:201–205.)

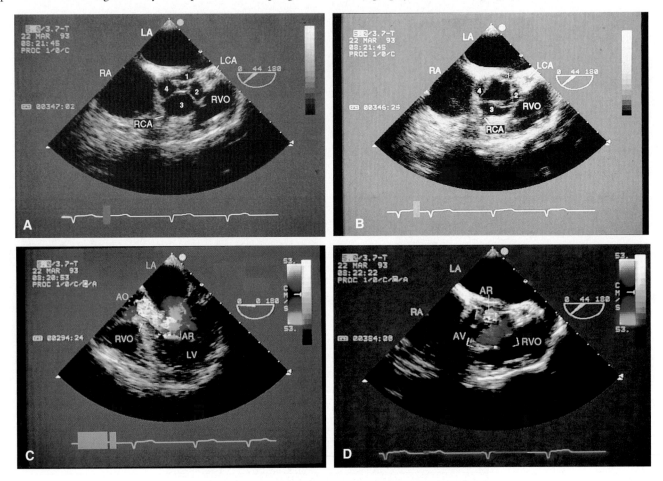

Figure 8.1.40. **Quadricuspid AV mimic**. A redundant tricuspid AV (systolic frame) that mimics a quadricuspid valve in diastole is shown. (Reproduced with permission from Patel JN, Osman K, Nanda NC, et al. Quadricuspid aortic valve diagnosed by multiplane transesophageal echocardiography. Echocardiography 1994;11:201–205.)

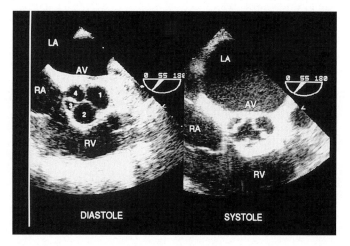

Figure 8.1.41. **Redundant AV**. A myxomatous AV appears to have multiple cusps in diastole (1–6), but in systole only three cusps are seen. Figures 8.1.40 and 8.1.41 underscore the importance of carefully examining the AV throughout the cardiac cycle for assessment of its morphology. (Reproduced with permission from Patel JN, Osman K, Nanda NC, et al. Quadricuspid aortic valve diagnosed by multiplane transesophageal echocardiography. Echocardiography 1994;11: 201–205.)

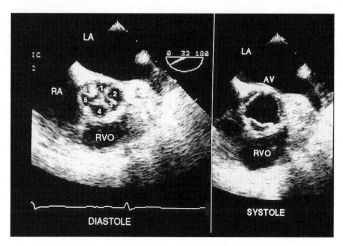

Figure 8.1.42. **Infected quadricuspid AV. A,B.** Transverse plane examination demonstrates four aortic cusps (1, 2, 3, and 4) and a saccular aneurysm (AN) of the noncoronary sinus of Valsalva communicating with the aortic root. **C,D.** The aneurysm also is visualized in the longitudinal plane views. **E.** Color Doppler examination shows mosaic signals completely filling the proximal portion of the LVOT in diastole, indicating the presence of severe AR. This was a 33-year-old man with past drug abuse who presented with a 1-month history of fever and increasing dyspnea on exertion. (Reproduced with permission from Finch A, Osman K, Kim KS, Nanda NC, Willman B, Soto B, Kirklin JK. Transesophageal echocardiographic findings of an infected quadricuspid aortic valve with an anomalous coronary artery. Echocardiography 1994;11:369–375.)

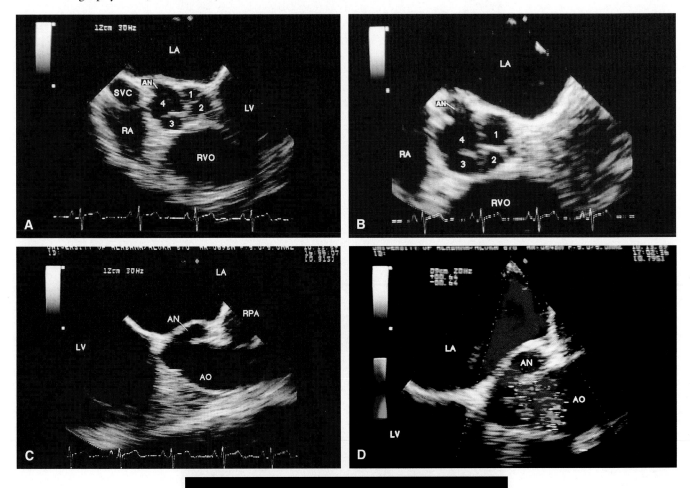

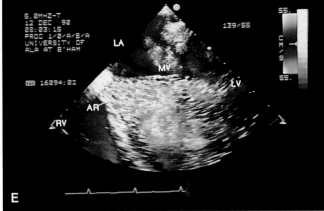

Figure 8.1.43. Infected quadricuspid AV: anomalous origin of right coronary artery from left main coronary artery. Same patient as in Fig. 8.1.42. **A**. Transverse plane aortic short-axis view demonstrates the left main coronary (LM) artery trifurcating into circumflex (CX), ramus (R), and left anterior descending (LAD) branches. **B.** A segment of the right coronary artery (RC) is seen between the aorta (AO) and the RVOT/main PA. Coronary arteriography demonstrated an anomalous right coronary artery arising from the left main coronary artery. (Reproduced with permission from Finch A, Osman K, Kim KS, Nanda NC, Willman B, Soto B, Kirklin JK. Transesophageal echocardiographic findings of an infected quadricuspid aortic valve with an anomalous coronary artery. Echocardiography 1994;11:369–375.)

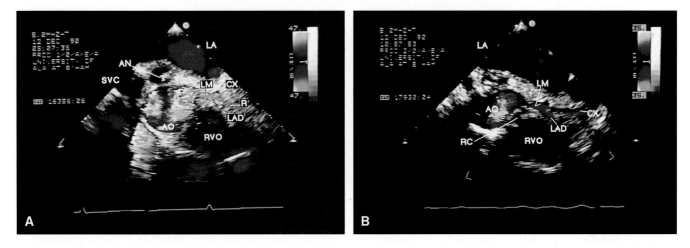

Figure 8.1.44. Unicommissural unicuspid AV. In the long-axis view, the unicuspid valve appears to have two separate leaflets, one large (posterior) and the other smaller (anterior). This appearance mimics a bicuspid aortic valve. (Reproduced with permission from Osman K, Nanda NC, Kim KS, et al. Transesophageal echocardiographic features of unicuspid aortic valve. Echocardiography 1994;11:469–473.)

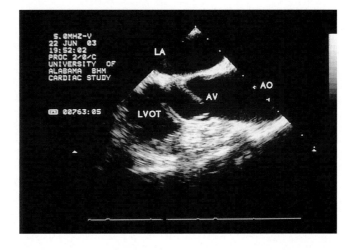

Figure 8.1.45. **Unicommissural unicuspid AV.** Same patient as in Figure 8.1.44. Short-axis view at the level of the AV demonstrates only one commissural attachment to the aortic wall. The inset shows the smallest orifice area. This measures 0.4 cm², indicative of severe stenosis, which was confirmed subsequently by the surgeon. (Reproduced with permission from Osman K, Nanda NC, Kim KS, et al. Transesophageal echocardiographic features of unicuspid aortic valve. Echocardiography 1994;11:469–473.)

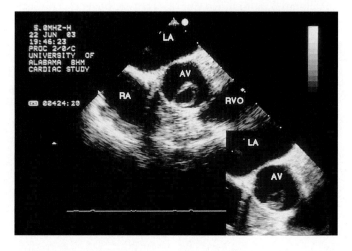

Figure 8.1.46. **Bicuspid AV mimicking unicommissural or acommissural AV. A.** Short-axis view clearly shows two commissural attachments in this patient with a stenotic bicuspid AV (left). In some views it mimicked a unicommissural AV, however, because only one commissural attachment was noted as a result of improper transducer angulation (right). **B.** Short-axis view in another patient with a stenotic bicuspid aortic valve does not show any distinct and convincing commissural attachment, raising the possibility of an acommissural aortic valve (left). This resulted from imaging the valve at the tip rather than the base (right), where the commissural attachments are typically seen. (Reproduced with permission from Osman K, Nanda NC, Kim KS, et al. Transesophageal echocardiographic features of unicuspid aortic valve. Echocardiography 1994;11:469–473.)

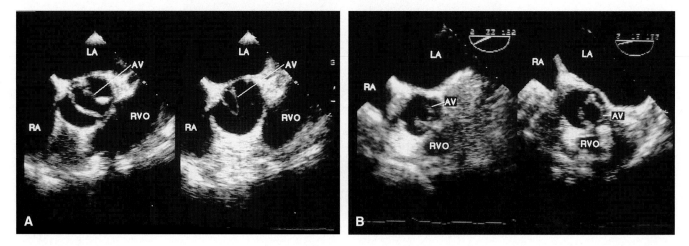

Figure 8.1.47A–M. AV stenosis. A–M. **B** demonstrates systolic doming of the AV consistent with stenosis. **C.** A narrow jet (arrowheads) originates from the AV in systole. **D.** Poststenotic dilatation of the ascending aorta. **E.** The numbers 1, 2, and 3 show the location of short-axis sections in subsequent frames. These sections are taken at the base (3), at the middle of the valve (2), and at the flow-limiting orifice at top of the domed valve (1). The corresponding short-axis views are shown in **F** and **G** (base); **H** and **I** (mid-level); and **J** and **K** (at the top of the domed valve). Note that the minimal valve area (0.83 cm²) is obtained at the flow-limiting orifice at the top of the domed valve and that it corresponds to the catheterization derived aortic valve area. **L.** Composite demonstrates cross-sectional areas at the different locations on the domed valve. **M.** Color Doppler examination shows turbulent flow signals appearing in the AV orifice. To obtain the correct area (flow-limiting orifice) the minimal area must be determined. To do this, the probe must be moved up and down the esophagus until the smallest short-axis area at the top of the domed AV is obtained. Color Doppler is useful in identifying the location of the aortic orifice in patients with calcified valves that do not move in systole. However, planimetry of the color jet overestimates valve area and should not be used. (**L** reproduced with permission from Kim KS, Maxted W, Nanda NC, et al. Comparison of multiplane and biplane transesophageal echocardiography in the assessment of aortic stenosis. Am J Cardiol 1997;79:436–441.)

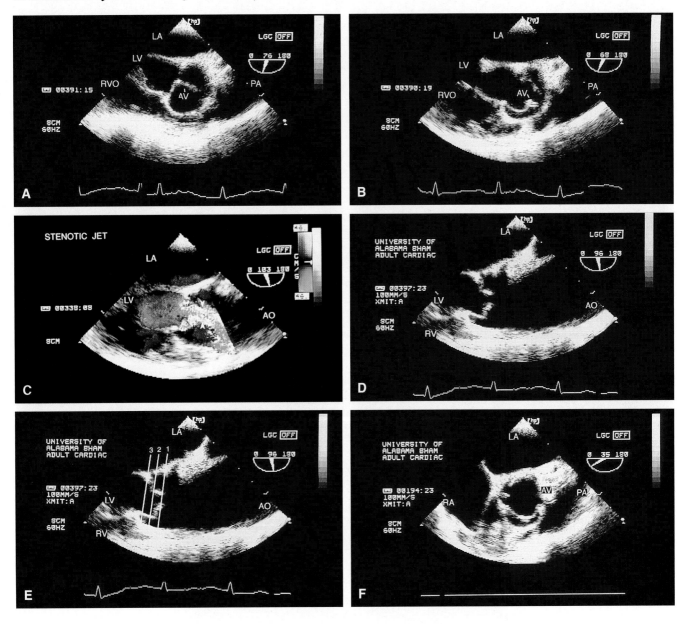

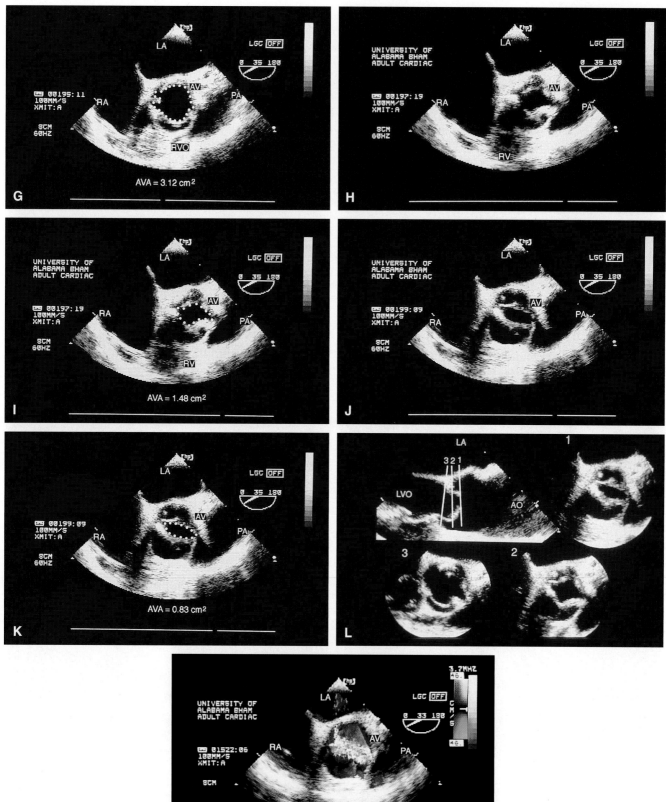

Figure 8.1.48. **Redundant bicuspid aortic valve.** The arrow in **A** points to mild systolic doming of the AV, but the valve appears to open well when viewed in short axis **(B)**, consistent with minimal stenosis. **C.** A late systolic frame shows mild preclosure, resulting in decreased cross-sectional area, which should not be confused with aortic stenosis. The arrow in **D** shows a redundant valve prolapsing into the LVOT, producing severe AR (arrowhead in **E**). **F,G.** Short-axis views show AV redundancy and noncoaptation with resultant AR (black arrows).

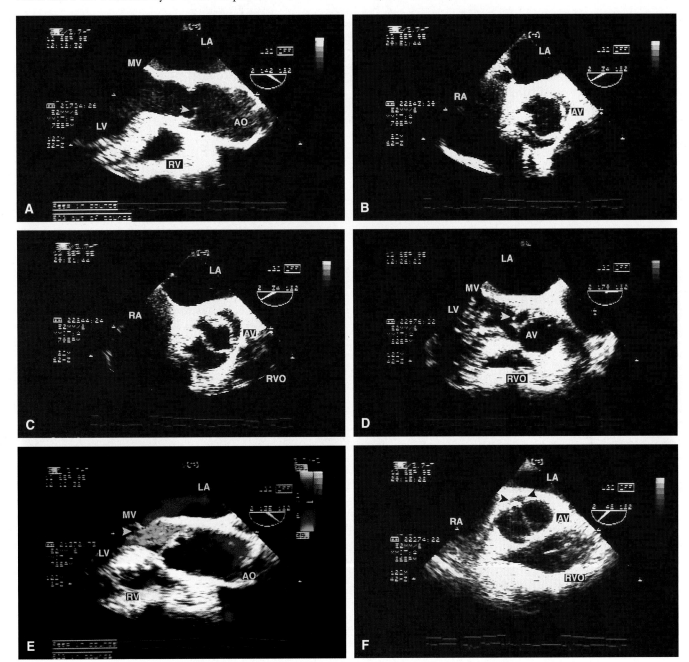

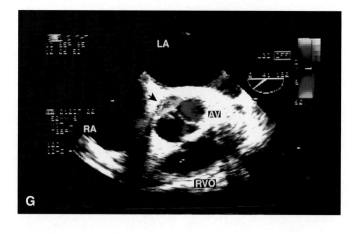

Figure 8.1.49. **Supravalvular aortic stenosis. A.** Narrowing of the aorta (AO; arrows) beyond the AV, producing turbulent flow. **B.** Supravalvular narrowing (arrow) in another patient. **C.** A narrowed, turbulent jet (arrows) in the area of stenosis in the same patient shown in **B.**

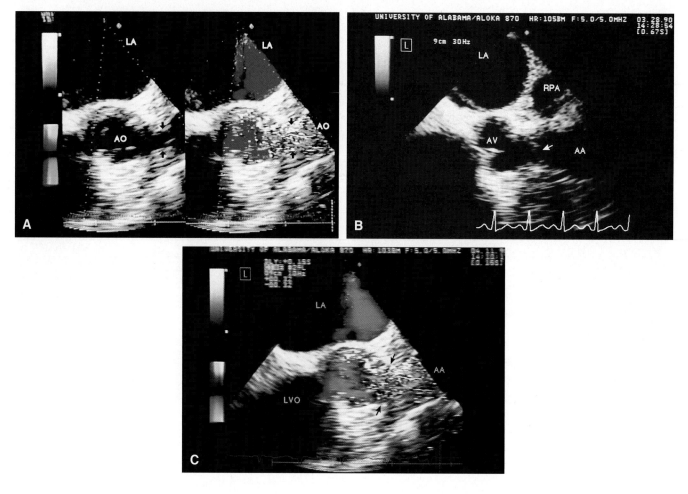

Figure 8.1.50. **Coarctation of the aorta. A.** Longitudinal plane examination in a 58-year-old man previously diagnosed with AV stenosis who presented with a 4-month history of progressive dyspnea and dizziness exacerbated by exertion. The coarcted segment (arrows) and poststenotic dilatation of the descending thoracic aorta (DA) distal (D) to the coarctation are shown. *Inset*: the coarctation site (arrows) on the aortogram. **B.** Color Doppler–guided high-pulse-repetition-frequency Doppler examination demonstrates a high velocity of 3.5 m/sec (equivalent to a peak pressure gradient of 49 mm Hg) across the coarctation (arrow). **C.** Collaterals (arrows) are present in the vicinity of the coarctation. *Inset*: a spectral tracing from a collateral vessel, which typically shows flow signals in systole and diastole. **D.** A large posterior intercostal artery (C) carries blood into the descending thoracic aorta beyond the coarctation site. This is demonstrated by color and pulsed Doppler (inset) examinations. **E.** Schematic shows longitudinal plane examination. The arrow points to the coarctation site. *DA(P)*, descending thoracic aorta proximal to the coarctation site. (Reproduced with permission from Ryan K, Sanyal RS, Pinheiro L, Nanda NC. Assessment of aortic coarctation and collateral circulation by biplane transesophageal echocardiography. Echocardiography 1992;9:277–285.)

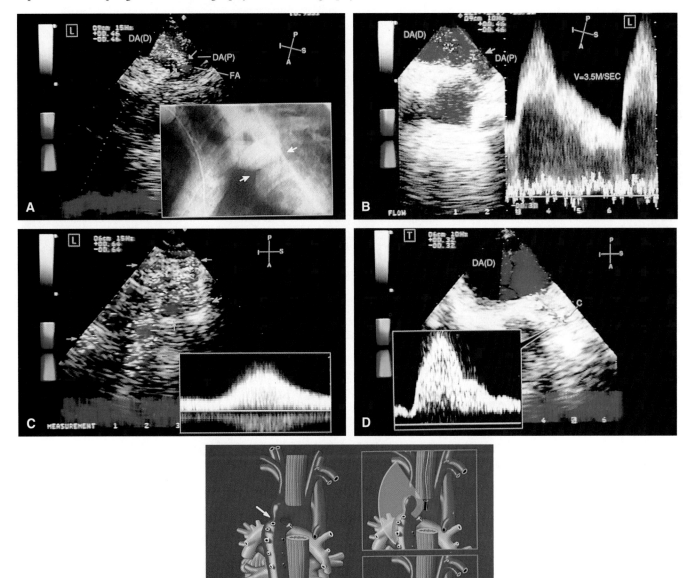

Figure 8.1.51. **Coarctation of the aorta associated with bicuspid AV and subaortic membranous stenosis.** **A,B.** Longitudinal plane examination in a 23-year-old woman with a 1-month history of shortness of breath and absent left radial and lower extremity pulses. The coarcted segment (arrows) and poststenotic dilatation of the descending aorta (DA) distal (D) to the coarctation are well seen. *FA* represents flow acceleration or convergence noted immediately proximal to the coarctation. **C.** Longitudinal plane examination demonstrates aliased signals in LVOT consistent with high flow velocity of approximately 2.5 m/sec (inset). **D.** Longitudinal plane examination demonstrates the subaortic membrane (horizontal arrows) and the bicuspid AV. Tethering of the left cusp of the AV to the membrane is also shown (right, oblique arrow). This finding was confirmed at surgery. **E.** Transverse plane examination demonstrates a thickened bicuspid AV with a raphe (arrow) in the open (left) and closed (right) positions. **F.** Transverse plane examination demonstrates eccentric closure of the bicuspid aortic valve as well as tethering (arrow) of the left aortic cusp to the subaortic membrane (M). (Reproduced with permission from Ryan K, Sanyal RS, Pinheiro L, Nanda NC. Assessment of aortic coarctation and collateral circulation by biplane transesophageal echocardiography. Echocardiography 1992;9:277–285.)

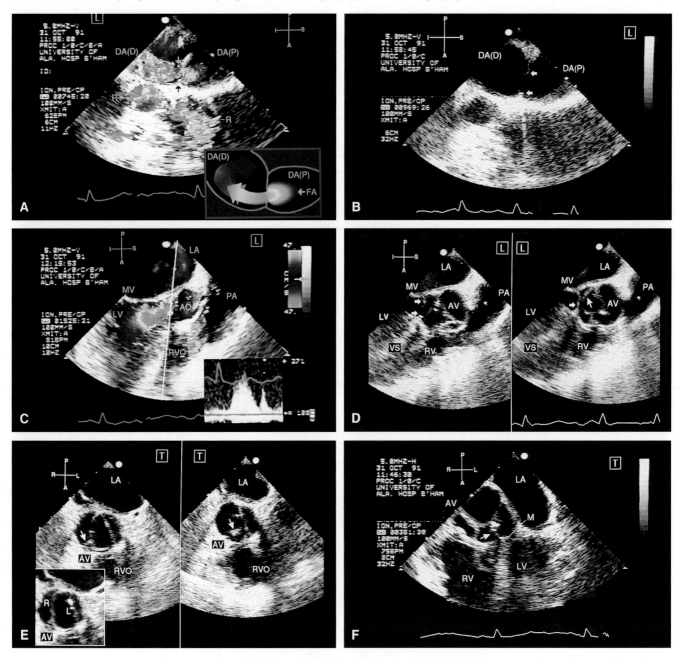

Figure 8.1.52. **Coarctation of the aorta.** **A.** Longitudinal plane examination in a 17-year-old-female with a 1-year history of dyspnea on exertion. The narrowed segment (arrows) as well as the poststenotic dilation of the descending thoracic aorta (DA) distal (D) to the coarctation site are well visualized. **B.** Transverse plane examination demonstrates a large collateral (C) vessel (dilated posterior intercostal artery) bringing flow to the descending thoracic aorta (DA) beyond the coarctation site. **C,D.** Color Doppler–guided pulsed Doppler interrogation of the collateral vessels shows prominent flow signals in systole and diastole. The collateral vessel in **D** probably represents a dilated bronchial artery. *DA(P)*, descending thoracic aorta proximal to coarctation. (Reproduced with permission from Ryan K, Sanyal RS, Pinheiro L, Nanda NC. Assessment of aortic coarctation and collateral circulation by biplane transesophageal echocardiography. Echocardiography 1992;9:277–285.)

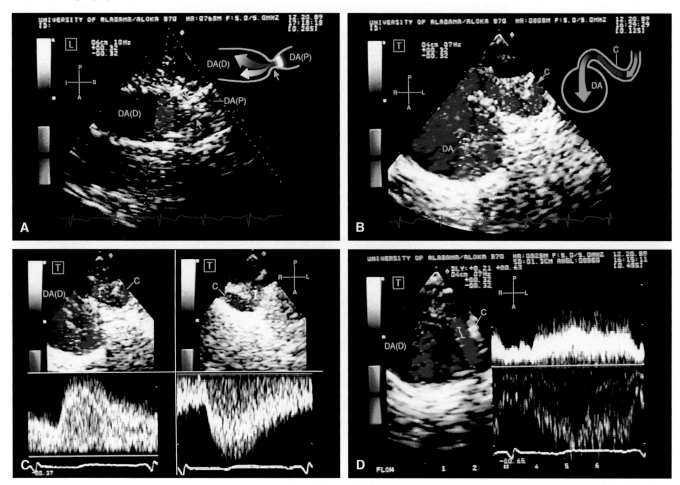

Figure 8.1.53. **Coarctation of the aorta.** Gross specimen shows coarctation of the aorta.

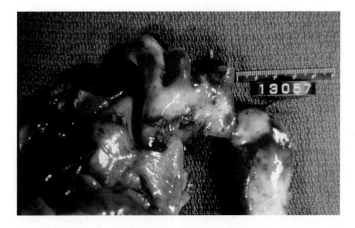

Figure 8.1.54. **RV trabeculation.** Prominent nonobstructing trabeculations (TB) are seen in the RVOT adjacent to the PV.

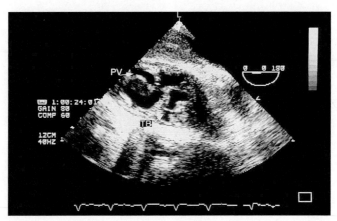

Figure 8.1.55. **Double-chambered RV. A.** A small ventricular septal defect (arrow). A prominent hypertrophied muscle band divides the RV into two chambers, C1 and C2 **(A,B). C.** Turbulent flow signals (arrow) consistent with obstruction are produced by the hypertrophied muscle bands running transversely through the RV body.

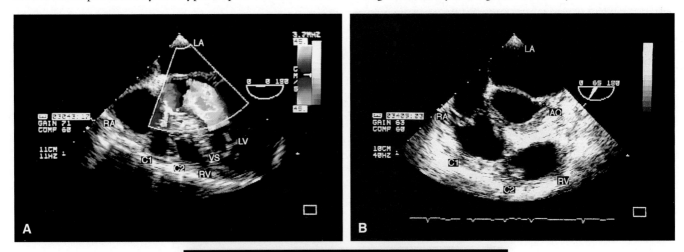

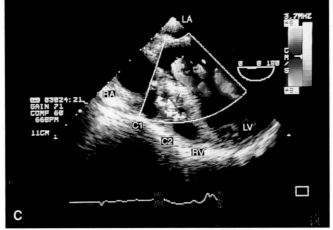

Figure 8.1.56. **Infundibular stenosis.** The arrows in **A** and **B** show narrowing of the RVOT below the pulmonary valve (PV), which is structurally normal. *P* in **A** points to a patch that had been used to close a ventricular septal defect. **C.** Turbulent flow signals (arrow) in the RVOT and pulmonary artery produced by infundibular stenosis.

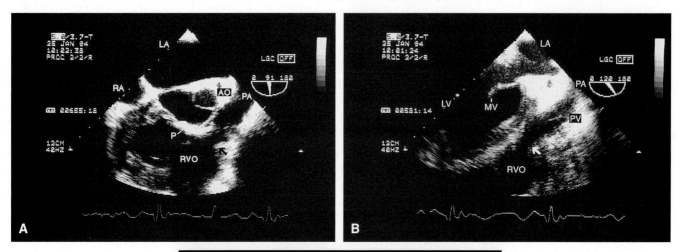

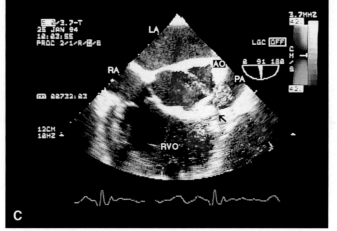

Figure 8.1.57. **Infundibular stenosis. A.** Marked narrowing of the RVOT (arrow) consistent with infundibular stenosis. **B,C.** Turbulent flow signals (arrows) produced by infundibular stenosis. **D.** Infundibular stenosis (arrows) in another patient. The PV is only mildly thickened.

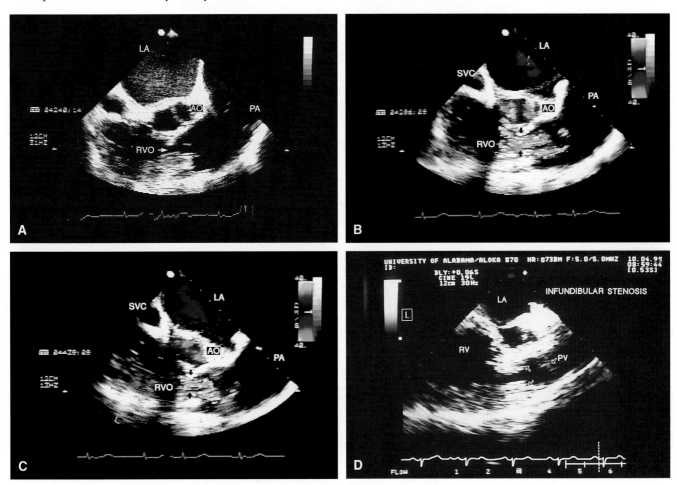

Figure 8.1.58.   **Bicuspid pulmonary valve**. Wide separation of the PV leaflets (arrowheads) in systole, indicative of absence of stenosis. The PV was bicuspid in this patient.

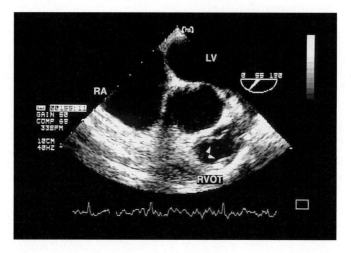

Figure 8.1.59.   **Pulmonary valve stenosis**. **A.** The PV shows restricted opening in systole, consistent with stenosis. The valve leaflets appear only mildly thickened. **B.** Color Doppler examination shows a narrow turbulent jet at the PV level, confirming the presence of severe stenosis.

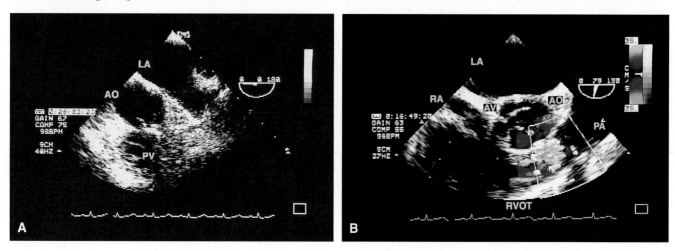

Figure 8.1.60. Bicuspid pulmonary valve stenosis associated with levotransposition or corrected transposition of the great arteries. Transverse (T) plane at the level of the great vessels in a 14-year-old boy. **A.** Diastolic frame shows the PV in the closed position. Note the transversely oriented commissure and the abnormal location of the valve posterior and to the right of the AV. **B.** Systolic frame shows markedly restricted motion of the PV leaflets and a very small orifice, indicative of severe stenosis. (Reproduced with permission from Finch AD, Snell DR, Sanyal RS, Nanda NC, Loungani RR. Transesophageal echocardiographic identification of a bicuspid pulmonary valve associated with congenitally corrected transposition of the great arteries. Echocardiography 1993;10:359–362.)

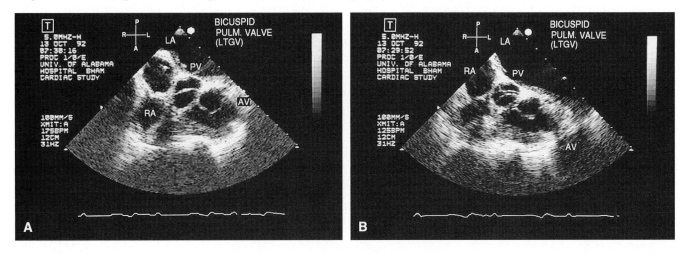

Figure 8.1.61. Idiopathic dilatation of the pulmonary artery. **A,B.** The pulmonary artery (PA) is markedly dilated. The PV is not thickened and opens normally. No other abnormality was detected in this adult, either clinically or on echocardiographic examination.

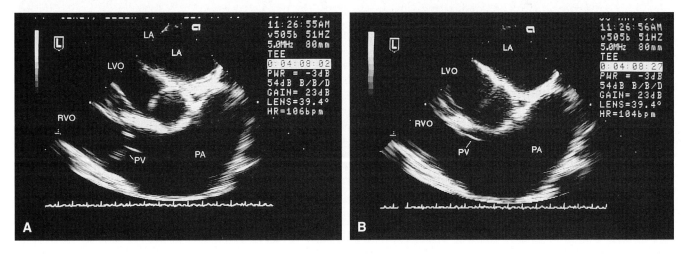

Figure 8.1.62. **Complete atrioventricular septal (canal) defect.** **A.** The four-chamber view in this elderly woman demonstrates both the atrial (open arrow; ASD) and ventricular (closed arrow) components of the atrioventricular septal (canal) defect. Shunting occurred only at the atrial level because the ventricular component was found closed by redundant septal TV leaflet tissue. Both atrial (D) and ventricular (open arrow) defects are well seen. **B–E.** Another patient with complete atrioventricular septal defect. The RV is markedly hypertrophied because of the presence of pulmonary hypertension. **C.** The open leaflets (arrows) of the common atrioventricular valve. **D.** Atrioventricular valve regurgitation jet (open arrows) straddling the interatrial septum (IAS). **E.** Two jets of regurgitation (R,R) are clearly seen originating from the common atrioventricular valve (closed arrow), one extending into the RA and the other into the LA. The open arrow points to the ventricular defect, through which left-to-right shunting is shown (blue signals). **F.** Another patient with a common atrioventricular septal defect demonstrating LV to RA shunt (arrow) as well as MR. Note the huge atrial defect and a much smaller ventricular defect.

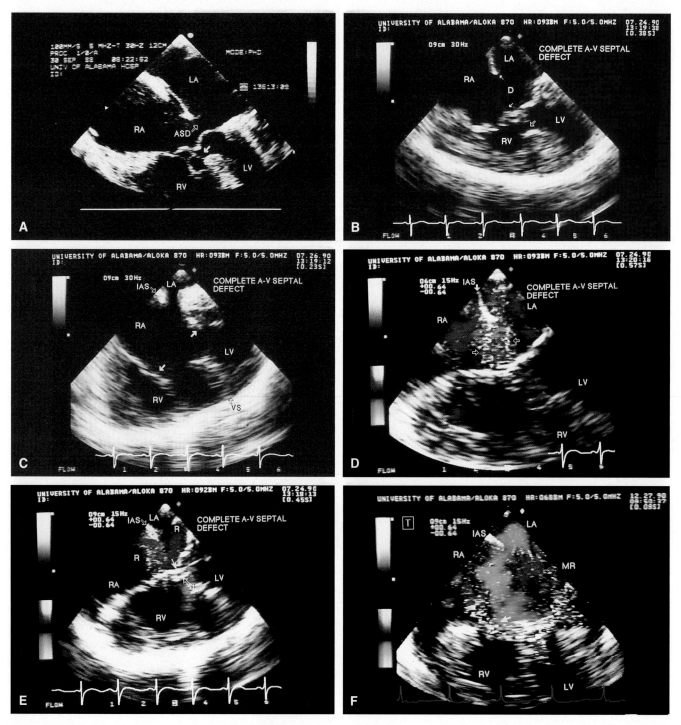

Figure 8.1.63.   Ebstein's anomaly. **A,B.** Transverse plane examination in a 24-year-old man shows the free **(A)** component of the anterior tricuspid leaflet as well as the part tethered (arrowheads) to the RV free wall. **B.** Marked displacement (arrows) of the septal (S) tricuspid leaflet. **C.** Longitudinal plane examination shows both the free (P) and tethered (arrowheads) components of the posterior (P) tricuspid leaflet. *A*, anterior TV leaflet. (Reproduced with permission from Maxted W, Nanda NC, Kim KS, et al. Transesophageal echocardiographic identification and validation of individual tricuspid valve leaflets. Echocardiography 1994;11:585–596.)

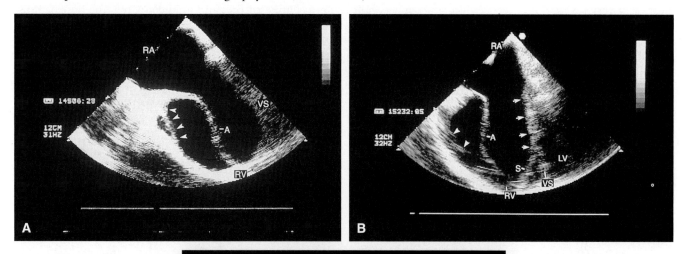

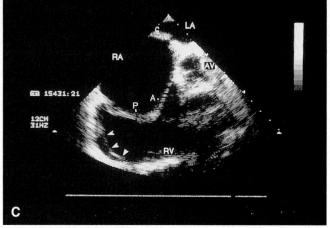

Figure 8.1.64. **Ebstein's anomaly. A,B.** The four-chamber view (at multiplane angulations of 180° and 0°) in a 72-year-old woman shows ventricular deviation (arrowheads) of a diminutive septal leaflet (S) of the TV. The anterior tricuspid leaflet has two portions—one freely mobile **(A)** and the other tethered (arrow in **B**) to the anterior wall of the RV. **C–E.** Multiplane angulations of 111° **(C)**, 93° **(D)**, and 90° **(E)** show free (P, A) and tethered (arrow in **C** and arrowheads in **D**) components of both posterior (P) and anterior (A) tricuspid leaflets. **F.** Color Doppler examination done at a plane angulation of 180° shows predominantly non-mosaic red flow signals filling a large portion of the huge RA in systole, indicative of very severe TR. Absence of mosaic signals reflects an insignificant pressure gradient across the noncoapting and, hence, very severely incompetent TV, with the RV and RA acting practically as one chamber. (Reproduced with permission from Maxted W, Nanda NC, Kim KS, et al. Transesophageal echocardiographic identification and validation of individual tricuspid valve leaflets. Echocardiography 1994;11:585–596.)

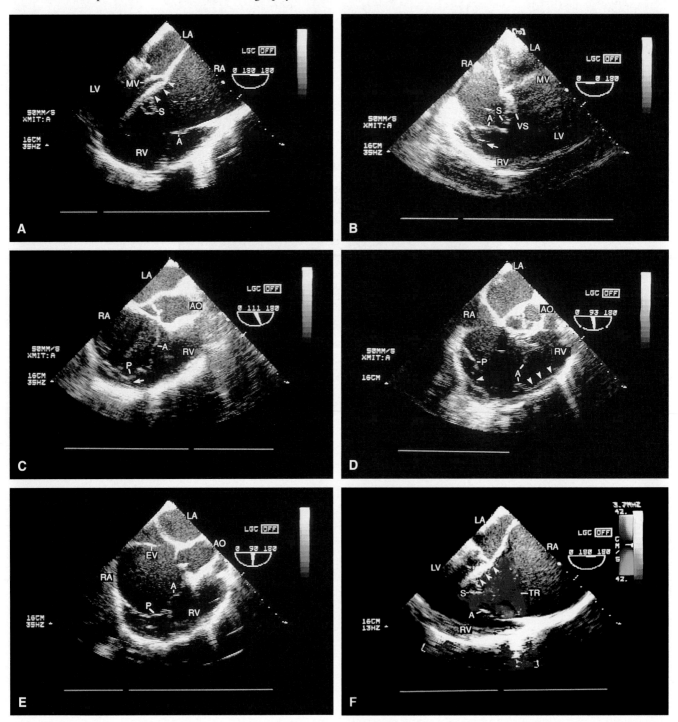

Figure 8.1.65. **Ebstein's anomaly with secundum atrial septal defect**. Transverse **(A)** plane examination in a 32-year-old female demonstrates marked ventricular deviation (arrowheads) of the septal (S) leaflet of the TV. The anterior (A) leaflet is elongated. Longitudinal plane **(B, C)** examination shows both free (P) and tethered (arrowheads) portions of the posterior (P) tricuspid leaflet. *D* in **C** denotes an associated secundum atrial septal defect. (Reproduced with permission from Maxted W, Nanda NC, Kim KS, et al. Transesophageal echocardiographic identification and validation of individual tricuspid valve leaflets. Echocardiography 1994;11:585–596.)

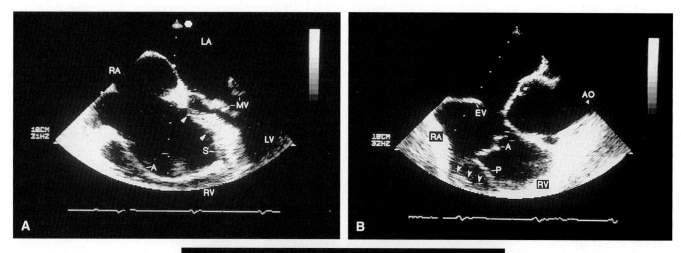

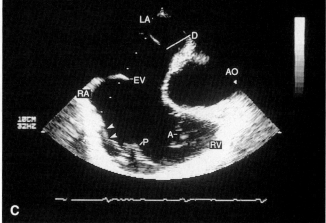

Figure 8.1.66. **Ebstein's anomaly. A–C.** Transverse plane four-chamber views in a 17-year-old male show the freely moving portion of the anterior tricuspid leaflet as well as the component tethered (arrowheads) to the RV anterior free wall. Two parts of the septal tricuspid leaflet (S) are also demonstrated—a small portion has a bubble-like appearance near the annulus, and the other, larger component shows marked inferior displacement (arrows) into the RV. The bubble-like appearance of the tethered portions of the anterior and septal leaflets results from nonuniform tethering of the leaflets to RV wall. **D.** Longitudinal plane examination shows two portions of the posterior leaflet—one freely moving (P) and the other tethered to the RV posterior (inferior) wall (arrowheads). **E,F.** Transgastric examination also shows both the freely moving (P) and the tethered portions (arrowheads) of the posterior tricuspid leaflet. **G.** Color Doppler examination in the four-chamber view demonstrates mosaic signals filling a large portion of the RA in systole, indicative of severe TR. (Reproduced with permission from Maxted W, Nanda NC, Kim KS, et al. Transesophageal echocardiographic identification and validation of individual tricuspid valve leaflets. Echocardiography 1994;11:585–596.)

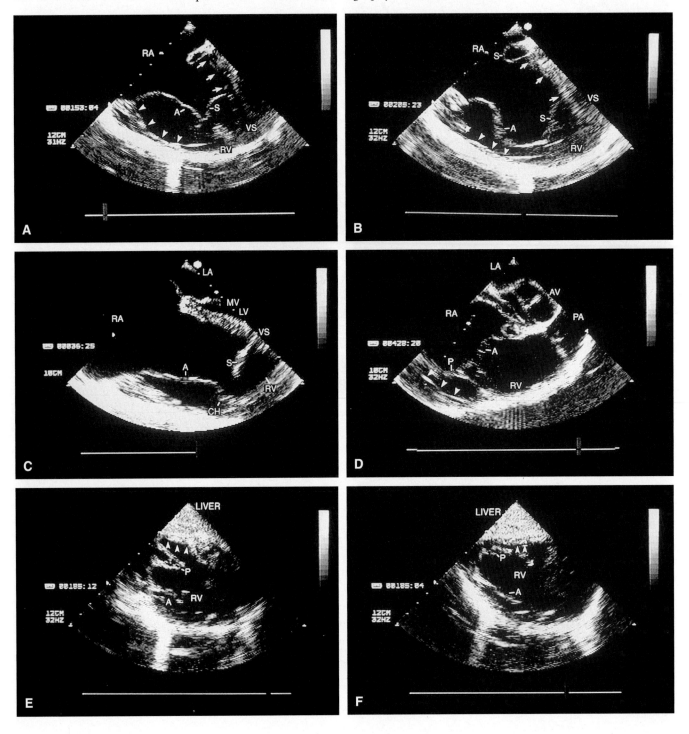

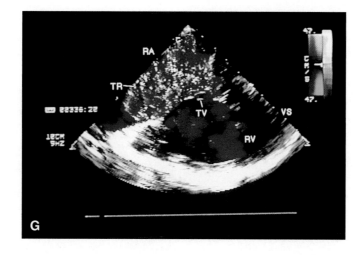

Figure 8.1.67. Corrected transposition of the great vessels with Ebstein's malformation of the left-sided atrioventricular valve. Transverse **(A)** and longitudinal **(B,C)** plane examinations in a 13-year-old boy show ventricular deviation (arrowheads) of both the septal (S) and posterior (P) leaflets of the left-sided TV. *A*, anterior TV leaflet; *CH*, chordae tendinae. (Reproduced with permission from Maxted W, Nanda NC, Kim KS, et al. Transesophageal echocardiographic identification and validation of individual tricuspid valve leaflets. Echocardiography 1994;11:585–596.)

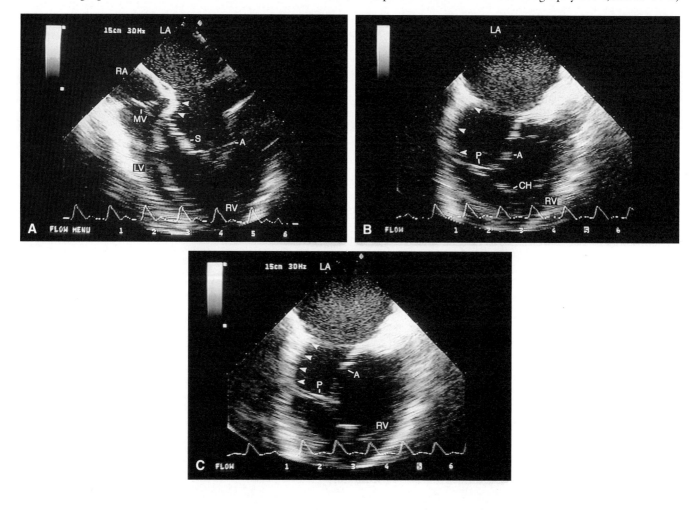

Figure 8.1.68. **Ebstein's anomaly. A.** Schematic shows Ebstein's anomaly with a secundum atrial septal defect. The anterior TV leaflet is elongated and the septal leaflet is plastered against the ventricular septum. The opening of the TV is displaced into the RV. **B.** Pathology specimen shows the septal leaflet of the TV plastered over the ventricular septum and the RV inferior wall.

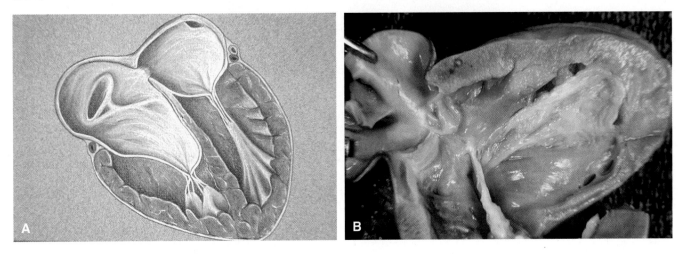

Figure 8.1.69. **Tricuspid atresia. A.** Schematic of tricuspid atresia. A thick, atretic TV is seen with a hypoplastic RV and both atrial and ventricular septal defects. **B.** Tricuspid atresia. Atretic tricuspid valve (ATV) and large atrial secundum (D) and ventricular septal defects (VSD) are shown. **C.** Color Doppler examination in the same patient shows shunt flow (open arrow) from the RA to the LA. The closed arrow points to the VSD.

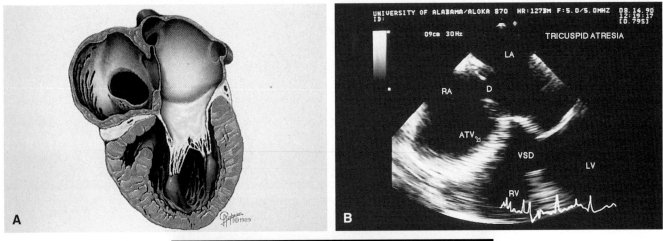

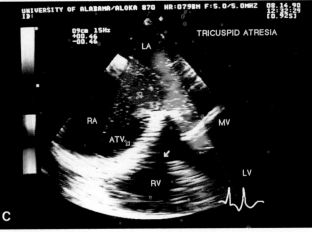

Figure 8.1.70. **Tricuspid atresia. A.** An atretic tricuspid valve (ATV) and a large ventricular septal defect (VSD) are seen in this adult patient. **B.** Shunt flow from RA/SVC to right pulmonary artery (RPA) via a direct surgical anastomosis is shown. The atrial septal defect, but not the VSD, has been closed. **C.** Pulsed Doppler examination shows shunt flow into RPA throughout the cardiac cycle.

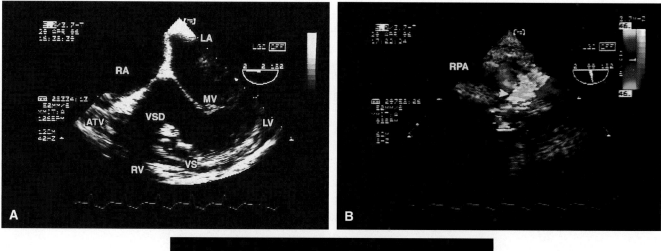

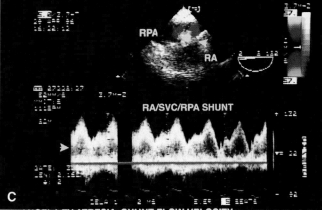

Figure 8.1.71. **Tetralogy of Fallot**. **A,B.** The aorta overriding the ventricular septum. The arrow points to the ventricular septal defect. **C,D.** Color Doppler examination shows shunt flow from the left to the RV through the ventricular septal defect. **E,F.** Another patient with tetralogy of Fallot. A large ventricular septal defect and infundibular stenosis (arrow) are imaged using longitudinal plane examination. **G.** A different patient with tetralogy of Fallot. Longitudinal plane study demonstrates a large ventricular septal defect (arrow) and severe infundibular stenosis (IS). The PV is only mildly thickened. **H.** Postoperative study in another patient shows the patch (arrow) used to close the ventricular septal defect. **I.** Gross specimen of tetralogy of Fallot shows the aorta partly arising from the RV. The ventricular septal defect is seen just below the AV.

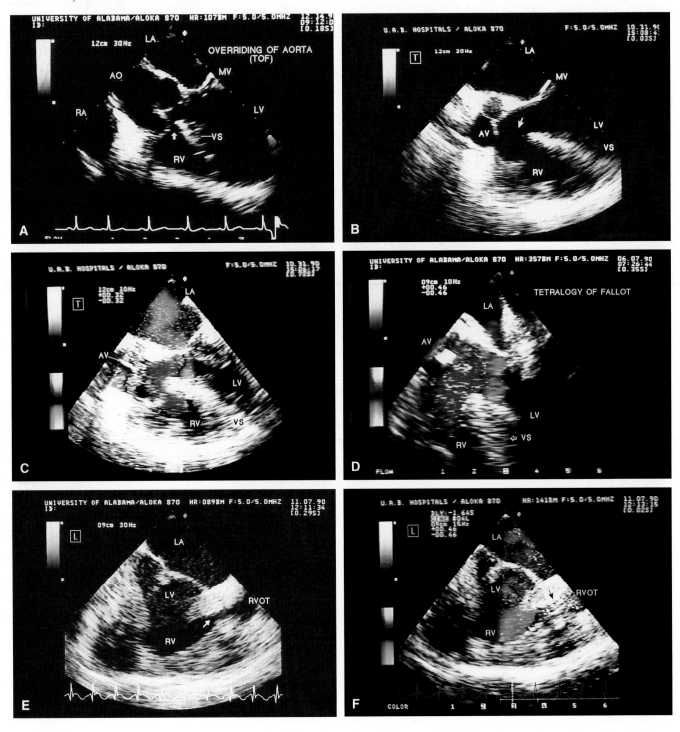

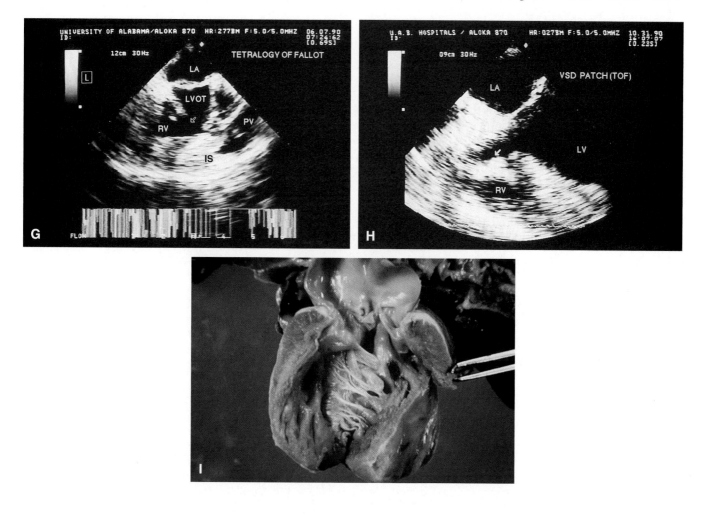

Figure 8.1.72. **Transposition of the great vessels. A.** The pulmonary artery arises from the LV and the aorta from the RV. **B–D.** Gross specimens showing the aorta arising from the RV **(B,D)** and the main and left pulmonary arteries arising from the LV **(C,D). E.** The pulmonary artery (PA) is located posterior and to the right of the aortic root (AO), indicative of transposition. The left main coronary artery (LMCA) can be seen arising from the aortic root. **F.** Another patient with transposition of the great vessels. The pulmonary artery (PA) is located posterior and to the left of the aorta (AO). The LMCA arises from the aortic root at about 12 o'clock and then courses to the left posterior to the PA. **G,H.** A different patient with transposition of the great vessels, status post–Mustard procedure. **G.** The intra-atrial baffle separating the pulmonary venous return from the systemic venous flow is well visualized. **H.** An M-mode study shows the motion pattern of the baffle. **I.** Obstruction (arrowhead) in the pulmonary venous portion (PVP) of the atrium in another patient with transposition of the great vessels who had undergone a Mustard procedure. *SVP,* systemic venous portion of the atrium.

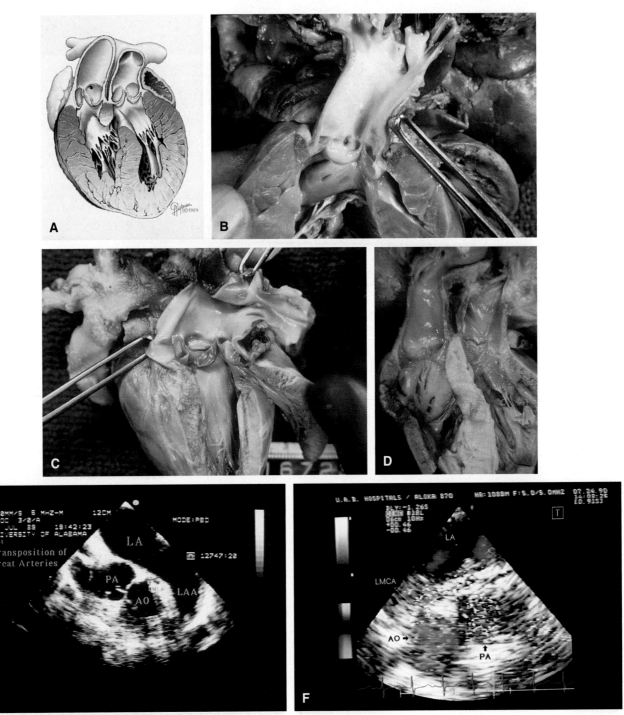

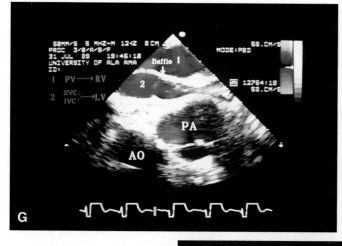

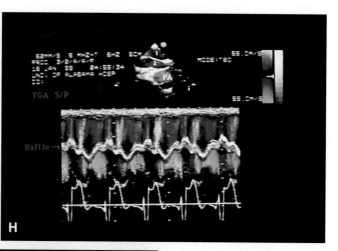

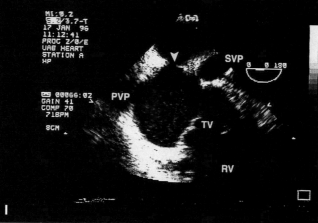

Figure 8.1.73. **Transposition of the great vessels**. **A.** The pulmonary artery (PA) is located posteriorly as compared to the aortic root and valve (AoV), typical of transposition of the great vessels. The arrow points to associated subpulmonic membranous obstruction, and *D* indicates a large ventricular septal defect. **B–H.** A 13-year-old boy with transposition of the great vessels demonstrating the posterior location of the pulmonary artery and valve (PV) as compared to the aorta and the aortic valve (AV). In **B**, the PV appears redundant and prolapses into the LVOT. **D, E,** and **H** show systolic doming of the PV, with turbulent flow signals in the PA consistent with stenosis. PV thickening is well seen in **F.** A large associated ventricular septal defect (arrowheads in **D** and **H** and *D* in **G**) also is visualized. **G.** Both the MV and TV are shown opening into the LV, typical of a double inlet LV. **H.** A secundum atrial septal defect (arrow) is present.

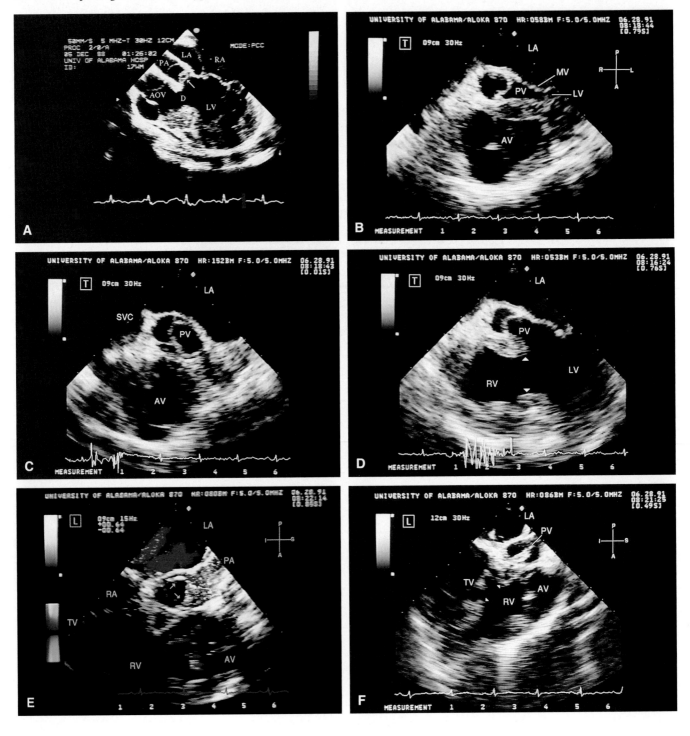

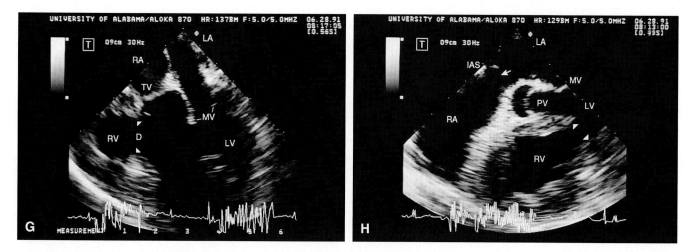

Figure 8.1.74. Double outlet right ventricle: juxtaposition of the atrial appendages. Both LAA and RAA are imaged on the left side and appear to have similar morphology. *C*, catheter in the LA.

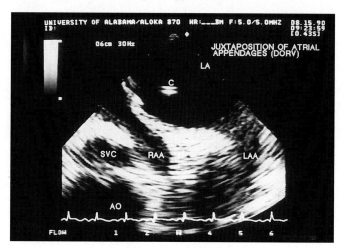

Figure 8.1.75. **Double outlet right ventricle.** **A–E.** Both the aorta and the pulmonary artery are shown arising from the RV in this 10-year-old boy. The TV straddles the ventricular system (VS). **C.** Large ventricular (VSD) and secundum atrial (D) septal defects are also noted. Pulsed Doppler examination of the VSD (noncommitted) shows flow signals moving into the RV from the LV throughout the cardiac cycle, except during atrial systole, when the shunt reverses. **E.** Short-axis view shows posterior location of the pulmonary artery (PA) as compared to the aorta (AO), indicative of transposition of the great vessels. **F.** Color Doppler examination in another patient with double outlet RV and transposition of the great vessels (PA is located posterior to AO), demonstrating flow signals (blue) moving into both outflow vessels during systole. *D*, ventricular septal defect.

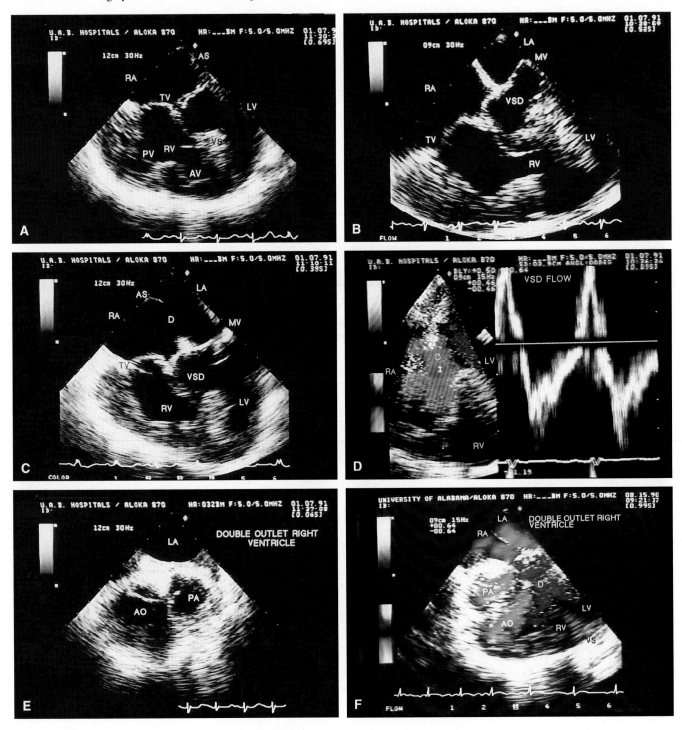

Figure 8.1.76. Tricuspid valve straddling the ventricular septum. The TV is shown straddling the ventricular septum (VS). Note the presence of a large ventricular septal defect.

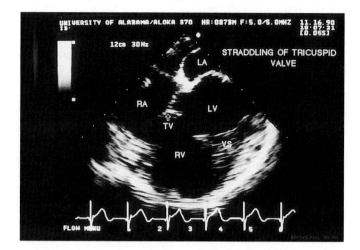

Figure 8.1.77. Single ventricle. **A.** A systolic frame shows the atrioventricular valves in the closed position. **B,C.** Both atrioventricular valves open into a large single ventricle. No ventricular septum is present.

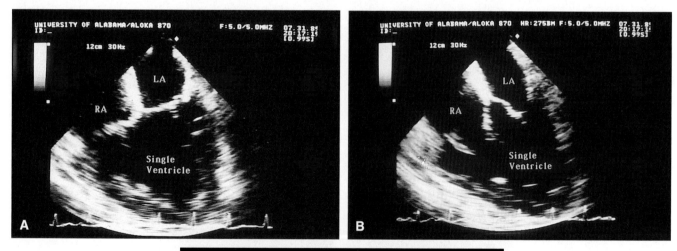

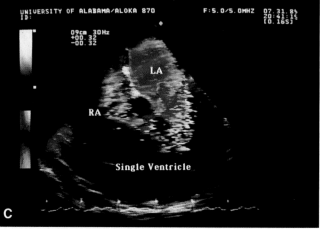

Figure 8.1.78. **Single ventricle: transposition of the great vessels.** **A–D.** This patient essentially has a large single ventricle located posteriorly (PO VEN). Both atrioventricular valves communicate with this ventricle. A small, rudimentary and thick-walled second ventricle also is seen anteriorly (AN VEN). There is prolapse of the anterior MV leaflet and septal and anterior TV leaflets (arrowheads in **B**). **E–J.** The PA is located posteriorly as compared to the AO, typical of transposition of the great vessels. In **F**, both great vessels are seen arising from the posterior ventricle. In **G** and **H**, the PV is shown to be bicuspid (BPV), whereas the AV is tricuspid (TAV). **I,J.** An associated secundum atrial septal defect (ASD) with flow signals moving into LA from RA (arrowhead in **J**). *VSD*, ventricular septal defect.

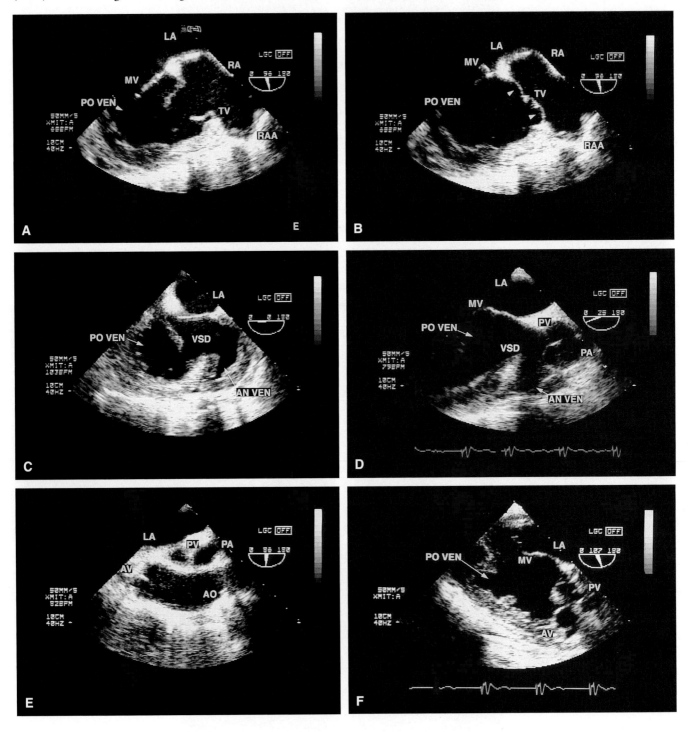

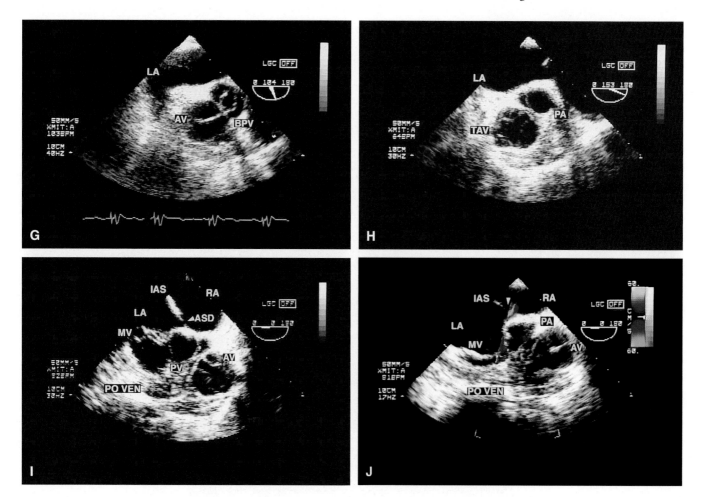

Figure 8.1.79. Dilatation of the sinuses of Valsalva. Three different patients with mildly dilated sinuses of Valsalva are shown. **A.** The sinuses (arrows) viewed in long axis. **B.** Mild dilatation of all three sinuses imaged in short axis in another patient. **C.** Localized dilatation (arrowhead) of the noncoronary sinus seen in the aortic short-axis view in a different patient.

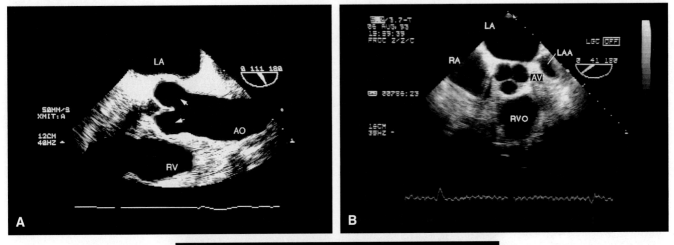

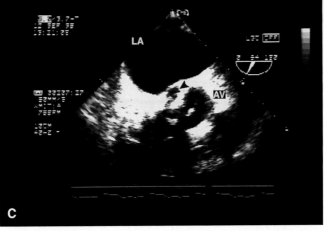

Figure 8.1.80.   **Sinus of Valsalva aneurysm.** A large aneurysm (arrowheads) involving the left coronary sinus.

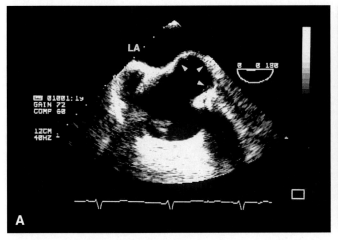

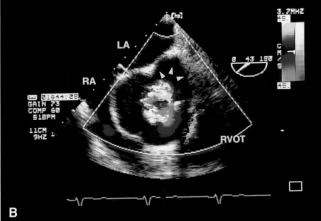

Figure 8.1.81. **Sinus of Valsalva aneurysm with rupture into the right ventricle. A.** The site of rupture (arrowhead) of the aneurysm into the RV just beneath the anterior (ATV) and septal (STV) leaflets of the TV. **B–D.** A huge aneurysm (arrowheads) involving the noncoronary sinus. **E,F.** The rupture is confirmed by color Doppler examination, which shows turbulent flow signals (arrowheads) moving from the aneurysm into the RV.

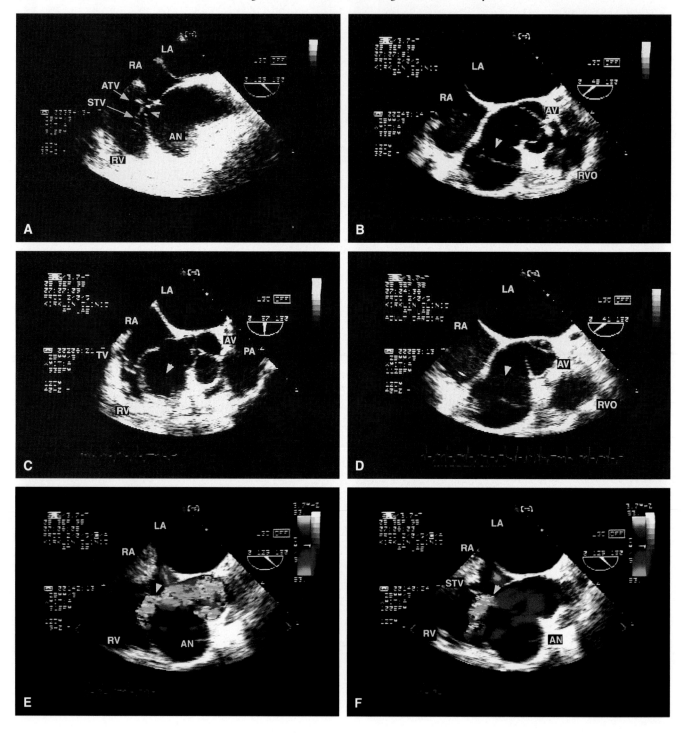

Figure 8.1.82. **Sinus of Valsalva aneurysm with rupture into the right ventricle**. The arrowheads in **A** and the arrow in **B** demonstrate a tubelike protrusion of the right sinus of Valsalva aneurysm into the RV. **C.** Short-axis view shows aneurysmal dilatation of the right coronary sinus. **D.** Color Doppler examination shows mosaic colored turbulent flow signals moving from the aneurysm into the RV indicative of rupture. Note the presence of prominent flow acceleration on the aortic side at the site of rupture.

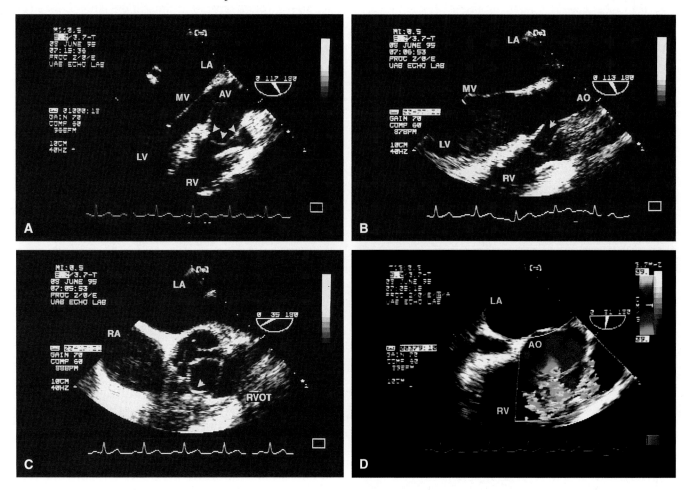

Figure 8.1.83. **Anomalous separate origin of left circumflex coronary artery from a separate ostium in the left coronary sinus.** A 62-year-old man evaluated before prosthetic replacement of a severely regurgitant AV. **A.** Aortic short-axis view. The left circumflex (LCX) and left anterior descending (LAD) coronary arteries arise from adjacent but separate orifices. **B.** Color M-mode echocardiography shows flow signals in both vessels. **C.** Coronary angiogram shows separate orifices of the two coronary arteries. (Reproduced with permission from Boogaerts J, Samdarshi TE, Nanda NC, Pinheiro L. Anomalous separate origin of left circumflex coronary artery from a separate ostium in the left coronary sinus: identification by transesophageal color Doppler echocardiography. Echocardiography 1990;7:165–167.)

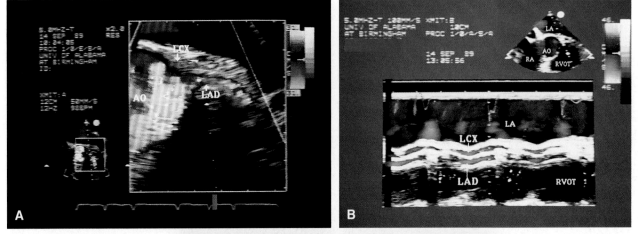

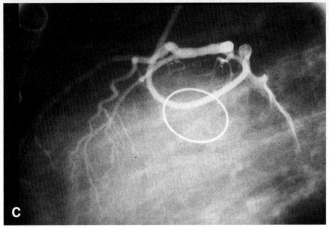

Figure 8.1.84. Anomalous origin of the left circumflex coronary artery from the right sinus of Valsalva. A 33-year-old woman with congenital bicuspid AV stenosis. Oblique aortic short-axis view demonstrates the right-sided origin of the anomalous vessel (CX), which then angles sharply posteriorly and subsequently takes a leftward course between the aorta (AO) and the LA. Note the presence of color flow signals within the vessel lumen. **B.** This view shows adjacent but separate origins of the circumflex (CX) and right coronary (RCA) arteries from the right sinus of Valsalva. **C.** The coronary artery arising from the left sinus of Valsalva courses anteriorly like a left anterior descending artery (LAD) and does not show any evidence of bifurcation. It is important to document this congenital anomaly, because it may contribute to myocardial infarction and sudden death. (Reproduced with permission from Samdarshi TE, Hill DL, Nanda NC. Transesophageal color Doppler diagnosis of anomalous origin of left circumflex coronary artery. Am Heart J 1991;122:571–573.)

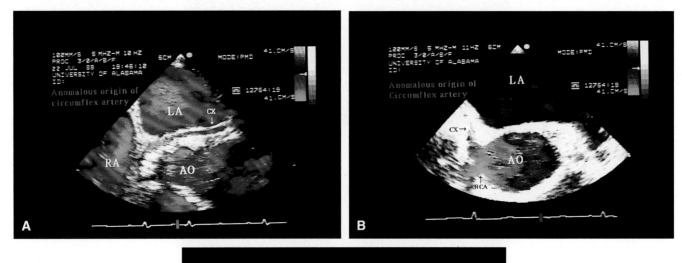

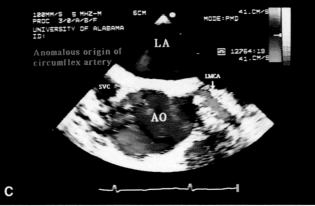

Figure 8.1.85. **Anomalous origin of the right coronary artery from the left anterior descending artery.** Aortic short-axis view demonstrates the right coronary artery (RCA) originating from the left anterior descending coronary vessel (LAD). The circumflex coronary artery (LCX) is imaged immediately anterior to the RCA.

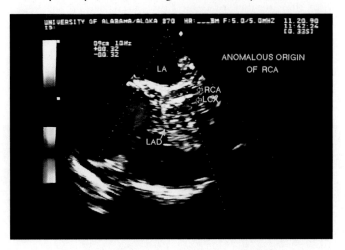

Figure 8.1.86. **Coronary artery aneurysms**. **A.** Left main coronary artery aneurysm. A large aneurysm (AN) involves the distal left main coronary artery in this patient. Its origin from the aorta (AO) and the proximal portion are uninvolved. **B,C.** Left anterior descending coronary artery (LAD) aneurysm. A large aneurysm containing a thrombus (TH) is seen in the distal LAD. The left main (LM) coronary artery and the proximal LAD are not dilated (insets in **B**). **D–F.** Right coronary artery aneurysm. The arrow in **D** points to the origin of the right coronary artery (RCA), which is aneurysmally dilated. **E,F.** Another patient with a proximal RCA aneurysm containing a thrombus (TH).

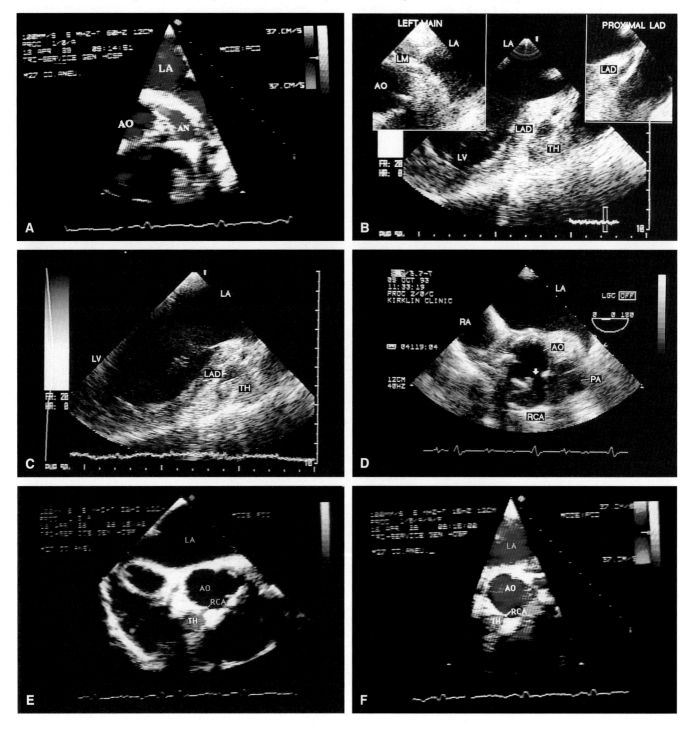

Figure 8.1.87. **Fistula of right coronary artery to coronary sinus.** This 46-year-old man presented with episodes of atrial flutter. **A.** The aortic short-axis view demonstrates a markedly enlarged right coronary artery (RCA; lumen width = 20 mm) with mosaic colored flow signals within it and in the aortic root (AO), indicative of turbulent blood flow. **B.** The RV inflow view demonstrates several large, bounded echo-free spaces containing mosaic colored signals indicating turbulent blood flow. These structures represent segments of the enlarged and tortuous right coronary artery viewed in the long-axis, short-axis, and oblique-axis planes. Mosaic flow signals from one of these structures are seen moving through an area of discontinuity into the grossly enlarged adjacent coronary sinus, near its entrance into the RA. **C.** After surgical obliteration of the fistulous connection, mosaic colored flow signals in the coronary sinus (CS) are replaced by blue signals indicative of laminar flow. *J*, jet from coronary sinus entering RA. (Reproduced with permission from Samdarshi TE, Mahan EF III, Nanda NC, Sanyal R. Transesophageal echocardiographic assessment of congenital coronary artery to coronary sinus fistulas in adults. Am J Cardiol 1991;68:263–266.)

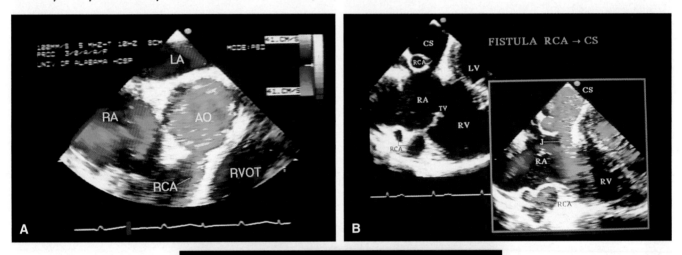

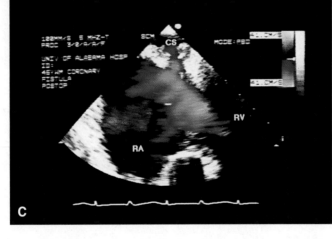

Figure 8.1.88. **Left circumflex coronary artery to coronary sinus fistula**. A 35-year-old woman with frequent ventricular ectopics. **A.** The aortic (AO) short-axis view demonstrates enlargement of the left main (LMC) and circumflex (LCX; lumen width = 16 mm) coronary arteries. **B.** Mosaic colored signals indicative of turbulent blood flow are seen moving from the left circumflex coronary artery into the coronary sinus (CS), near its entrance into the RA. Large circular and linear bounded spaces also were noted in this patient adjacent to the coronary sinus and represented the enlarged and tortuous LCX segments viewed in long and short axis. **C.** Color Doppler–guided pulsed Doppler interrogation of the communication (C) site demonstrates aliased high-velocity signals throughout the cardiac cycle. *SV,* Doppler sample volume. (Reproduced with permission from Samdarshi TE, Mahan EF III, Nanda NC, Sanyal R. Transesophageal echocardiographic assessment of congenital coronary artery to coronary sinus fistulas in adults. Am J Cardiol 1991;68:263–266.)

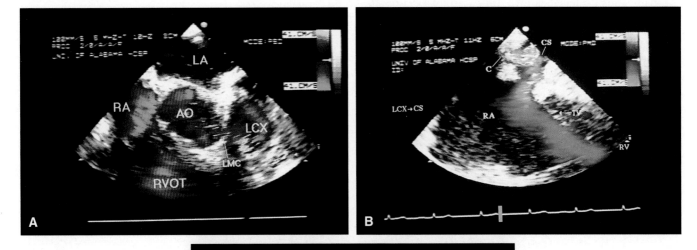

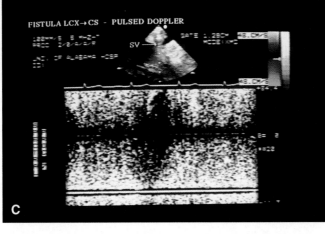

Figure 8.1.89. **Left circumflex coronary artery to coronary sinus fistula**. This 53-year-old woman presented with nonanginal chest pain. **A,B.** The aortic (AO) short-axis view demonstrates marked enlargement of the left circumflex (LCX; lumen width = 13 mm) coronary artery (CA). There is also enlargement of the left main CA (LMCA; lumen width = 12 mm), with a prominent atherosclerotic plaque (P) noted within its lumen. **C.** The LCX CA is shown communicating with another structure, located in the usual position of the coronary sinus (CS) in this plane and adjacent to a left-sided pulmonary vein (LPV). **D,E.** After surgical obliteration of the fistula, mosaic colored turbulent flow signals within the coronary sinus are replaced by laminar flow signals (blue), except at its entrance into the RA, where the fenestrated (F) thebesian valve results in persistence of turbulent blood flow. (Reproduced with permission from Samdarshi TE, Mahan EF III, Nanda NC, Sanyal R. Transesophageal echocardiographic assessment of congenital coronary artery to coronary sinus fistulas in adults. Am J Cardiol 1991;68:263–266.)

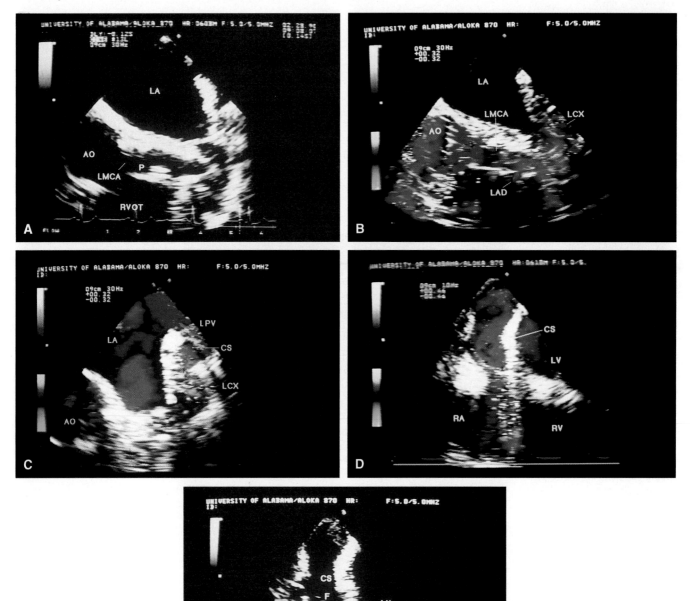

Figure 8.1.90.   **Aortopulmonary communication**. A 7-month-old infant with truncus arteriosus. **A.** A high basal view demonstrates a short main pulmonary artery (MPA) arising from the truncal vessel (TRV) and dividing into right (RPA) and left (LPA) branches, which appear to be normal in size. **B.** Color flow signals are noted arising from the truncal vessel and entering the pulmonary artery. **C.** The five-chamber view demonstrates the truncal vessel overriding the interventricular septum. The arrow points to the ventricular septal defect. **D.** Color flow signals are seen in the right (RV) and left (LV) ventricles and in the ventricular septal defect. **E,F.** Postoperative study demonstrates the valved bovine pericardial extracardiac conduit (C) connecting the RV to the pulmonary arteries. Note the absence of communication between the truncal vessel (now the neo-aorta, AO) and the main pulmonary artery. With two-dimensional imaging only **(F)**, a false impression of restriction at the distal conduit anastomosis is created as a result of the plane of scan through the oversewn stump of the main pulmonary. The arrow points to the detached and oversewn stump of the main pulmonary artery. *HV*, homograft valve in the conduit; *SV*, semilunar valve. (Reproduced with permission from Samdarshi TE, Morrow WR, Nanda NC, et al. Transesophageal echocardiography in aortopulmonary communications. Echocardiography 1991;8:383–395.)

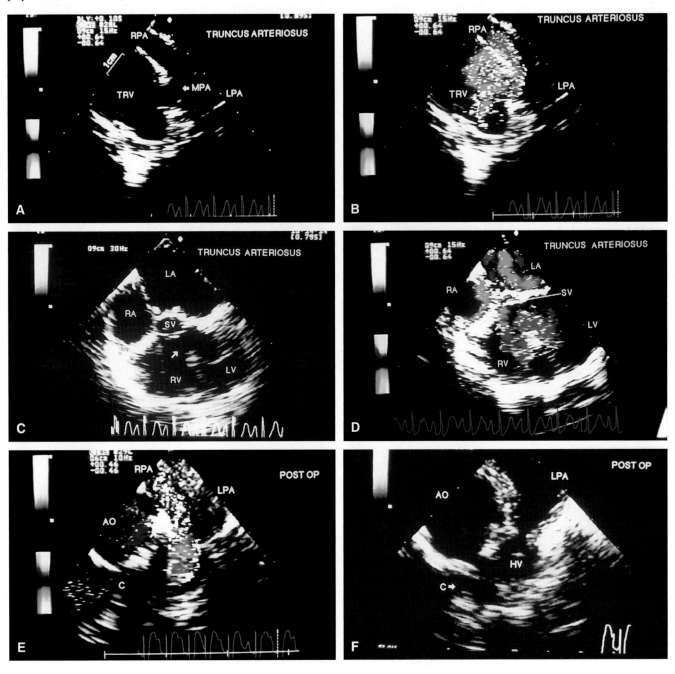

Figure 8.1.91. **Aortopulmonary communication**. A 7-month-old infant with an aortopulmonary window. **A.** A large (13-mm) defect is seen between the ascending aorta (AO) and the main pulmonary artery (MPA). **B.** Prominent color flow signals are seen moving from the aorta (AO) into the main pulmonary artery (MPA) and the proximal right (RPA) and left (LPA) branches through the defect. The pulmonary valve (PV) is clearly seen. **C.** The postoperative study demonstrates the patch (P) used to close the defect. (Reproduced with permission from Samdarshi TE, Morrow WR, Nanda NC, et al. Transesophageal echocardiography in aortopulmonary communications. Echocardiography 1991; 8:383–395.)

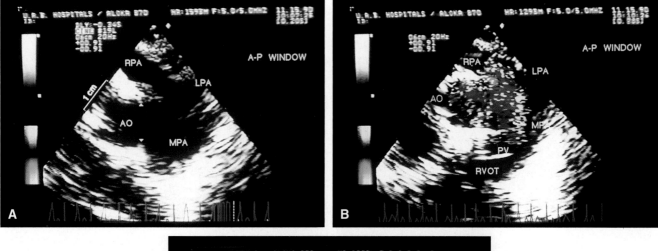

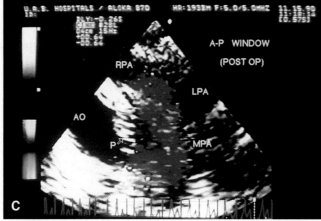

Figure 8.1.92. **Aortopulmonary communication**. A 4-year-old patient with transposition of the great arteries and pulmonary atresia. **A.** The high basal short-axis view demonstrates color flow signals representing flow from the aorta (AO) into the right pulmonary artery (RPA) through the Waterston shunt (D). **B.** High-pulse-repetition-frequency Doppler interrogation of the shunt reveals a peak velocity of 3.77 m/sec across the shunt. (Reproduced with permission from Samdarshi TE, Morrow WR, Nanda NC, et al. Transesophageal echocardiography in aortopulmonary communications. Echocardiography 1991;8:383–395.)

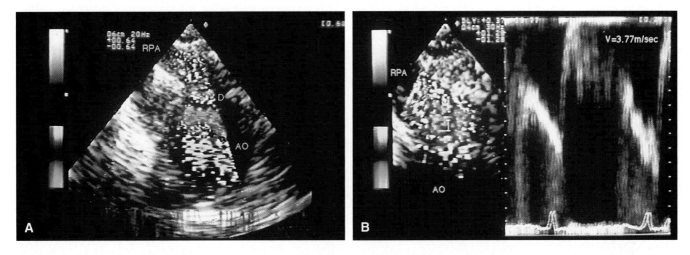

Figure 8.1.93. **Aortopulmonary communication**. A 1-year-old child with tetralogy of Fallot and complete atrioventricular septal defect. **A.** *Left*: Prominent color flow signals are noted representing flow from the aorta (AO) into the main pulmonary artery (MPA) through a surgically created central shunt (S). Flow is encoded as mosaic because of turbulence and frequency aliasing. *Right*: High-pulse-repetition-frequency Doppler interrogation of the shunt demonstrates continuous flow from the aorta to pulmonary artery with a high velocity throughout the cardiac cycle. **B.** High-pulse-repetition-frequency Doppler interrogation of the left-sided Blalock-Taussig shunt (BT) also shows continuous flow. *LPA*, left pulmonary artery; *RPA*, right pulmonary artery. (Reproduced with permission from Samdarshi TE, Morrow WR, Nanda NC, et al. Transesophageal echocardiography in aortopulmonary communications. Echocardiography 1991;8:383–395.)

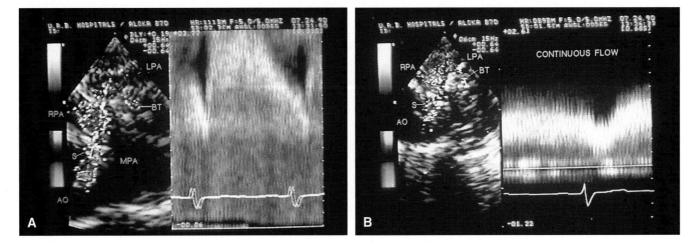

Figure 8.1.94. **Aortopulmonary communication**. A 10-year-old patient with tetralogy of Fallot, pulmonary atresia, and nonconfluent pulmonary arteries. **A.** Color signals are seen depicting flow from the lateral wall of the aorta (AO) into the distal right pulmonary artery (RPA) through the Waterston shunt (S). **B.** Pulsed Doppler interrogation of the shunt reveals flow throughout the cardiac cycle. **C.** Postoperative study demonstrates the proximal anastomosis of the Gore-Tex conduit (C), which carries blood from the RV to the right and left pulmonary arteries. **D.** Pulsed Doppler interrogation of the conduit demonstrates predominantly laminar systolic flow. *CF*, conduit flow. (Reproduced with permission from Samdarshi TE, Morrow WR, Nanda NC, et al. Transesophageal echocardiography in aortopulmonary communications. Echocardiography 1991;8:383–395.)

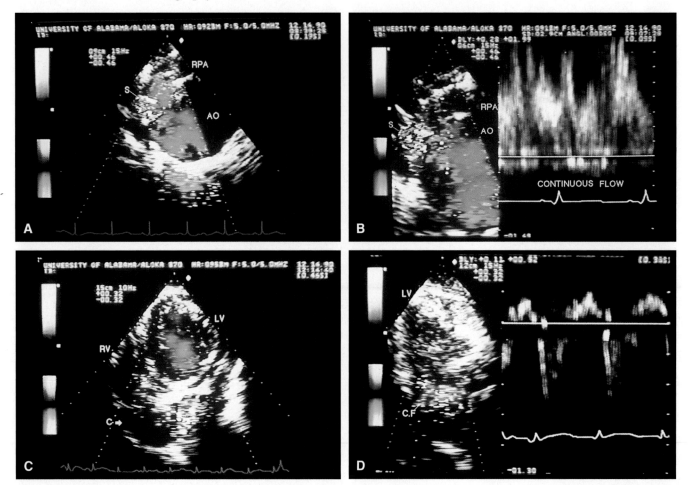

Congenital Heart Disease **395**

Figure 8.1.95. **Aortopulmonary communication.** A 10-year-old patient with double outlet right ventricle and pulmonary artery banding. **A,B.** Prominent flow signals are seen moving from the aorta (A) into the right (RPA) and main (MPA) pulmonary arteries through the Waterston shunt (D, arrow). The shunt measures 4 mm in diameter. **C.** *Left:* Longitudinal plane imaging demonstrates discrete narrowing of the main pulmonary artery produced by banding. *Right:* High-pulse-repetition-frequency Doppler interrogation reveals a high velocity (V) of 3.04 m/sec across the narrowed segment. **D.** Postoperative study demonstrates closure of the Waterston shunt and unrestricted pulmonary artery bifurcation. **E.** Postoperative study. *Left:* The anastomosis (size by color Doppler = 1 cm) between the superior vena cava (SVC) and the right pulmonary artery (RPA) is seen. *Right:* Pulsed Doppler interrogation of the right pulmonary artery reveals continuous flow throughout the cardiac cycle. *LPA,* left pulmonary artery. (Reproduced with permission from Samdarshi TE, Morrow WR, Nanda NC, et al. Transesophageal echocardiography in aortopulmonary communications. Echocardiography 1991;8:383–395.)

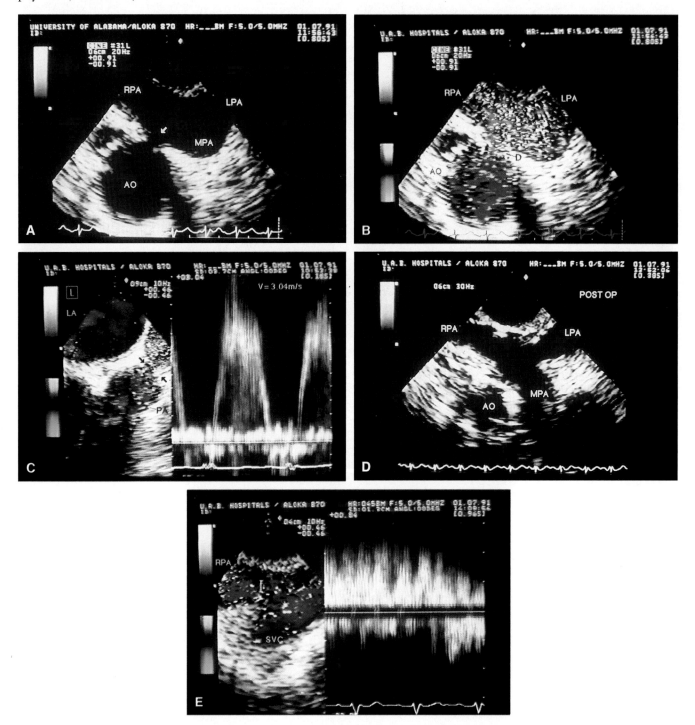

Figure 8.1.96. **LV diverticulum. A–C.** A large diverticulum (arrowheads) involves the LV inferior wall. This was confirmed at surgery.

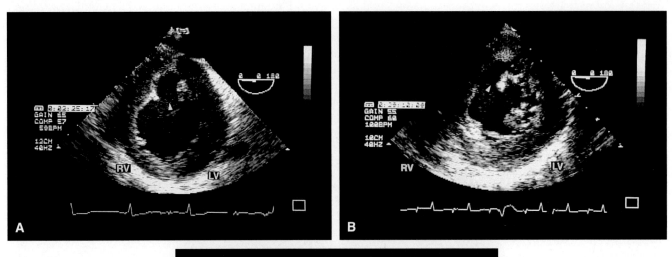

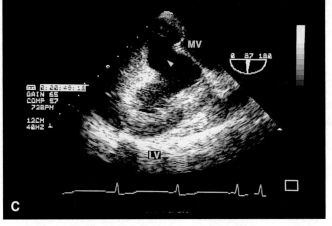

Figure 8.1.97. **Multiple LV papillary muscles.** Three papillary muscles (arrowheads) visualized in the LV short-axis view. This is not a specific finding, because normal papillary muscles may have more than one head, which can result in a similar picture.

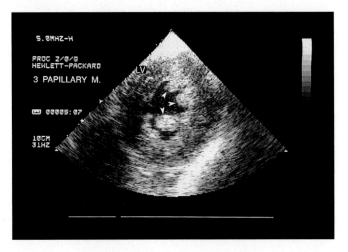

SUGGESTED READINGS

Alboliras ET, Gotteiner NL, Berdusis K, et al. Transesophageal echocardiographic imaging for congenital lesions of the left ventricular outflow and the aorta. Echocardiography 1996;13:439–446.

Andrade A, Vargas-Baron J, Rijlaarsdam M, et al. Utility of transesophageal echocardiography in the examination of adult patients with patent ductus arteriosus. Am Heart J 1995;130:543–546.

Ascione L, Caso P, De Leva F, et al. Transesophageal color flow echocardiographic evaluation of supra valve mitral ring in an adult period. Echocardiography 1994;11:231–235.

Benheim A, Karr SS, Sell JE, et al. Routine use of transesophageal echocardiography and color flow imaging in the evaluation and treatment of children with congenital heart disease. Echocardiography 1993;10:583–593.

Benson MJ, Cahalan MK. Cost-benefit analysis of transesophageal echocardiography in cardiac surgery. Echocardiography 1995;12:171–183.

Blackshear JL, Safford RE, Lane GE, et al. Unruptured noncoronary sinus of Valsalva aneurysm: preoperative characterization by transesophageal echocardiography. J Am Soc Echocardiogr 1991;4:485–490.

Boogaerts J, Samdarshi TE, Nanda NC, Pinheiro L. Anomalous separate origin of left circumflex coronary artery from a separate ostium in the left coronary sinus: identification by transesophageal color Doppler echocardiography. Echocardiography 1990;7:165–167.

Chang RY, Kuo CH, Rim RS, et al. Transesophageal echocardiographic image of double-chambered right ventricle. J Am Soc Echocardiogr 1996;9:347–352.

Child JS. Echocardiographic assessment of adults with tetralogy of Fallot. Echocardiography 1993;10:629–640.

Cox D, Taylor J, Nanda NC. Refractory hypoxemia in right ventricular infarction from right-to-left shunting via a patent foramen ovale: efficacy of contrast transesophageal echocardiography. Am J Med 1991;91:653–655.

Cyran S, Kimball TR, Meyer RA, et al. Efficacy of intraoperative transesophageal echocardiography in children with congenital heart disease. Am J Cardiol 1989;63:594–598.

Dhar PK, Fyfe DA, Sharma S. Multiplane transesophageal echocardiographic evaluation of defects of the atrioventricular septum: the crux of the matter. Echocardiography 1996;13:663–676.

Dobbertin A, Warnes CA, Seward JB. Cor triatriatum dexter in an adult diagnosed by transesophageal echocardiography: a case report. J Am Soc Echocardiogr 1995;8:952–957.

Duch PM, Chandrasekaran K, Mulhern CB, et al. Transesophageal echocardiographic diagnosis of pulmonary arteriovenous malformation. Role of contrast and pulsed Doppler echocardiography. Chest 1994;105:1604–1605.

Essop MR, Skudicky D, Sareli P. Diagnostic value of transesophageal versus transthoracic echocardiography in discrete subaortic stenosis. Am J Coll Cardiol 1992;70:962–963.

Finch A, Osman K, Kim KS, Nanda NC, Willman B, Soto B, Kirklin JK. Transesophageal echocardiographic findings of an infected quadricuspid aortic valve with an anomalous coronary artery. Echocardiography 1994;11:369–375.

Finch AD, Snell DR, Sanyal RS, Nanda NC, Loungani RR. Transesophageal echocardiographic identification of a bicuspid pulmonary valve associated with congenitally corrected transposition of the great arteries. Echocardiography 1993;10:359–362.

Folk TG, Kon ND, Nomeir AM, Kitzman DW. Coincidental finding of cor triatriatum by intraoperative transesophageal echocardiography in a patient with severe mitral regurgitation from myxomatous degeneration. Echocardiography 1994;11:579–583.

Fyfe DA. Multiplane transesophageal echocardiography for congenital heart disease: leveling the playing field. Echocardiography 1996;13:651–652.

Fyfe DA, Kline CH. Transesophageal echocardiography for congenital heart disease. Echocardiography 1991;8:573–584.

Fyfe DA, Ritter SB, Snider AR, et al. Guidelines for transesophageal echocardiography in children. J Am Soc Echocardiogr 1992;5:640–644.

Georgeson S, Neibart RM. Quadricuspid aortic valve diagnosed by transesophageal echocardiography. Am Heart J 1996;132:1292–1293.

Goldberg N, Schifter D, Aron M, et al. Double orifice mitral and tricuspid valves. Echocardiography 1996;13:85–90.

Hashimoto H. Double-orifice mitral valve with three papillary muscles. Chest 1993;104:1616–1617.

Hoppe UC, Dederichs B, Deutsch HJ, et al. Congenital heart disease in adults and adolescents: comparative value of transthoracic and transesophageal echocardiography and MR imaging. Radiology 1996;199:669–677.

Justo RN, Nykanen DG, Boutin C, et al. Clinical impact of transcatheter closure of secundum atrial septal defects with the double umbrella device. Am J Cardiol 1996;77:889–892.

Kichura GM, Castello R. Abnormalities of the interatrial septum as a potential cardiac source of embolism: patent foramen ovale and atrial septal aneurysm. Echocardiography 1994;10:441–449.

Kim KS, Maxted W, Nanda NC, et al. Comparison of multiplane and biplane transesophageal echocardiography in the assessment of aortic stenosis. Am J Cardiol 1997;79:436–441.

Krauss D, Weinert L, Lang RM. The role of multiplane transesophageal echocardiography in diagnosis PDA in an adult. Echocardiography 1996;13:95–97.

Kronzon I, Tunick PA, Freedberg RS, et al. Transesophageal echocardiography is superior to transthoracic echocardiography in the diagnosis of sinus venosus atrial septal defect. J Am Coll Cardiol 1991;17:537–542.

Lam J, Neirotti RA, Nijveld A, et al. Transesophageal echocardiography in pediatric patients: preliminary results. J Am Soc Echocardiogr 1991;4:43–50.

Lin FC, Chang HJ, Chern MS, et al. Multiplane transesophageal echocardiography in the diagnosis of congenital coronary artery fistula. Am Heart J 1995;130:1236–1244.

Lloyd TR, Vermilion RP, Zamora R, et al. Influence of echocardiographic guidance on positioning of the buttoned occluder for transcatheter closure of atrial septal defects. Echocardiography 1996;13:117–121.

Maxted W, Finch A, Nanda NC, et al. Multiplane transesophgeal echocardiographic detection of sinus venosus atrial septal defect. Echocardiography 1995;12:139–143.

Maxted W, Nanda NC, Kim KS, et al. Transesophageal echocardiographic identification and validation of individual tricuspid valve leaflets. Echocardiography 1994;11:585–596.

Mehta RH, Helmcke F, Nanda NC, et al. Transesophageal Doppler color flow mapping assessment of atrial septal defect. J Am Coll Cardiol 1990;16:1010–1016.

Mehta RH, Jain SP, Nanda NC, et al. Isolated partial anomalous pulmonary venous connection: echocardiographic diagnosis and a new color Doppler method to assess shunt volume. Am Heart J 1991;122:870–873.

Miller DS, Schwartz SL, Geggel RL, et al. Detection of partial anomalous right pulmonary venous return with an intact atrial septum by transesophageal echocardiography. J Am Soc Echocardiogr 1995;8:924–927.

Monducci I, Tomasi C, Bacchi M, Menozzi C. Usefulness of biplanar transesophageal echocardiography in arrhythmogenic right ventricular dysplasia: clinical experience with seven cases. Echocardiography 1996;13:1–8.

Morimoto K, Matsuzaki M, Tohma Y, et al. Diagnosis and quantitative evaluation of secundum-type atrial septal defect by transesophageal Doppler echocardiography. Am J Cardiol 1990;66:85–91.

Mugge A, Daniel WG, Klopper JW, Lichtlen PR. Visualization of patent foramen ovale by transesophageal color-coded Doppler echocardiography. Am J Cardiol 1988;62:837–838.

Muhiudeen I, Silverman N. Intraoperative transesophageal echocardiography using high resolution imaging in infants and children with congenital heart disease. Echocardiography 1993;10:599–608.

Nanda NC, Pinheiro L, Sanyal R, et al. Transesophageal echocardiographic examination of left-sided superior vena cava and azygos and hemiazygos veins. Echocardiography 1991;8:731–740.

Obeid AI, Carlson RJ. Evaluation of pulmonary vein stenosis by transesophageal echocardiography. J Am Soc Echocardiogr 1995;8: 888–896.

Osman K, Nanda NC, Kim KS, et al. Transesophageal echocardiographic features of unicuspid aortic valve. Echocardiography 1994;11: 469–473.

Pascoe RD, Oh JK, Warnes CA, et al. Diagnosis of sinus venosus atrial septal defect with transesophageal echocardiography. Circulation 1996;94:1049–1055.

Patel JN, Osman K, Nanda NC, et al. Quadricuspid aortic valve diagnosed by multiplane transesophageal echocardiography. Echocardiography 1994;11:201–205.

Pearson AC, Nagelhout D, Camp A, et al. Atrial septal aneurysm and stroke: a transesophageal echocardiographic study. J Am Coll Cardiol 1991;18:1223–1229.

Podolsky LA, Jacobs LE, Schwartz M, et al. Transesophageal echocardiography in the diagnosis of the persistent left superior vena cava. J Am Soc Echocardiogr 1992;5:159–162.

Rainer RS, Wanat FE, Nanda NC, Chang LK. Multiple secundum type atrial septal defects: identification by transthoracic color Doppler echocardiography. Echocardiography 1990;7:567–569.

Ritter SB. Transesophageal real-time echocardiography in infants and children with congenital heart disease. J Am Coll Cardiol 1991;18: 569–580.

Ritter SB. Transesophageal echocardiography in children: new peephole to the heart (editorial). J Am Coll Cardiol 1990;16:447–450.

Ryan K, Sanyal RS, Pinheiro L, Nanda NC. Assessment of aortic coarctation and collateral circulation by biplane transesophageal echocardiography. Echocardiography 1992;9:277–285.

Samdarshi TE, Hill DL, Nanda NC. Transesophageal color Doppler diagnosis of anomalous origin of left circumflex coronary artery. Am Heart J 1991;122:571–573.

Samdarshi TE, Mahan EF III, Nanda NC, Sanyal R. Transesophageal echocardiographic assessment of congenital coronary artery to coronary sinus fistulas in adults. Am J Cardiol 1991;68:263–266.

Samdarshi TE, Morrow R, Helmcke FR, Nanda NC, Bargeron LM Jr, Pacifico AD. Assessment of pulmonary vein stenosis by transesophageal echocardiography. Am Heart J 1991;122:1495–1498.

Samdarshi TE, Morrow WR, Nanda NC, et al. Transesophageal echocardiography in aortopulmonary communications. Echocardiography 1991;8:383–395.

Santini F, Bonato R, Pittarello D, et al. Intraoperative transesophageal echocardiography during surgery for congenital heart disease. Cardiovasc Imag 1992;4:127–132.

Sanyal RS, Nanda NC, Snell D, et al. Transesophageal echocardiographic findings of complete unilateral anomalous pulmonary venous connection of right lung to right atrium. Echocardiography 1994;11:93–100.

Schneider B, Hanrath P, Vogel P, Meinertz T. Improved morphology characterization of atrial septal aneurysm by transesophageal echocardiography: Relation to cerebrovascular events. J Am Coll Cardiol 1990;16:1000–1009.

Schurger D, Bartel T, Muller S, et al. Multiplane transesophageal echocardiography is the only definitive ultrasound approach in adult supra valvular aortic stenosis. Int J Cardiol 1996;53:305–309.

Scott PJ, Blackburn ME, Wharton GA, et al. Transesophageal echocardiography in neonates, infants and children: applicability and diagnostic value in everyday practice of a cardiothoracic unit. Br Heart J 1992;68:488–492.

Seward JB. Ebstein's anomaly: ultrasound imaging and hemodynamic evaluation. Echocardiography 1993;10:641–664.

Seward JB, Tajik AJ. Transesophageal echocardiography in congenital heart disease. Am J Cardiac Imaging 1990;4:215–222.

Sharma S, Stamper T, Dhar P, et al. The usefulness of transesophageal echocardiography in the surgical management of older children with subaortic stenosis. Echocardiography 1996;13:653–661.

Shirani J, Woo D, Gotsi W, et al. Mitral stenosis, sinus venosus atrial septal defect, and partial anomalous pulmonary venous return: diagnosis by multiplane transesophageal echocardiography. Echocardiography 1996;13:635–637.

Sloth E, Hasenkam JM, Sorensen KE, et al. Pediatric multiplane transesophageal echocardiography in congenital heart disease: new possibilities with a miniaturized probe. J Am Soc Echocardiogr 1996;9: 626–628.

Staffen RN, Davidson WR. Echocardiographic assessment of atrial septal defects. Echocardiography 1993;10:545–552.

Stern H, Erbel R, Schreiner G, et al. Coarctation of the aorta: quantitative analysis by transesophageal echocardiography. Echocardiography 1987;4:387–395.

Stumper OFW, Elzenga NJ, Hess J, Sutherland GR. Transesophageal echocardiography in children with congenital heart disease: an initial experience. J Am Coll Cardiol 1990;16:433–441.

Stumper OFW, Fijlaarsdam M, Vargas-Barron J, et al. The assessment of juxtaposed atrial appendages by transesophageal echocardiography. Int J Cardiol 1990;29:365–371.

Stumper O, Sutherland GR, Geuskens R, et al. Transesophageal echocardiography in evaluation and management after a Fontan procedure. J Am Coll Cardiol 1991;17:1152–1160.

Subahi SA, Al-Damegh S, Akhtar MJ, et al. Acquired intercostal arteriovenous fistulas: transesophageal Doppler echocardiography diagnosis. Echocardiography 1996;13:639–641.

Wang KY, Hsieh K, Yang M, et al. The use of transesophageal echocardiography to evaluate the effectiveness of patent ductus arteriosus ligation. Echocardiography 1994;10:53–57.

Weintraub R, Shiota T, Elkadi T, et al. Transesophageal echocardiography in infants and children with congenital heart disease. Circulation 1992;86:711–722.

Willens HJ, Levy R, Perez A. Diagnosis of accessory mitral valve tissue by transesophageal echocardiography. Echocardiography 1994;11: 39–45.

Williams RG. Echocardiography in the management of single ventricle: fetal through adult life. Echocardiography 1993;10:331–342.

Xu J, Shiota T, Ge S, et al. Intraoperative transesophageal echocardiography using high-resolution biplane 7.5 MHz probes with continuous-wave Doppler capability in infants and children with tetralogy of Fallot. Am J Cardiol 1996;77:539–542.

Zboyovsky KL, Nanda NC, Jain H. Transesophageal echocardiographic identification of atrial septal aneurysm. Echocardiography 1991;8: 435–437.

Part 2
TRANSESOPHAGEAL SEQUENTIAL ANALYSIS OF CARDIOVASCULAR SEGMENTS IN DIAGNOSIS OF COMPLEX CONGENITAL HEART DISEASE

INTRODUCTION

Echocardiographic diagnosis of complex congenital heart disease requires a systematized study that is most logical if based on the sequential identification of the principal cardiovascular segments. It is advisable to begin the echocardiographic exploration with an evaluation of the atrial segments, followed by the ventricles and, finally, the great vessels. With the information obtained it is possible to define the types of intersegmental connections, i.e., atrioventricular (A-V) and ventriculoarterial (V-A) connections.

When the atrial segment is examined, situs should be determined. Atrial situs indicates the morphology of the atria. When the atria have different morphologies, situs is solitus or inversus. The situation in which both atria have the same morphology is known as right or left atrial isomerism.

There are various methods of recognizing atrial situs, such as electrocardiography and, particularly, bronchial morphology observed in radiologic studies. Examination of other viscera, specifically the main lobe of the liver, is of no value, because in about half of patients with complex congenital heart disease there is a discrepancy between atrial situs and visceral situs.

At present the identification of atrial situs is considered reliable if it is based on a morphologic examination of the atrial appendages. Transesophageal echocardiography has facilitated noninvasive diagnosis of atrial situs by permitting visualization of the appendages and of systemic and pulmonary venous return or other anatomic signs originating from embryonic remains.

There are four possible variants of atrial situs: 1) situs solitus, in which the morphologically right atrium is found on the right and the morphologically left atrium on the left; 2) situs inversus, in which the right atrium is located on the left and the left on the right; and 3) right or 4) left atrial isomerism, also known as situs ambiguous, in which both atria have a right or left morphology.

Once the atrial situs is determined the ventricles must be identified to establish the A-V connection. Two well-developed ventricles can exist, or there may be one main ventricle and a rudimentary one, or, less frequently, a true single ventricle. When there are two well-developed ventricles, the tricuspid valve always accompanies the morphologically right ventricle and the mitral valve the morphologically left ventricle.

After the atrial and ventricular segments have been identified, the type of A-V connection can be established.

The possible variations include the following: (1) concordant A-V connection, in which the right atrium is connected to the right ventricle and the left atrium with the left ventricle, regardless of their spatial relationships; (2) discordant A-V connection, in which the right atrium is connected to the left ventricle and vice versa; (3) ambiguous A-V connection, in which in the presence of right or left isomerism the separate atrial cavities or a common atrial chamber connect with the two ventricles; (4) double ventricular inlet, in which the two atria are connected to the same ventricular cavity; and (5) absence of right or left A-V connection, in which a single A-V valve connects an atrium with the main ventricular cavity and the other atrium has no ventricular connection.

In addition to identifying the type of A-V connection, echocardiographic exploration helps define the mode of this connection. The connection between atria and ventricles can be made 1) by means of two perforate valves, 2) by one perforate valve and one imperforate valve, or 3) by an overriding and straddling A-V valve.

The next step is to identify the great vessels and establish the type of ventriculoarterial (V-A) connection. The identification of the great vessels can be achieved by examining their anatomy and trajectory as they emerge from the heart using two-dimensional imaging. The aorta continues cephalad, parallel to the sternum, until it reaches the aortic arch, from which the supraaortic vessels originate. In contrast, the pulmonary artery has a short course, because it takes a posterior direction and rapidly bifurcates. The possible variations are as follows: 1) concordant V-A connection, in which the left ventricle is connected to the aorta and the right ventricle to the pulmonary artery; 2) discordant V-A connection, in which the left ventricle is connected to the pulmonary artery and the right ventricle to the aorta; 3) double ventricular outlet, in which both semilunar orifices are connected in more than 50% of their diameter with one ventricle, usually the morphologically right ventricle; and 4) univentricular outlet, in which a single artery emerges from the heart, as in the case of truncus arteriosus or pulmonary or aortic atresia.

Once the echocardiographic diagnosis of V-A connection has been established, the mode of connection—which can be with two perforate valves, with one perforate valve and one imperforate valve, with overriding valves, or with a common valve—also should be clarified.

The rest of this chapter discusses the use of transesophageal echocardiography in the study of congenital malformations of the heart, using sequential segmental diagnosis in the description.

ATRIAL SITUS

Situs Solitus

Transesophageal studies in transverse and longitudinal planes allow identification of the cardiac structures and chambers.

The right atrial appendage has a triangular morphology with a large implantation base connecting it to the atrial cavity (1). (Fig. 8.2.1). In transverse plane images the crista terminalis of the right atrium can be seen as a prominence separating the appendage, with its pectineal musculature, from the smooth atrial portion (Fig. 8.2.1). The right atrium receives the systemic venous return, and the connection with the superior vena cava can be observed in progressive sections in the transverse plane (Fig. 8.2.2). It is possible to see the connections of both venae cavae with images in the longitudinal plane. Transgastric recordings show the connection of the suprahepatic veins to the inferior vena cava and its communication with the right atrium.

Starting with a four-chamber image, posterior angulation of the probe allows visualization of the coronary sinus, which crosses from left to right and connects to the right atrium (2) (Fig. 8.2.3). The eustachian valve appears as a linear structure crossing the right atrial cavity. Injection of a solution in a peripheral vein opacifies the right-sided atrial cavity.

The left atrial appendage can be identified with recordings in transverse and longitudinal planes by its finger-shaped form with a narrow base (Fig. 8.2.4). This last finding may disappear with volume overload of the atrial cavity.

The pulmonary veins are connected to the atrium situated on the left. With color Doppler their flow is coded

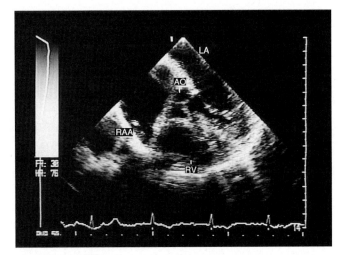

Figure 8.2.1. Situs solitus. Transverse plane image demonstrates the normal morphology of the right atrial appendage (RAA).

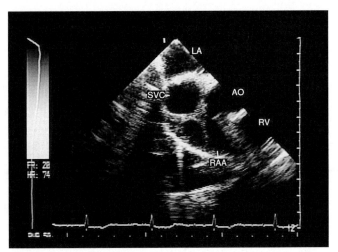

Figure 8.2.2. Situs solitus. In this transverse plane image the connection of the superior vena cava (SVC) to the right atrium can be observed.

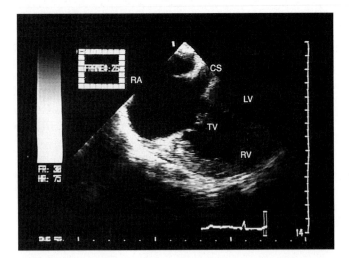

Figure 8.2.3. Situs solitus. Transverse plane image of the four chambers with posterior angulation demonstrates the normal drainage of the coronary sinus (CS) into the right atrium (RA).

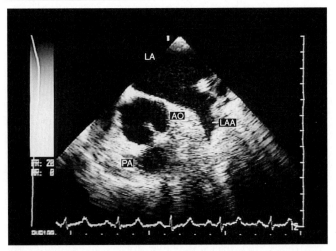

Figure 8.2.4. Situs solitus. Transverse plane view at the atrial level. The normal morphology of the left atrial appendage (LAA) can be identified.

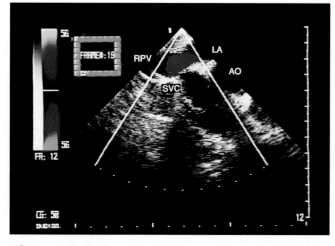

Figure 8.2.5. **Situs solitus.** Atrial situs solitus, showing connection of the right pulmonary vein (RPV) with the left atrium (LA). The superior vena cava (SVC) drains into the right atrium.

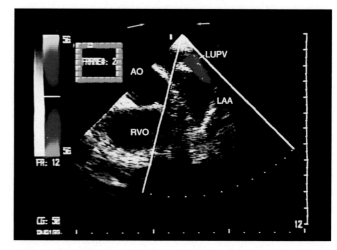

Figure 8.2.6. **Situs solitus.** Transverse plane imaging with color Doppler demonstrates the left upper pulmonary vein (LUPV) behind the left atrial appendage (LAA) and its connection with the left atrium.

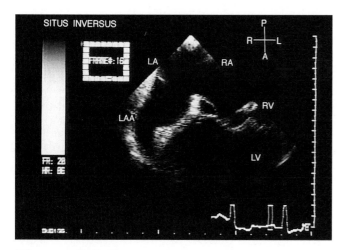

Figure 8.2.7. **Atrial situs inversus.** The anatomically left atrial appendage (LAA) is located on the right.

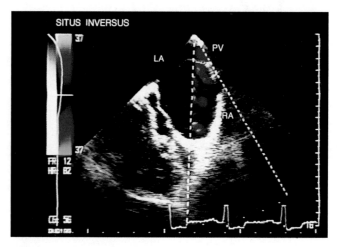

Figure 8.2.8. **Atrial situs inversus.** The presence of atrial situs inversus is demonstrated by the anatomically right atrial appendage (RAA) located on the left. The pulmonary veins (PV) drain into the left atrium (LA), found on the right.

in red (Figs. 8.2.5 and 8.2.6) because the flow is directed posteriorly and forward in relation to the transducer.

Situs Inversus

In situs inversus, the right-sided appendage has the characteristics of an anatomically left appendage (Fig. 8.2.7), whereas the left-sided appendage has the characteristics of an anatomically right appendage (Fig. 8.2.8). The atrial cavity on the right is connected to the pulmonary veins (Fig. 8.2.9), whereas the atrial cavity on the left is connected to the venae cavae and receives the coronary sinus. When contrast studies are performed, the atrial chamber situated on the left is opacified (Fig. 8.2.10). The

eustachian valve can be recognized in the atrium situated on the left (Fig. 8.2.11). The connection of the suprahepatic veins to the inferior vena cava and its drainage into the atrium situated on the left can be observed in transgastric recordings (Fig. 8.2.12).

Findings provided for identifying atrial situs should complement the information obtained from conventional transthoracic and abdominal recordings. These findings can be completed with transgastric recordings; rotation of the transducer directing the beam posteriorly allows evaluation of the position of the inferior vena cava and aorta in relation to the spinal column. In situs solitus the inferior vena cava is found to the right of the column and the aorta to the

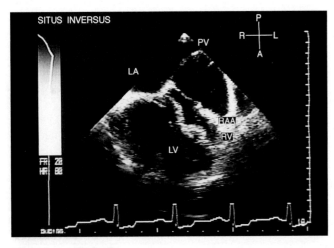

Figure 8.2.9. **Atrial situs inversus.** Transverse plane imaging with color-coded Doppler. The left pulmonary veins (PV) drain into the left atrium (LA), located on the right.

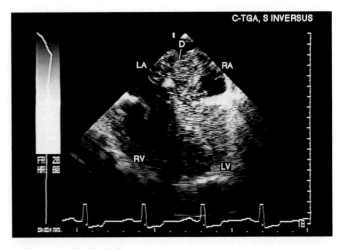

Figure 8.2.10. **Situs inversus and atrioventricular discordance.** A contrast study shows the microbubbles first reaching the right atrium (RA) located on the left, then crossing an interatrial septal defect (D) into the left atrium (LA) and left ventricle (LV).

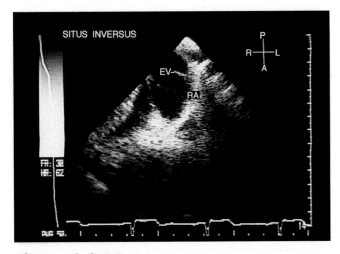

Figure 8.2.11. **Situs inversus.** The right atrium (RA), situated on the left, is identified by the presence of the eustachian valve (EV).

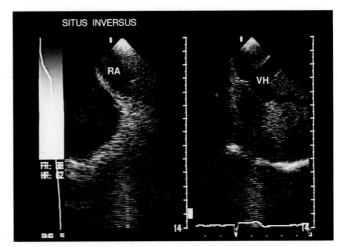

Figure 8.2.12. **Atrial situs inversus.** Situs inversus with progressively superior imaging in the transverse plane. The connection of the hepatic veins (HV) to the left-sided inferior vena cava and right atrium (RA) can be demonstrated in this patient.

left. The aorta can be recognized by its pulsations, and Doppler recordings show systolic flow. Flow in the inferior vena cava is both systolic and diastolic and of lower velocity.

Following the course of the inferior vena cava in longitudinal sections, its connection with the hepatic veins can be identified, as can its drainage into the right atrium.

In situs inversus a mirror image appears, with the inferior vena cava to the left of the spine and the aorta to the right.

Atrial Isomerism

The term *atrial isomerism* refers to the absence of anatomic lateralization of the atria, which confers ambiguous

characteristics on atrial situs. In right isomerism, transesophageal recordings show that both atrial appendages are of right morphology, i.e., they are triangular with broad bases (Fig. 8.2.13). In left isomerism, both atrial appendages are elongated with narrow implantations into their atrial cavities (Fig. 8.2.14).

When atrial isomerism occurs, alterations of systemic and pulmonary venous return often coexist. Because of the important implications such anomalies may have for determining surgical approach, the patterns of venous connection to the heart must be defined before surgical correction.

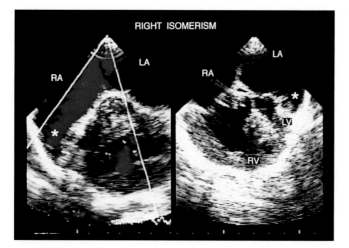

Figure 8.2.13. **Right atrial isomerism.** Transverse plane images. Both atrial appendages (*) have a right morphology.

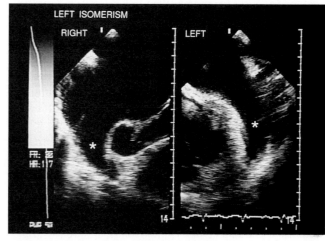

Figure 8.2.14. **Left atrial isomerism.** Transverse plane images. Both atrial appendages (*) have a left morphology.

Although the alterations vary, when a patient presents with right isomerism, it is necessary to check for two superior venae cavae draining directly into both atrial cavities, abnormal connections of hepatic veins to the inferior vena cava, and abnormalities in the pulmonary venous connections, among other anomalies. When left isomerism is present, it is common to find an interrupted inferior vena cava with azygos or hemiazygos continuation, bilateral superior venae cavae, and pulmonary venous return with two veins connected to the atrium located on the right and two to the atrium on the left (2).

Because of the proximity of the transesophageal transducer to the sites of venous return and to the atrial chambers, this technique using the standard transverse axis scan planes may permit a more accurate evaluation of these cardiac structures than is obtained by the transthoracic approach.

The existence of a left persistent superior vena cava can be documented by high left atrial views; the course of the vessel running anterior to the left pulmonary artery and interposed between the left-sided pulmonary veins and left-sided atrial appendage and draining into the roof of the left-sided atrium or connected to the coronary sinus is demonstrated by combining cross-sectional imaging and color flow mapping (Fig. 8.2.15).

The azygos and hemiazygos veins can be demonstrated only in cases in which these vessels are dilated. An azygos vein is sought by combined two-dimensional images and color Doppler posterior and to the right of the right atrium and the right pulmonary artery. The hemiazygos vein is sought posterior to the left atrium and next to the descending aorta (2).

Images similar to those observed with the transducer in subcostal position at the level of the tenth thoracic vertebra can be obtained with transgastric recordings. Right isomerism is diagnosed by visualizing the aorta and the

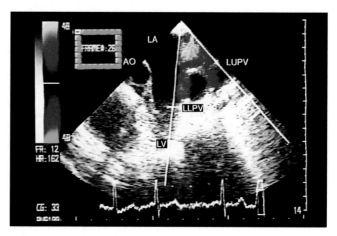

Figure 8.2.15. **Left isomerism.** Left persistent superior vena cava (LSVC) is demonstrated in transverse plane image.

inferior vena cava on the same side of the spine (aortocaval juxtaposition). In this condition, the inferior vena cava is anterolateral in relation to the aorta.

When levoisomerism is present, transesophageal recording makes it possible to document the interruption of the inferior vena cava, an abnormality that occurs in 85% of the cases. In addition, total anomalous connection of hepatic veins can be established and, as described earlier, the azygos and hemiazygos veins can be visualized.

Abnormalities of the right superior vena cava such as absence or anomalous connection also can be demonstrated with transesophageal recordings. The use of the longitudinal plane in biplane imaging offers substantial additional value in the evaluation of systemic venous connections. However, it contributes little in the assessment of pulmonary venous connections, which are discussed in the section on shunts later in this chapter.

Juxtaposed Atrial Appendages

Juxtaposition is an uncommon malformation in which the two atrial appendages are located on the same side of the great vessels. Left juxtaposition is six times more frequent than right and usually is associated with discordant V-A connection, which may be isolated or may be combined with absence of right A-V connection. The identification of this malformation is important, particularly when a procedure such as a Rashkind septostomy or a Mustard, Senning, or Fontan-type surgery is planned.

Recognition of juxtaposition with transthoracic echocardiography can be difficult in older children or patients with poor acoustic windows. Its angiographic identification requires an intense contrast in both atria and the juxtaposed atrial appendages. Transesophageal echocardiography is considered the technique of choice for identifying this anomaly. The transesophageal features of left juxtaposition of the atrial appendage include 1) right lateral deviation of the inferior and posterior portion of the atrial septum; 2) a more frontal orientation of the anterosuperior part of the atrial septum, forming the floor and the posterior wall of the junction of the right-sided atrial appendage with the venous component of the atrial cavity (Fig. 8.2.16); 3) the two atrial appendages, each with its own morphology, visualized on the same side, either in superior-inferior positions or side to side (Figs. 8.2.16 and 8.2.17); and 4) the association of one or various septal defects of the ostium secundum type, which may be difficult to recognize.

The abnormal orientation of the atrial septum may give the false impression of an atrial septal defect located at the site of the junction of the atrial appendage with the venous cavity (3).

VENTRICULAR IDENTIFICATION

In transesophageal recordings the right ventricle is recognized by a number of features. A more apical insertion of the tricuspid septal leaflet in the interventricular septum than of the mitral septal leaflet is present (Fig. 8.2.18). When a perimembranous ventricular septal defect with posterior extension is present, the two A-V valves are inserted at the same level. A muscular structure known as the moderator band can be observed in the inferior portion of the ventricular cavity. The tricuspid subvalvular apparatus has insertions into the interventricular septum (inlet septum) (Fig. 8.2.19). These three characteristics can be identified in the four-chamber transesophageal image.

In transverse transgastric images the two ventricles can be visualized, showing the left ventricle with two papillary muscles and a circular shape and the right ventricle with a crescent-moon shape and muscular trabeculations (Fig. 8.2.20). These recordings are also useful for identifying rudimentary chambers, which is not always possible with transesophageal imaging.

The presence of the infundibulum in the right ventricle and the fibrous continuity between the mitral valve (left ventricle) and the semilunar valve are other criteria in ventricular identification that can be seen with biplanar transesophageal recordings. Their discriminatory value is lost in congenital heart disease with bilateral infundibulum.

ATRIOVENTRICULAR CONNECTION

After atrial situs and ventricular position have been identified, the type and mode of A-V connection should be clarified. In the past, injection of saline solution in a peripheral vein was used to demonstrate the type of A-V connection according to the opacification of the atria and ventricles; today intersegmental connection is established with transesophageal recordings using color Doppler.

Concordant A-V Connection

Once the atria and ventricle are identified, a Doppler study (spectral analysis or color) from a four-chamber trans-

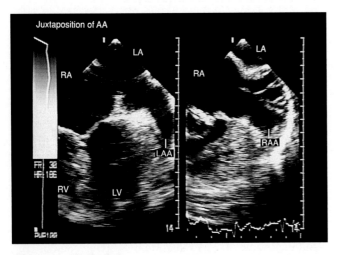

Figure 8.2.16. Juxtaposition of atrial appendages. Transverse plane imaging shows both atrial appendages (LAA, RAA) located on the left side.

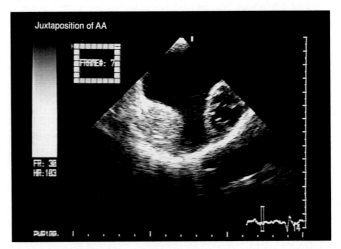

Figure 8.2.17. Juxtaposition of atrial appendages. The right atrial appendage is imaged more anteriorly as compared to the left atrial appendage (LAA).

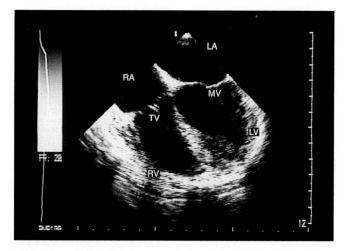

Figure 8.2.18. Concordant atrioventricular connection. The insertion of the tricuspid septal leaflet (TV) into the interventricular septum is more apical than the insertion of the mitral septal leaflet (MV). This information is useful in identifying the ventricles.

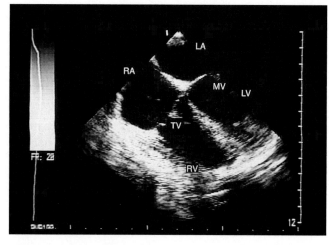

Figure 8.2.19. Concordant atrioventricular connection. The anatomically right ventricle (RV) can be identified by demonstrating the insertion of the tricuspid subvalvular apparatus (TV) into the interventricular septum.

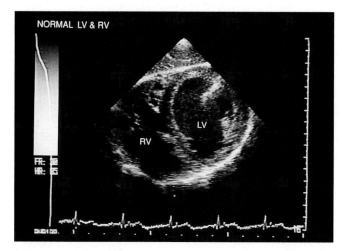

Figure 8.2.20. Concordant atrioventricular connection. Transgastric study shows the right ventricle (RV) to have a crescent-moon shape and multiple trabeculae. The left ventricle (LV) has a circular shape and two papillary muscles.

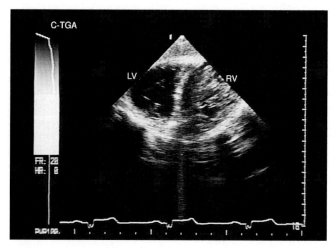

Figure 8.2.21. Discordant atrioventricular connection. In a patient with atrioventricular and ventriculoarterial discordance, the anatomic left ventricle (LV) is located on the right and the anatomic right ventricle (RV) on the left.

esophageal image shows that right atrial flow passes through the tricuspid valve into the anatomically right ventricle and left atrial flow crosses the mitral valve into the anatomically left ventricle.

Discordant A-V Connection

The diagnosis of discordant A-V connection can be established with transesophageal studies in both situs solitus and situs inversus, as well as in levocardia, mesocardia, and dextrocardia, based on the findings discussed in the following paragraphs (4).

In patients with situs solitus, after ensuring that the anatomically right atrium is actually on the right, color

Doppler is used to confirm that it connects with an anatomically left ventricle located on the right (Fig. 8.2.21). The moderator band and more apical insertion of the tricuspid septal leaflet in the interventricular septum observed in the four-chamber image as anatomic markers of the right ventricle are found in the ventricle located on the left (Fig. 8.2.22).

In the presence of discordant A-V connection, most patients have a perimembranous ventricular septal defect with extension to the inlet portion, which causes the insertion of both A-V valves in the septum to occur at the same level.

The insertion of the tricuspid chordae tendineae in the interventricular septum is perhaps the most reliable sign

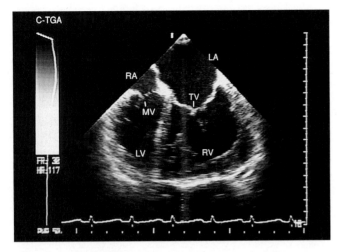

Figure 8.2.22. Discordant atrioventricular connection. Four-chamber study of a patient with situs solitus and atrioventricular discordance. The insertion of the tricuspid septal leaflet (TV) is more apical than the insertion of the mitral septal leaflet (MV).

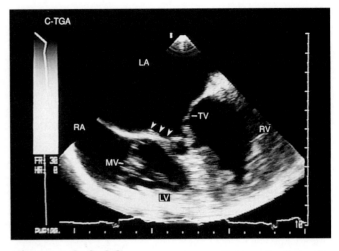

Figure 8.2.23. Discordant atrioventricular connection. Situs solitus and atrioventricular discordance. Tethering of the tricuspid septal leaflet to the ventricular septum is present (arrows).

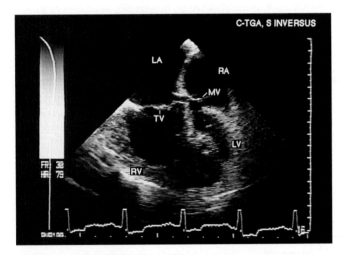

Figure 8.2.24. Discordant atrioventricular connection. Four-chamber image shows atrioventricular discordance and situs inversus.

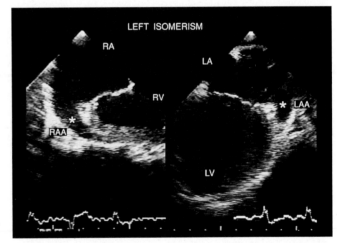

Figure 8.2.25. Ambiguous atrioventricular connection. In the presence of left atrial isomerism, both atrial appendages (*) have anatomically left morphology.

for identifying the right ventricle located on the left. It is relatively easy to demonstrate this in the four-chamber transesophageal image.

In patients with discordant A-V connection the V-A connection usually is also discordant—i.e., the condition corresponds to the anomaly known as corrected transposition of the great vessels. Occasionally, the tricuspid valve is tethered to the ventricular wall, a finding known as left-sided Ebstein's anomaly, which is easily recognized in transesophageal recordings (Fig. 8.2.23).

When situs inversus is present, the A-V discordance is demonstrated on observing that the left atrium situated on the right is connected to the anatomically right ventricle situated on the right, and the right atrium situated on the left is connected to the anatomically left ventricle situated on the left (Fig. 8.2.24).

Apart from the ventricular septal defect in patients with corrected transposition of the great vessels, subvalvular pulmonary obstruction is another commonly associated malformation. It is best identified by visualizing the left ventricular outlet using transesophageal longitudinal plane examination.

Ambiguous A-V Connection

In ambiguous A-V connection, transesophageal visualization of the atrial appendages shows that both have a right or left morphology, i.e., that there is right or left isomerism (Fig. 8.2.25). Color Doppler shows that each atrium is connected with a different ventricle. The term "ambiguous A-V connection" does not indicate the position of the ventricles. The criteria described above are applied for identifying the position of the ventricles.

The concordant, discordant, and ambiguous A-V connections are biventricular. Double inlet ventricle and absence of right or left A-V connection, discussed in the following paragraphs, correspond to univentricular A-V connection.

In contrast to biventricular A-V connection, in univentricular A-V connection the atrial segment is connected to a single ventricular chamber called the main ventricle. In most cases another ventricle is present. It is, by definition, rudimentary, and because it has no A-V connection it lacks the greater part of its inlet. The main ventricular chamber may have a left morphology with a rudimentary right ventricle, a right morphology with a rudimentary left ventricle, or indeterminate morphology with no rudimentary ventricle (true univentricular heart).

Ventricular morphology is identified by noting the position of the rudimentary ventricle in relation to the main ventricle. In cases of left ventricular main chamber, the trabecular septum has a forward deviation and does not reach the crux of the heart, so that the rudimentary right ventricle always has an anterosuperior position distant from the crux. When the main ventricle is of right ventricular morphology, the trabecular septum has a more posterior position than normal and extends to the crux of the heart. Consequently, the rudimentary left ventricle always is postero-inferior and is found close to the crux of the heart. The rudimentary ventricle can be located on the right or left of the main ventricle, depending on bulboventricular loop.

Double Inlet Ventricle

The double inlet most commonly corresponds to the anatomically left ventricle. The features discussed in the following paragraphs can be detected by echocardiography.

In the four-chamber transesophageal image, the two A-V valves open into the same ventricular cavity, and their septal leaflets approximate each other during diastole because of the lack of septal tissue between them. A common A-V valve may exist.

In transesophageal recordings the two A-V valves are visualized within a large ventricular cavity. Their anatomy is variable; often both have only two leaflets.

The rudimentary ventricular cavity can be identified with transgastric recordings in the transverse plane. Its position is anterior in relation to the main ventricular cavity. A ventricular septal defect of variable size communicating with the main ventricle and the rudimentary ventricle also can be identified (Fig. 8.2.26).

Occasionally one of the A-V valves can be seen in the four-chamber view; it may demonstrate a domeshaped opening owing to its insertion into a single papillary muscle (parachute valve) (Fig. 8.2.27).

Overriding of the anterior A-V valve over the interventricular septum is not unusual. It is sometimes accompanied by insertion of its chordae tendineae in the rudimentary ventricle, and should be looked for with transesophageal echocardiography using biplane or multiplane imaging.

The trabecular septum is seen to deviate forward in different biplane sections. Portions of the atrial septum point toward the left ventricular cavity because of malalignment with the interventricular septum.

Recordings with the different Doppler techniques allow the diagnosis of stenosis or regurgitation of the A-V valves

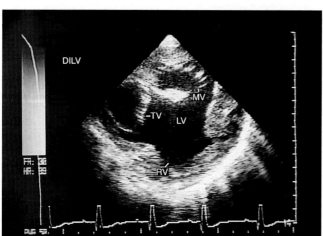

Figure 8.2.26. **Double inlet ventricle.** Transgastric transverse plane image of a patient with double inlet left ventricle. Both atrioventricular valves (TV, MV) can be seen in the left ventricular cavity (LV), which is located posteriorly. The right ventricle (RV) is rudimentary and in an anterior position.

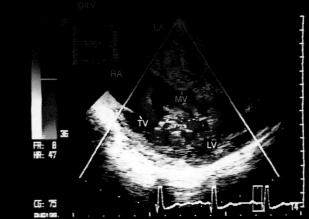

Figure 8.2.27. **Double inlet ventricle.** Transverse plane imaging with color Doppler shows the connection of both atria (RA, LA) to a single ventricular cavity (LV). The mitral valve (MV) opening is restricted by congenital stenosis.

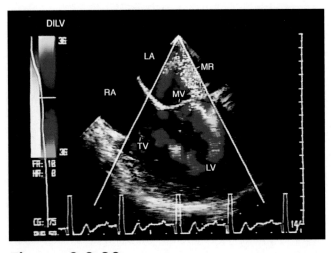

Figure 8.2.28. **Double inlet ventricle.** Four-chamber imaging with color Doppler demonstrates mitral regurgitation (MR) in a patient with double inlet left ventricle (DILV).

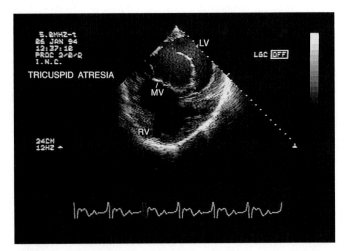

Figure 8.2.29. Absence of atrioventricular connection. Transgastric view in a patient with a large ventricular septal defect. Only one atrioventricular valve, the mitral valve (MV), exists. The anterior rudimentary chamber corresponds to the right ventricle (RV).

(Fig. 8.2.28). They also help to recognize defects of the interatrial septum or its absence (common atrium).

The echocardiographic characteristics of double inlet of the right ventricle have a great deal in common with those of double inlet of the left ventricle, with the difference that the two A-V valves, or the common A-V valve, are always visualized in a position anterior to the trabecular septum. The rudimentary ventricle is posterior in relation to the main ventricle. The posterior A-V valve often straddles the interventricular septum with insertions in the rudimentary ventricle.

Absence of A-V Connection

Right-sided absence, or classic tricuspid atresia, is characterized by a lack of continuity between the right cavities. The floor of the right atrium is muscular and is separated from the right ventricle by fibrous tissue from the A-V sulcus. There are rare cases of true tricuspid atresia in which the right chambers have a potential connection through an imperforate valvular membrane.

In patients with absence of right A-V connection (classic tricuspid atresia), the signs discussed in the following paragraphs can be observed with transesophageal echocardiography.

Absence of movement of the tricuspid valve can be seen, with ample diastolic mobility of the mitral valve (Fig. 8.2.29). In the four-chamber image a line of dense echoes can be seen below the right atrial floor, which represents the fibrous tissue of the A-V sulcus (Fig. 8.2.30). The presence of a small right ventricle and a dilated and hypertrophied left ventricle is confirmed by biplanar transgastric and transesophageal recordings (Fig. 8.2.31).

Because of the loss of alignment of the interatrial and interventricular septa resulting from anterior displacement

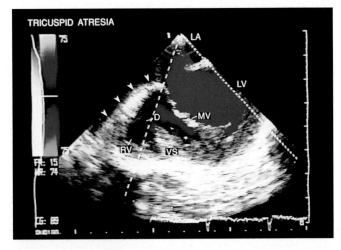

Figure 8.2.30. Absence of atrioventricular connection. Transverse plane image. Dense echoes (arrows), which separate the right-sided cavities, are seen. Color Doppler identifies left ventricular filling. A large ventricular septal defect (D) can also be observed.

of the interventricular septum, the right atrium can be seen to project to a greater or lesser degree on the left ventricle in four-chamber images. Color-coded Doppler recordings show the obligatory atrial septal defect (Fig. 8.2.32). In cases in which one of the great vessels is connected to the rudimentary ventricle, a defect of the trabecular portion of the ventricular septum also can be identified. Doppler spectral analysis aids in detecting possible gradients through the septal defects when one of these is restrictive. Atrioseptostomy is indicated when an important gradient is generated through the atrial septal defect.

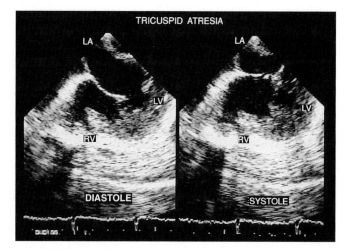

Figure 8.2.31. Absence of atrioventricular connection. Four-chamber image reveals the absence of right atrioventricular connection. There is malalignment between the interatrial and interventricular septa, and a large ventricular septal defect is evident.

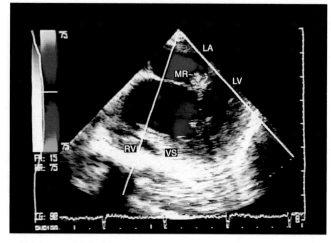

Figure 8.2.33. Absence of atrioventricular connection. In tricuspid atresia, color Doppler is useful in determining the severity of mitral regurgitation (MR). This is important in preoperative evaluation.

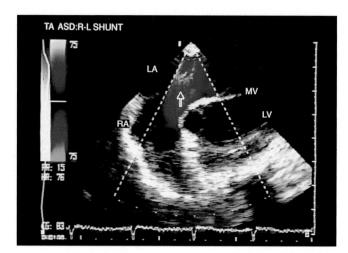

Figure 8.2.32. Absence of atrioventricular connection. Tricuspid atresia. Color-coded Doppler identifies the large secundum atrial septal defect with obligatory right-to-left shunting (arrow).

The study of left ventricular function should be included to evaluate the feasibility of a Fontan-type procedure and to check for the presence of mitral regurgitation (Fig. 8.2.33).

In the absence of left A-V connection, fibrous tissue from the A-V sulcus separates the left atrium from the left ventricle. The floor of the left atrium rests, to a variable degree, on the right ventricle because of the posterior deviation of the interventricular septum.

Another congenital malformation is mitral atresia with imperforate membrane, which usually forms part of the hypoplastic left heart syndrome. This is also characterized by hypoplasia of the aortic root.

In patients with absence of left A-V connection there is absence of movement of the mitral valve with ample mobility of the tricuspid valve. In the four-chamber image, a line of hyperreflectant echoes from the fibrous tissue of the A-V sulcus can be seen on the atrial floor. The left ventricle is seen to be rudimentary, and the right ventricle dilated and hypertrophied, in transthoracic and transesophageal biplanar images. In the four-chamber image the left atrium can be seen to rest, to a greater or lesser degree, on the right ventricle. This results from a posterior displacement of the interventricular septum, which leads to the loss of alignment of the interatrial and interventricular septa.

Color Doppler shows the left-to-right shunt at the atrial level and left ventricular filling through a ventricular septal defect. In addition, the absence of inflow to the left ventricle is confirmed.

Crossed A-V Connection

Crossed A-V connection is not a specific type of connection; it corresponds, rather, to an alteration in the spatial relation between the atria and ventricles. The atrium situated on the right is connected to a ventricle located on the left; the left-sided atrium is connected to a ventricle positioned on the right. The A-V connection may be concordant or discordant. It is not easy to establish the diagnosis with transesophageal echocardiography in the transverse plane using monoplanar transducers, because the normal parallel relationship of the inlet chambers of the two ventricles is lost; in general, the abnormal spatial orientation of the A-V valves makes it difficult to observe both in the same sector.

Color Doppler can be useful in demonstrating that the ventricular filling flows cross each other (Figs. 8.2.34

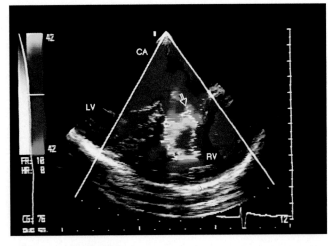

Figure 8.2.34. **Crossed atrioventricular connection.** Two-dimensional and color Doppler study in a patient with criss-cross heart. The right portion of the common atrium (arrow) is connected to the anatomically right ventricle located on the left (RV).

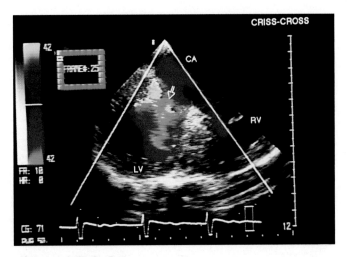

Figure 8.2.35. **Crossed atrioventricular connection.** When a crossed atrioventricular connection exists, the left portion of the common atrium (CA) connects (arrow) to the anatomically left ventricle located on the right.

and 8.2.35). Transesophageal and transgastric images in the longitudinal plane are of greater utility for aligning along the long axes of both ventricular filling flows.

After the type of A-V connection has been identified, echocardiographic exploration should include examination of the mode of connection. It is important to determine whether there are two perforate valves, if one is imperforate, if there is a common A-V valve, or if one of the valves straddles the interventricular septum.

TRANSESOPHAGEAL ECHOCARDIOGRAPHY AND FONTAN-TYPE SURGERY

In some complex congenital cardiac malformations, such as tricuspid atresia or left ventricular double inlet, the diverse Fontan-type surgical techniques, which are based on a redistribution of systemic venous return with increased pulmonary arterial flow, have improved the clinical condition of these patients. This type of surgery includes anterior or posterior connection of the right atrium directly to the pulmonary artery or through a valved conduit, connection of the right atrium and ventricle with valved or nonvalved conduit, or connection of the venae cavae to the pulmonary artery. A significant percentage of patients who undergo this type of surgery present residual lesions or develop lesions in the postoperative period that are not easily identified with transthoracic imaging, particularly in adolescents and adults.

The transesophageal examination of these patients should follow a protocol, and ideally should be performed with biplanar or multiplanar transducers (5,6). Each study should include transgastric recordings to evaluate the connection of the hepatic veins to the infe-

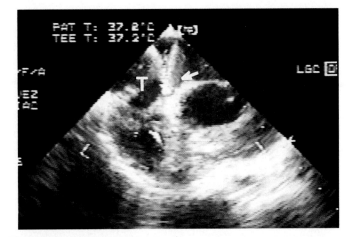

Figure 8.2.36. **Fontan-type surgery.** Transverse plane image at the level of the atrial septum shows the integrity of the tunnel wall (T). Red and yellow represent flow greater than expected through the obligatory atrial septal defect (arrow).

rior vena cava and the latter to the right atrium. As the transducer is withdrawn into the esophagus, the progressive transverse sections permit exploration of the entire right atrium. When these recordings are complemented with longitudinal plane images, it is possible to evaluate the integrity of the interatrial septum as well as the intra-atrial patch used in total cavopulmonary connections (Figs. 8.2.36 and 8.2.37A). Likewise, the connection of the right atrium to the right ventricle or to the pulmonary arterial circulation can be directly visualized with multiple images in both planes.

When the connections are of a posterior type, transesophageal study allows their complete evaluation. How-

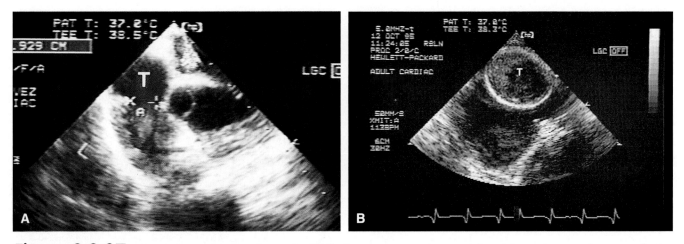

Figure 8.2.37. **Fontan-type procedure. A.** High short-axis view in a patient with total cavopulmonary deviation. There is a large defect, which permits a venoarterial shunt, in the wall of the intraatrial patch or tunnel (T). **B.** Transesophageal echocardiogram in a patient with total cavopulmonary anastomosis and thrombosis of the atrial tunnel (T).

ever, if they are located in an anterior position their analysis is difficult, and precordial recordings can be more useful.

Images in longitudinal planes have diminished the difficulties involved in visualizing the pulmonary artery and the proximal portion of its branches. In transverse section the right branch is seen posterior to the superior vena cava and the left branch anterior to the descending aorta.

The presence of intracavitary thrombi or thrombosis involving prosthetic conduits should be looked for in various two-dimensional images (Fig. 8.2.37B). If a thrombus is present or if it is absent but spontaneous contrast echoes are noted, administration of thrombolytic agents should be considered.

The echocardiographic study should include visualization of the sites of connection of the four pulmonary veins. Evaluation of function of both ventricles usually can be achieved with conventional precordial recordings; its analysis can be complemented with transverse plane transgastric recordings. Both conventional and color Doppler modalities are very useful and allow identification of residual atrial shunts. The spectral curves obtained in the pulmonary arteries with Doppler vary according to the type of surgery. In cases of cavopulmonary deviation flow is continuous, of low velocity, and demonstrates marked respiratory variation. In the pulmonary arteries of patients who underwent atriopulmonary connection there is biphasic (systolic and diastolic) forward flow. Retrograde flow in the distal third of the pulmonary branches can be seen when arterial hypertension exists. In patients with atrioventricular connection the forward flow in the pulmonary artery is limited to systole; in these cases, retrograde diastolic flow seems to occur, because during this phase of the cardiac cycle the ventricle functions as a reservoir without pulmonary valve closure.

The morphology of flow in the pulmonary veins is related to the pressures in the left cavities; Doppler study shows it to be biphasic regardless of the type of surgery performed.

When obstruction of a pulmonary arterial branch exists, the pulmonary veins on the same side show elevated peak retrograde velocity and diminished systolic and diastolic flow, reflecting to-and-fro flow in the pulmonary veins of the obstructed side.

Transesophageal echocardiography provides ample information in adult patients who have undergone one of the Fontan surgical techniques, and can be considered the most valuable adjunct in mid-term and long-term follow up (7).

Identification of the Great Vessels

Once the A-V connection has been determined, the aorta and pulmonary artery must be identified to establish the V-A connection. With the transducer in the patient's esophagus, the pulmonary artery usually is recognized in transverse and longitudinal plane images by its bifurcation. In contrast, the aorta has a long course until it forms the aortic arch.

Visualization of the origin of the coronary arteries in a transverse section close to the level of the semilunar plane identifies the vessel as the aorta. In this plane the spatial relationship of the great arteries also can be recognized. The aorta normally is posterior and to the right of the pulmonary artery. The point at which the great vessels cross can be observed in biplanar transesophageal images (8).

VENTRICULOARTERIAL CONNECTIONS

Concordant V-A Connection

In concordant V-A connections, each of the vessels is connected with its corresponding ventricle. The outlet of the right ventricle and the pulmonary arteries with their bifurcation surrounding the aorta can be observed with transesophageal echocardiography and biplanar recordings. The connection of the left ventricle with the aorta and the right ventricle with the pulmonary artery is confirmed using color Doppler.

Discordant Ventriculoarterial Connection

Ventriculoarterial discordance, or complete transposition of great vessels, is the condition in which the aorta is connected to the right ventricle and the pulmonary artery to the left ventricle, while the A-V connection is concordant. In this anomaly the aorta is located in front and to the right of the main pulmonary artery. However, this abnormal spatial relationship of the semilunar vessels is not constant; in about 20% of cases the aorta is found in different positions depending on the orientation of the infundibular septum.

The echocardiographic diagnosis of this malformation should include both morphologic and functional aspects. Following segmental sequence, situs and type of A-V connection should be clarified. V-A discordance should be established with conventional transthoracic recordings and transesophageal exploration used to aid in clarifying some specific alterations. Conditions discussed in the following paragraphs can be detected with this technique.

In images in the transverse plane at the level of the great arteries, the vessel that is anterior and to the right can be seen to correspond to the aorta and the posterior left vessel to the main pulmonary artery (Fig. 8.2.38). In these images, confirmation that the aorta is connected to the ventricle that receives systemic venous return is obtained by demonstrating that the anterior vessel opacifies when saline solution is injected into a peripheral vein. In progressively superior sections the posterior vessel can be recognized as corresponding to the pulmonary artery because it bifurcates early. It is easy to demonstrate valvular or subvalvular pulmonary stenosis, or both, using color Doppler (Figs. 8.2.39 and 8.2.40).

In recordings in the longitudinal plane, the anterior vessel (aorta) can be seen to maintain a long anterior

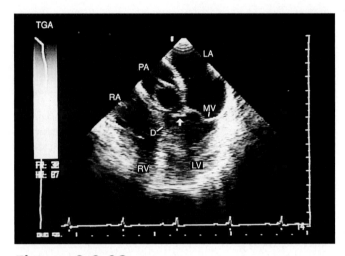

Figure 8.2.39. Discordant ventriculoarterial connection. Transposition of the great arteries exists. The transverse plane image shows mitral-pulmonary continuity. A pulmonary subvalvular obstruction (arrow) is seen secondary to the anomalous insertion of the mitral subvalvular apparatus in the ventricular septum. Stenosis of the pulmonary valve coexists.

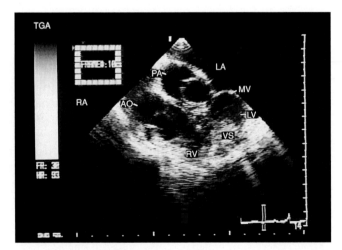

Figure 8.2.38. Discordant ventriculoarterial connection. In the presence of transposition of the great arteries, transverse plane imaging makes it possible to recognize the connection of the right ventricle (RV) with the aorta (AO) and the left ventricle (LV) with the pulmonary artery (PA). An anomalous insertion of the mitral valve (MV) produces subvalvular pulmonary obstruction. The pulmonary valve opening is also restricted.

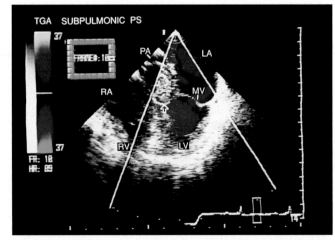

Figure 8.2.40. Discordant ventriculoarterial connection. The connection of the left ventricle (LV) with the pulmonary artery (PA) is identified with transverse plane imaging and color-coded Doppler. Subvalvular pulmonary stenosis (arrow) is also seen, together with the dome-shaped opening of the pulmonary valve, which indicates the presence of the coexisting pulmonary valvular stenosis.

course without bifurcating. From this type of section, rotation of the transducer to the left shows the pulmonary artery, which runs parallel to the aorta in a posterior position (Fig. 8.2.41). In images of the right cavities in the longitudinal plane, the aortic valve is normally seen very close to the tricuspid valve. When transposition of great vessels occurs, the aortic valve is found away from the tricuspid valve.

The mitral-pulmonary fibrous continuity can be recognized in transverse and longitudinal images. These views also are useful for recognizing abnormal systolic movement of the mitral valve toward the interventricular septum, which may result in dynamic subpulmonary obstruction.

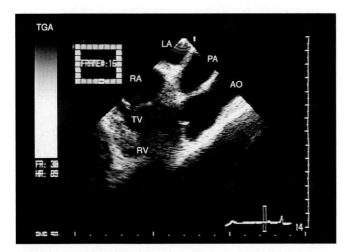

Figure 8.2.41. **Discordant ventriculoarterial connection.** Transposition of the great arteries (TGA) exists. The right ventricle (RV) is connected to the anterior vessel, which corresponds to the aorta (AO). This is identified in longitudinal plane imaging.

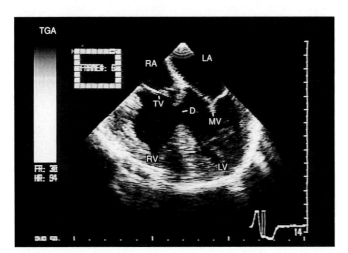

Figure 8.2.42. **Discordant ventriculoarterial connection.** Four-chamber image from a patient with transposition of the great arteries. A large ventricular septal defect (D) is noted.

Ventricular septal defect occurs in approximately 40% of cases. Because the location of the defect is predominantly subpulmonary (2 out of 3 cases), transesophageal exploration of this area in biplanar or multiplanar recordings should be included in the study of every patient with transposition (Fig. 8.2.42). Likewise, evaluation of interatrial shunts, some of which are augmented by the Rashkind septostomy, should be included in the analysis of biplanar or multiplanar two-dimensional images with color Doppler.

In view of the possibility of exploring the principal coronary arteries with transesophageal echocardiography, abnormalities of their origin and distribution should be investigated in these cases.

STUDY OF ATRIAL BAFFLE FUNCTION AFTER MUSTARD OR SENNING PROCEDURES

The transesophageal approach allows the assessment of the entire systemic and pulmonary venous pathways after atrial corrective surgery (5). The relative shape and size of each baffle component are variable, according to the surgical technique used.

The proximal portions of the superior and inferior venae cavae, as well as their respective unions with the superior and inferior baffle limbs of the systemic venous atrium, are visualized using multiple short-axis scans with rotations and probe tip angulations. By advancing and rotating the probe, the individual sites of drainage of all four pulmonary veins and the entire pulmonary venous pathway are scanned (Fig. 8.2.43). A morphologic and hemodynamic evaluation of both venous atria is performed using two-dimensional imaging in combination with Doppler color flow mapping and pulsed wave spectral analysis. Flow

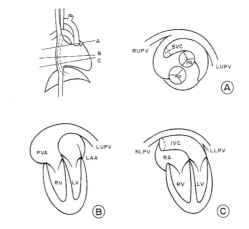

Figure 8.2.43. **Atrial switch procedure.** Transesophageal interrogation with progressively higher sections (from C to A) allows imaging of the entire inferior limb of the systemic venous atrium (C), the pulmonary venous atrium (B), and the superior limb of the systemic venous atrium near the great arteries (A). The pulmonary veins appear in a posterior position.

patterns in both systemic and venous limbs, in the pulmonary venous pathway, and in each of the pulmonary veins are obtained.

Transesophageal exploration is definitely superior to precordial investigation of superior or inferior limb obstructions and mid-baffle obstructions. With this technique individual pulmonary vein velocity profiles can be recognized, as can mid-pulmonary venous atrium obstruction. With color flow mapping, definite evidence of baffle leakage also is obtained (9).

The echocardiographic study also should include the search for late complications such as right ventricular dysfunction, tricuspid insufficiency, and progressive left ventricular outflow tract obstruction.

CONGENITALLY CORRECTED TRANSPOSITION

In congenitally corrected transposition, both the A-V and the V-A connections are discordant. Associated defects, especially ventricular septal defect, either isolated or with pulmonary valve stenosis, are common, occurring in 70% to 90% of cases. Cardiac malpositions also are commonly associated and can make it difficult to obtain satisfactory transthoracic recordings. The study of these patients should include transesophageal and transgastric recordings, and the main findings are discussed in the following paragraphs (4).

Atrioventricular discordance is established by identifying atrial situs and the position of the ventricles using the criteria discussed at the beginning of the chapter. The most reliable way of identifying the atria is through the morphology of the atrial appendages. The principal signs used for identification of the ventricles are the different levels of implantation of the mitral and tricuspid septal leaflets (when ventricular septal defect is absent) and insertion of the tricuspid chordae tendineae in the interventricular septum. In addition, the ventricular morphology evident in the four-chamber image facilitates recognition—the right ventricular chamber has a triangular shape and the left ventricular chamber an ellipsoid form. These characteristics are independent of the ventricular spatial relationship.

In ventriculoarterial discordance, identification of the great arteries is based on the bifurcation of the pulmonary artery. The parallel positions of the two vessels can be observed with monoplanar recordings taken at the level of the semilunar valves. When situs is solitus, the aorta is anterior and to the left and the main pulmonary artery posterior and to the right (Fig. 8.2.44). In situs inversus the aorta is anterior but to the right of the main pulmonary artery.

Direct visualization of the connection of the ventricles to the great vessels is facilitated by the use of biplanar transducers. In images in the longitudinal plane it is possible to visualize the connection of the posterior vessel (pulmonary artery) with the left ventricle, to corroborate mitral-pulmonary continuity and to demonstrate the connection between the anterior outflow tract (right ventricular) and the aorta.

It is possible to identify cardiac position from the transesophageal four-chamber image. The apex of the ventricles points to the left in levocardia, to the right in dextrocardia, and toward the midline in mesocardia. Moreover, the subpulmonary outflow tract of the left ventricle is deeply wedged between the mitral and tricuspid valves, which generates malalignment of the atrial and ventricular septum and prominent anterior recess in the morphologically left ventricle.

Transesophageal study is superior to transthoracic study for visualizing the frequently associated ventricular septal defect. The defect usually is a wide perimembranous type in subpulmonary position. It can be visualized directly in transverse or longitudinal planes.

Obstruction of left ventricular emptying can be determined with transesophageal recording. In most cases there is mixed pulmonary stenosis, both subvalvular and valvular (10). The capacity to explore the subvalvular pulmonary area is one of the principal advantages of the transesophageal technique. The various causes of subpulmonary obstruction, such as narrowing of the outflow tract, abnormal tissue tags, and discrete pulmonary membrane (rare), can be recognized in images in the longitudinal plane. It is also possible to recognize nonobstructive bulging of the membranous septum into the subpulmonary outflow tract.

Abnormalities of the A-V valves are not uncommon; the tricuspid valvular anomaly known as left-sided Ebstein's anomaly is noteworthy. In patients with this anomaly, it is possible to recognize tethering of the septal leaflet to the interventricular septum in the transesophageal four-chamber image and to evaluate the severity of valvular regurgitation with color Doppler (Figs. 8.2.45 and 8.2.46).

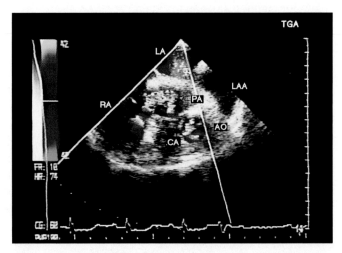

Figure 8.2.44. **Ventriculoarterial discordance.** Transverse plane image. The aorta (AO) is identified by the origin of the right coronary artery (CA). The pulmonary artery (PA) is located behind and to the right of the aorta, and its turbulent flow is secondary to the coexistence of subvalvular pulmonary stenosis.

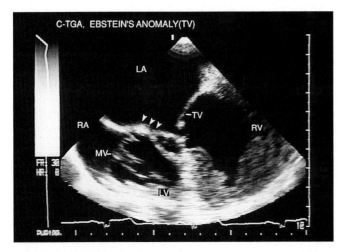

Figure 8.2.45. Left-sided Ebstein's anomaly. Four-chamber image in a patient with corrected transposition of the great arteries (C-TGA). Tethering of the tricuspid septal leaflet to the ventricular septum is present (arrows). The anterior tricuspid leaflet (TV) shows ample movement.

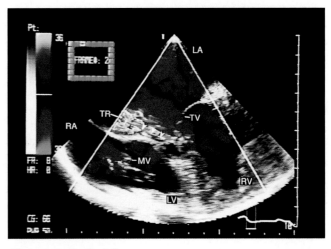

Figure 8.2.46. Left-sided Ebstein's anomaly. Corrected transposition of the great arteries is seen coexisting with an Ebstein-type anomaly of the tricuspid valve. Color Doppler shows the presence of tricuspid regurgitation (TR).

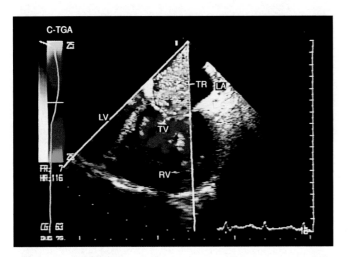

Figure 8.2.47. Corrected transposition of the great arteries. Two-dimensional imaging with color Doppler demonstrates significant tricuspid regurgitation (TR).

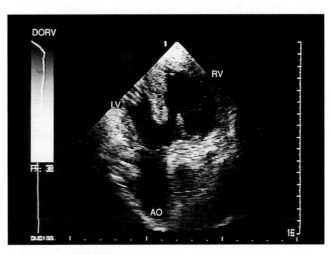

Figure 8.2.48. Double outlet right ventricle. Transgastric view shows aortic (AO) septal override.

Because of the prognostic implications and importance in making the surgical decision, an evaluation of right ventricular function should be included in the transesophageal study. Ventricular dysfunction is most common in patients with significant long-term tricuspid regurgitation (Fig. 8.2.47).

Right Ventricular Double Outlet

In right ventricular double outlet both great arteries arise mainly or completely from the right ventricle. Any type of A-V connection can coexist. The position of the vessels is variable. When they are side to side or the aorta is anterior, the emergence of the vessels is parallel. When the aorta is posterior and right, the great arteries cross in space. Often

the underlying anomaly is tetralogy of Fallot with aortic overriding of more than 50%.

In the past, double infundibulum was considered a prerequisite for the diagnosis. However, it has been established that the presence of fibrous continuity between the posterior vessel and the mitral valve does not preclude the type of V-A connection being a double outlet.

The principal findings observed with transesophageal echocardiography are discussed in the following paragraphs.

Overriding of more than 50% of the posterior vessel over the interventricular septum is evident in recordings of both transverse and longitudinal planes (Fig. 8.2.48). The connection of both vessels with the right ventricle can be observed in longitudinal images (Figs. 8.2.49 and 8.2.50). When only monoplanar recordings can be obtained, multiple sections at various levels should be visualized to demonstrate that the great arteries are located on the same side of the interventricular septum (Fig. 8.2.51).

The examination of the ventricular outflow tracts should include images in transverse and longitudinal planes to look for subpulmonary obstructions and to investigate the relationship between the ventricular septal defect and the great vessels.

Color Doppler study demonstrates that the flow that crosses the ventricular septal defect is directed preferentially toward the vessel with which the defect is associated. The defect can be subaortic or subpulmonary, can be related to both arteries, or can have no relation with either (Fig. 8.2.52).

Truncus Arteriosus

When only one artery emerges from the heart, the V-A connection is defined as single outlet. Three possibilities exist: truncus arteriosus, pulmonary atresia or aortic atresia. In truncus arteriosus, the vessel emerging from the heart originates the systemic, pulmonary, and coronary circulation. Images in the longitudinal plane obtained with a biplanar or multiplanar transducer show the truncus arteriosus straddling the interventricular septum (Fig. 8.2.53). The absence of right ventricular infundibulum is evident in transverse and longitudinal sections, and multiple images in both planes show the ventricular septal defect due to the absence of the infundibular septum. Transverse sections also show supernumerary truncal leaflets.

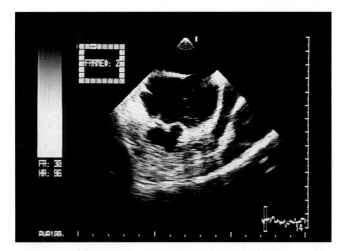

Figure 8.2.49. Double outlet right ventricle and pulmonary stenosis. Longitudinal plane examination shows both semilunar valves arising from one chamber, which is the right ventricle.

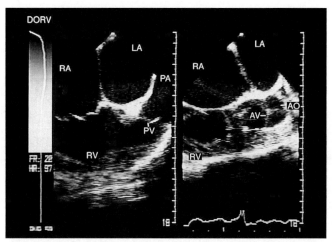

Figure 8.2.50. Double outlet right ventricle. Images in the longitudinal plane show that the pulmonary artery (PA) and the aorta (AO) are connected to the right ventricle (RV).

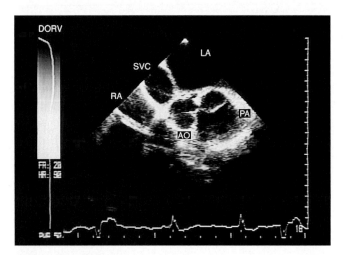

Figure 8.2.51. Double outlet right ventricle. Transverse plane image. The great arteries (AO, PA) have a side-to-side relationship.

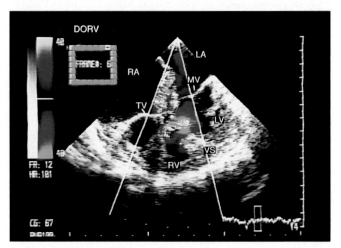

Figure 8.2.52. Double outlet right ventricle. Color Doppler shows tricuspid valve regurgitation and a large ventricular septal defect.

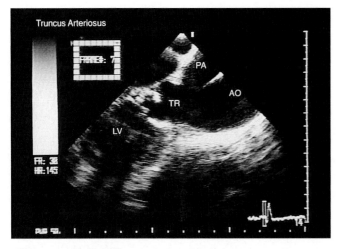

Figure 8.2.53. **Truncus arteriosus.** Images in the longitudinal plane confirm that the pulmonary artery (PA) originates from the posterior wall of the truncus arteriosus (TR). Dysplasia of the truncal valve also can be visualized.

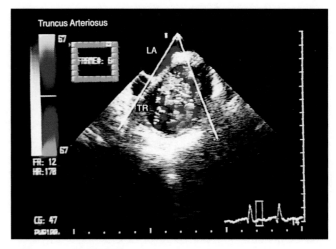

Figure 8.2.54. **Truncus arteriosus.** Transverse plane image at the level of the common truncus arteriosus (TR) below the origin of the pulmonary circulation.

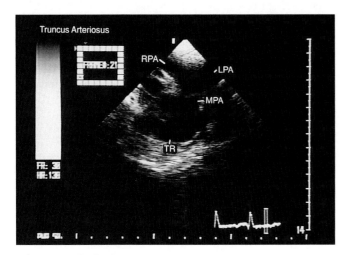

Figure 8.2.55. **Truncus arteriosus.** The origin of the main pulmonary artery (MPA) and its branches (RPA, LPA) from the posterior portion of the common truncus arteriosus (TR) can be identified in images in the transverse plane.

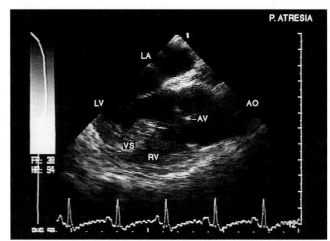

Figure 8.2.56. **Pulmonary atresia.** Longitudinal plane view. Overriding of the aortic valve (AV) over the ventricular septum (VS) can be seen.

As the transducer is withdrawn to a plane slightly superior to the truncal valve, an attempt should be made to identify the emergence of the pulmonary artery or its branches from the posterior or lateral walls of the truncus arteriosus (Figs. 8.2.54 and 8.2.55).

Color Doppler aids in detecting stenosis or regurgitation of the truncal valve.

Pulmonary Atresia With Ventricular Septal Defect

The anatomic characteristic of pulmonary atresia with ventricular septal defect is complete obstruction of the right ventricular outflow tract. The obstruction can vary from an imperforate pulmonary valve with hypoplastic pulmonary artery to total atresia of the ventricular infundibulum and pulmonary artery. Echocardiographic findings help to establish diagnosis as described in the following paragraphs.

Variable aortic overriding of the interventricular septum is seen (Fig. 8.2.56). Transverse and longitudinal sections at the aortic valve level show a normal or hypoplastic infundibulum that terminates blindly. In these recordings the proximal portion of the pulmonary artery at a variable distance from the atretic pulmonary valve can be seen (Fig. 8.2.57). An attempt should be made to measure the diameters of the pulmonary branches, but this may not be possible, particularly with the left branch.

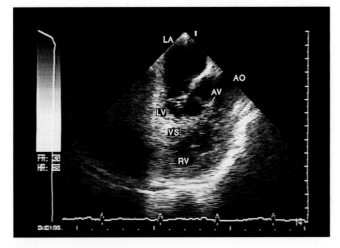

Figure 8.2.57. **Pulmonary atresia.** In a patient with pulmonary atresia, a single vessel (AO) that connects to both ventricles can be observed in longitudinal plane images. No connection exists between the pulmonary circulation and the right ventricle (RV).

Doppler demonstrates the absence of forward flow in the pulmonary artery. The characteristics of the ductus arteriosus should be investigated with a color-coded Doppler study. On rare occasions, a portion of the collateral circulation can be visualized.

REFERENCES

1. Stümper OFW, Sreeram N, Elzenga NJ, et al. Diagnosis of atrial situs by transesophageal echocardiography. J Am Coll Cardiol 1990; 16:442–446.
2. Stümper O, Vargas-Barron J, Rijlaarsdam M, et al. Assessment of anomalous systemic and pulmonary venous connections by transesophageal echocardiography in infants and children. Br Heart J 1991;66: 411–418.
3. Stümper O, Rijlaarsdam M, Vargas-Barron J, et al. The assessment of juxtaposed atrial appendages by transesophageal echocardiography. Int Cardiol 1990;29:365–371.
4. Stümper O, Hess J, Godman MJ, et al. Transesophageal echocardiography in congenital heart disease. Cardiol Young 1993;3:3–12.
5. Stümper O, Sutherland GR, Geuskens R, et al. Transesophageal echocardiography in evaluation and management after a Fontan procedure. J Am Coll Cardiol 1991;17:1152–1160.
6. Fyfe DA, Kline ChH, Sade RM, Gillette PC. Transesophageal echocardiography detects thrombus formation not identified by transthoracic echocardiography after the Fontan operation. J Am Coll Cardiol 1991;18:1733–1737.
7. Lam J, Neirotti RA, Lubbers WJ, et al. Usefulness of biplane transesophageal echocardiography in neonates, infants and children with congenital heart disease. Am J Cardiol 1993;72:699–706.
8. Kaulitz R, Stümper OFW, Geuskens R, et al. Comparative values of the precordial and transesophageal approaches in the echocardiographic evaluation of atrial baffle function after an atrial correction procedure. J Am Coll Cardiol 1990;16:686–694.
9. Finch AD, Snell DR, Sanyal RS, Nanda NC, Loungani RR. Transesophageal echocardiographic identification of a bicuspid pulmonary valve associated with congenitally corrected transposition of the great arteries. Echocardiography 1993;10:359–362.

Part 3

TRANSESOPHAGEAL ECHOCARDIOGRAPHY IN CONGENITAL HEART DISEASE

ATRIAL SEPTAL DEFECT

The most common type of atrial septal defect is ostium secundum, located in the middle portion of the interatrial septum. The ostium primum type defect is located in the most inferior portion of the septum, near the crux of the heart. The sinus venosus type of defect can be found in the superior portion of the septum and often is associated with partial anomalous connection of the pulmonary veins.

In most patients with atrial septal defect transthoracic studies provide sufficient information to indicate surgical correction without cardiac catheterization. Indications for a transesophageal echocardiogram, particularly in adult patients, are limited to situations in which conventional transthoracic images do not definitively establish the diagnosis (e.g., obesity, thoracic deformity), when a sinus venosus type defect is suspected (Figs. 8.3.1 and 8.3.2), or when a paradoxic embolism through a patent foramen ovale must be excluded in a patient who has had a stroke (Fig. 8.3.3).

The information obtained from transesophageal two-dimensional recordings should include the following: (1) the exact location of the defect or presence of various defects (Fig. 8.3.4); (2) the size of the septal defect, with calculation of its area; (3) calculation of the shunt flow volume, as well as the ratio of pulmonary to systemic blood flow; (4) the site of connection of the four pulmonary veins; and (5) any associated defects.

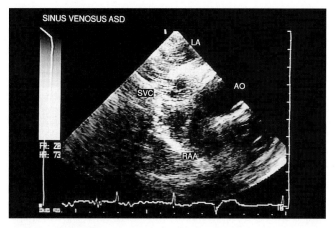

Figure 8.3.2. **Atrial septal defect.** Microbubbles are seen flowing from the superior vena cava into the right atrium and from there into the left atrium through a sinus venosus septal defect.

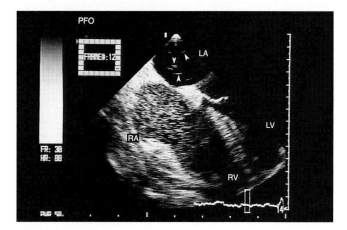

Figure 8.3.3. **Patent foramen ovale.** A contrast study confirms the flow of microbubbles from the right atrium into the left atrium (arrows).

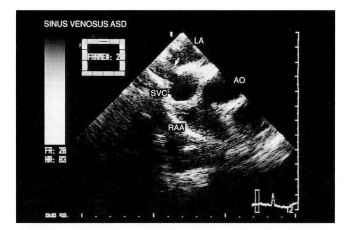

Figure 8.3.1. **Atrial septal defect.** Transverse plane image at the atrial level demonstrates a sinus venosus type of atrial septal defect (arrow), located near the connection of the superior vena cava (SVC) to the right atrium.

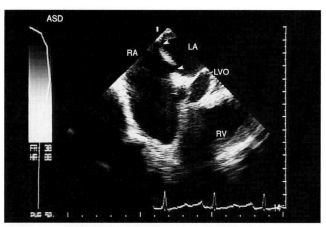

Figure 8.3.4. **Atrial septal defect.** Transverse plane image at the level of the atrial septum. The arrows point to two atrial septal defects.

Multiplane images make it possible to determine the exact location of the atrial septal defect. The diameters of the defect can be measured, and the characteristics of the atrial cavity can be examined. Moreover, embryonic structures such as the eustachian valve can be identified (Figs. 8.3.5–8.3.7).

It has been shown that the dimensions of ostium secundum type defect determined from transverse images correlate well with those obtained in the operating room, as follows:

$$r = 0.92; P < .001 \text{ for horizontal width}$$
$$r = 0.85; P < .01 \text{ for vertical length}$$

The diameter and area of the septal defect also can be calculated from the maximum color flow jet width at the defect site. The defect is assumed to be circular, and comparison with values obtained with those estimated in surgery has shown a fair correlation:

$$r = 0.73; P = .004$$

The volume of the shunt is calculated as the product of the area of the defect, mean velocity, flow duration, and heart rate.

A good correlation exists between shunt flow volume calculated by transesophageal echocardiography and that obtained by cardiac catheterization, as follows:

$$r = 0.91; P < .001$$

The comparison of shunt flow volume calculated by transesophageal echocardiography with the pulmonary to systemic blood flow ratio calculated by cardiac catheterization has also shown good correlation:

$$r = 0.84; P < .001$$

Once the diagnosis of atrial septal defect is established, the Qp:Qs ratio can be calculated from the flow that crosses the pulmonary valve in systole (Qp) and the aortic or mitral valve (Qs).

A semiquantitative estimation of mixed shunts is achieved with simultaneous M-mode and color Doppler transesophageal recordings, or by examination of the positive and negative deflections (spectral analysis) of the flow curve crossing the septum. The planimetry of the positive curve has a certain relationship with the venoarterial shunt, as does the planimetry of the negative curve with the arteriovenous shunt.

Other pathologies of the interatrial septum exist, such as lipomatous hypertrophy or septal aneurysms, which are identified with relative ease using transesophageal imaging.

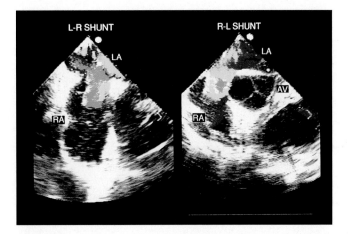

Figure 8.3.5. Atrial septal defect. Two-dimensional images with color-coded Doppler at the atrial level. The variations in the shunt through a large septal defect are demonstrated.

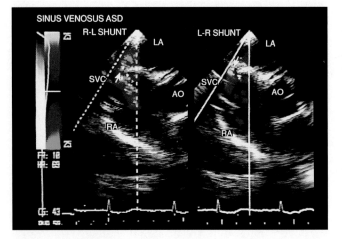

Figure 8.3.6. Atrial septal defect. In a patient with a sinus venosus type of atrial septal defect, transverse plane images with color Doppler show a bidirectional shunt through the septal defect (arrow).

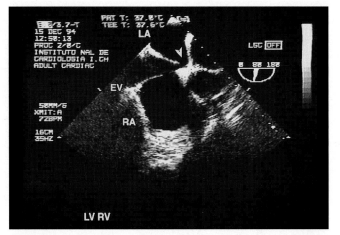

Figure 8.3.7. Atrial septal defect. Echocardiogram taken with multiplanar transducer shows a fossa ovalis type atrial septal defect (arrow). *EV*, eustachian valve; *RA*, right atrium; *LA*, left atrium.

In lipomatous hypertrophy, the transesophageal images show diffuse thickening of the septum. In patients with septal aneurysms the two signs required for diagnosis are (1) bulging of the fossa ovalis region >15 mm beyond the plane of the atrial septum or >15 mm phasic excursion during the cardiorespiratory cycle and (2) the base of the aneurysm measuring >15 mm in diameter (Figs. 8.3.8 and 8.3.9). Shunting has been detected in up to 83% of aneurysms of the interatrial septum studied by transesophageal imaging using echocardiographic contrast imaging in combination with color flow mapping, and in 41% when only transthoracic examination was performed. Moreover, transesophageal recordings have confirmed that the aneurysms are thrombogenic, which explains their frequent association with paradoxic embolism.

Transesophageal studies also have served to evaluate the existence of interatrial shunts secondary to percutaneous mitral valvulotomy with balloon catheter, or as a guide in the closure of atrial septal defects with an umbrella-type patch introduced through a catheter.

PARTIAL ANOMALOUS PULMONARY VENOUS CONNECTION

The most useful noninvasive technique in diagnosis of anomalous pulmonary venous connections currently available is transesophageal echocardiography. The pattern of pulmonary venous drainage in relation to the atrial septum is best defined with transverse axis imaging (Figs. 8.3.10 and 8.3.11). Transesophageal echocardiography

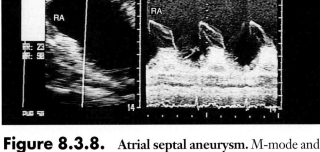

Figure 8.3.8. Atrial septal aneurysm. M-mode and two-dimensional images in the transverse plane demonstrate the movement of the interatrial septum (IAS) toward the left atrium in systole and toward the right atrium in diastole.

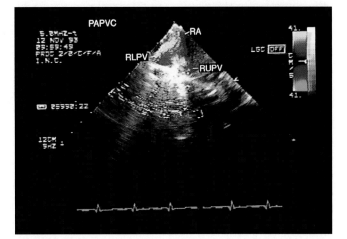

Figure 8.3.10. Partial anomalous connection of the pulmonary veins. Transverse plane image in a patient with anomalous connection of the pulmonary veins with the right atrium.

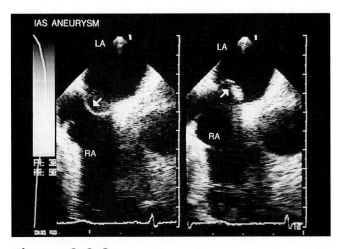

Figure 8.3.9. Atrial septal aneurysm. Longitudinal plane views demonstrate both atria. The arrows indicate the aneurysmal movement of the interatrial septum.

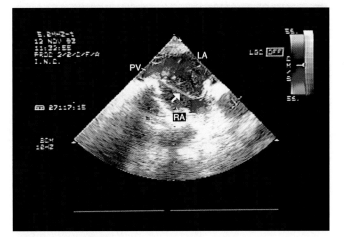

Figure 8.3.11. Partial anomalous connection of the pulmonary veins. Postoperative study after correction of anomalous connection of the right pulmonary veins. Pulmonary venous return has been connected to the left atrium. The arrow points to the intact interatrial septum.

has a sensitivity and specificity close to 100% in the detection of anomalous pulmonary venous connections.

Partial anomalous connections often accompany sinus venosus-type atrial septal defects. The most common form is connection of the right pulmonary veins with the superior vena cava. Less often these veins are found to be connected to the right atrium or the inferior vena cava (Figs. 8.3.12 and 8.3.13); even less common is the connection of left pulmonary veins with the innominate vein. Direct visualization of anomalous connections, especially of pulmonary veins, has been facilitated by the advent of multiplane transesophageal probes (Fig. 8.3.14). Contrast studies visualize the clearing of microbubbles in the right atrium by anomalous pulmonary venous flow (Fig. 8.3.15).

TOTAL ANOMALOUS CONNECTION OF PULMONARY VEINS

In total anomalous connection of the pulmonary veins the connection between the four pulmonary veins and left atrium is absent. The veins drain into the right atrium, either directly or through systems of venous tributaries.

Three types of anomalous connection exist: 1) supracardiac, in which the connection is to the superior vena cava or the innominate vein; 2) cardiac, in which the pulmonary venous return connects to the coronary sinus or directly to the right atrium; and 3) infracardiac, in which the anomalous connection is established with the inferior vena cava or the portal vein. Mixed anomalous connections that include at least two of the types.

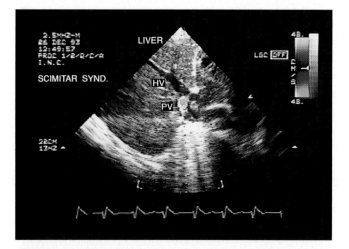

Figure 8.3.12. **Partial anomalous connection of the pulmonary veins.** With transgastric images and color-coded Doppler it is possible to identify the site of anomalous pulmonary venous drainage (PV) into the inferior vena cava. *HV*, hepatic vein.

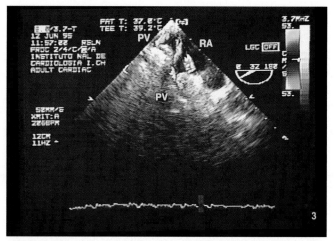

Figure 8.3.14. **Partial anomalous connection of the pulmonary veins.** Preoperative transesophageal echocardiogram in a patient with anomalous pulmonary venous connection to the right atrium (RA).

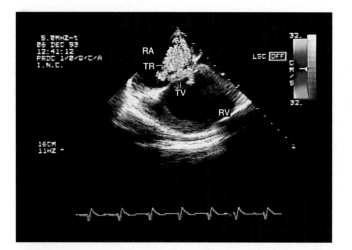

Figure 8.3.13. **Partial anomalous connection of the pulmonary veins.** Transverse plane image shows dilatation of the right heart cavities and functional tricuspid regurgitation (TR) secondary to anomalous pulmonary venous drainage.

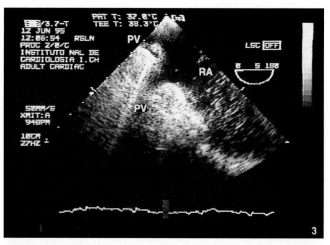

Figure 8.3.15. **Partial anomalous connection of the pulmonary veins.** Transesophageal echocardiogram with contrast shows the effect of clearing of microbubbles in the right atrium (RA) by pulmonary venous flow.

The sites to which anomalous connections occur are, in decreasing frequency, the innominate vein, by way of a left vertical vein; the coronary sinus; the right superior vena cava; the right atrium; and the inferior vena cava.

In four-chamber transesophageal images, dilatation of the right cavities can be demonstrated and the lack of connection of the pulmonary veins to the left atrium confirmed. The use of transverse plane images makes it possible to recognize the characteristics of the obligatory atrial septal defect (Fig. 8.3.16). In addition, the small size of the left ventricle can be detected, a finding that has been considered a prognostic index in those patients who undergo surgical correction. When the two-dimensional images are complemented with color Doppler and spectral analysis, the magnitude of the venoarterial interatrial shunt becomes evident, and when flow is recorded in the anomalous pulmonary venous channel it is seen to be forward both in systole and diastole. The appearance of a color mosaic with increased flow velocity corresponds to venous obstruction, a situation of considerable clinical significance.

In anomalous connections of the supracardiac type, transesophageal studies complement the information obtained with suprasternal imaging. In the latter examination, the most common form of supracardiac anomalous connection is well demonstrated: the vertical vein (persistent left superior vena cava) drains into the innominate vein, and from there the venous flow connects with the superior vena cava and finally reaches the right atrium. In contrast, when the anomalous connection is with the right superior vena cava, transesophageal echocardiography shows that the pulmonary veins form a venous confluence posterior to the left atrium that points toward and connects with the posterior portion of the vena cava.

Pulmonary venous anomalous connection can be demonstrated with greatest facility at the cardiac level in transesophageal images. When the connection is with the coronary sinus, images in the transverse plane show that

the pulmonary veins form a retrocardiac confluence, which drains into the coronary sinus at the level of the atrioventricular sulcus. The coronary sinus is very dilated and has an abnormal vertical position (Fig. 8.3.17).

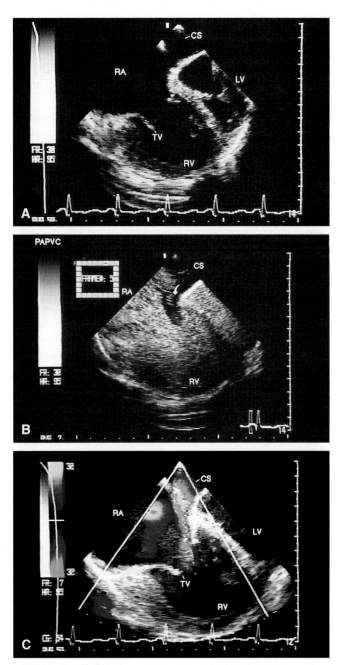

Figure 8.3.17. **Total anomalous connection of the pulmonary veins. A.** Four-chamber image with posterior angulation. There is dilatation of right heart chambers and the coronary sinus secondary to the anomalous pulmonary venous connection. **B.** When saline solution is injected through a peripheral vein, all four chambers become opaque. The arrow indicates the washout effect of the anomalous pulmonary venous flow from the coronary sinus into the right atrium. **C.** Color Doppler demonstrates increased coronary sinus flow as a consequence of anomalous pulmonary venous connection.

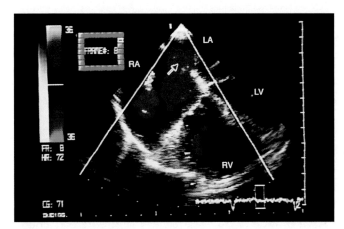

Figure 8.3.16. Total anomalous connection of the pulmonary veins. In a patient with total anomalous pulmonary venous connection, color Doppler demonstrates the obligatory atrial septal defect (arrow).

If the anomalous connection is with the right atrium, transesophageal recordings make it possible to establish whether the connection occurs through a large common pulmonary vein or through two to four pulmonary veins that drain separately into the posterior-inferior portion of the atrium (Figs. 8.3.18 and 8.3.19).

In anomalous infracardiac connections, the four pulmonary veins form a common confluence that descends in front of the esophagus, crosses the diaphragm through the esophageal hiatus, and drains into the inferior vena cava, hepatic or portal vein, or a persistent ductus venosus. Diagnosis of this type of anomaly can be established with subcostal recordings. Low transesophageal and transgastric recordings are very useful, especially when drainage is into the inferior vena cava or hepatic veins.

Transesophageal echocardiography, when performed in the cardiac catheterization laboratory, can avoid the excessive use of angiocardiographic contrast medium. In the operating room it can aid in planning the type of corrective surgery and in the identification of mixed anomalous connections.

VENTRICULAR SEPTAL DEFECT

The echocardiographic diagnosis of ventricular septal defect in children usually can be established with conventional transthoracic recordings. When technical difficulties in obtaining adequate images exist, especially in adolescents and adults, the transesophageal technique is a good alternative method that, with the advent of biplanar recordings, can confirm the diagnosis and determine the size and location of the defect with precision. The interventricular septum is made up of four principal segments: 1) membranous or perimembranous; 2) inlet; 3) outlet; and 4) trabecular. Septal defects can exist in one or more of these segments. They produce the features discussed in the following paragraphs in transesophageal echocardiographic studies.

A defect of the membranous septum is the most common. On the right ventricular side it is located beneath and behind the supraventricular crest (infracristal). On the left ventricular side it is located in the subaortic portion, near the commissure of the right and noncoronary leaflets. Diagnosis can be established with transesophageal images in transverse and longitudinal planes (Fig. 8.3.20). In the former, the shunt is seen close to the tricuspid valve and in front of the aorta (at the 8 o'clock position). In longitudinal recordings the defect is located in the basal (superior) third of the septum in a small subaortic portion.

A defect of the posterior or inlet septum may be found behind the tricuspid valve and between it and the mitral valve. It often forms part of a malformation of the endocardial cushions and often is associated with atrioventricu-

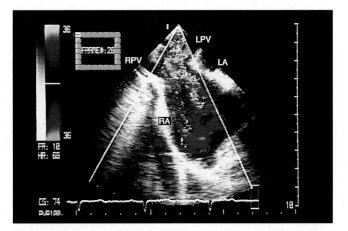

Figure 8.3.19. **Total anomalous connection of the pulmonary veins.** Transverse plane imaging with color Doppler shows flows from both pulmonary veins moving into the right atrium.

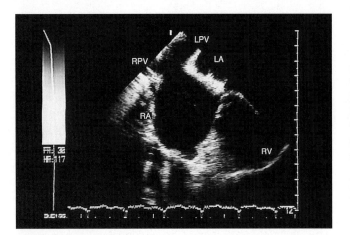

Figure 8.3.18. **Total anomalous connection of the pulmonary veins.** Transesophageal study demonstrates anomalous pulmonary venous drainage directly into the right atrium.

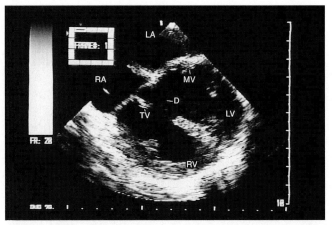

Figure 8.3.20. **Ventricular septal defect.** Four-chamber view with a large perimembranous-inlet ventricular septal defect (D).

lar valve defects. The shunt is located with color Doppler, usually in a four-chamber transesophageal image in the transverse plane.

A defect of the infundibular or outlet septum is another possibility. On the right ventricular side it is located below the pulmonary leaflets; on the left side, it is inferior to the aortic leaflets. Transesophageal recordings in the transverse plane are not useful for recognizing the exact characteristics of the defect. In longitudinal images, however, it is possible to see the ventricular outflow tracts and, with color Doppler, to demonstrate the shunt crossing the defect.

A defect of the trabecular septum is located in an anterior and inferior portion of the septum. Occasionally, multiple trabecular defects are present (Fig. 8.3.21). This type of defect usually is small, although it can be very large.

Such a defect can be difficult to demonstrate in the transverse plane when it is small; identification usually requires biplanar recordings.

In patients with ventricular septal defects the flow crossing the defect can affect tricuspid structures, and this valvular trauma can promote the development of infective endocarditis. When this occurs, transesophageal recordings with color Doppler aid in identifying the location and magnitude of the ventricular septal defect, the characteristics of the vegetations adhering to the tricuspid leaflets, the existence and severity of the lesions of the leaflets themselves, and the extension of the infectious process to other cardiovascular structures (Figs. 8.3.22–8.3.24).

One of the principal contributions of transesophageal studies in the evaluation of patients with ventricular septal

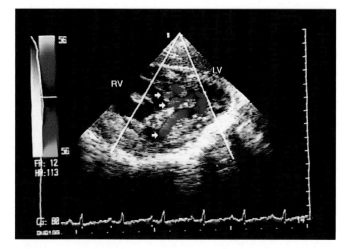

Figure 8.3.21. Ventricular septal defect. Transgastric imaging with color Doppler demonstrates multiple ventricular septal defects (arrows).

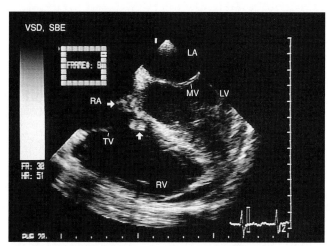

Figure 8.3.23. Ventricular septal defect. Infective vegetations involving the tricuspid valve (arrows) are seen in a patient with a ventricular septal defect.

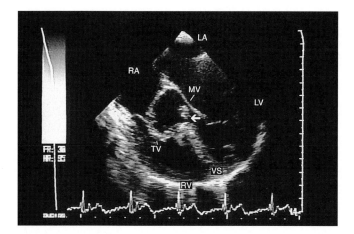

Figure 8.3.22. Ventricular septal defect. Transverse plane image shows a trabecular ventricular septal defect (arrow). The insertion of the tricuspid subvalvular apparatus in the ventricular septum (VS) also is observed.

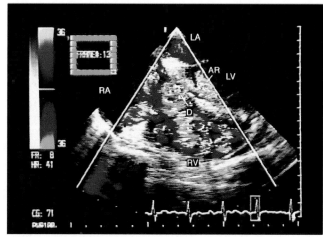

Figure 8.3.24. Ventricular septal defect. Color Doppler shows a ventricular septal defect (VSD) and also documents aortic regurgitation.

defects is visualization of overriding of the atrioventricular valve rings or straddling of subvalvular structures that cross the interventricular defect and insert in the contralateral ventricle (Fig. 8.3.25).

Transesophageal echocardiography also has been used in the intraoperative evaluation of surgical closure of ventricular septal defects. It is more useful than epicardial recordings. However, when a patch of synthetic material is used to cover the defect, the patch can produce ultrasonic shadowing in the right ventricle that makes color Doppler evaluation difficult and demonstration of residual shunts impossible. This interference can be avoided by using "high" (i.e., at the level of the right ventricular outflow tract and the aorta) transesophageal recordings complemented with contrast echocardiography.

COMMON ATRIOVENTRICULAR CANAL

The common atrioventricular canal is the extreme form of endocardial cushion defects, also called atrioventricular septal defects. In this malformation there is a common A-V valve, a defect of the lower portion of the interatrial septum (ostium primum), and a defect of the high, posterior portion of the interventricular septum (inlet).

The A-V valve is formed by five leaflets, three of which correspond to the left ventricle—lateral, anterior, and posterior; and two of which correspond to the right ventricle—one anterior and the other lateral.

The left anterior and posterior leaflets cross the crest of the interventricular septum toward the right ventricle. These have been called "bridging leaflets" and have variable degrees of tethering to both ventricles (Fig. 8.3.26).

In addition, the characteristics of these bridging leaflets determine whether one or two atrioventricular orifices exist. If the bridging leaflets are separate, there is only one A-V orifice, whereas if the leaflets are joined by fibrous tissue, there are two A-V orifices.

In infants and children transthoracic and subcostal echocardiograms are of sufficient quality to clarify the characteristics of the malformation. Transesophageal studies should be limited to those situations in which it is not possible to obtain satisfactory transthoracic recordings, particularly in adults or during intraoperative evaluation of surgical correction of the defect.

The transesophageal echocardiographic study should demonstrate the morphology of the atrioventricular valve. With transesophageal four-chamber images and transgastric transverse plane images it is possible to determine whether there is a single A-V orifice or two orifices (Fig. 8.3.27). When two-dimensional recordings are complemented with color-coded Doppler, existing shunts can be

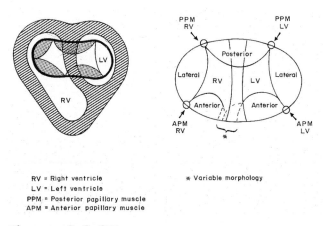

RV = Right ventricle
LV = Left ventricle
PPM = Posterior papillary muscle
APM = Anterior papillary muscle

* Variable morphology

Figure 8.3.26. **Common atrioventricular canal defect.** Diagram of transesophageal recordings in a patient with Rastelli type A common atrioventricular canal, in which the left anterior leaflet crosses the ventricular septum and inserts in a medial papillary muscle of the right ventricle. *PPM,* posterior papillary muscle; *APM,* anterior papillary muscle.

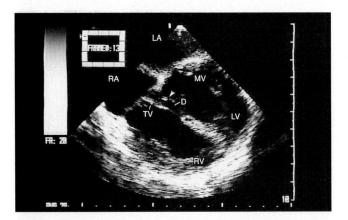

Figure 8.3.25. **Ventricular septal defect.** Systolic frame shows insertion of the tricuspid valve into the interventricular septum. In systole the tricuspid tissue protrudes toward the left ventricular outlet (arrow). *D,* defect.

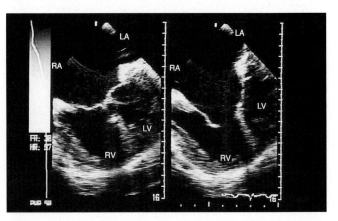

Figure 8.3.27. **Common atrioventricular canal defect.** Four-chamber images in a complete atrioventricular canal or septal defect. The anterior mitral component of the common A-V valve can be seen to insert into the free edge of the the ventricular septum.

seen. Patients with two A-V orifices usually have a single shunt at the atrial level. Patients with a single A-V orifice present with both interatrial and interventricular shunts. The Doppler study also aids in determining the existence and degree of regurgitation of the mitral and tricuspid components of the common A-V valve (Fig. 8.3.28).

In four-chamber and longitudinal plane images it is important to identify the atrial and ventricular components of the A-V septum, the size of both ventricles, and, particularly, the characteristics of the left anterior bridging leaflet, which defines the most common variants of this malformation according to Rastelli's classification. In type A the left anterior bridging leaflet crosses the interventricular septum and inserts in the medial papillary muscle of the right ventricle. Valvular mobility is limited by the insertions in the crest of the interventricular septum. In types B and C, "crossing" of the left anterior leaflet is greater. In type B, after crossing the septum, the leaflet reaches the medial papillary muscle, which is located in an abnormally apical position. In type C, the leaflet crosses and inserts in the anterior papillary muscle of the right ventricle.

In patients with separate A-V valve orifices, transesophageal study helps to demonstrate that the left anterior and left posterior bridging leaflets are joined by a band of fibrous tissue that divides the common orifice.

A "goose-neck" image can be observed in recordings in the longitudinal plane at the level of the left ventricular outlet. This results from the outlet being longer and abnormally far from the interventricular septum because of the more vertical orientation of the A-V valve annulus. Obstructions of the left ventricular outlet can be recognized and quantified with the various Doppler techniques.

Transesophageal echocardiography is particularly useful in the operating room because the information it provides allows better planning of the type of corrective surgery, and in the immediate postoperative period it helps to identify residual shunts and valvular regurgitation.

PATENT DUCTUS ARTERIOSUS

Patent ductus arteriosus involves abnormal communication between the descending aorta and the proximal portion of the left branch of the pulmonary artery. In premature and term infants it can be diagnosed with relative ease using conventional transthoracic recordings. In older children and adults it presents a broad spectrum of clinical manifestations, which vary from the asymptomatic patient with a continuous precordial murmur to a patient with signs of severe pulmonary hypertension.

Transesophageal echocardiography is an alternative when satisfactory transthoracic recordings cannot be obtained. It is difficult to visualize the ductus directly in the transverse plane; it may be suspected when there is retrograde systolic and diastolic flow in the pulmonary artery (Figs. 8.3.29 and 8.3.30). The diagnosis is established with biplanar or multiplanar transducers using recordings in the

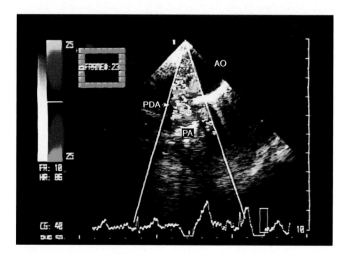

Figure 8.3.29. Patent ductus arteriosus. In a high transverse section, color Doppler demonstrates flow through the patent ductus arteriosus (PDC).

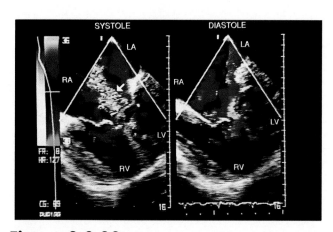

Figure 8.3.28. Common atrioventricular canal defect. When a common atrioventricular valve exists, a color Doppler study aids in recognizing the degree of valvular regurgitation (arrow).

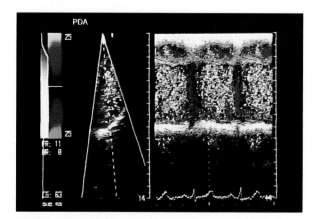

Figure 8.3.30. Patent ductus arteriosus. Simultaneous two-dimensional and color M-mode images show increased velocity of systolic and diastolic flows at the level of the pulmonary artery secondary to a patent ductus arteriosus (PDA).

longitudinal plane. In this plane the descending thoracic aorta should be recorded at the postductal level. The transducer then is withdrawn slowly to obtain sections progressively superior with slight rotation to the right (Fig. 8.3.31). Doppler shows the shunt as a mosaic of colors connecting the aorta to the pulmonary artery (Fig. 8.3.32). Flow with increased velocity in both systole and diastole is recorded in spectral analysis (Fig. 8.3.33).

Another application of transesophageal echocardiography in patients with patent ductus arteriosus (PDA) is for evaluation of the effectiveness of surgical ligation of the ductus. Likewise, in patients with calcification or hypertrophy of the walls of the ductus, residual shunts can exist and can be detected with color Doppler during surgery.

The transesophageal technique also has been used as an aid during interventional procedures. During percutaneous oc-

clusion of patent ductus arteriosus with the double umbrella device, transesophageal echocardiography shows the precise position of the device, and, before the device is released, the completeness of occlusion assessed by color Doppler.

In some of the various complications that can occur with patent ductus arteriosus, transesophageal studies provide information useful for therapeutic management of the patient. These include pulmonary hypertension and infective endarteritis of the pulmonary artery.

Because of the left-to-right shunt and the transmission of systemic pressure to the pulmonary circulation, pulmonary vascular disease develops; the shunt diminishes as pulmonary resistance increases. In this situation it has been recommended that transesophageal echocardiography, complemented by provocative maneuvers designed to lower pulmonary vascular resistance, such as the use of 100% inspired oxygen, should be used for the echocardiographic diagnosis of patent ductus arteriosus with pulmonary hypertension. We believe that another alternative method in these patients is transesophageal contrast echocardiography. When glucose solution is injected in a peripheral vein, microbubbles can be observed in the descending thoracic aorta as evidence of the venoarterial shunt through the ductus (Fig. 8.3.34). A slight rotation of the transducer shows that there are no microbubbles in the left chambers or in the aortic root, thus confirming that the shunt is not intracardiac (Figs. 8.3.35 and 8.3.36).

When it is not possible to obtain adequate transthoracic recordings, transesophageal recordings can be an alternative method of diagnosis for detection of vegetations in the pulmonary artery. It is possible to demonstrate the size, shape, and mobility of the vegetations that develop at the site at which the patent ductus flow hits the intima of the pulmonary artery (Figs. 8.3.37 and 8.3.38). The infective process also can involve the pulmonary valve (Fig. 8.3.39).

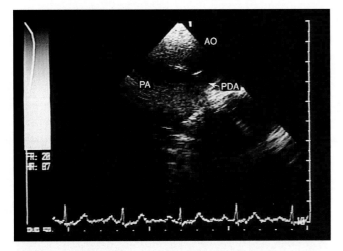

Figure 8.3.31. Patent ductus arteriosus. Longitudinal plane imaging at the level of the great arteries directly visualizes the ductus arteriosus (PDA).

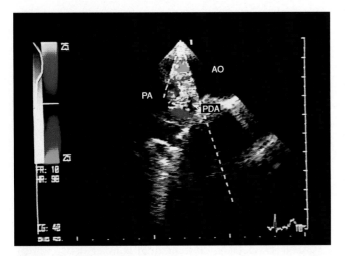

Figure 8.3.32. Patent ductus arteriosus. The shunt between the aorta (AO) and the pulmonary artery (PA) is corroborated by color Doppler in longitudinal plane imaging.

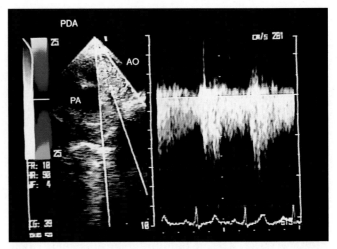

Figure 8.3.33. Patent ductus arteriosus. Longitudinal plane images with color Doppler and spectral analysis demonstrate continuous flow from the ductus arteriosus. *PDA*, patent ductus arteriosus.

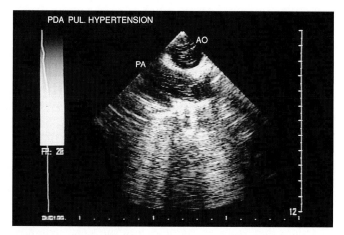

Figure 8.3.34. Patent ductus arteriosus. Contrast study shows microbubbles in both the left pulmonary branch and the descending thoracic aorta, confirming the patency of the ductus arteriosus.

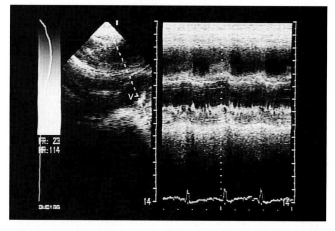

Figure 8.3.37. Patent ductus arteriosus. A vegetation adhering to the anterior wall of the pulmonary branch (V) is observed in a patient with patent ductus arteriosus.

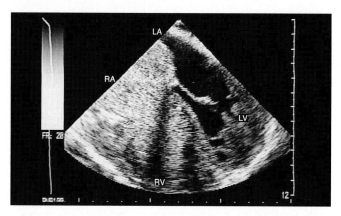

Figure 8.3.35. Patent ductus arteriosus. In a patient with severe arterial hypertension, a contrast study shows the presence of microbubbles only in the right heart cavities, ruling out the existence of an intracardiac shunt.

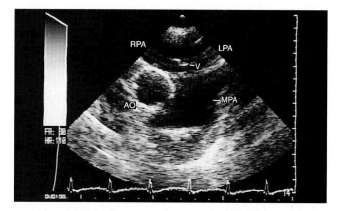

Figure 8.3.38. Patent ductus arteriosus. Infective endarteritis (V) at the level of the bifurcation of the pulmonary artery in a patient with patent ductus arteriosus is evident in this transverse plane image.

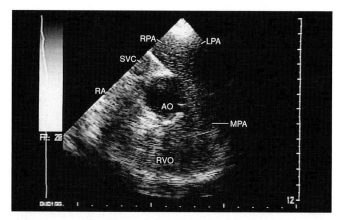

Figure 8.3.36. Patent ductus arteriosus. Transverse plane image at the level of the great arteries. With contrast the course of the microbubbles is visualized from the superior vena cava to the right atrium, right ventricular outlet, pulmonary artery, and pulmonary branches. No microbubbles appear in the aortic root.

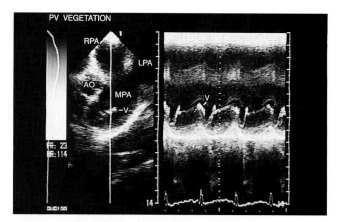

Figure 8.3.39. Patent ductus arteriosus. M-mode and two-dimensional images in the longitudinal plane show vegetations at the level of the pulmonary leaflets (V).

AORTOPULMONARY WINDOW

Patent ductus arteriosus is the most common cause of continuous murmur detected on the anterior wall of the chest. However, other causes of continuous or systolic-diastolic murmurs, such as aortic insufficiency with ventricular septal defect, aortopulmonary window, rupture of an aneurysm of the sinus of Valsalva into the cardiac cavities, or coronary fistula, are not unusual.

Aortopulmonary window is characterized by a communication between the ascending portion of the aorta and the main pulmonary artery with two well-formed semilunar valves. The orifice is usually large and oval and is located on the left lateral wall of the ascending aorta, near the origin of the left coronary artery. The communication less commonly occurs in a more distal position between the ascending aorta and the union of the right branch of the pulmonary artery with the main trunk.

Echocardiographic diagnosis of this malformation requires evidence of signs of volume overload of the left cavities. It usually is possible to visualize the aortopulmonary defect directly with transthoracic and subcostal two-dimensional images and corroborate the shunt with color Doppler. When transesophageal echocardiography is performed because the diagnosis cannot be demonstrated with transthoracic recordings, the images in both planes show the lack of septation between the aorta and the pulmonary artery above the level of the valve plane (Fig. 8.3.40). When two-dimensional images are complemented with color Doppler or contrast studies, the shunt is demonstrated and the size of the defect can be assessed (Fig. 8.3.41).

CONGENITAL ANEURYSM OF SINUS OF VALSALVA

Congenital aneurysms of the sinus of Valsalva are relatively rare malformations. In the course of their evolution they tend to rupture into cavities of the heart. A few years ago congenital aneurysms without rupture could be diagnosed only by angiography. Now they can be detected using noninvasive ultrasound (Fig. 8.3.42).

When the aneurysm ruptures, two-dimensional echocardiography with color Doppler is useful for clarifying its presence, size, and location. When rupture occurs in adult patients, transesophageal echocardiography is superior to conventional transthoracic echocardiography for demonstrating the ruptured aneurysm because of better acoustic window (Figs. 8.3.43 and 8.3.44). It is possible to identify deformities of the aortic root with abnormal echoes in the ruptured sinus of Valsalva with biplane or multiplane transducers, using primarily images in the transverse plane.

When the aneurysm ruptures into the right atrium or ventricle, the sinuses of Valsalva usually affected are the noncoronary and the right coronary sinus, respectively.

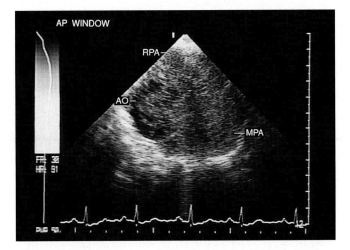

Figure 8.3.41. **Aortopulmonary window.** Contrast study confirms the flow of microbubbles from the aorta into the pulmonary circulation.

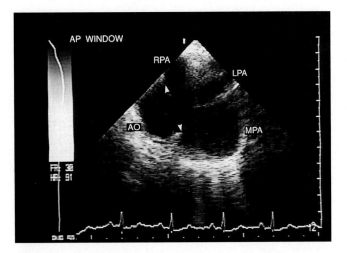

Figure 8.3.40. **Aortopulmonary window.** Transverse plane image of the great arteries demonstrates a large communication between the aorta and the pulmonary artery.

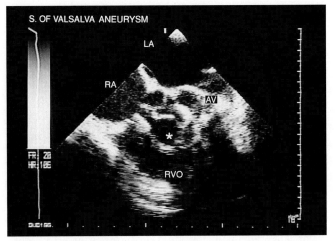

Figure 8.3.42. **Congenital aneurysm of the sinus of Valsalva.** Transverse plane image of the aorta. Aneurysmal dilatation of the right coronary sinus of Valsalva (*) can be seen.

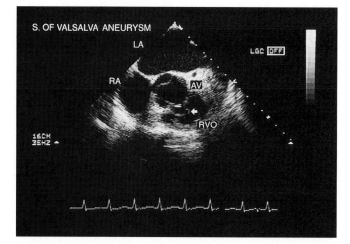

Figure 8.3.43. **Congenital aneurysm of the sinus of Valsalva.** Transverse plane image in a patient with aneurysm of the right coronary sinus of Valsalva (arrow) with rupture into the right ventricle.

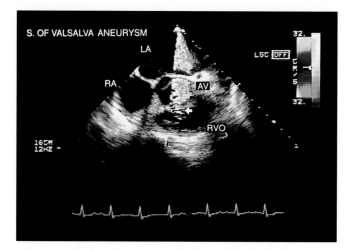

Figure 8.3.44. **Congenital aneurysm of the sinus of Valsalva.** Rupture of an aneurysm of the sinus of Valsalva (arrow) into the right ventricle is demonstrated with transverse plane imaging and color Doppler.

When the pulsed Doppler sample volume is placed in the cavity connected to the ruptured sinus of Valsalva, turbulent flow with increased velocity is recorded in both phases of the cardiac cycle.

Transesophageal images make it possible to differentiate sinus of Valsalva aneurysms from aneurysms of the interventricular septum, coronary aneurysms, or coronary fistulas. The association of two-dimensional studies and color Doppler recording is useful for characterizing flow patterns in the heart chambers, detecting the site of an arteriovenous shunt, and discovering associated lesions such as ventricular septal defects and aortic valve regurgitation.

CORONARY ARTERY FISTULA

Traditionally, coronary artery fistulas have been diagnosed by coronary angiography. They can be diagnosed with transthoracic echocardiography and color Doppler, although the information provided is limited to the demonstration of a coronary artery dilated in its origin with turbulent flow (mosaic of colors) in the cavity into which the fistula drains. With the advent of transesophageal echocardiography, especially with biplane and multiplane transducers, the diagnosis of these anomalies has been facilitated.

With images in the transverse plane it is possible to identify the origin of the fistula from one of the coronary ostia as well as the distal portion of the fistula (Fig. 8.3.45). The left-to-right shunt is visualized as a high-velocity mosaic jet arising from the fistula and extending into a cardiac chamber or main pulmonary artery. Pulsed-wave Doppler interrogation of the fistula reveals a continuous systolic-diastolic flow disturbance (Fig. 8.3.46). Images in the longitudinal plane have been described as useful in

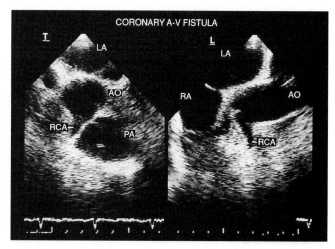

Figure 8.3.45. **Coronary artery fistula.** The dilated proximal portion of a fistula between the right coronary artery (RCA) and right ventricle can be seen in transverse (T) and longitudinal (L) plane images.

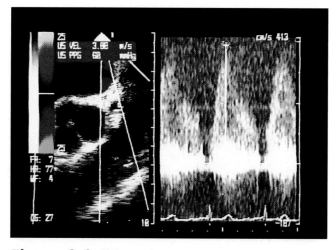

Figure 8.3.46. **Coronary artery fistula.** Longitudinal plane view complemented with Doppler study of flow in the coronary fistula. Spectral analysis shows increased flow velocity in both systole and diastole.

visualizing the fistula along its entire course (Fig. 8.3.47). Currently, transesophageal echocardiography seems to be the noninvasive diagnostic procedure that provides the most information in patients with coronary fistulas.

CORONARY ANEURYSMS

Although coronary aneurysms are not congenital malformations, we have included the coronary aneurysms seen in patients with Kawasaki's disease in this chapter because they occur primarily in children and their transesophageal echocardiographic evaluation has great relevance. The cardiovascular alterations that can be detected by echocardiography, in addition to the aneurysms themselves, are dilatation of the left ventricle, with deterioration of its systolic function, and pericardial effusion.

Two-dimensional transthoracic and subcostal echocardiography are very useful in the study of children with Kawasaki's disease. The use of additional scanning planes has increased the success rate of delineating the coronary artery anatomy in these patients.

The feasibility of using transesophageal recordings to explore some coronary segments with greater clarity clearly justifies these studies in the follow-up of children or adults with Kawasaki's disease. The transesophageal technique has been particularly useful for visualizing thrombi formed in the aneurysmal coronary arteries. Recordings in the transverse plane show proximal aneursyms, whereas more of the course of a coronary artery can be visualized in longitudinal plane images (Figs. 8.3.48–8.3.50).

Transesophageal echocardiography probably is the noninvasive technique of choice in the detection and follow-up of coronary aneurysms in which transthoracic studies are not satisfactory.

AORTIC COARCTATION

Echocardiographic diagnosis of coarctation of the aorta does not require transesophageal recordings; the vascular

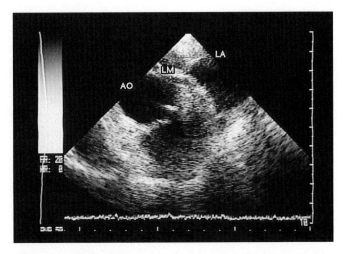

Figure 8.3.48. Coronary aneurysm. Transverse plane image shows the normal origin of the left coronary artery (LM).

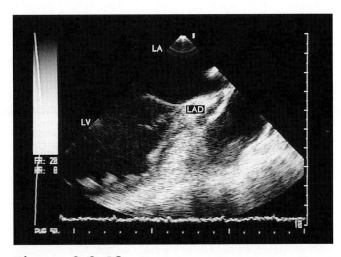

Figure 8.3.49. Coronary aneurysm. Aneurysmal dilatations are seen at the level of the proximal portion of the left anterior descending coronary artery (LAD).

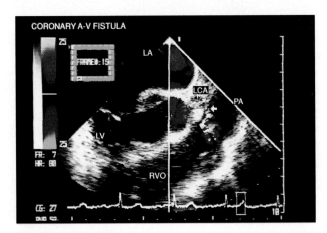

Figure 8.3.47. Coronary artery fistula. Longitudinal plane image with color Doppler shows the course of the fistula between the left coronary artery (LCA) and the pulmonary artery (PA).

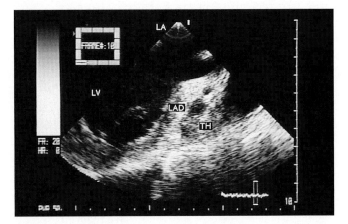

Figure 8.3.50. Coronary aneurysm. Longitudinal plane image shows an aneurysm of the left anterior descending coronary artery (LAD). A thrombus (TH) can be seen inside it.

obstruction can be identified and quantified with suprasternal images and continuous wave Doppler. In transesophageal echocardiography, the use of transverse scanning probes reveals some overestimation of angiographically calculated diameters, perhaps because of an oblique scanning plane, because the proximal descending aorta is a curved structure rather than a vertical cylinder. Fortunately, it is possible to visualize the coarcted zone with greater clarity using biplane or multiplane transducers (Fig. 8.3.51). Perhaps the principal application of transesophageal echocardiography in patients with aortic coarctation is as a guide in the dilatation of the coarctation with a balloon catheter.

DOUBLE AORTIC ARCH

In the double aortic arch malformation, two aortic arches that surround the trachea and esophagus split from the ascending aorta. Later they unite to form the descending aorta.

Both arches can be identified with suprasternal and subcostal echocardiography. In most cases the ipsilateral carotid and subclavian arteries originate from them. Transesophageal recordings make it possible to visualize the origin of the two arches from the ascending aorta. The pulmonary artery with its bifurcation should then be shown to be connected to the right ventricle (Figs. 8.3.52 and 8.3.53).

AORTIC STENOSIS

Transthoracic echocardiography aids in diagnosis and estimation of the severity of congenital obstruction of the aortic valve. Transesophageal imaging has been used to monitor interventional cardiac catheterization. The routine use of transesophageal monitoring adds additional safety to the procedure and helps reduce both the amount of radiation and the contrast material required.

During aortic valvuloplasties, transesophageal imaging allows a more precise measurement of the aortic valve an-

nuli and provides a detailed assessment of the valvular morphology, both before and after dilatation. It also aids in correcting malposition of the guidewire and the balloon catheter and in the rapid detection of aortic regurgitation following each inflation of the balloon. Left ventricular function can be evaluated during inflation of the balloon. The balloon is deflated when ventricular contraction is almost abolished, and the next inflation is performed only when contractility is restored. The images obtained by a transesophageal monoplane transducer are inadequate to determine the spatial position of the balloon catheter. This information is more completely obtained using biplane or multiplane transducers. Likewise, if continuous wave Doppler can be used, the residual transvalvular gradients can be determined.

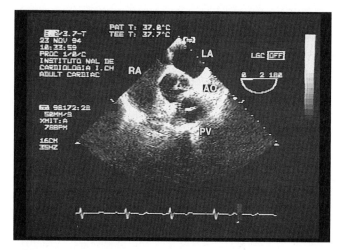

Figure 8.3.52. Double aortic arch. In this echocardiogram taken with a multiplane probe in a patient with a double aortic arch, the normal relationship between aortic (AO) and pulmonic (PV) valves can be observed.

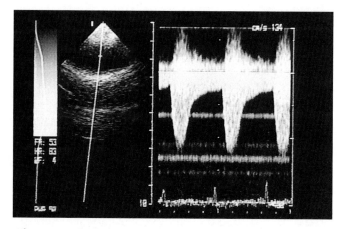

Figure 8.3.51. Coarctation of the aorta. Continuous wave Doppler analysis in a patient with coarctation of the aorta (COA) shows characteristic flow distal to the obstruction.

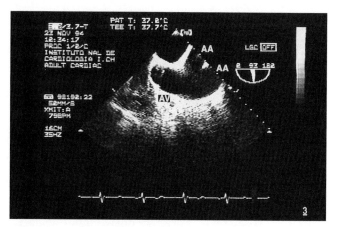

Figure 8.3.53. Double aortic arch. Transesophageal study shows the aortic valve (AV) and two aortic arches (AA) splitting off the ascending aorta.

Multiplane transducers facilitate recognition of bicuspid valves and provide the exact systolic area of the aortic valves (Fig. 8.3.54).

In our experience, transesophageal echocardiography also has been useful in transoperative monitoring of pulmonary valve autograft in the aortic position with placement of a bioprosthesis or homograft in the pulmonary position (Ross procedure) (Fig. 8.3.55). The principal purpose of this type of surgery is to provide a "permanent" valve replacement in children and adolescents. Placement of a mechanical prosthesis in the aortic position would expose these patients to many years of risk of embolic or hemorrhagic events and the necessity of continuous cardiologic supervision, as well as one or more replacements of the bioprosthesis. Transesophageal echocardiography provides invaluable information in the study of these patients, allowing determination of the diameters of the semilunar valve rings. It is particularly useful in the immediate postoperative evaluation because it permits identification of unsatisfactory results and the necessity of replacing the aortic valve with a prosthesis.

SUBVALVULAR AORTIC STENOSIS

Subvalvular aortic stenosis can be dynamic or fixed. In the former type, the obstruction is caused by systolic anterior movement of mitral valve structures and is seen in obstructive cardiomyopathy (Fig. 8.3.56). The latter type of obstruction is caused by a subaortic membrane (discrete obstruction) or, less frequently, by a fibromuscular tunnel.

Transesophageal study of patients with discrete subaortic stenosis is limited to cases in which an adequate transthoracic study cannot be obtained or as an intraoperative control during surgical resection of the membrane. Visualization of the obstruction with monoplane recordings provides only partial information about the membrane or ring. Images with color Doppler also offer information about the co-

existence of aortic valve regurgitation and the not infrequent association of a ventricular septal defect. The information obtained with recordings in the longitudinal plane is more complete, because it is possible to explore all of the left ventricular outlet and reliably quantify the subaortic pressure gradient with continuous wave Doppler (Figs. 8.3.57 and 8.3.58). Other causes of left ventricular outlet obstruction that can be detected with transesophageal imaging include accessory mitral tissue and malalignment of the trabecular septum (Figs. 8.3.59 and 8.3.60).

CONGENITAL MALFORMATIONS OF THE MITRAL VALVE

Parachute Mitral Valve   The parachute mitral valve is a congenital heart defect that represents between 1% and

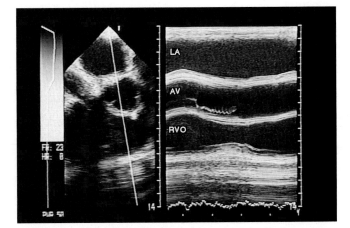

Figure 8.3.55. Ross procedure. M-mode and two-dimensional longitudinal plane images in a patient who underwent a Ross procedure. The pulmonary valve (PV) autograft in the aortic position shows normal motion.

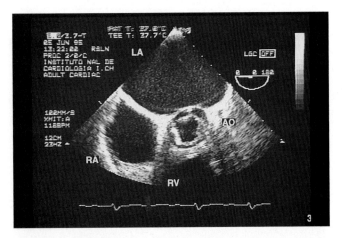

Figure 8.3.54. Aortic stenosis. Transesophageal echocardiogram taken with multiplanar probe shows a bicuspid aortic valve (AO).

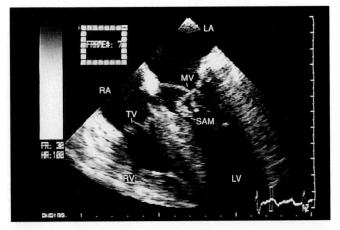

Figure 8.3.56. Subvalvular aortic stenosis. Transverse plane image shows significant hypertrophy of the ventricular septum and systolic anterior movement (SAM) of the mitral valve (MV) producing dynamic subvalvular aortic obstruction.

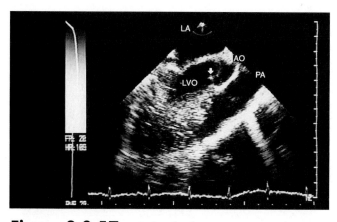

Figure 8.3.57. Subvalvular aortic stenosis. Longitudinal plane image in a patient with a subaortic membrane (arrow).

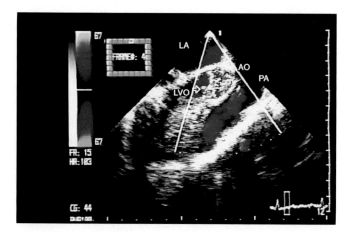

Figure 8.3.58. Subvalvular aortic stenosis. In this longitudinal plane imaged with color Doppler, the arrow points to accelerated flow in the left ventricular outlet, which appears as a mosaic of colors and is secondary to subvalvular aortic obstruction.

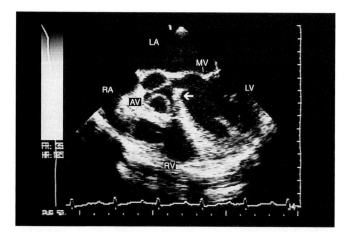

Figure 8.3.59. Subvalvular aortic stenosis. Transverse plane image of the left ventricular outlet. A malalignment exists between the trabecular and infundibular portions of the ventricular septum, which produces subvalvular aortic obstruction (arrow).

2% of malformations of the heart. It can be associated with diverse types of obstruction to left ventricular emptying. Parachute mitral valve is the most common variety of congenital obstructive mitral lesion. The existence of a single papillary muscle in the left ventricle into which the chordae tendineae insert can be demonstrated in transgastric echocardiographic studies in transverse and longitudinal planes. Because of this, the mitral valve has limited diastolic displacement. In four-chamber and left ventricular long-axis transesophageal images, the dome-shaped valvular opening can be seen (Fig. 8.3.61). These recordings and color Doppler demonstrate that obstruction is more significant at the subvalvular level than

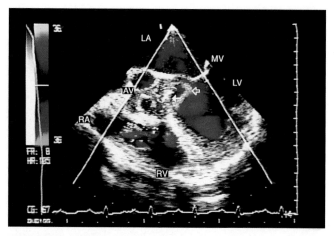

Figure 8.3.60. Subvalvular aortic stenosis. Four-chamber image shows severe subvalvular aortic obstruction secondary to posterior deviation of the trabecular portion of the ventricular septum (lower arrow). With color Doppler, accelerated flow in the left ventricular outlet (upper arrow) can be seen. There is a coexisting ventricular septal defect.

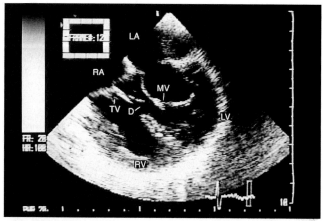

Figure 8.3.61. Parachute mitral valve. Four-chamber image shows a congenital stenosis of the mitral valve (dome-shaped opening) and tricuspid subvalvular structures crossing a ventricular septal defect (D).

at the level of the ring (Fig. 8.3.62). In some cases two papillary muscles can exist, but because of their extreme closeness they function as a single muscle.

Duplication of the Mitral Orifice

Two mitral valve openings can be identified with transesophageal echocardiography, especially with multiplanar probes. The characteristics of the subvalvular apparatus, including accessory papillary muscles, can be defined, and associated defects identified. When the examination is complemented with color Doppler, stenosis or regurgitation of one of the valvular components can be demonstrated (Figs. 8.3.63–8.3.67).

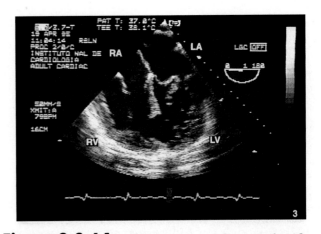

Figure 8.3.64. Duplication of the mitral orifice. Multiplane transesophageal study shows the mitral valve with two orifices. There is a large ventricular septal defect.

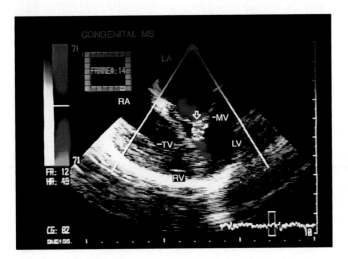

Figure 8.3.62. Parachute mitral valve. Congenital mitral stenosis. The dome-shaped opening of the leaflets (MV) can be seen, and color Doppler demonstrates turbulent flow (arrows).

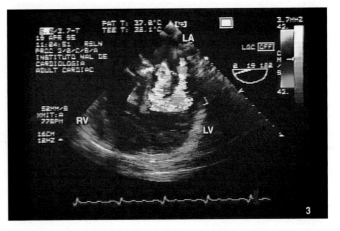

Figure 8.3.65. Duplication of the mitral orifice. Transesophageal echocardiogram with color Doppler shows the left ventricular inflow through both orifices.

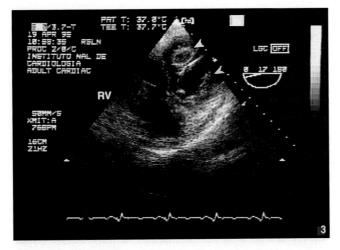

Figure 8.3.63. Duplication of the mitral orifice. Transgastric study with multiplanar transducer in a patient with mitral valve with double opening (arrows).

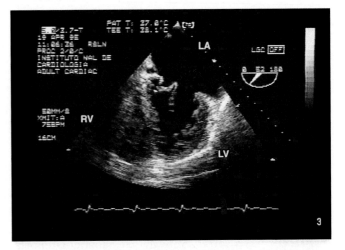

Figure 8.3.66. Duplication of the mitral orifice. Transesophageal echocardiographic image at 52° makes it possible to observe the anteroposterior relationship of the two mitral orifices.

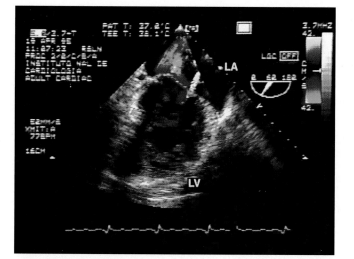

Figure 8.3.67. Duplication of the mitral orifice. The color Doppler image in systole shows minimal regurgitation from the anterior mitral opening (arrows).

Accessory Mitral Tissue

The presence of accessory mitral tissue in the aortic subvalvular region can create hemodynamically significant obstruction to left ventricular outflow (Fig. 8.3.68). This anomaly may go unnoticed in angiographic studies and even during cardiac surgery. In these patients transesophageal studies, especially with biplane transducers, are very useful because they provide information about the state of the mitral leaflets, aid in clarifying the site of implantation of accessory mitral tissue, and demonstrate anomalies of the chordae tendineae or papillary muscles. They also allow identification of associated malformations. This information is a great help to the surgeon for planning adequate corrective surgery.

Anomalous Insertion of Mitral Chordae Tendineae in the Interventricular Septum

Anomalous insertion of the mitral chordae tendineae in the interventricular septum can create obstruction of the left ventricular outflow tract and should be differentiated from subaortic stenosis caused by a subvalvular membrane because the surgical management is different. Transverse plane images make it possible to identify the left ventricular outflow tract obstruction, and longitudinal sections with multiplane transducers help to determine the mechanism (Fig. 8.3.69).

COR TRIATRIATUM

Cor triatriatum, or subdivided left atrium, is a cardiac malformation produced by a defect in the incorporation of the common pulmonary vein in the left atrium. The defect consists of a fibromuscular membrane, which divides the left atrium into two chambers: a superior chamber that receives the pulmonary veins, and an inferior chamber, or

true atrium, that includes the atrial appendage and the mitral valve, a finding which permits differentiation from a supravalvular mitral ring. The membrane usually inserts in the interatrial septum near the fossa ovalis and extends to the lateral wall of the left atrium.

Although the malformation may be diagnosed in newborns and infants with transthoracic recordings, in older patients, transesophageal echocardiography is the noninvasive diagnostic technique that offers the most information. The features discussed in the following paragraphs are demonstrated with transverse and longitudinal plane recordings complemented with continuous wave and color Doppler.

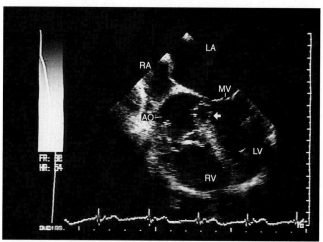

Figure 8.3.68. Accessory mitral tissue. Accessory mitral tissue (arrow) produces obstruction in the left ventricular outlet.

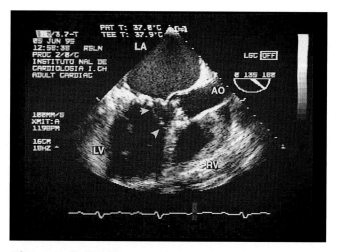

Figure 8.3.69. Anomalous insertion of the mitral chordae tendinae. Transesophageal echocardiographic image at 132° demonstrates the abnormal insertion of mitral chordae tendinae (arrows) in the anteropseptal portion of the left ventricle.

A membrane is seen that divides the left atrium into two cavities (Fig. 8.3.70). The pulmonary veins drain into the posterosuperior atrial cavity; the atrial appendage and mitral valve are included in the anteroinferior cavity (Figs. 8.3.71 and 8.3.72). In about half of cases an atrial septal defect is observed and can coexist with a patent formen ovale.

The site of communication between the two atrial portions can be recognized with color Doppler, and spectral analysis of flow shows whether the atrial membrane is obstructive (Fig. 8.3.73). The right cardiac cavities are dilated, and there is tricuspid regurgitation. Pulmonary hypertension can be quantified with Doppler.

The information provided by transesophageal echocardiography is complete enough that patients with cor triatriatum can undergo corrective surgery without requiring cardiac catheterization.

EBSTEIN'S ANOMALY

Ebstein's malformation is characterized by abnormal insertion of the tricuspid valve, which is tethered from the atrioventricular ring along the endocardium of the right ventricle. This creates an atrialized portion of the right ventricle located between the true valve ring and the area corresponding to the abnormal attachment of the tricuspid

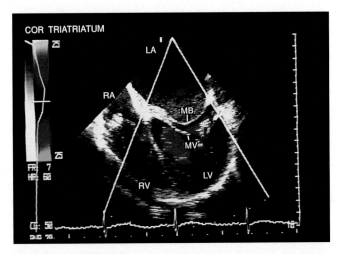

Figure 8.3.70. Cor triatriatum. Four-chamber image of a patient with cor triatriatum. The superior chamber of the left atrium is dilated with spontaneous echo contrast within it; the inferior portion communicates with the mitral valve. MB = cor triatriatum membrane.

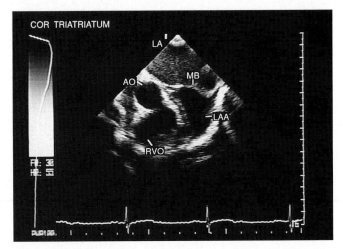

Figure 8.3.72. Cor triatriatum. Transverse plane image. The inferior chamber of the left atrium includes the implantation of the left atrial appendage. MB = cor triatum membrane.

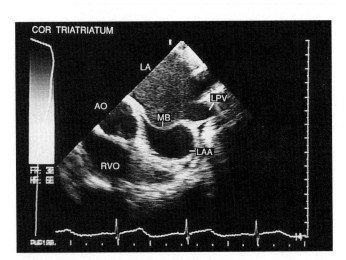

Figure 8.3.71. Cor triatriatum. The left atrium is divided by a membrane (MB). The upper chamber of the left atrium shows spontaneous echo contrast because of low blood-flow velocity and also receives the dilated pulmonary veins (LPV).

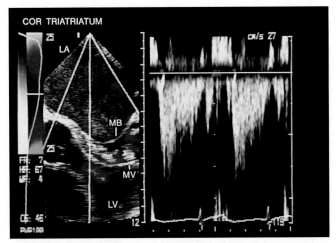

Figure 8.3.73. Cor triatriatum. Transverse plane recordings with color Doppler and spectral analysis. The hole in the atrial membrane (MB) can be identified. Flow is predominantly diastolic.

leaflets. The degree of attachment is variable. In the mild form, only the proximal portions of the septal and posterior leaflets are tethered, to the interventricular septum and ventricular wall, respectively. Usually the anterior leaflet is elongated, with an abnormally posterior insertion into the edge of the junction of the right ventricular inlet and trabecular portion. The tricuspid valve often is insufficient and occasionally is stenotic.

Two-dimensional echocardiography has replaced angiography as the procedure of choice for the diagnosis of Ebstein's anomaly. Patients with this anomaly have been studied by transthoracic two-dimensional echocardiography using parasternal, apical, and subcostal imaging. The four-chamber apical view is particularly valuable for determining the dimensions of the tricuspid valve ring, the atrialized portion of the right ventricle, and the functional right ventricle. On the basis of these findings, the indices of anatomic severity of the lesion have been described. It is also possible to observe the elongation of the anterior leaflet and its exaggerated movement, as well as the ventricular attachment of the septal leaflet. With this information, the most appropriate type of surgery can be chosen.

In adult patients with Ebstein's malformation, transesophageal echocardiography is the most useful diagnostic technique available. Using monoplanar transesophageal recordings, it is possible to determine the characteristics of the septal and anterior tricuspid leaflets and visualize the atrialized portion of the right ventricle in a four-chamber image (Figs. 8.3.74 and 8.3.75). The degree of tricuspid regurgitation and associated atrial septal defects can be evaluated with color Doppler (Fig. 8.3.76). In transgastric images the three tricuspid leaflets can be visualized and the attachment of the posterior leaflet to the ventricular wall evaluated from the apex to the tricuspid ring.

With biplanar transesophageal recordings, particularly with right ventricular longitudinal images, multiple data can be obtained, including partial attachment of the leaflet to the infundibulum or the trabecular portion of the right ventricle and adequate imaging of the right ventricular outflow tract and pulmonary arterial tree. In addition, the dimensions of the atrialized and functional portions of the right ventricle can be determined. Likewise, with recordings in two planes with color Doppler, more information on the degree of tricuspid regurgitation is available, and the interatrial septum can be explored completely and the

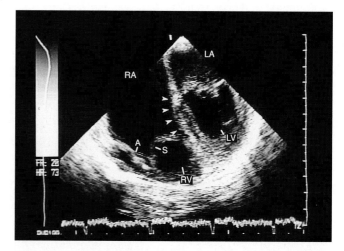

Figure 8.3.75. Ebstein's anomaly. Transverse plane image in a patient with Ebstein's malformation. There is tethering of both the anterior (A) and septal (S) leaflets of the tricuspid valve. The functional right ventricle (RV) is moderately reduced in size.

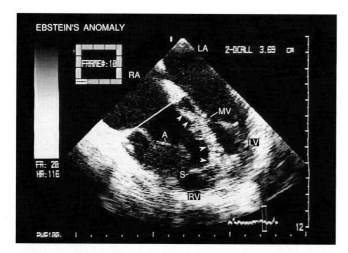

Figure 8.3.74. Ebstein's anomaly. Four-chamber image shows tethering (arrows) of the tricuspid septal leaflet (S). The movement of the anterior leaflet (A) is large, and the diameter of the tricuspid ring is increased (37 mm).

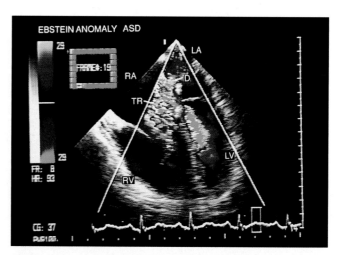

Figure 8.3.76. Ebstein's anomaly. Color Doppler aids in evaluating the degree of tricuspid regurgitation (TR) as well as the coexistence of an atrial septal defect (ASD).

type of septal defect identified with precision (Figs. 8.3.77 and 8.3.78).

With the development of new corrective surgical techniques for Ebstein's malformation, echocardiographic studies have served to guide reconstructive surgical management (valvuloplasty) or tricuspid replacement. Transesophageal biplanar or multiplanar imaging is the optimal type of study for evaluating the anatomic and functional status of each of the tricuspid leaflets and their subvalvular apparati as well as the size of the atrialized and functional portions of the right ventricle.

PULMONARY VALVULAR STENOSIS

Pulmonary valvular stenosis may be isolated or may form one part of complex congenital heart disease. When

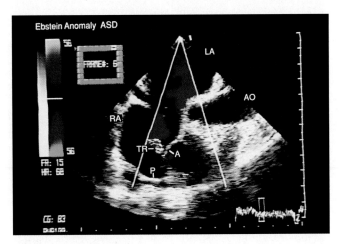

Figure 8.3.77. Ebstein's anomaly. Longitudinal plane image with color Doppler shows tethering of the posterior tricuspid leaflet (P). Large movement of the anterior leaflet (A) can be seen. Color Doppler demonstrates mild tricuspid regurgitation (TR).

it is isolated, the diagnosis and severity of the obstruction can be established with transthoracic recordings. Transesophageal images have been used during interventional procedures in the hemodynamic laboratory to reduce the length of exposure to x-rays and the quantity of contrast material required.

The use of transesophageal recordings only in the transverse plane has limitations because it does not offer adequate visualization of the right ventricular outflow tract, and even analysis of the leaflets themselves is incomplete. With biplane or multiplane transducers, the monitoring of balloon pulmonary valvuloplasties provides an assessment of the morphology both before and after dilatation. It is particularly useful for avoiding a malposition of the balloon or guidewire, which can provoke a tricuspid valve lesion. Doppler evaluation of the postdilatation transvalvular pressure gradient has limitations, however, because of the difficulty of aligning the Doppler beam to the direction of blood flow. With color Doppler an immediate estimation of the presence and magnitude of valvular regurgitations is available (Fig. 8.3.79).

Transesophageal study with biplanar images also is useful for recognizing the three pulmonary leaflets (right, left, and anterior). It helps to identify bicuspid valves and, most importantly, allows differentiation of valvular and infundibular obstructions or identification of their coexistence (Figs. 8.3.80 and 8.3.81).

TETRALOGY OF FALLOT

Tetralogy of Fallot is caused by an alteration in the development of the embryonic conus. The anterior displacement of the ventricular infundibulum produces pulmonary subvalvular stenosis (in two thirds of patients, stenosis also is valvular). There is a large ventricular septal defect, which is usually below the aortic valve and anterior to the membranous portion of the interventricular septum, although it

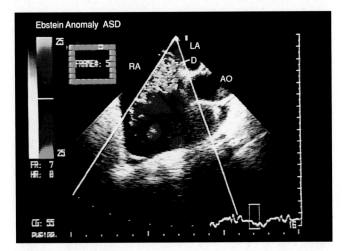

Figure 8.3.78. Ebstein's anomaly. Longitudinal plane examination complemented with color Doppler demonstrates regurgitation as well as an atrial septal defect (ASD).

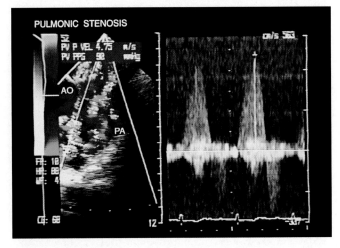

Figure 8.3.79. Pulmonary valve stenosis. Color Doppler–guided continuous wave Doppler demonstrates a peak transvalvular gradient of 90 mm Hg.

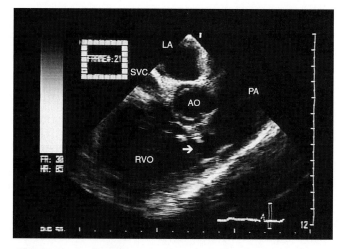

Figure 8.3.80. **Pulmonary valve stenosis.** It is possible to recognize subvalvular pulmonary obstruction (arrow) in the longitudinal plane image. Pulmonary valve leaflets are thickened as well.

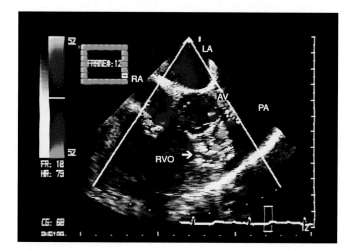

Figure 8.3.81. **Pulmonary valve stenosis.** Significant stenosis of the right ventricular infundibulum (arrow) is demonstrated by color Doppler in longitudinal plane imaging.

With transgastric images in the transverse plane or transesophageal images in the longitudinal plane, dextroposition of the aorta overriding the interventricular septum is recognized. When these images are complemented with color Doppler, the characteristics of the interventricular shunt and the degree of obstruction to right ventricular outflow can be appreciated.

Subvalvular or mixed pulmonary stenosis requires images in the longitudinal plane. With these, the ventricular infundibulum can be explored, the characteristics of the pulmonary valves clarified, and the diameters of the principal pulmonary arterial branches determined, information of great utility for selecting palliative or corrective surgery. With biplane or multiplane transducers, the de-

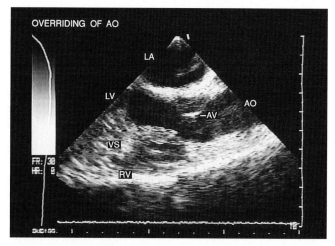

Figure 8.3.82. **Tetralogy of Fallot.** Longitudinal plane imaging in tetralogy of Fallot (TOF). The aorta (AO) overrides the ventricular septum (VS).

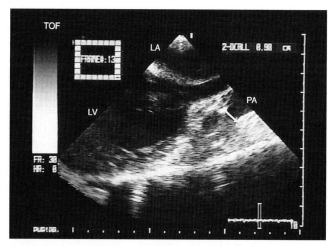

Figure 8.3.83. **Tetralogy of Fallot.** In this longitudinal plane image it is possible to identify stenosis of the right ventricular infundibulum (arrow). The pulmonary valve annulus is small.

can extend to other portions of the interventricular septum. The aorta is biventricular, because it overrides the interventricular septum. Approximately 10% of patients with tetralogy of Fallot have anomalies of the coronary arteries.

In infants and children, conventional transthoracic echocardiography allows diagnosis of tetralogy of Fallot, and, in most cases, the indication for cardiac surgery, without requiring cardiac catheterization. Transesophageal echocardiography is the noninvasive technique of choice in adolescents and adults for recognizing the diverse abnormalities found in these patients. Recordings in transverse and longitudinal planes are indispensable for evaluating these abnormalities (Figs. 8.3.82 and 8.3.83).

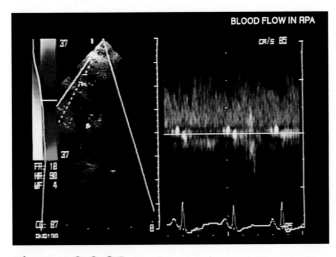

Figure 8.3.84. **Pulmonary atresia.** In a patient with pulmonary atresia, color Doppler and spectral analysis identify systolic and diastolic flow from a systemic-pulmonary fistula.

gree of right ventricular hypertrophy can also be defined, as can the courses of the coronary arteries. Continuous wave and color Doppler study offers information about the degree of obstruction to right ventricular outflow. Moreover, it allows differentiation of tetralogy of Fallot with very severe pulmonary stenosis from pulmonary atresia with ventricular septal defect. In the former, flow in the pulmonary artery is turbulent and systolic, whereas in pulmonary atresia the flow that reaches the pulmonary artery comes from the aorta through a patent ductus arteriosus and appears in both phases of the cardiac cycle, predominantly in diastole.

Transesophageal echocardiography is particularly important for transoperative and late postoperative evaluation of surgical results. Biplane or multiplane imaging provides assessment of the operated subvalvular, valvular, and proximal supravalvular pulmonary anatomy; of ventricular-to-pulmonary conduits; and of the adequacy of the ventricular septal patch. In patients with palliative shunts it is possible to recognize the lack of patency of the fistula or diminished flow because of increased pulmonary vascular resistance with Doppler studies (Fig. 8.3.84).

REFERENCES

1. Andrade A, Vargas-Barron J, Romero-Cardenas A, et al. Transthoracic and transesophageal echocardiographic study of pulmonary autograft valve in aortic position. Echocardiography 1994;11:221–226.
2. Arazoza EA, Bowser M, Obeid AI. Coronary artery fistula: diagnosis by biplane transesophageal echocardiography. J Am Soc Echocardiogr 1992;5:277–280.
3. Calafiore PA, Raymond R, Schiavone WA, Rosenkranz ER. Precise evaluation of a complex coronary arteriovenous fistula: the utility of transesophageal color Doppler. J Am Soc Echocardiogr 1989; 2:337–341.
4. Child JS. Echocardiographic assessment of adults with tetralogy of Fallot. Echocardiography 1993;10:629–640.
5. Goldfarb A, Weinreb J, Daniel WG, Kronzon I. A patient with right and left atrial membranes: the role of transesophageal echocardiography and magnetic resonance imaging in diagnosis. J Am Soc Echocardiogr 1989;2:350–353.
6. Hellenbrand WE, Fahey JT, McGowan FX, et al. Transesophageal echocardiographic guidance of transcatheter closure of atrial septal defect. Am J Cardiol 1990; 6:207–213.
7. Kindman LA, Wright A, Tye T, et al. Lipomatous hypertrophy of the interatrial septum: characterization by transesophageal and transthoracic echocardiography, magnetic resonance imaging and computed tomography. J Am Soc Echocardiogr 1988;1:450–454.
8. Kronzon I, Tunick PA, Freedberg RS, et al. Transesophageal echocardiography is superior to transthoracic echocardiography in the diagnosis of sinus venosus atrial septal defect. J Am Coll Cardiol 1991;17: 537–542.
9. Lin SL, Ting CT, Hsu TL, et al. Transesophageal echocardiographic detection of atrial septal defect in adults. Am J Cardiol 1992;69: 280–282.
10. Ludomirsky A, Erickson Ch, Vick GW, Cooley DA. Transesophageal color flow Doppler evaluation of cor triatriatum in an adult. Am Heart J 1990;120:451–455.
11. Mehta RH, Helmcke F, Nanda NC, et al. Transesophageal Doppler color flow mapping assessment of atrial septal defect. J Am Coll Cardiol 1990;16:1010–1016.
12. Minich LL, Snider AR. Echocardiographic guidance during placement of the buttoned double-disk device for atrial septal defect closure. Echocardiography 1993;10:567–572.
13. Morimoto K, Matsuzaki M, Tohma Y, et al. Diagnosis and quantitative evaluation of secundum type atrial septal defect by transesophageal echocardiography. Am J Cardiol 1990;66:85–91.
14. Oh JK, Seward JB, Khandheria BK, et al. Visualization of sinus venosus atrial septal defect by transesophageal echocardiography. J Am Soc Echocardiogr 1988;1:275–277.
15. Oniki T, Hashimoto Y, Aerbajinai W, et al. Transesophageal echocardiographic recognition of a fistula between a coronary artery and the left atrium. J Am Soc Echocardiogr 1992;5:628–630.
16. Pearson AC, Nagelhout D, Castello R, et al. Atrial septal aneurysm and stroke: a transesophageal echocardiographic study. J Am Coll Cardiol 1991;18:1223–1229.
17. Ritter SB. Transesophageal real-time echocardiography in infants and children with congenital heart disease. J Am Coll Cardiol 1991;18:569–580.
18. Roberson DA, Muhiudeen IA, Silverman NH, et al. Intraoperative transesophageal echocardiography of atrioventricular septal defect. J Am Coll Cardiol 1991;18:537–545.
19. Romero-Cardenas A, Vargas-Barron J, Rylaarsdam M, et al. Total anomalous pulmonary venous return: diagnosis by transesophageal echocardiography. Am Heart J 1991;121:1831–1834.
20. Schlüter M, Burkhart A, Langenstein BA, et al. Transesophageal two dimensional echocardiography in the diagnosis of cor triatriatum in the adult. J Am Coll Cardiol 1983;2:1011–1015.
21. Schneider B, Hanrath P, Vogel P, Meinertz T. Improved morphological characterization of atrial septal aneurysm by transesophageal echocardiography: relation to cerebrovascular events. J Am Coll Cardiol 1990;16:1000–1009.
22. Schwinger ME, Gindea AJ, Freedberg RS, Kronzon I. The anatomy of the interatrial septum: a transesophageal echocardiographic study. Am Heart J 1990;119:1401–1405.
23. Stern H, Erbel R, Schreiner G, et al. Coarctation of the aorta: quantitative analysis by transesophageal echocardiography. Echocardiography 1987;4:387–395.
24. Stümper OFW, Elzenga NJ, Hess J, Sutherland GR. Transesophageal echocardiography in children with congenital heart disease: an initial experience. J Am Coll Cardiol 1990;16:433–441.
25. Stümper O, Elzenga NJ, Sutherland GR. Obstruction of the left ventricular outflow tract in childhood improved diagnosis by transesophageal echocardiography. Int J Cardiol 1990;28:107–109.

26. Stümper O, Hess J, Godman MJ, Sutherland GR. Transesophageal echocardiography in congenital heart disease. Cardiol Young 1993; 3:3–12.

27. Stümper O, Kaulitz R, Elzenga NJ, et al. The value of transesophageal echocardiography in children with congenital heart disease. J Am Soc Echocardiogr 1991;4:164–176.

28. Stümper O, Kaulitz R, Sreeram N, et al. Intraoperative transesophageal versus epicardial ultrasound in surgery for congenital heart disease. J Am Soc Echocardiogr 1990;3:392–401.

29. Stümper O, Vargas-Barron J, Rijlaarsdam M, et al. Assessment of anomalous systemic and pulmonary venous connection by transesophageal echocardiography in infants and children. Br Heart J 1991;66: 411–418.

30. Stümper O, Witsenburg M, Sutherland GR, et al. Transesophageal echocardiographic monitoring of interventional cardiac catheterization in children. J Am Coll Cardiol 1991;18:1506–1514.

31. Szulc M, Ritter SB. Patent ductus arteriosus in an infant with atrioventricular septal defect and pulmonary hypertension: diagnosis by transesophageal color flow echocardiography. J Am Soc Echocardiogr 1991;4:194–198.

32. Takenata K, Sakamoto T, Shiota T, et al. Diagnosis of patent ductus arteriosus in adults by biplane transesophageal color Doppler flow mapping. Am J Cardiol 1991;68:691–693.

33. Tapia MM, Rijlaarsdam M, Romero CA, et al. Obstrucción de la vía de salida del ventrículo izquierdo por tejido valvular mitral accesorio. Arch Inst Cardiol Mex 1991;61:325–330.

34. Tumbarello R, Sanna A, Cardu G, et al. Usefulness of transesophageal echocardiography in the pediatric catheterization laboratory. Am J Cardiol 1993;71:1321–1325.

35. Vargas-Barron J, Rijlaarsdam M, Romero-Cardenas A, et al. transesophageal echocardiography in adults with congenital cardiopathies. Am Heart J 1993;126:426–432.

36. Wang KY, Hsieh KS, Yang MW, et al. The use of transesophgeal echocardiography to evaluate the effectiveness of patent ductus arteriosus ligation. Echocardiography 1993;10:53–57.

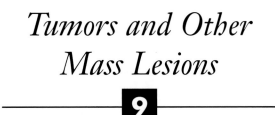

Tumors and Other Mass Lesions

9

Although cardiac tumors often can be seen on transthoracic echocardiography, their location, size, and relation to surrounding structures are better defined by transesophageal echocardiography.

The most common primary cardiac tumor is the myxoma. This tumor rarely metastasizes, but it can cause obstruction and frequently embolizes, making its immediate removal mandatory. These tumors also can cause regurgitation by interfering with valve function, and they can cause a variety of constitutional symptoms. Myxomas usually are solitary and most commonly are located in the left atrium. However, because they can occur in any chamber and may be multiple, a careful transesophageal echocardiographic investigation of all the cardiac chambers should be conducted preoperatively to be certain that all tumors have been detected and are removed. Myxomas characteristically have cystic spaces caused by hemorrhages and areas of calcification. The base of the tumor may be either broad or narrow, and a careful search should be made for the attachment point. In one patient we studied there was massive calcification that involved the left atrial free wall and protruded into the left atrial cavity, mimicking a myxoma. Heavy mitral annular calcification also may produce a confusing picture, especially if some areas are soft and mobile. Lipomas are characteristically more refractile than a noncalcified myxoma, which may help in distinguishing between them. Tumors such as a leiomyoma or leiomyosarcoma may arise from the wall of a blood vessel and cause obstruction to blood flow. Fibroelastomas often present as irregular mobile masses on valves or chamber walls, emanating from narrow stalks. Because of their embolic potential they should be surgically removed. Large mobile vegetations attached to valves may mimic fibroelastoma or a small myxoma on a valve, but the associated clinical picture, which is suggestive of infective endocarditis, helps in differentiating between them. Myxomatous thickening or nodules involving the mitral valve also may simulate a small tumor.

Thrombus can mimic tumor, and the distinction often cannot be made by echocardiography. As with tumors, identifying the point of attachment is important in surgical planning. Although low flow velocities often are present (and, indeed, causative) when a thrombus is found, this may not always be the case, and thrombi can occur in the absence of an identifiable precipitating factor. Interestingly, during transesophageal examination we have visualized thrombi, subsequently confirmed by both surgery and pathology, attached to the mitral valve and in the region of papillary muscles in the normally functioning left and right ventricles, with no clinically or echocardiographically discernible cause. Right-sided tumors must be differentiated from normal structures such as hypertrophied trabeculations in the right atrium or right ventricle and prominent or hypertrophied right ventricular papillary muscles. A prominent eustachian or thebesian valve and Chiari network, as well as a prominent crista terminalis visualized at the junction of the superior vena cava and the right atrium, also may be mistaken for a tumor mass. Abnormal thickening of normal structures, such as lipomatous hypertrophy of the interatrial septum or nonspecific thickening of the "Q-tip" (i.e., left atrial wall invagination or infolding separating the appendage from the left upper pulmonary vein) also may mimic tumor infiltration.

Malignant tumors of the heart are unusual but, when present, tend to metastasize early. They often can be recognized based on the fact that they deform the walls of the heart. Other tumors, such as melanoma, may produce bloodborne metastases to the heart. Mediastinal tumors such as a leiomyosarcoma may compress or invade the heart, either directly or through vascular accesses such as the pulmonary veins. Because these tumors are vascular, multiple small blood vessels may be imaged within the tumor by color Doppler, especially if the Nyquist limit is kept low. Sclerosing mediastinitis producing narrowing of systemic and pulmonary veins at their junction with the heart may simulate an extracardiac tumor. Postoperative hematomas also must be differentiated from extracardiac tumor masses.

Figure 9.1. **Left atrial myxoma. A–F.** A huge LA myxoma (M) with a broad attachment on the atrial septum (AS, arrow in **B**). **C.** An area of calcification (closed arrow) in the tumor and an echolucency caused by hemorrhage (open arrow). **D.** M-mode study of the tumor. **E.** Associated mild MR (arrow). **F.** Postoperative study after removal of the myxoma shows persistence of mild MR.

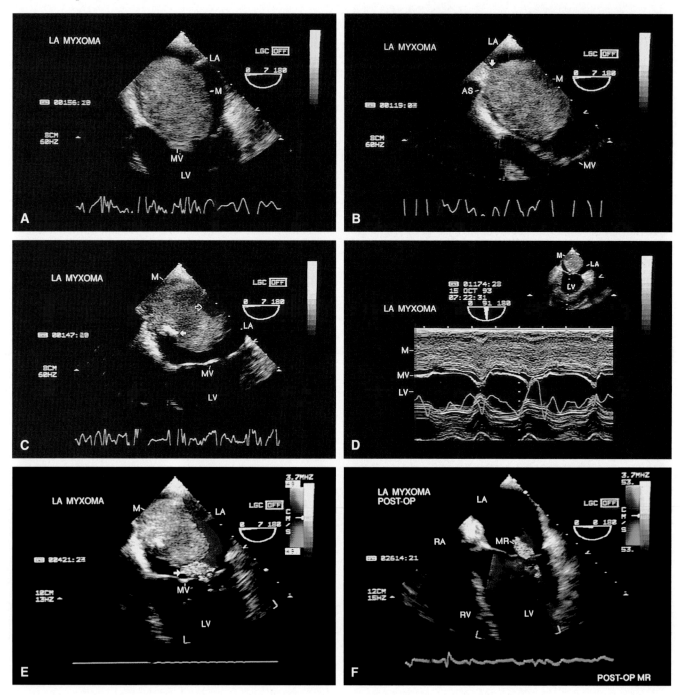

Figure 9.2. Left atrial myxoma. A–D. A huge myxoma (M) is seen in the LA obstructing the mitral orifice in diastole (D).

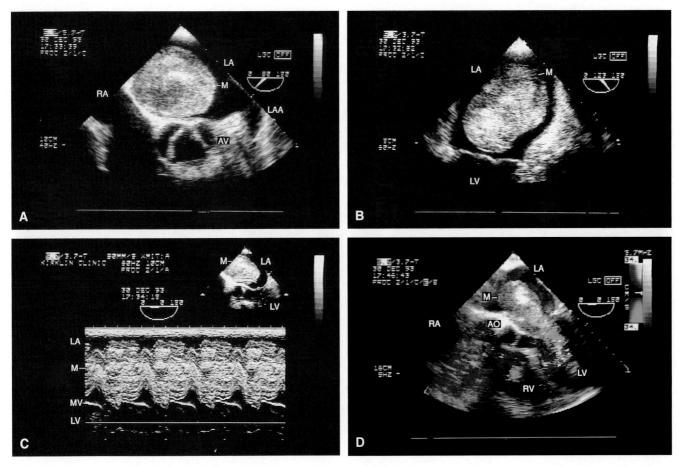

Figure 9.3. **A-K. Left atrial myxoma. A.** The myxoma (MYX) is seen attached to the base of the atrial septum. **B.** Another myxoma (M) is seen attached to the lower portion of the atrial septum, with a longer stalk (arrow) than the myxoma in **A**. **C–E.** Another patient with a huge myxoma (M) that has a very broad attachment (arrows in **C**) to the atrial septum (AS). **C,D.** A calcified area (C) in the tumor. In this patient, systolic anterior motion (SAM) of the mitral valve and septal thickening and narrowing of the LVOT also were present, consistent with hypertrophic cardiomyopathy. **F.** Schematic of an LA myxoma obstructing the mitral orifice. **G.** Specimen of an LA myxoma attached to the LA free wall. **H.** Specimen of a hemorrhagic, calcified myxoma that was resected. **I–K.** Another patient with a large lobulated LA myxoma (arrowheads in **I** and **J**). The figure shows the myxoma after surgical removal. **L–S. LA leiomyosarcoma.** A large mass is seen in the LA (arrowheads in **L**, M in **M**). **N.** The mass (arrowheads) invading the LA from the right upper pulmonary vein (RUPV). **O.** A narrow flow jet (arrow) shows RUPV obstruction. **P.** A markedly dilated left upper pulmonary vein and its tributaries (arrow). **Q.** The leiomyosarcoma (M) is seen invading the mediastinum in the vicinity of the right pulmonary artery (PA) and the SVC. **R,S.** Multiple blood vessels (arrowheads) within the tumor mass (T) characteristic of vascular tumors such as the leiomyosarcoma. (**A** and **F** reproduced with permission from Nanda NC, Mahan EF III. Transesophageal echocardiography. AHA Council on Clinical Cardiology Newsletter 1990;Summer:3–22.)

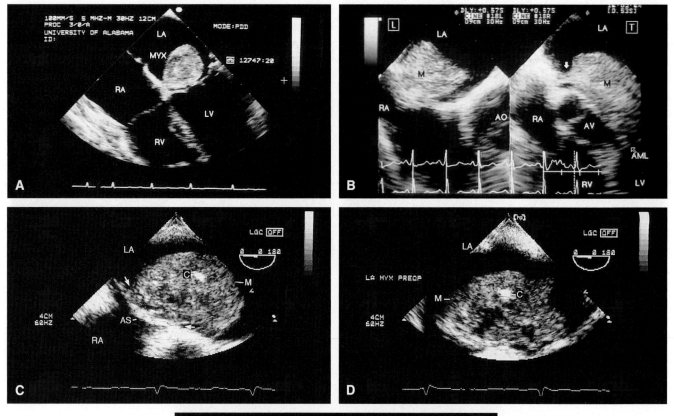

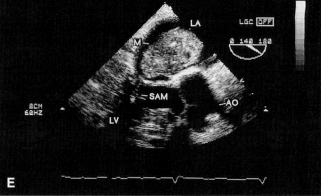

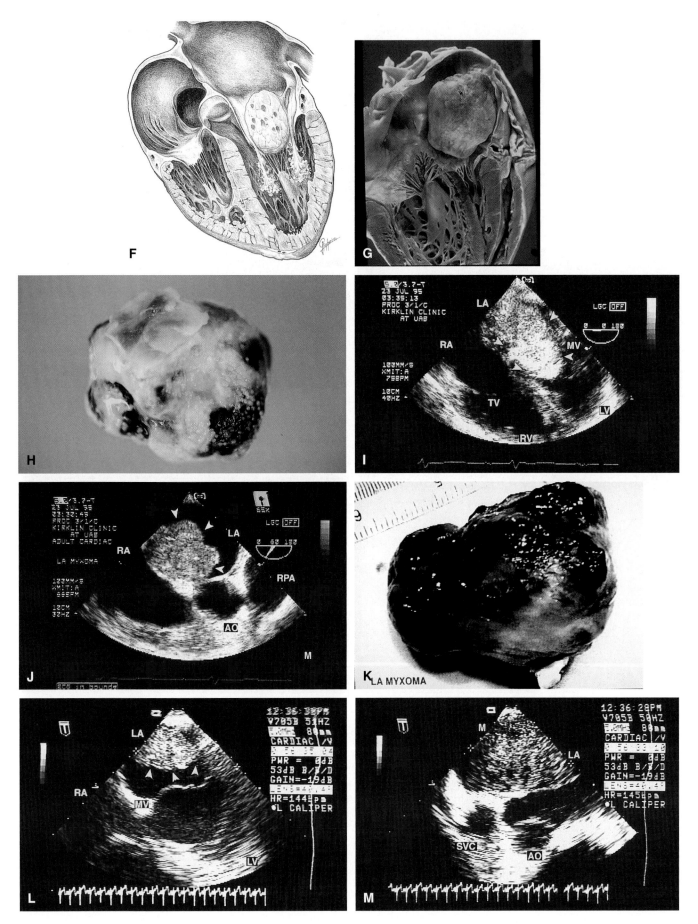

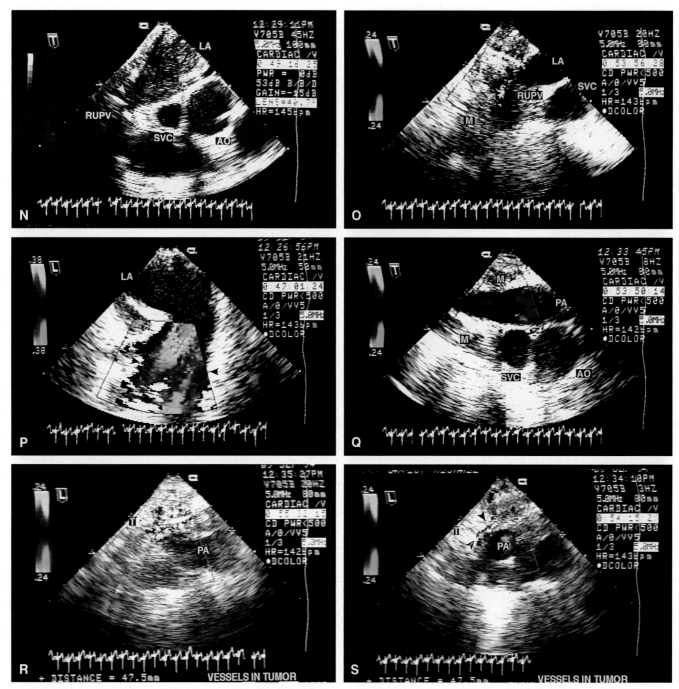

Figure 9.4.   **Left atrial tumor mimic. A,B.** A huge non-mobile mass (arrowheads) consistent with a tumor in the LA. It appeared to have a broad attachment to the LA free wall **(B). C.** Spontaneous contrast echoes in LA next to the mass, which was successfully removed. **D.** The suture line (arrowheads) repairing the LA wall following its resection. **E.** The resected mass, which was found to be a thrombus and not a tumor at pathology. No etiologic factors were identified.

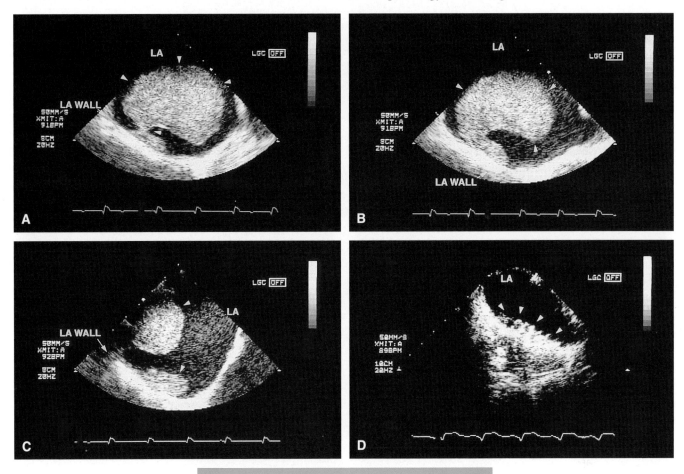

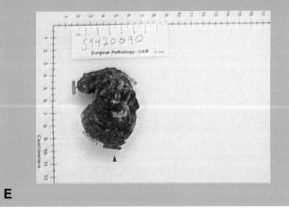

Figure 9.5. **Left atrial tumor.** A small mass consistent with a tumor is seen at the base of the LA appendage in this patient, who presented with symptoms of an embolic stroke.

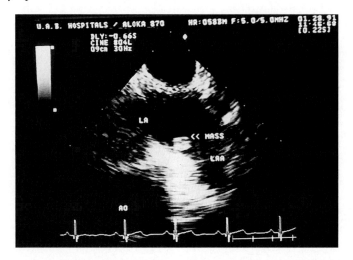

Figure 9.6. **Left atrial thrombus/calcification. A.** Two large thrombi (TH) are seen in the LA. These could be distinguished from tumor by their mobility and the presence of spontaneous contrast echoes seen in other views. **B,C.** In another patient, heavy calcifications (arrows) involving the LA free wall are seen protruding into the LA cavity and mimicking a tumor. The findings were verified at surgery and by pathological examination.

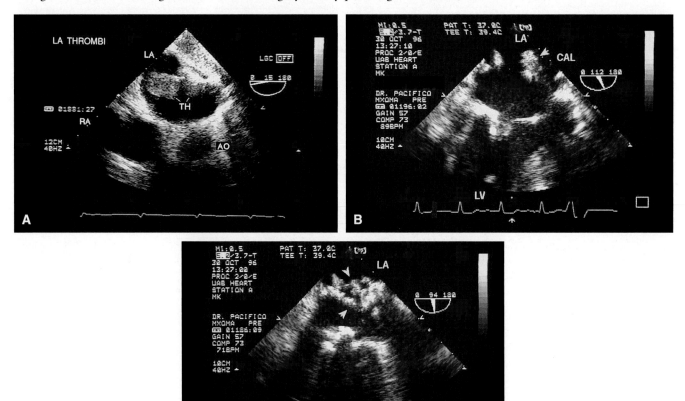

Figure 9.7. Left atrial tumor mimic. **A,B.** Nonspecific thickening (arrows) of the invaginated/infolded part of the LA free wall ("Q-tip") mimicking a tumor. LA wall infolding is a normal finding at the site where the LUPV enters into the LA and appears as a "septum" separating the LUPV from the LAA.

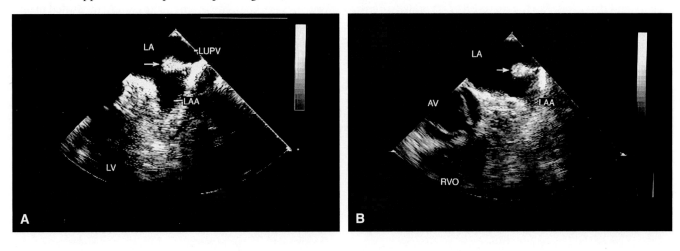

Figure 9.8. Mitral valve myxoma. **A,B.** A large tumor (arrows) attached to the atrial aspect of the anterior mitral leaflet. The multiple tiny echolucencies seen within the tumor suggest the presence of hemorrhage, often seen in myxomas. **C.** The resected specimen.

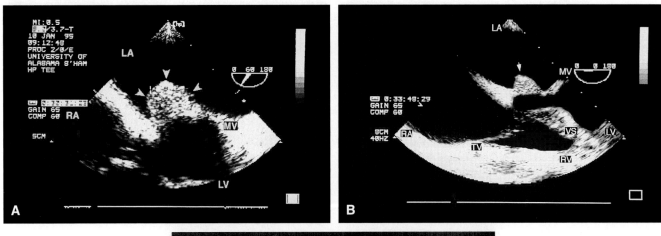

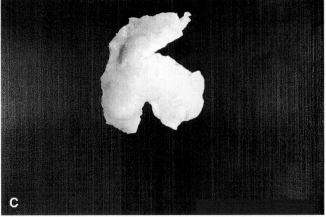

Figure 9.9. **Mitral valve thrombus/myxomatous degeneration. A–C.** The prominent echodensity involving the posterior mitral leaflet was identified as a thrombus at surgery and on pathological examination. **B.** Mild MR is noted. The arrowheads in **D, E,** and **G** show two other patients with masses involving the MV that were found to be thrombi at surgery and pathology. **F,H.** The resected thrombi from these two patients. No predisposing factors were identified in any of the three patients shown here. **I–K.** A different patient with a small rounded mass (arrowheads) attached to the base of the posterior MV leaflet. The MV showed prolapse and mild MR (arrow in **K**). Pathological examination of the resected mass showed myxomatous degenerative changes and no evidence of tumor. *AML,* anterior mitral leaflet; *PML,* posterior mitral leaflet.

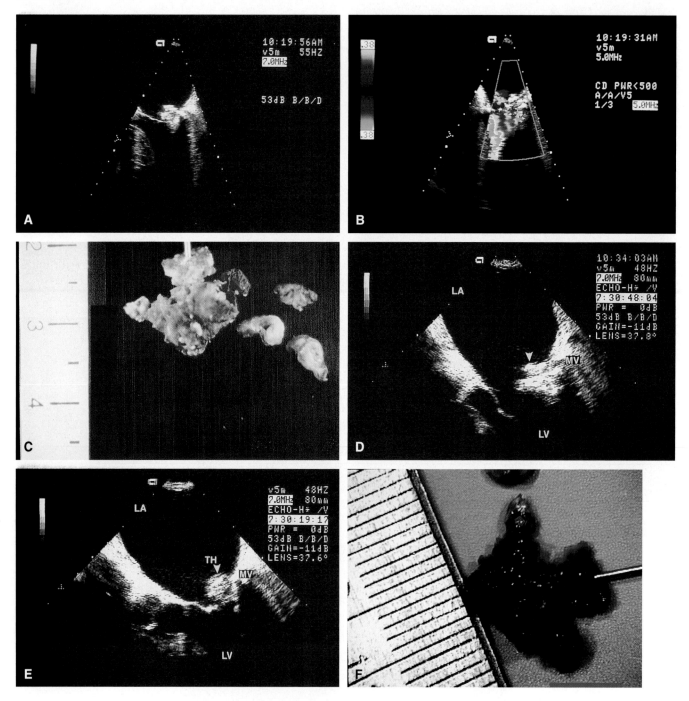

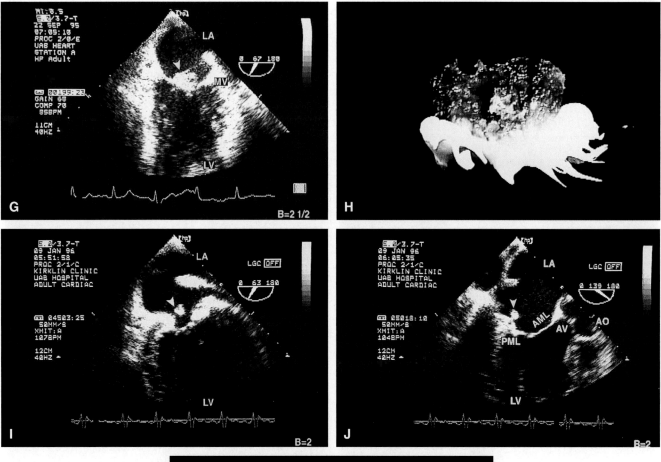

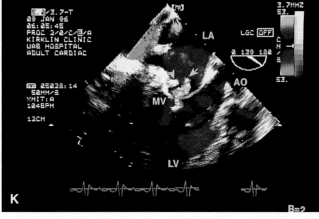

Figure 9.10. **Left ventricular myxoma. A–C.** A large mass (M) in the LA that appears to be attached to the anterior mitral leaflet. **D–F.** Further examination showed that the mass actually arose from the LV and was attached by a long stalk (S) to a papillary muscle (PM). **G.** In the short-axis view, two separate masses (M1 and M2) together with two separate stalks (arrows) were identified in the region of the papillary muscles. **H.** An M-mode study demonstrates the mass in the left atrium only during systole. Note a large arc-like side-lobe (SL) artifact in **C**. Because of the long stalk, one of the myxomas intermittently prolapsed into the left atrium, sometimes becoming trapped in that chamber. These tumors were successfully resected. *AML*, anterior mitral leaflet; *PML*, posterior mitral leaflet. (**A** and **G** reproduced with permission from Samdarshi TE, Mahan III EF, Nanda NC, et al. Transesophageal echocardiographic diagnosis of multicentric left ventricular myxomas mimicking a left atrial tumor. J Thorac Cardiovasc Surg 1992;103:471–474.)

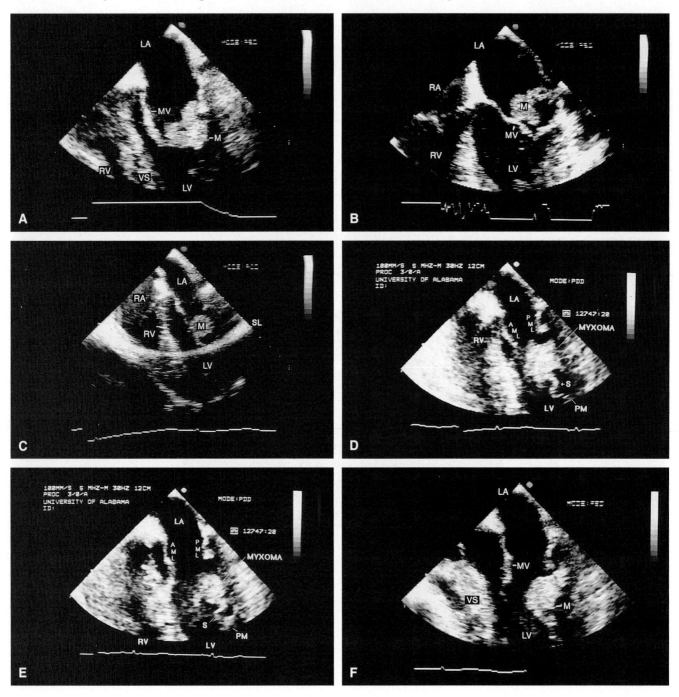

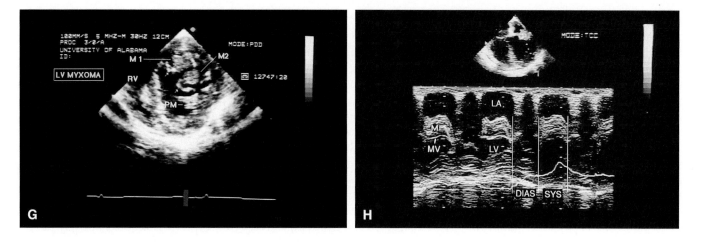

Figure 9.11. **Left ventricular myxoma.** A large mass (M; arrows) arising from the apex. Pathology examination demonstrated it to be a myxoma. *AL,* anterior mitral leaflet; *PL,* posterior mitral leaflet. (Reproduced with permission from Nanda NC, Pinheiro L, Sanyal RS, Storey O. Transesophageal biplane echocardiographic imaging: technique, planes, and clinical usefulness. Echocardiography 1990;7:771–788.)

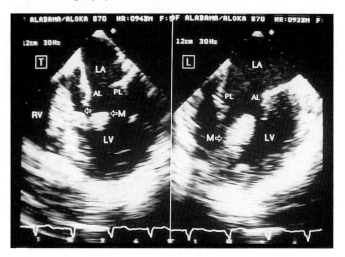

Figure 9.12.   **Left ventricular lipoma. A.** The lower arrow shows a bright, highly echogenic and generally homogenous mass arising from the apical portion of the ventricular septum. The mass (arrow, T) was also well seen in the two-chamber **(B)** and short-axis **(C)** views. This elderly female patient underwent angioplasty of the proximal LAD subsequent to an episode of chest pain, and the mass was discovered on a follow-up two-dimensional echocardiogram. Consequently, thrombus was considered in the differential diagnosis, along with myxoma and lipoma. There were no obvious wall motion abnormalities. The mass was surgically removed and found to be a lipoma. **D.** Patch repair (arrow) of the apical ventricular septum following lipoma resection. **E,F.** Mild turbulence (arrows) is seen in the region of the patch, but no defect is present. The resected lipoma and a myxoma removed from another patient were studied in vitro by suspending them in a water bath using the same transesophageal probe used for the in vivo study. At the same instrument settings and similar distance from the transducer surface, the lipoma **(G)** appeared to be significantly hyperrefractile compared to the myxoma **(H)**, except for the areas of calcifications (C in frame **I**) in the myxoma. **I.** S indicates the string that suspended the myxoma in the water bath. This study suggests that, in the absence of calcification, a very hyperrefractile mass may be a lipoma rather than a myxoma. (**A**, **B**, and **G** through **I** reproduced with permission from Mehta R, Nanda NC, Osman K, et al. Left ventricular lipoma by transesophageal and in vitro echocardiographic studies. Echocardiography 1995;12:283–288.)

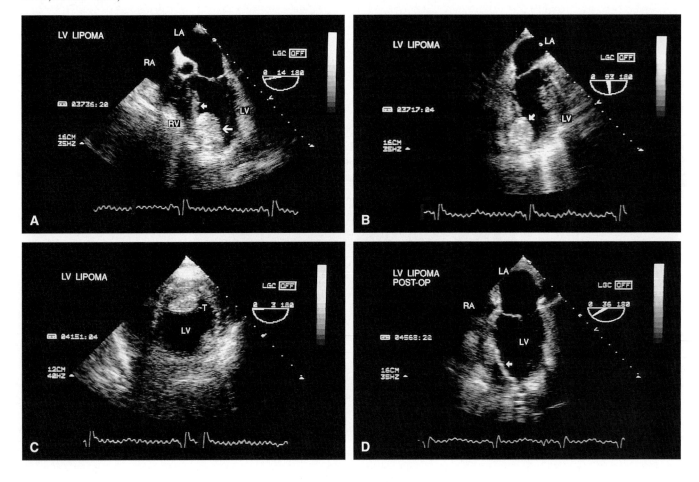

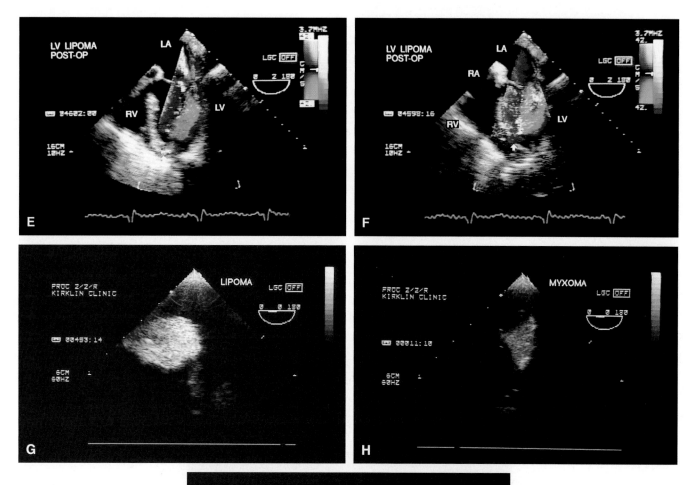

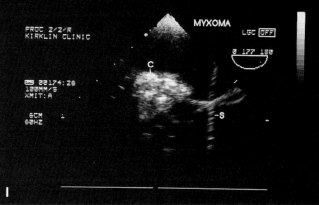

Figure 9.13. **Left ventricular thrombus. A–C.** A mass (arrowheads) attached to a papillary muscle in the LV in a patient with aortic stenosis. This mass was found to be a thrombus (TH) at surgery.

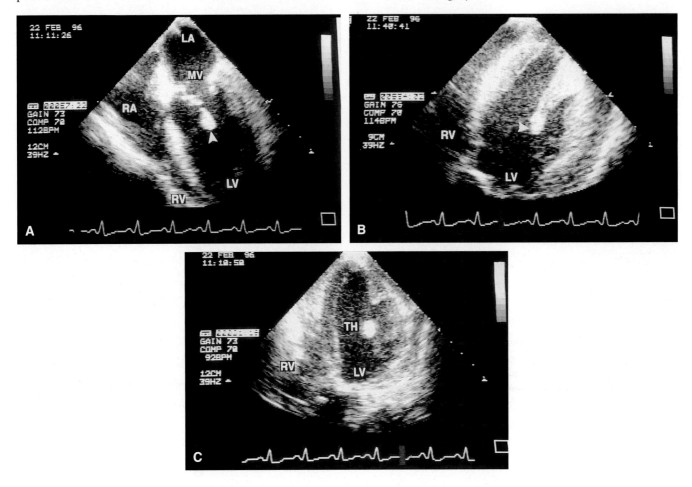

Figure 9.14. **Aortic valve fibroelastoma.** A small irregular mass (arrow in **B**, T in **C**) is seen attached to the left coronary leaflet of the AV by a short stalk **(A)**. There was no clinical evidence of endocarditis or significant AR in this patient. The mass was resected and found to be a fibroelastoma. **D.** Schematic shows a fibroelastoma.

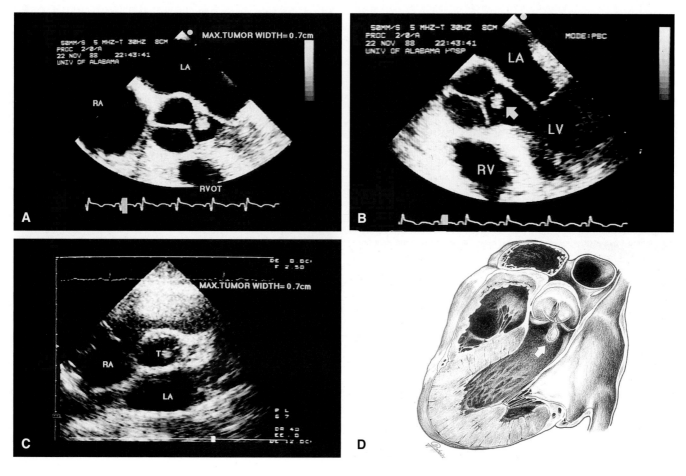

Figure 9.15. **Aortic valve mass. A–D.** The mass-like lesion (T) attached to the noncoronary cusp of the AV in this patient mimics a tumor but is actually a vegetation with typical clinical findings of endocarditis. Note associated severe AR **(C)**.

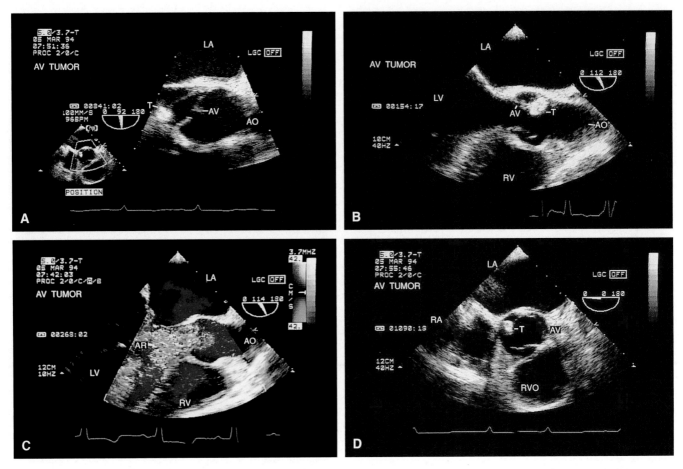

Figure 9.16. **Aortic leiomyosarcoma. A–F.** A mass (arrowheads) in the descending thoracic aorta (DA). Color Doppler examination shows prominent flow signals in the unobstructed portion of the aorta. This makes thrombus unlikely, because associated spontaneous contrast echoes caused by a low flow state usually are present. Also, no dissection flap is identified. The arrows in **A** through **C** and **E** through **H** show a large echogenic mass outside the aorta, consistent with hematoma. **G,H.** A hematoma is seen extending on both sides of the descending aorta (DA, AO), even where the tumor mass is not present. At surgery the mass was found to be a leiomyosarcoma that involved the aortic wall, resulting in perforation that caused the hematoma.

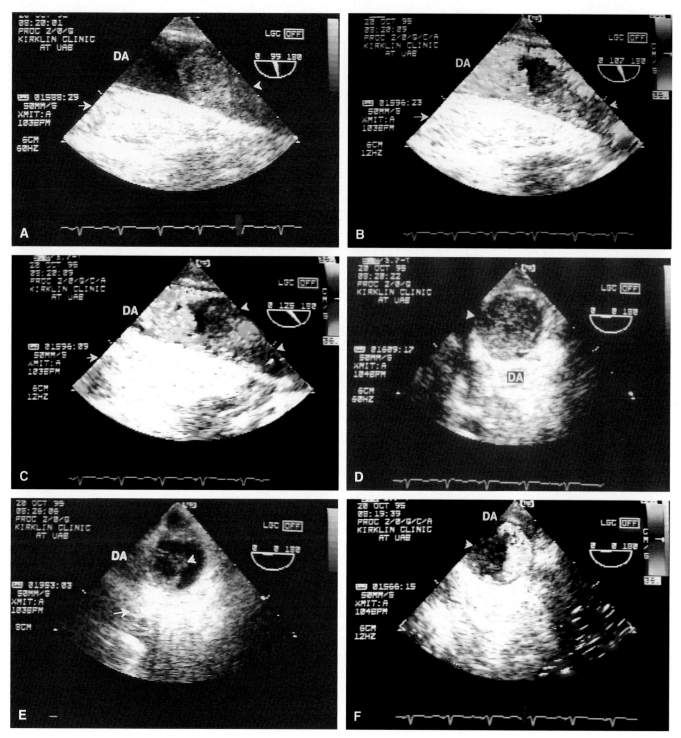

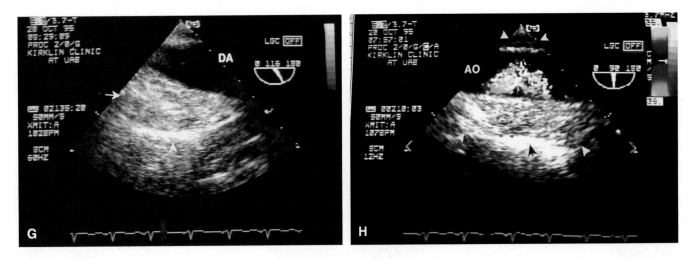

Figure 9.17.   **Primary leiomyoma of the inferior vena cava**. **A,B.** The subcostal transverse planes show the large tumor mass (T) clearly attached (S) in the IVC. **B,C.** The portion of the tumor protruding into the RA is highly echogenic, indicative of calcific involvement, whereas the IVC portion has very few highly refractile echo densities, suggesting paucity of calcific deposits. **D.** Longitudinal plane examination also demonstrates the tumor (T) protruding into the RA. *L*, liver. (Reproduced with permission from Loungani RR, Nanda NC, Sanyal RS, et al. Transesophageal echocardiographic findings in primary leiomyoma of inferior vena cava. Echocardiography 1993;10:623–627.)

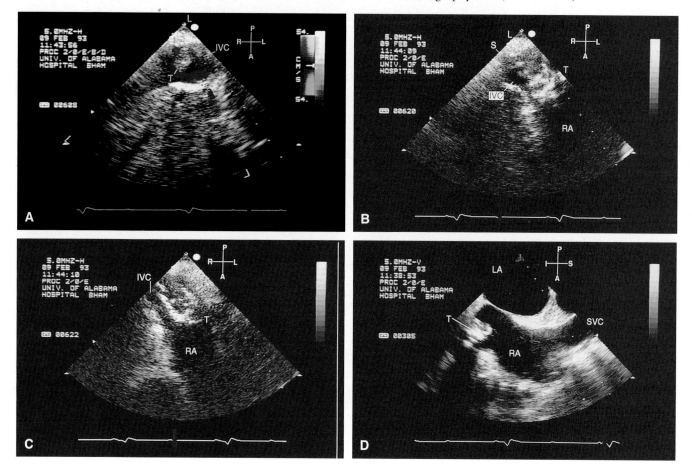

Figure 9.18. **Primary leiomyoma of the inferior vena cava.** Surgically resected tumor from the patient shown in Figure 9.17. (Reproduced with permission from Loungani RR, Nanda NC, Sanyal RS, et al. Transesophageal echocardiographic findings in primary leiomyoma of inferior vena cava. Echocardiography 1993;10:623–627.)

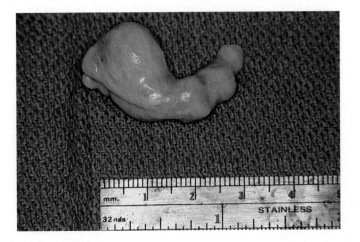

Figure 9.19.   **Right atrial myxoma. A,B.** A large mass (M) is seen attached by a short stalk (arrow in **B**) to the RA free wall. At surgery it was found to be a myxoma. **C, D,** and **E.** Two other patients with huge myxomas (arrowheads) in the RA. The echolucencies within the tumor represent hemorrhagic areas.

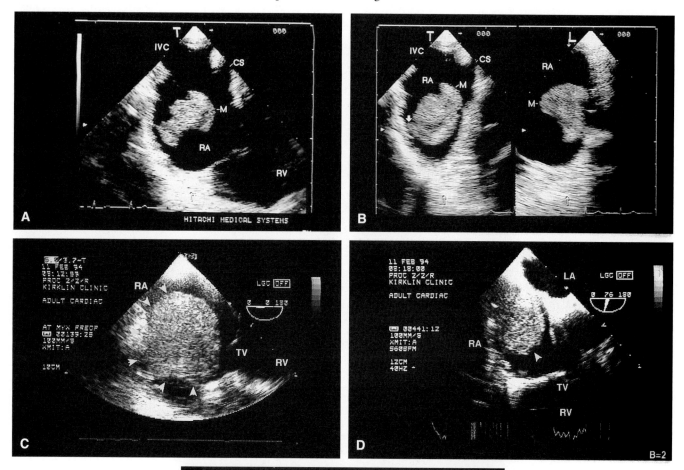

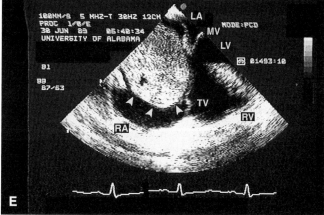

Figure 9.20. **Right atrial myxoma. A.** Another patient with a mass (M) in the RA is shown. **B.** The mass is attached by a broad stalk to the RA free wall near the entrance of the IVC. At surgery it was identified as a myxoma and was successfully removed.

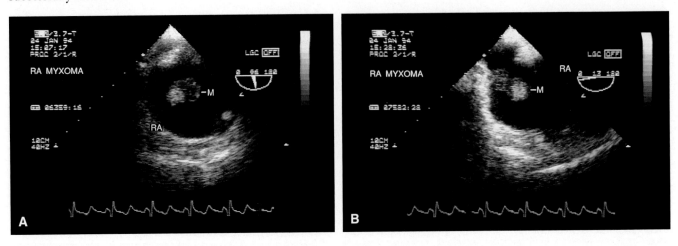

Figure 9.21. **A–E. Right atrial thrombus. A.** Multiple masses consistent with thrombus (TH) are seen in the RA. **B–D.** Further examination shows them to be components of a single thrombus. The elongated shape of the thrombus suggests a possible origin in the leg veins. **D.** Bulging of the atrial septum into the LA (arrowheads) indicates elevated RA pressure. **E.** A portion of the thrombus is seen in the left atrium, presumably having crossed over through a patent foramen ovale. **F–L.** Impending paradoxic embolus: right atrial thrombus wedged in the foramen ovale and extending into the left atrium. The multiple echo densities seen in the RA in **F** are parts of the large elongated thrombus (TH) seen in **G** (left panel). The right panel in **G** shows attachment of a portion of the thrombus to the eustachian valve (EV). **H,I.** The thrombus crosses into the LA (arrow in **H**). **J–L.** Gross specimens of the surgically resected thrombus. *AS*, atrial septum. (Courtesy of Drs. Vasu Goli [Birmingham, AL] and T. Narain Srivastava [Jackson, MS].)

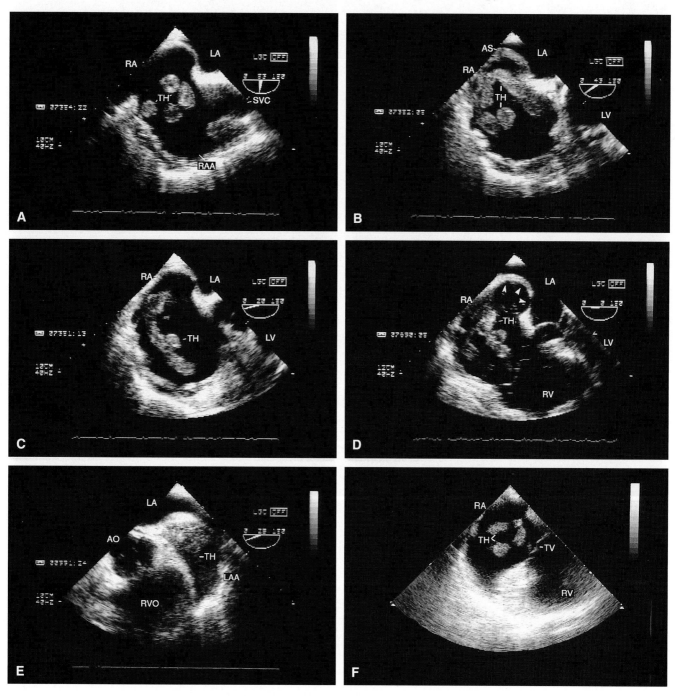

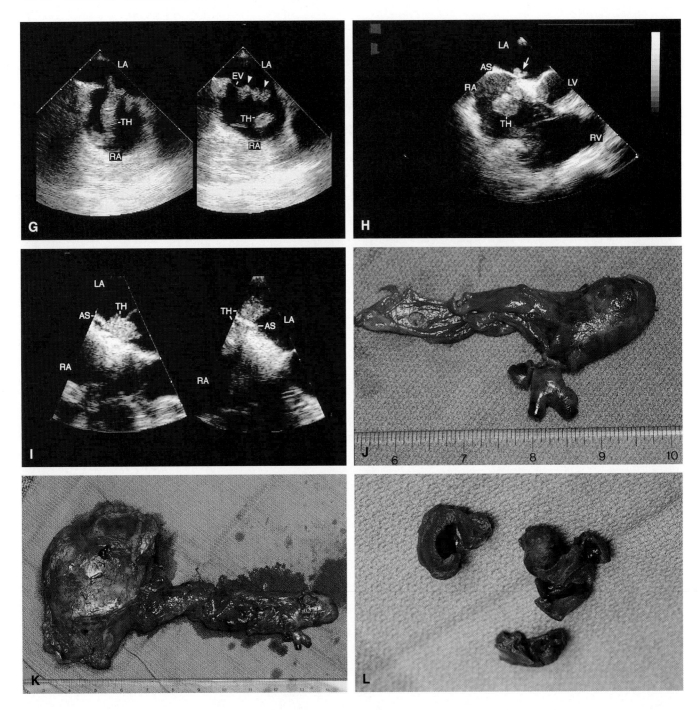

Figure 9.22.   **Right atrial thrombus.** An elongated thrombus (M) is seen in the RA. *EV*, Eustachian valve.

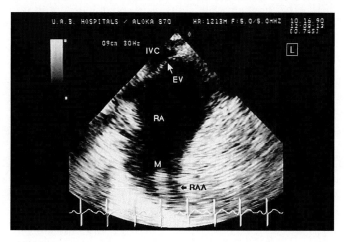

Figure 9.23. **Lipomatous hypertrophy of the atrial septum. A–C.** The arrows in **A** and **C** point to thickening of the atrial septum (AS) that spares the foramen ovale. This is caused by fatty infiltration of the septum and usually has no clinical sequelae. *EV,* eustachian valve. **D,E.** Massive lipomatous hypertrophy (arrowheads) affects the entire atrial septum and occupies most of the RA in another patient. **F.** A third patient with extensive lipomatous involvement of the atrial septum. (**D** and **E** courtesy of Dr. Allan Schwadron, Dothan, AL.)

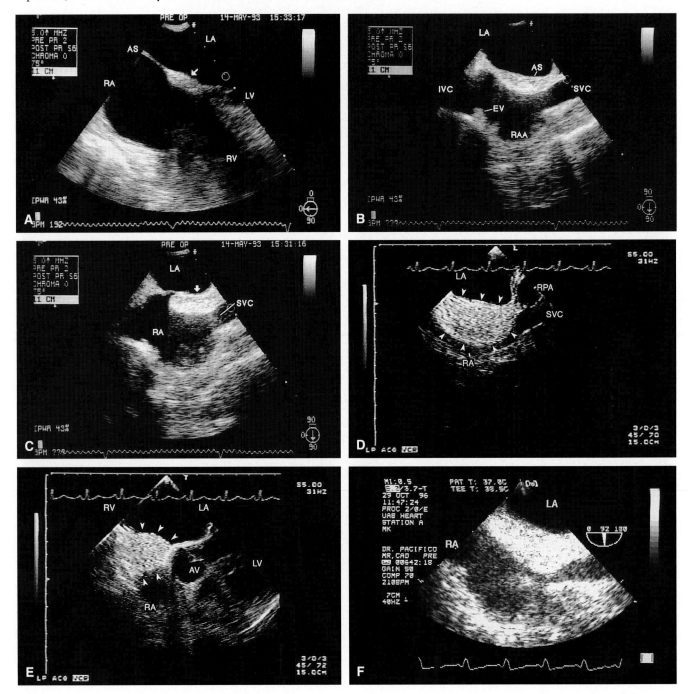

Figure 9.24. Papillary fibroelastoma of the tricuspid valve. **A,B.** Transverse plane four-chamber view shows the tumor (T, M) in the RA in the vicinity of the septal (SL) tricuspid leaflet, but the exact site of attachment of the tumor is not clear. **C,D.** Longitudinal plane (LP) examination clearly shows the tumor (T, M) arising from the posterior leaflet (PL). These findings were confirmed at surgery. *AL*, anterior tricuspid leaflet; *S*, tumor stalk. (Reproduced with permission from Maxted W, Nanda NC, Kim KS, et al. Transesophageal echocardiographic identification and validation of individual tricuspid valve leaflets. Echocardiography 1994;11:585–590.)

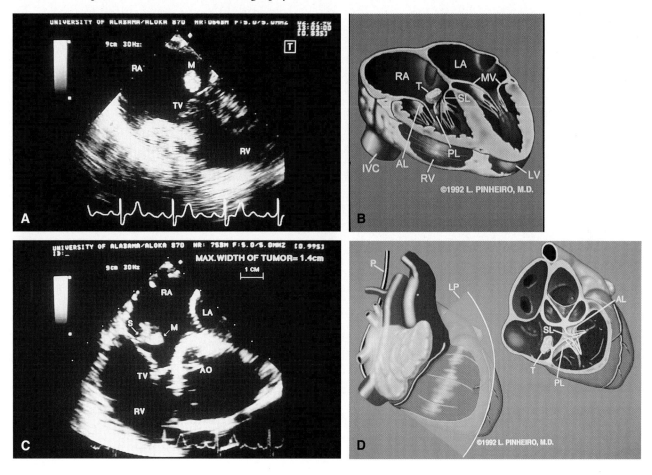

Figure 9.25. **Myxoma of the tricuspid valve. A, B.** A large mass (M) is seen attached to the anterior leaflet of the TV by a short stalk. Rounded areas of echolucency in the mass suggest hemorrhagic areas within the tumor, characteristic of a myxoma. These findings were confirmed at surgery, and the tumor was successfully removed.

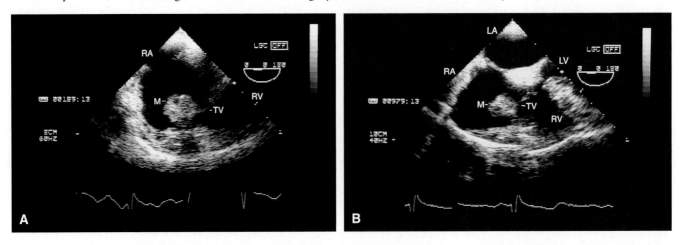

Figure 9.26. Metastatic melanoma involving the right ventricle. **A–G.** A huge tumor mass (M,T) is noted in the RV reaching up to the PV. The arrows in **B** and **F** show narrowing of the systolic flow signals in the RVO produced by obstruction caused by the tumor. **G.** Color Doppler–guided pulsed Doppler demonstrates a high velocity of 2.02 m/sec in the RVOT. **H. Right ventricular thrombus.** A thrombus (arrowheads) in the RV imaged from the transgastric approach, in another patient.

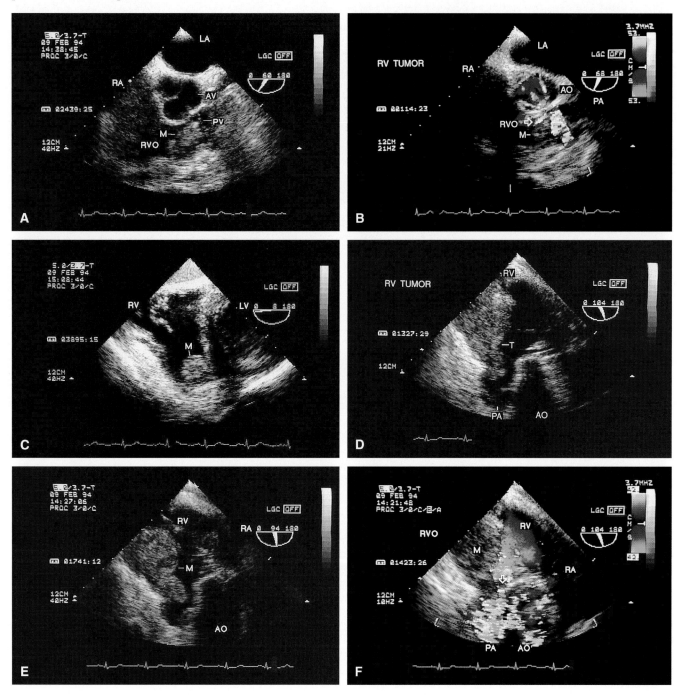

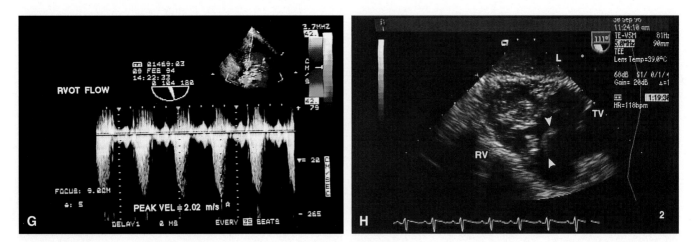

Figure 9.27. **Thrombus in the pulmonary artery. A–C.** Large thrombi (M, C) are noted in the SVC and the right pulmonary artery (RPA) in this patient with an infusion catheter, which acted as the nidus for the thrombus. **D,E.** A large thrombus (arrowheads in **D**, arrow in **E**) is seen in the right pulmonary artery (RPA) in another patient.

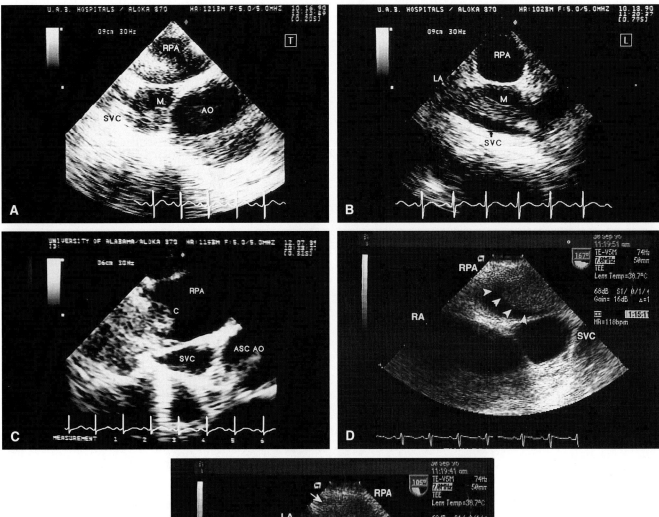

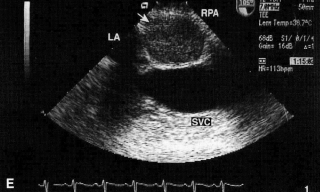

Figure 9.28. **A-G. Extracardiac tumor. A–C.** A tumor (T) is seen posterior to the aortic root bulging into the LA. **D.** Narrowing (arrows) of the left pulmonary vein (LPV) at its entrance into the LA. **E.** Unrestricted flow through unobstructed right lower (RLPV) and upper (RUPV) pulmonary veins. **F.** The tumor wedged between the esophagus and the right pulmonary artery (RPA). **G.** Narrowing (arrow) of the SVC flow jet at its entrance into the RA.

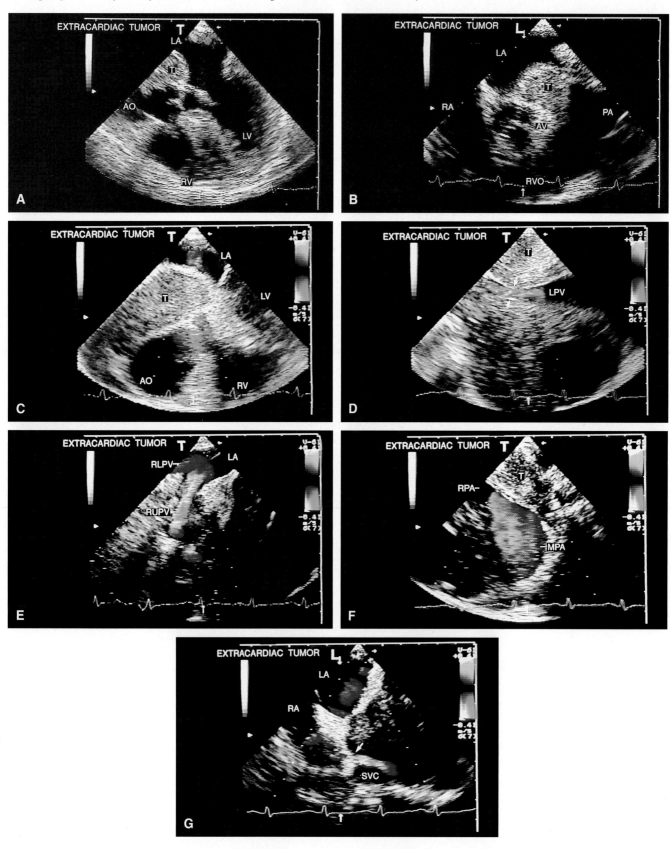

Figure 9.29. Mediastinal metastasis from ductal carcinoma of the breast. **A**. A large mediastinal mass (M) compresses the RUPV and produces aliased flow signals in a 39-year-old woman. **B**. High-pulse-repetition-frequency Doppler interrogation demonstrates a high peak velocity of 1.5 m/sec with little phasic variation. (Reproduced with permission from Samdarshi TE, Morrow WR, Helmcke FR, Nanda NC, Bargeron LM Jr, Pacifico AD. Assessment of pulmonary vein stenosis by transesophageal echocardiography. Am Heart J 1991;122:1495–1498.)

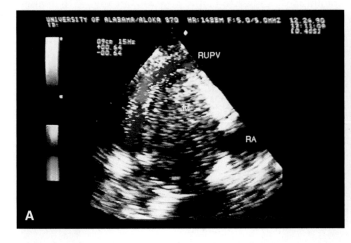
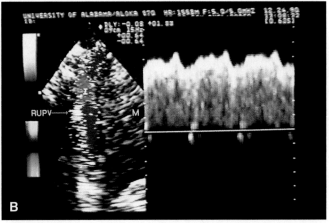

Figure 9.30. **Pulmonary vein obstruction following lung transplantation.** The arrows in **A, C,** and **D** show localized narrowing of the right upper (RUPV) and lower (RLPV) pulmonary veins following right lung transplantation. In **C** the narrowing is better seen with than without color Doppler. **B.** Pulsed Doppler examination shows a high velocity of 1.82 m/sec, with spectral broadening consistent with some obstruction to flow. **E.** Doppler examination of the nonobstructed LUPV shows lower velocities and less spectral broadening. Mild obstruction of the right pulmonary veins in this patient resulted in increased flow through the normal left-sided pulmonary veins, producing flow velocity higher than normal and spectral broadening. This patient did not require surgical intervention and was managed conservatively.

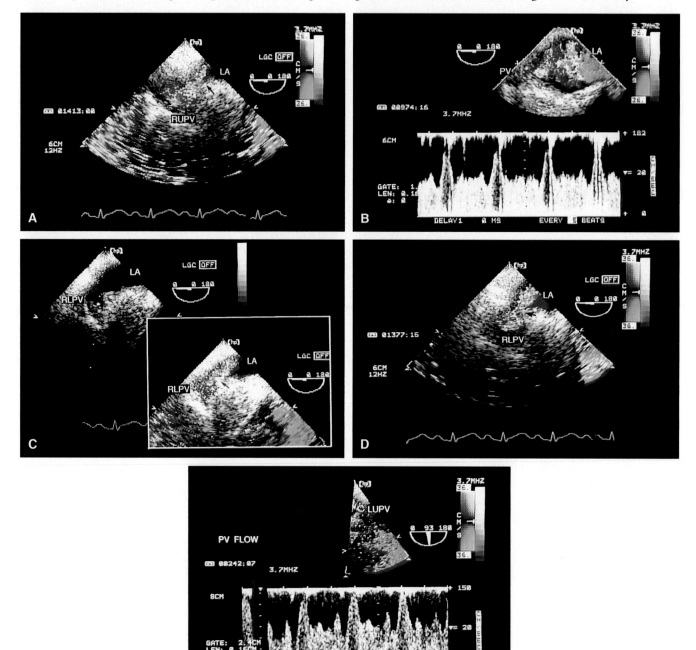

Figure 9.31. **Sclerosing mediastinitis**. This 43-year-old man presented with respiratory failure. **A.** Contrast-enhanced chest CT scan at the level of the right upper lobe bronchus. There are bilateral pleural effusions. Abnormal soft tissue is noted between the right upper lobe bronchus, left main stem bronchus, and ascending aorta (AO), as well as the superior vena cava (C). This abnormal tissue also separates the ascending aorta from the superior vena cava. There is dense opacification of the azygous vein (AZ), indicating superior vena caval obstruction and collateral flow. *PA*, main pulmonary artery. **B.** Contrast-enhanced chest CT scan at the level of the aortic root. Abnormal soft tissue (m) is noted all around the LA. This tissue extends around the interatrial septum on the right and involves the venoatrial junctions of the right and left lower lobe pulmonary veins (arrow). Note the opacification of enlarged azygous (A) and hemiazygous (H) veins resulting from collateral flow. (Reproduced with permission from Kovach TA, Nanda NC, Kim KS, et al. Transesophageal echocardiographic findings in sclerosing mediastinitis. Echocardiography 1996;13:103–108.)

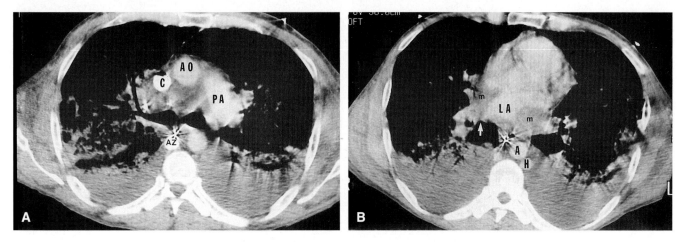

Figure 9.32. **Sclerosing mediastinitis**. Same patient as in Figure 9.31. **A.** A mass (M) surrounds the LA, right pulmonary artery (RPA), and SVC. **B,C.** The mass appears to infiltrate and invaginate into the LA and extends up to the base of the LAA. This resembles an intracardiac tumor. (Reproduced with permission from Kovach TA, Nanda NC, Kim KS, et al. Transesophageal echocardiographic findings in sclerosing mediastinitis. Echocardiography 1996;13:103–108.)

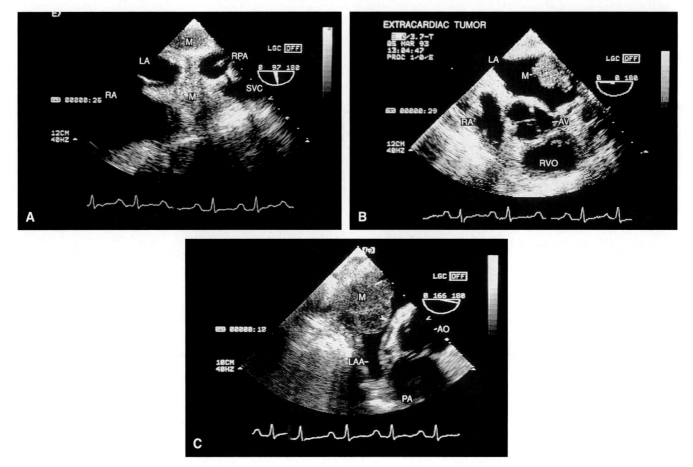

Figure 9.33. Sclerosing mediastinitis. Same patient as in Figures 9.31 and 9.32. **A,B.** Both the right lower (RLPV) and upper (RUPV) pulmonary veins demonstrate obstruction near their entrance into the LA. The exact sites of obstruction in the lower and upper pulmonary veins, shown by the arrow and the arrowhead, respectively, mark the transition from laminar (red) to disturbed (mosaic) flow. **C.** Pulsed Doppler interrogation of the mosaic flow reveals a high velocity of 2.58 m/sec, indicative of obstruction. (Reproduced with permission from Kovach TA, Nanda NC, Kim KS, et al. Transesophageal echocardiographic findings in sclerosing mediastinitis. Echocardiography 1996;13:103–108.)

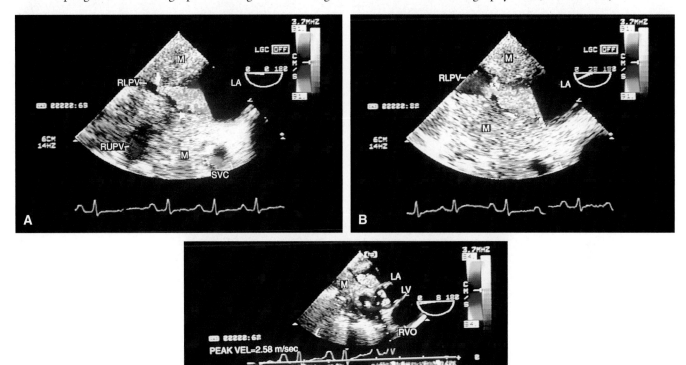

Figure 9.34. **Sclerosing mediastinitis**. Same patient as in Figures 9.31 through 9.33. **A,B.** The arrow points to the site of obstruction in the SVC near its junction with the RA. Color Doppler examination shows a thin mosaic flow jet in **B**, indicative of obstruction. **C.** Pulsed Doppler interrogation reveals a high velocity of at least 1.61 m/sec. (Reproduced with permission from Kovach TA, Nanda NC, Kim KS, et al. Transesophageal echocardiographic findings in sclerosing mediastinitis. Echocardiography 1996;13:103–108.)

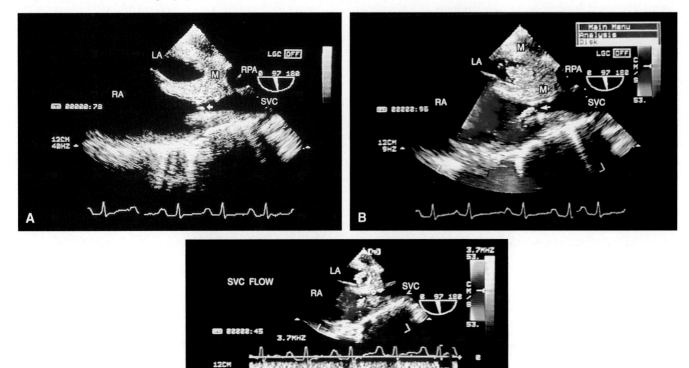

Figure 9.35.   **Sclerosing mediastinitis**. Histology of mediastinal biopsy tissue from the same patient shown in Figures 9.31 through 9.34. **A.** Photomicrograph of sclerosing process impinging on mediastinal adipose tissue (Congo red, original magnification ×125). **B.** Photomicrograph of collagenization of blood vessel wall with narrowing of the lumen (center), a region of cellular fibrosis (above), and a region of acellular fibrosis (below) (hematoxylin and eosin, original magnification 125). (Reproduced with permission from Kovach TA, Nanda NC, Kim KS, et al. Transesophageal echocardiographic findings in sclerosing mediastinitis. Echocardiography 1996;13:103–108.)

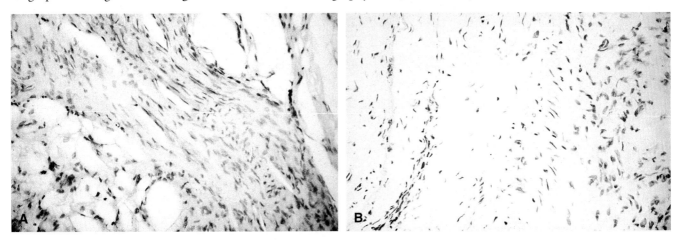

Figure 9.36. **Hematoma following surgery.** A large hematoma (H) is noted in the interatrial septum between the RA and LA in **A** and between the SVC (arrowheads) and the LA in **B** and **C**. This developed immediately following AV replacement but did not cause any hemodynamic compromise. The patient had an uneventful course.

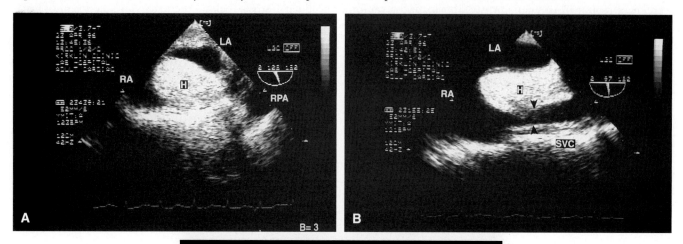

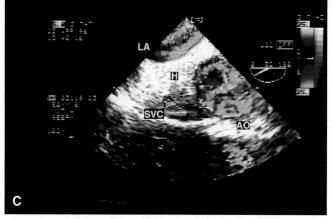

Figure 9.37. **Hematoma following cardiac surgery.** Two different patients with hematoma (H in **A**, arrowheads in **B**) that developed around the aortic root following aortic valve replacement are shown. Both had a benign course.

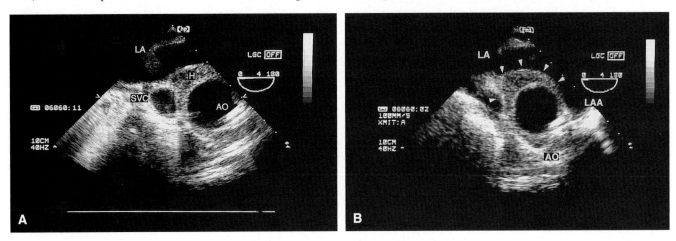

Figure 9.38. **Hematoma compressing the RA.** A huge hematoma (H) compressing the RA and producing tricuspid inflow obstruction (arrowheads in **A,B**). This developed after replacement with a porcine aortic valve that appeared to be functioning normally. Because of hemodynamic deterioration and severe hypotension, the hematoma was surgically evacuated.

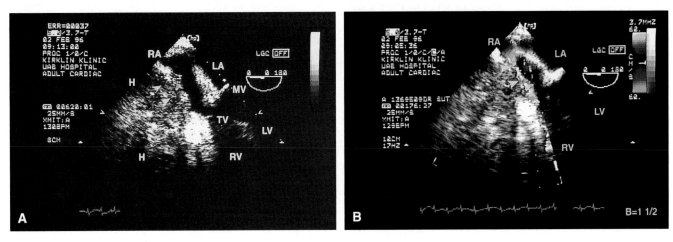

SUGGESTED READING

Artel B, Colvin SB, Kronzon I. Rapid growth rate of an apical left ventricular myxoma. Am Heart J 1996;131:820–822.

Chow WH, Chow TC, Cheung H, et al. Mediastinal liposarcoma causing left ventricular inflow tract obstruction. Echocardiography 1993;10:141–143.

de Virgilio C, Dubrow TJ, Robertson JM, et al. Detection of multiplane cardiac papillary fibroelastomas using transesophageal echocardiography. Ann Thorac Surg 1989;48:119–121.

Faletra F, Ravini M, Moreo A, et al. Transesophageal echocardiography in the evaluation of mediastinal masses. J Am Soc Echocardiogr 1992;5:178–186.

Gandhi AK, Pearson AC, Orsinelli DA. Tumor invasion of the pulmonary veins: a unique source of systemic embolism detected by transesophageal echocardiography. J Am Soc Echocardiogr 1995;8:97–99.

Hicks KA, Kovach JA, Frishberg DP, et al. Echocardiographic evaluation of papillary fibroelastoma: a case report and review of the literature. J Am Soc Echocardiogr 1996;9:353–360.

Hsu TL, Hsiung MC, Ling SL, et al. The value of transesophageal echocardiography in the diagnosis of cardiac metastasis. Echocardiography 1992;9:1–7.

Joffe II, Jacobs LE, Owen AN, et al. Noninfective valvular masses: review of the literature with emphasis on imaging techniques and management. Am Heart J 1996;131:1175–1183.

Kindman LA, Wright A, Tye T, et al. Lipomatous hypertrophy of the interatrial septum: characterization by transesophageal and transthoracic echocardiography, magnetic resonance imaging, and computed tomography. J Am Soc Echocardiogr 1988;1:450–454.

Kovach TA, Nanda NC, Kim KS, et al. Transesophageal echocardiographic findings in sclerosing mediastinitis. Echocardiography 1996;13:103–108.

Kuecherer HF, Lee E, Schiller NB. Enhanced detection of intracardiac masses by transesophageal echocardiography. Am J Cardiac Imaging 1990;4:180–186.

Leibowitz G, Keller NM, Daniel WG, et al. Transesophageal versus transthoracic echocardiography in the evaluation of right atrial tumors. Am Heart J 1994;139:1224–1227.

Loungani RR, Nanda NC, Sanyal RS, et al. Transesophageal echocardiographic findings in primary leiomyoma of inferior vena cava. Echocardiography 1993;10:623–627.

Maxted W, Nanda NC, Kim KS, et al. Transesophageal echocardiographic identification and validation of individual tricuspid valve leaflets. Echocardiography 1994;11:585–590.

Mehta R, Nanda NC, Osman K, et al. Left ventricular lipoma by transesophageal and in vitro echocardiographic studies. Echocardiography 1995;12:283–288.

Micali ID, Jacobs LE, Ioli A, et al. Mediastinal tumor presenting as expanding aortic aneurysm diagnosed by transesophageal echocardiography. Echocardiography 1996;13:627–629.

Milano A, Dan M, Bortolotti U. Left atrial myxoma: excision guided by transesophageal cross-sectional echocardiography. Int J Cardiol 1990;27:125–127.

Mugge A, Daniel WG, Haverich A, Lichtlen PR. Diagnosis of noninfective cardiac mass lesions by two-dimensional echocardiography: comparison of the transthoracic and transesophageal approaches. Circulation 1991;83:70–78.

Nanda NC, Mahan EF III. Transesophageal echocardiography. AHA Council on Clinical Cardiology Newsletter 1990;Summer:3–22.

Nanda NC, Pinheiro L, Sanyal RS, Storey O. Transesophageal biplane echocardiographic imaging: technique, planes, and clinical usefulness. Echocardiography 1990;7:771–788.

Obeid AI, Marvasti M, Parker F, Rosenberg J. Comparison of transthoracic and transesophageal echocardiography in diagnosis of left atrial myxoma. Am J Cardiol 1989;63:1006–1008.

Rankin JM, Hartland GD, Ireland MA. Right atrial thrombus mimicking myxoma in a heart transplant recipient. Am Heart J 1996;132:452–454.

Reeder GS, Khandheria BK, Seward JB, Tajik AJ. Transesophageal echocardiography and cardiac masses. Mayo Clin Proc 1991;66:1101–1109.

Samdarshi TE, Mahan III EF, Nanda NC, et al. Transesophageal echocardiographic diagnosis of multicentric left ventricular myxomas mimicking a left atrial tumor. J Thorac Cardiovasc Surg 1992;103:471–474.

Samdarshi TE, Morrow WR, Helmcke FR, Nanda NC, Bargeron LM Jr, Pacifico AD. Assessment of pulmonary vein stenosis by transesophageal echocardiography. Am Heart J 1991;122:1495–1498.

Schecter SO, Fyfe B, Pou R, Goldman ME. Intramural left atrial hematoma complicating mitral annular calcification. Am Heart J 1996;132:455–457.

Tardof KC, Taylor K, Pandian NG, Schwartz S, Rastegar H. Right ventricular outflow tract and pulmonary artery obstruction by postoperative mediastinal hematoma: delineation by multiplane transesophageal echocardiography. J Am Soc Echocardiogr 1994;7:400–404.

Tighe DA, Rousou JA, Kenia S, et al. Transesophageal echocardiography in the management of mitral valve myxoma. Am Heart J 1995;130:627–629.

Vargas-Barron J, Romero-Cardenas A, Villegas M, et al. Transthoracic and transesophageal echocardiographic diagnosis of myxomas in the four cardiac cavities. Am Heart J 1991;121:931–933.

Vilacosta I, Zamorano J, Ramos JM, et al. Infected myxomas: report of a case and review of the literature. Echocardiography 1994;11:29–33.

Willens HJ, Chaddo S, Levy R, et al. Redundant mitral valve simulating an intracardiac mass on transesophageal echocardiography. Echocardiography 1994;11:227–230.

Yang SS, Wagner P, Dennis C. Images in cardiovascular medicine. Hiatal hernia masquerading as left atrial mass. Circulation 1996;93:836.

Miscellaneous Lesions

10

This section discusses a number of miscellaneous lesions, including pericardial effusion, pericardial cyst, pleural effusion, right heart catheters and associated thrombus, pacemaker wires, pacemaker vegetations, artifacts and contrast effects during cardiac surgery, and intra-aortic balloon pumps.

Figure 10.1. **Pericardial effusion**. **A–C.** Transgastric views demonstrate pericardial effusion (PE) behind the right ventricle. The pericardium (P) is mildly thickened. *AL*, anterior papillary muscle; *PM*, posterior papillary muscle. **D.** Pericardial effusion (PE) around the LAA.

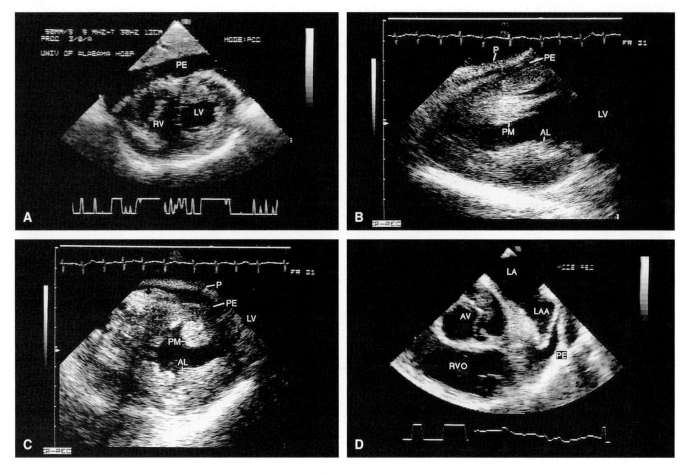

Figure 10.2. **Pericardial cyst. A–C.** A large pericardial cyst (PC) located anteriorly with compression of the RV **(C). D.** Intraoperative examination in another patient shows a large pericardial cyst (C) located lateral to the LA and RA. This frame was taken after cardioplegic arrest of the heart, when the cardiac chambers were empty and collapsed. **E–I.** An 18-year-old man had a pericardial hydatid cyst (C) compressing the LV lateral wall (arrowheads in **G**). The linear echoes in the cyst represent the laminated hydatid membrane. Prominent intramyocardial coronary arteries (arrowheads in **H**) with high velocity flow were imaged within the compressed LV lateral wall, consistent with coronary flow obstruction. This was confirmed by coronary angiogram, which showed systolic emptying of the first marginal branch of the circumflex coronary artery. The cyst was surgically resected. **I.** Microscopic examination of the hydatid cyst fluid shows typical scolices, one of which contains hooklets.

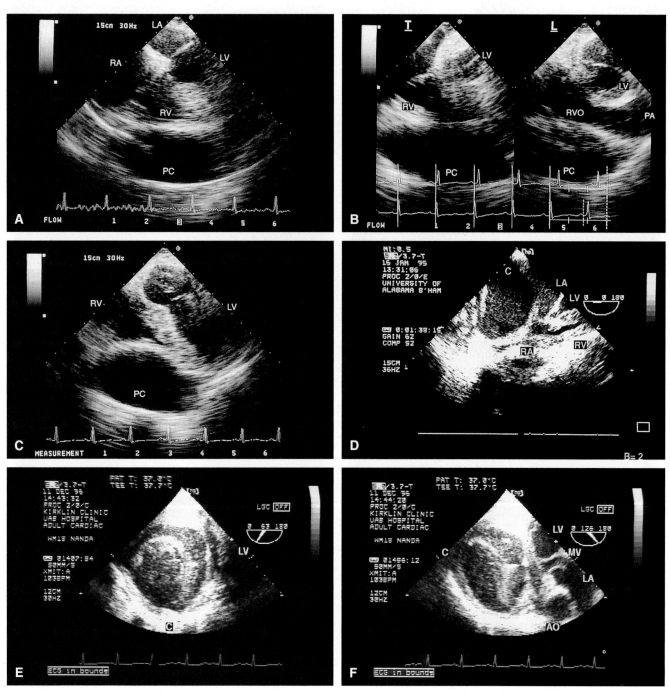

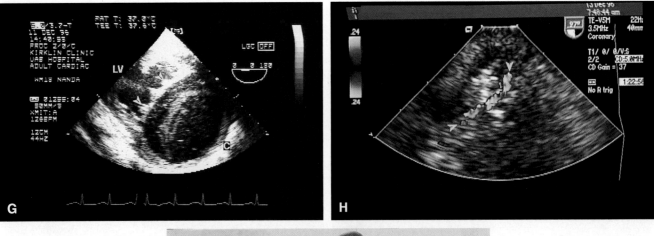

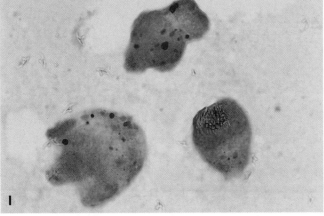

Figure 10.3. Pleural effusion. **A.** A large left pleural effusion (PLE) with a villus (VI) is present behind the descending thoracic aorta (DA). **B,C.** Large left pleural effusions (PLE) in two other patients are imaged behind the aorta (AO) in short-axis **(B)** and long-axis **(C)** views. **D.** A right pleural effusion (RPE) in another patient.

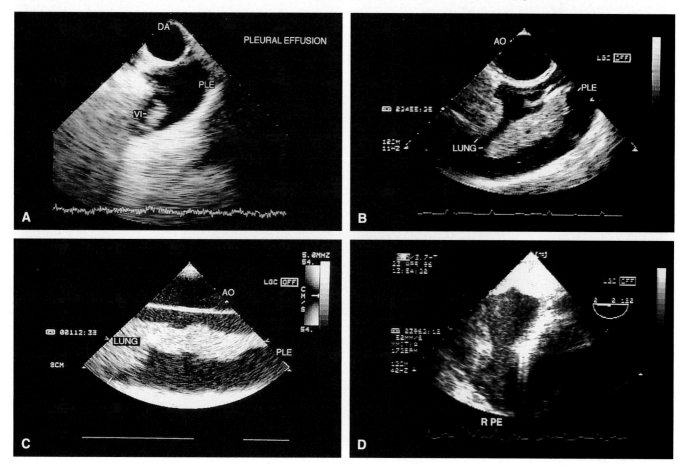

Figure 10.4. **Right heart catheter.** C in **A** and arrowheads in **B** and **C** indicate a long segment of a Swan-Ganz catheter in the right heart.

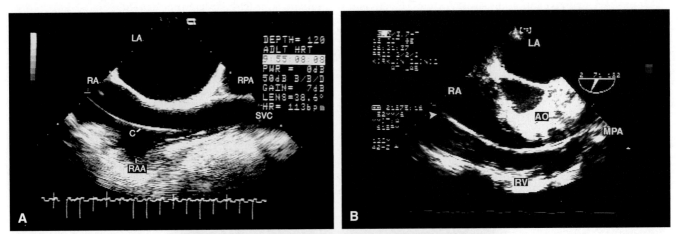

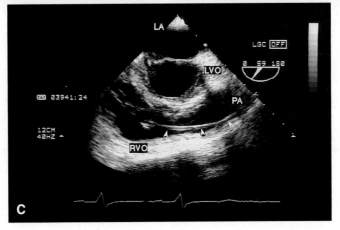

Figure 10.5.   **Right heart catheter thrombus. A–C.** A large mass (M) is noted in the RA. **D.** Further examination demonstrated a catheter (arrow) embedded in the mass, leading to the diagnosis of catheter-induced thrombus.

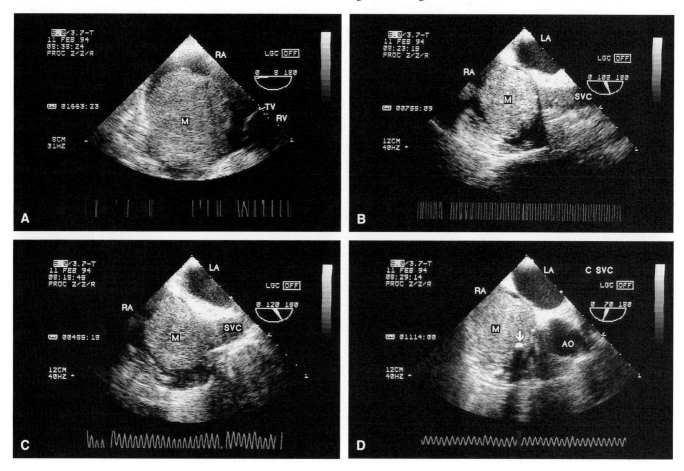

Figure 10.6. **Denver peritoneovenous shunt thrombus.** A 41-year-old man with Laennec's cirrhosis and a Denver peritoneovenous shunt presented with recurrent episodes of syncope whenever he sat up or stood. The Denver shunt and the massive thrombus were successfully removed surgically. **A.** Longitudinal plane examination demonstrates a large right atrial mass (maximum size, 5.5 × 4.5 cm) attached to the anterior wall of the superior vena cava (SVC) near its entrance into the right atrium (RA). The arrow points to a portion of the Denver shunt that is seen embedded in the mass. The inferior vena cava was not involved. **B.** Transverse plane examination also visualized the mass well and demonstrated a portion of it protruding into the right ventricle through the tricuspid orifice. The relationship of the mass to the superior vena cava could not be visualized in this plane, however. There were prominent echo-free spaces in the tumor mass. (Reproduced with permission from Holman WL, Coghlan CH, Dodson MR, Ballal R, Nanda NC. Removal of massive right atrial thrombus guided by transesophageal echocardiography. Ann Thorac Surg 1991;52:313–315.)

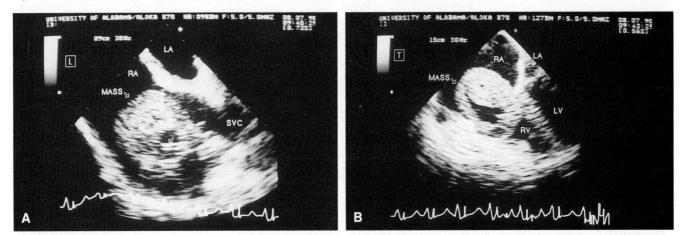

Figure 10.7. **Right heart catheter thrombus**. The bright echoes in the RA in **A** and **B** are caused by the infusion catheter (C). This is the typical appearance of a catheter, which appears thicker in **A** than its real size because of the presence of reverberations. Catheter-induced thrombus in the RA is well seen (M in **A–C** and arrow in **D**). The arrowhead in **C** shows an attachment of the thrombus to the RA wall near the eustachian valve. **E.** Gross specimen shows a catheter-induced thrombus in the RA.

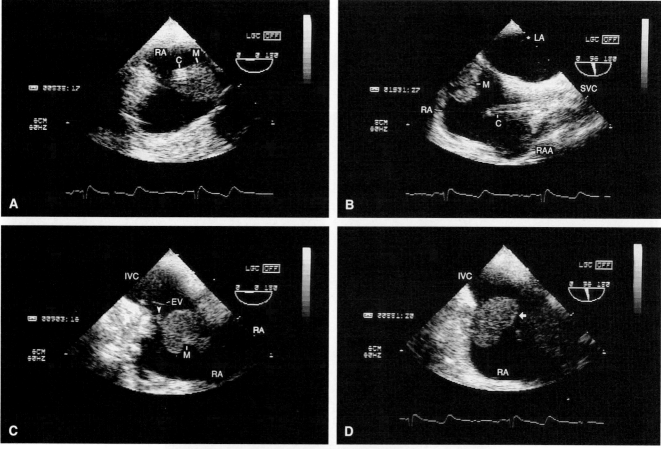

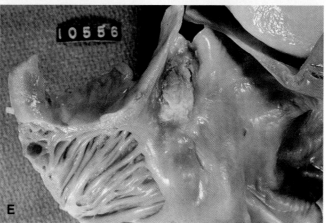

Figure 10.8. **Pacer lead in the right ventricle.** The pacer lead (P) is seen in the RA and RV in the four-chamber view **(A,B)**, but the location of its tip in the RV apex (arrowhead in **D**) is identified only using the transgastric approach **(D,E)**. The metal in the electrode tip produces prominent reverberations (black arrowheads in **E**) that assist in locating it. Other portions of the pacer also may produce reverberations (white arrowheads in **C**).

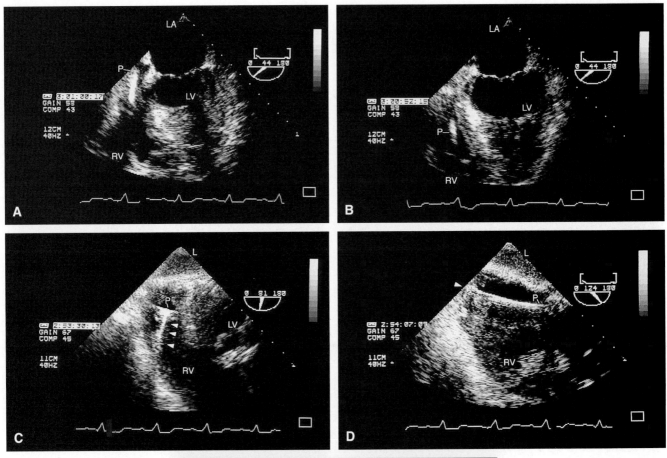

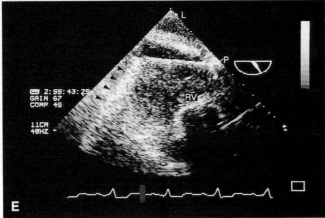

Figure 10.9. **Right heart pacer: endocarditis. A.** A large, mobile vegetation (arrow) on the right atrial portion of the pacing wire (C). **B.** Another patient with a vegetation (VEG) attached to a pacing wire in the RA. (**A** reproduced with permission from Nanda NC, Pinheiro L, Sanyal RS, Storey O. Transesophageal biplane echocardiographic imaging: Technique, planes, and clinical usefulness. Echocardiography 1990;7:771–783.)

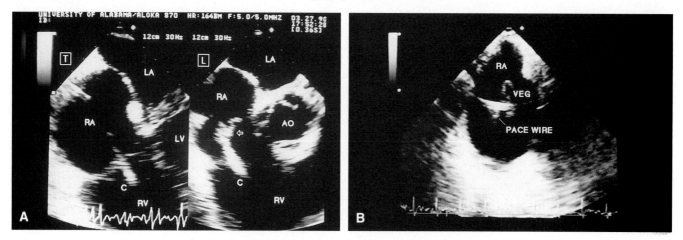

Figure 10.10. **Artifacts. A.** A large artifact (arrowheads) partially obscuring the LV. **B,C.** Multiple curved artifacts produced by electrocautery.

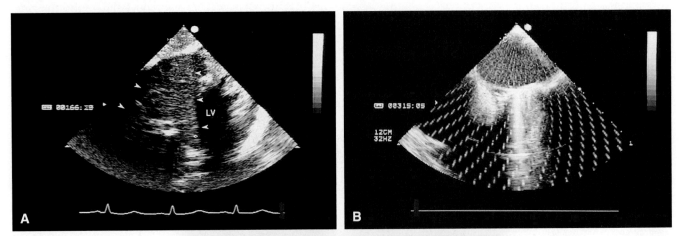

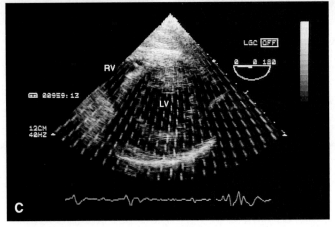

Figure 10.11. A–E. **Mirror image from a left atrial line mimicking a catheter in the LV.** *1*, true image of the left atrial line recorded in the LA. The arrowhead points to a reverberatory tail. *2*, artifactual image of the left atrial line visualized **(B,C)** in the left ventricle (LV). The arrowhead **(C)** points to a reverberatory tail. Note that this image is not recorded on the scan lines that include the true atrial line, but is placed more medially **(B–D)**, making it difficult to recognize it as an artifact. *3*, a second artifactual image of the left atrial line recorded in the aorta **(E)**. Unlike image 2, this image is recorded on the scan lines that include the true atrial line and therefore is easily recognized as a mirror-image artifact. (Reproduced with permission from Pothula AR, Nanda NC, Agarwal G, et al. Mirror image from a left atrial line mimicking a catheter in the left ventricle during transesophageal echocardiography. Echocardiography 1997;14:165–167.)

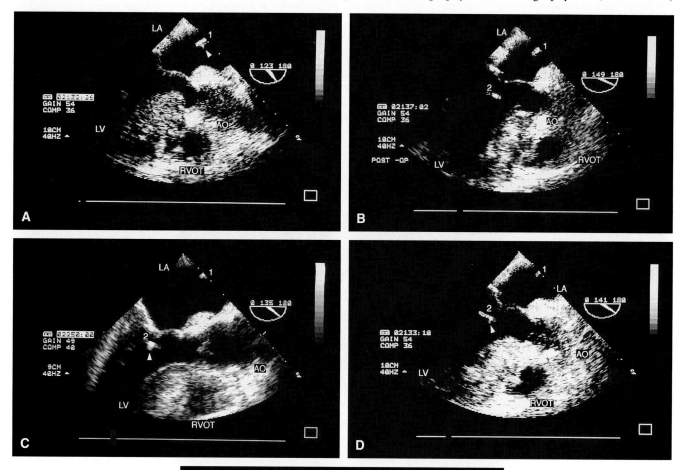

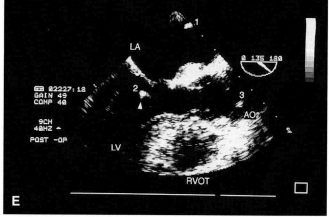

Figure 10.12. **Cardioplegia solution. A.** Contrast echoes are caused by the cardioplegia solution introduced during heart surgery. **B.** The cardioplegia solution (arrowheads) is seen crossing the aortic valve into the LVOT because of valve incompetence produced by cardiac standstill. **C.** The cardioplegia needle/catheter (arrowheads) imaged in the ascending aorta (A) in another patient.

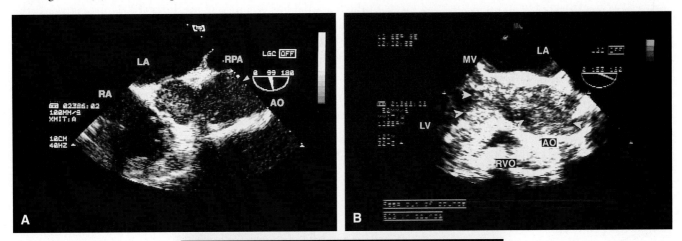

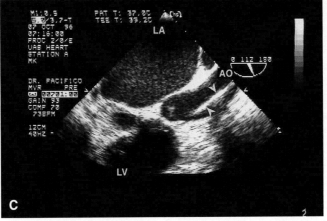

Figure 10.13. **A. Spontaneous contrast echoes in the left atrium.** Stasis of blood in the LA post-bypass causes spontaneous contrast echoes (SC). **B. Left ventricle venting.** Balloon-tipped catheter (arrowheads) in the LV used for de-airing in the immediate post-bypass period. This patient underwent prosthetic replacement (P) of a degenerated heterograft.

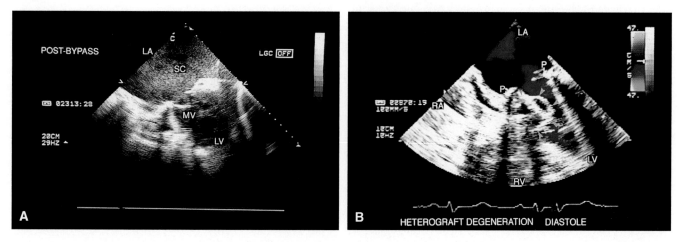

Figure 10.14. **A,B. Left heart air bubbles. A.** Contrast echoes (arrowheads) fill the left heart as a result of the presence of air, which enters when the left ventricle is opened during surgery. Intraoperative study is useful in helping the surgeon de-air the left heart to prevent air embolization. **B.** Another patient with air in the left heart imaged as the patient was coming off bypass following prosthetic (MP) replacement of the mitral valve. **C.** De-airing of the left ventricle. *F* is an image of the finger of a surgeon who is holding and "shaking" the heart to de-air it.

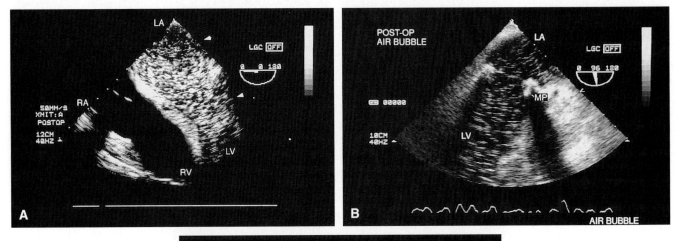

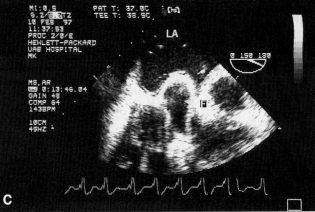

Figure 10.15. **Intra-aortic balloon pump**. An intra-aortic balloon pump (arrows) in the descending aorta imaged in the short-axis (top) and long-axis (bottom) views.

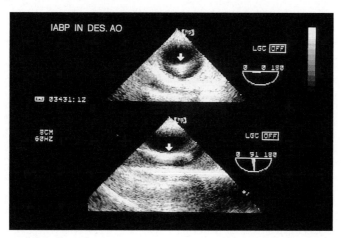

SUGGESTED READINGS

Asinger RW, Herzog CA, Dick CD, Michaud L. Echocardiography in the evaluation of cardiac sources of emboli: the role of transthoracic echocardiography. Echocardiography 1993;10:373–396.

Cohen GI, Klein AL, Chan KL, et al. Transesophageal echocardiographic diagnosis of right-sided cardiac masses in patients with central lines. Am J Cardiol 1992;70:925–929.

Dellsperger KC. Transthoracic echocardiography for evaluation of hypertensive heart disease. Echocardiography 1993;10:295–302.

Ducart A, Broka S, Collard E, et al. Regional increment in myocardial reflectivity after aortic valve replacement—early detection of air and assessment of treatment by transesophageal echocardiography. J Cardiothorac Vasc Anesth 1996;10:926–927.

Falcone RA, Morady F, Armstrong WF. Transesophageal echocardiographic evaluation of left atrial appendage function and spontaneous contrast formation after chemical and electrical cardioversion of atrial fibrillation. Am J Cardiol 1996;78:435–439.

Feinberg MS, Davila-Roman VG, Hopkins WE, et al. Successful withdrawal of biventricular assist devices after assessment of left ventricular function by transesophageal echocardiography and automatic border detection. Echocardiography 1994;11:575–578.

Fishel RS, Merlino JD, Felner JM. Diagnosis of main-stem pulmonary thromboemboli by transesophageal echocardiography. Echocardiography 1994;11:189–195.

Gomez CR, Tulyapronchote R. Neurologists perspective in the evaluation of ischemic stroke. Echocardiography 1994;10:367–372.

Gutterman DD, Ayres RW. Use of echocardiography in detecting cardiac sources of embolus. Echocardiography 1993;10:311–320.

Holman WL, Bourge RC, Fan P. Influence of left ventricular assist on valvular regurgitation. Circulation 1993;88:309–318.

Holman WL, Coghlan CH, Dodson MR, Ballal R, Nanda NC. Removal of massive right atrial thrombus guided by transesophageal echocardiography. Ann Thorac Surg 1991;52:313–315.

Hutchison SJ, Smalling RG, Albornoz M, et al. Comparison of transthoracic and transesophageal echocardiography in clinically overt or suspected pericardial heart disease. Am J Cardiol 1994;74:962–965.

Kamp O, De Cock C, Visser CA. High quality stress echocardiography using simultaneous transesophageal echocardiographic imaging and atrial pacing. Echocardiography 1995;12:43–48.

Katz WE, Jafar MZ, Mankad S, et al. Transesophageal echocardiographic identification of a malpositioned extracorporeal membrane oxygenation cannula. J Heart Lung Transplant 1995;14:790–792.

Kay GN, Holman WL, Nanda NC. Combined use of TEE and endocardial mapping to localize the site of origin of ectopic atrial tachycardia. Am J Cardiol 1990;65:1284–1286,

Klein AL, Cohen GI, Pietrolungo JF, et al. Differentiation of constrictive pericarditis from restrictive cardiomyopathy by Doppler transesophageal echocardiographic measurements of respiratory variations in pulmonary venous flow. J Am Coll Cardiol 1993;22:1935–1943.

Klein AL, Stewart WC, Cosgrove DM III, et al. Visualization of acute pulmonary emboli by transesophageal echocardiography. J Am Soc Echocardiogr 1990;3:412–415.

Kochar GS, Jacobs LE, Kotler MN. Right atrial compression in postoperative cardiac patients: detection by transesophageal echocardiography. J Am Coll Cardiol 1990;16:511–516.

Kronzon I, Tunick PA, Freedberg RS, et al. Transesophageal echocardiography in pericardial disease and tamponade. Echocardiography 1994;11:493–505.

Labovitz AJ. The increasing role of transesophageal echocardiography in unexplained cerebral ischemia. Echocardiography 1993;10:363–365.

Maxted W, Finch A, Nanda NC, et al. Multiplane transesophageal echocardiographic detection of sinus venosus atrial septal defect. Echocardiography 1995;12:139–143.

Nanda NC, Pinheiro L, Sanyal RS, Storey O. Transesophageal biplane echocardiographic imaging: technique, planes, and clinical usefulness. Echocardiography 1990;7:771–783.

Nellessen U, Daniel WG, Matheis G, et al. Impending paradoxical embolism from atrial thrombus: correct diagnosis by transesophageal echocardiography and prevention by surgery. J Am Coll Cardiol 1985;5:1002–1004.

Neskovic AN, Popovic AD, Babic R, et al. Color Doppler transesophageal echocardiography in detection of massive pulmonary embolism. Echocardiography 1996;13:631–633.

Nixdorff U, Erbel R, Drexler M, Meyer J. Detection of thromboembolus of the right pulmonary artery by transesophageal two-dimensional echocardiography. Am J Cardiol 1988;61:488–489.

Oh JK, Seward WC, Khandheria BK, et al. Transesophageal echocardiography in critically ill patients. Am J Cardiol 1990;66:1492–1495.

Oka Y, Inoue T, Hong Y, et al. Retained intracardiac air: transesophageal echocardiography for definition of incidence and monitoring removal by improved techniques. J Thorac Cardiovasc Surg 1986;91:329–337.

Omoto R, Kyo S, Matsumura M, et al. Variomatrix—a newly developed transesophageal echocardiography probe with a rotating matrix biplane transducer. Echocardiography 1993;10:79–84.

Pearson AC, Labovitz AJ, Tatineni S, Gomez CR. Superiority of transesophageal echocardiography in detecting cardiac source of embolism in patients with cerebral ischemia of uncertain etiology. J Am Coll Cardiol 1991;17:66–72.

Pop G, Sutherland GR, Koudstaal PJ, et al. Transesophageal echocardiography in the detection of intracardiac embolic sources in patients with transient ischemic attacks. Stroke 1990;21:560–565.

Pothula AR, Nanda NC, Agarwal G, et al. Mirror image from a left atrial line mimicking a catheter in the left ventricle during transesophageal echocardiography. Echocardiography 1997;14:165–167.

Rosenzweig BP, Glassman L, Kronzon I. Images in cardiovascular medicine. Impending paradoxical embolus. Circulation 1996;93:387.

Rosenzweig BP, Guarneri E. Transesophageal echocardiography in the evaluation of aortic trauma. Echocardiography 1996;13:247–257.

Roudaut R, Durandet J, Leherissier A, et al. Spontaneous echo contrast in patients with sinus rhythm but poor atrial contraction. Echocardiography 1993;10:5–10.

Roudaut R, Lartigue MC, Dartigues JF, et al. Meta-analysis of positive blood cultures during transesophageal echocardiography. Echocardiography 1993;10:289–292.

Sarnoski J, Bajwa T, Deshpande S, et al. Transesophageal echocardiography during radiofrequency ablation of left-sided free wall atrioventricular accessory pathways in Wolff-Parkinson-White Syndrome. Echocardiography 1994;11:461–467.

Simon P, Owen AN, Moritz A, et al. Transesophageal echocardiographic evaluation in mechanically assisted circulation. Eur J Cardiothorac Surg 1991;5:492–497.

Snoddy BD, Nanda NC, Holman WL, et al. Usefulness of transesophageal echocardiography in diagnosed and guiding correct placement of a right ventricular assist device malpositioned in the left atrium. Echocardiography 1996;13:159–163.

Tighe DA, Tejada LA, Kirchhoffer JB, et al. Pacemaker lead infection: detection by multiplane transesophageal echocardiography. Am Heart J 1996;131:616–618.

Topol EJ, Humphrey LS, Borkon AM, et al. Value of intraoperative left ventricular microbubbles detected by transesophageal two-dimensional echocardiography in predicting neurologic outcome after cardiac operations. Am J Cardiol 1985;56:773–775.

Vilacosta I, Sarria C, San Ramon JA, Jimenez J, et al. Usefulness of transesophageal echocardiography for diagnosis of infected transvenous permanent pacemakers. Circulation 1994;89:2684–2687.

Voller H, Schroder K, Spielberg C, et al. Does cardiac function modify left heart opacification with transpulmonary echo contrast agents? Echocardiography 1993;10:41–47.

Wellford AL, Lawrie G, Zoghbi W. Transesophageal echocardiographic features and management of retained intracardiac air in two patients after surgery. J Am Soc Echocardiogr 1996;9:182–186.

Yao FS, Barbut D, Hager DN, et al. Detection of aortic emboli by transesophageal echocardiography during coronary artery bypass surgery. Cardiothorac Vasc Anesth 1996;10:314–317.

Index

■

Abscess(es). *(see also)* Endocarditis
  of aortic homograft, *239, 241*
    subaortic obstruction with, *245*
  aortic valve, *128*
    with vegetation, *127*
  with Bjork-Shiley aortic prosthesis, *221*
  with Ionescu-Shiley porcine prosthesis
    prolapse, *237*
  with Medtronic-Hall prosthesis, *224-*
    225, 226, 227
  mitral valve, *64, 93*
    with vegetation, *95, 96*
  of porcine aortic prosthesis, *235-236*
    in patient with heterograft, *236*
  with vegetation
    postoperative two-chamber view, *95, 96*
    preoperative study, *95, 96*
Accessory mitral tissue, *437, 437*
Acute myocardial infarction
  cardiac rupture following, *261*
    ventricular, *263*
  left ventricular apical aneurysm follow-
    ing, *258, 259*
Aneurysm(s)
  abdominal aortic
    graft replacement with suspicion of
      suture dehiscence in, *160*
  of annulus fibrosa, *100*
    in mitral and aortic valve endocardi-
      tis, *98, 99*
    pericardial patch for, *100*
  aortic
    ascending, *132-134, 132-134*
    descending, *134*
  aortic arch
    with thrombus, *134*
  atrial septal, 305, *305-306*
  of coronary arteries, 387, *387*, 432, *432*
    left anterior descending artery, 432, *432*
    longitudinal image with color
      Doppler, 432, *432*
    normal origin of left coronary artery,
      432, *432*
    transverse image of, 432, *432*
  left atrial, *79, 79*
  left ventricular apical, 258, *258-259*
  at mitral-aortic junction, *100*
  with rupture into right ventricle, 430, *431*

of sinus of Valsalva, 381, *381*
  congenital, *430*
  with rupture into right ventricle,
    382-383, *382-383*
ventricular septal, 326, *326*
Annuloplasty
  aortic, *247*
  for coronary leaflet tear, *122*
  in left atrial aneurysm
    residual mitral regurgitation follow-
      ing, *79*
  mitral, *87*
    for chordal rupture and mitral regur-
      gitation, *84*
  for redundant aortic valve, *119-120*
Annuloplasty rings
  mitral, *199-203*
    assessment of, 182
    Carpentier, *199*
    Duran, *199*
Annulus fibrosa
  aneurysm of, 100, *100*
    in mitral and aortic valve endocardi-
      tis, *98, 99*
Anterior mitral leaflet
  mitral regurgitation into, *75*
  perforation of, *73*
  prolapse of, *76*
  redundancy of, *77*
  rupture of, *74*
Aorta
  anatomy of
    transesophageal echocardiography
      definition of, *104*
  aneurysm of, *132*
    ascending, *132-133*
    descending, *134*
  atherosclerosis of, *104, 161-166*
  dissections of, *104, 135-138, 140-160*
Aortic annuloplasty, *247*
Aortic arch
  atherosclerosis of, *164, 165*
    ulcerations in, *164-165*
  left-sided superior vena cava behind,
    317, *317*
  longitudinal plane examination of, *10,*
    11, 12
  pulsed Doppler interrogation of, *9*
  transverse plane examination of, *9, 10*
  from upper esophagus, *14-15*
  vessels of
    identification of, *11*

Aortic atherosclerosis, 161-166, *161-166*
  in ascending aorta, *162*
  in ascending aorta and arch
    hematoma in, *165*
    intimal thickening of, *165*
  in descending aorta, *161, 166*
  mobile and immobile plaques in, *164*
  plaque types in, *163*
Aortic cusp
  in oblique plane, *19*
Aortic dissection, 135-138, *135-138, 141-*
  160, 143-152, 154, 156, 159-160
  of ascending aorta, *135*
    long-axis view, *138*
    short-axis view, *138*
  ascending aortic true lumen in, *149*
  with associated aortic regurgitation, *141*
  from atherosclerotic plaque, *146*
  atrial regurgitation in, *104*
  communications in
    in descending aorta, *144*
    between true and false lumens, *141,*
      142, 144
  DeBakey type I, *104*
  DeBakey type II, *104, 147*
  DeBakey type III, *148*
  of descending thoracic aorta, *148*
    graft repair of, *159*
    graft rupture contained, *159*
  diagnosis of, *104*
  versus double aortic valve, *144*
  extension of
    into descending thoracic aorta, *141,*
      142, 145
    into left main coronary artery, *135, 136*
    into right coronary artery, *135, 136*
  false lumen in
    thrombosed, *149*
  flap in
    in aortic root and ascending aorta, *147*
    versus aortic valve leaflets, *141*
    close to aortic valve leaflets, *143*
    extension into right and left main
      coronary arteries, *145*
    near left main coronary artery, *135, 136*
    prolapse with aortic regurgitation, *135*
  from graft dehiscence
    aortic-right ventricular fistula in, *156,*
      158
    transverse and longitudinal planes,
      156, 157, 158
  impingement on aortic leaflets, *135*

507

Aortic dissection—*Continued*
 from intraluminal tube graft dehiscence, *152-153, 154-155*
 intramural, *138*
 pectinate muscles in, *21*
 pleural effusion associated with, *148*
 rupture of
   into mediastinum, *149*
   into right ventricle, *150*
 short axis view of
   communication between true and
     false lumens, *135, 136*
   thrombus and, *135, 136*
 thrombus formation in, *144*
Aortic endocarditis, 98-99, *98-99*
 with aneurysm of annulus fibrosa, *98*
 perforation of anterior mitral leaflet
   in, *91*
 workup for
   transesophageal echocardiography
     in, 103
Aortic graft
 for abdominal aortic dissection, *160*
   descending thoracic, *160*
 dehiscence of, *156, 157*
 distal, *156, 158*
 to left main coronary artery, *151*
 of proximal aorta, *151*
Aortic orifice
 Doppler location of, 349
Aortic prosthesis(es), 181
 Bjork-Shiley, *220-221*
 CarboMedics, *218-219*
 homograft, *239-245.* (*see also*) Homograft aortic prosthesis
 porcine, *229, 229-238, 232-233, 235,
   237-238*
 St. Jude, *216-217*
 Starr-Edwards, *222-223*
Aortic regurgitation, 115, *115-116*
 in aortic valve endocarditis, *92*
   five-chamber view of, *92, 93*
 from aortic valve thickening, *114*
 in aortic valve vegetation with abscess
   formation, *127*
 assessment of, 103-104
   Nyquist limit in, 104, *115, 116*
 causes of, 103
 eccentric, pandiastolic
   on color M-mode, *115*
 effect on
   with change of Nyquist limit, *115, 116*
 in flail aortic valve, *122*
 with infected quadricuspid aortic valve,
   346
 with ionescu-Shiley porcine prosthesis,
   238
 between left and right cusps, *115*
 mild, *115*
 in mitral and aortic valve endocarditis, *91*
 moderately severe, *115, 116*

prosthetic
 assessment of, 181
 with Medtronic-Hall valve, *224, 226*
 in redundant aortic valve, *118, 119,
   120, 121*
 severe, *115, 116*
 with ventricular septal defects, *425,
   425-426, 426*
Aortic root
 with advancement of probe from ascending aorta and arch, *19*
 and ascending aorta
   longitudinal plane examination of, *27*
 dissection flap in, *147*
 extracardiac tumor posterior to, *478*
 on five-chamber view, *39*
 flow acceleration and turbulence into,
   105, 106
 imaging planes with multiplane probe, *6*
 in left sinus of Valsalva dissection
   longitudinal examination of, *139*
   transverse examination of, *139*
 transgastric view of, *57*
Aortic stenosis, 105, *105-113*, 107, *109-113*
 with associated left ventricular hypertrophy
   in transgastric view, *112*
 bicuspid, *109*
   gross specimens of, *109*
   mimicking tricuspid, *110*
   severe and calcified, *110*
 coexistent with hypertrophic cardiomyopathy, *113*
 determination of flow-limiting orifice
   in, 349
 gross specimens of, *107, 108*
 hypertrophic cardiomyopathy with, 103
 longitudinal image of, *435*
   four-chamber image of, *435*
 mitral stenosis and, *70*
 in patients with fixed stenotic orifices, *111*
 planimetry of, *107, 109*
 poststenotic dilatation of ascending
   aorta and, 349, *349*
 pulmonary, 295-296
 severe, *105, 106*
   calcific, *105*
   eccentric, *110*
 on short axis, *107*
 significant, *105, 106*
 subvalvular, 295-296, 434, *434-435*
   transverse image of, *434, 435*
 supravalvular, 103, 352, *352*
   in familial homozygous hypercholes-
     terolemia, *114*
 on transesophageal echocardiography,
   103
 transesophageal echocardiography of,
   433-434
   during aortic valvuloplasties, 433
   multiplanar probe in, 434

 in transoperative monitoring of pulmonary valve autograft, 434, *434*
 tricuspid
   appearing as bicuspid, *110*
Aortic valve. (*see also*) Prosthetic valve(s),
   aortic
 abscess of, *128*
   communication with left ventricular
     outflow tract, *128*
   extension into right atrium, *128*
 assessment of
   morphologic, 345, *345*
 bicuspid
   redundant, 343, *343*, 351, *351*
   unicommissural unicuspid mimic of,
     347, *347*
   vertically and obliquely oriented,
     343, *343*
 endocarditis of, *91-92, 98-99*
   with perforation of valve, *92, 93*
 eversion of, *123*
 fibroelastoma of, *461*
 flail, *122, 124-125*
   in hypertrophic cardiomyopathy,
     122-123, 124-125
 gross specimen of
   in systemic lupus erythematosus, *124*
 leaflets of
   with advancement of probe from as-
     cending aorta and arch, *19*
   in ascending aortic aneurysm, *132*
 multiplane probe examination of, 103
 myxomatous, 345, *345*
 preclosure of
   in hypertrophic cardiomyopathy, *276*
 prosthetic artifact from versus aortic
   dissection, *151*
 quadricuspid, 344, *344*. (*see also*)
   Quadricuspid aortic valve
   infected, 346, *346, 347, 347*
   mimic of, 345, *345*
 redundant, 117-121, *117-121*, 345, *345*
   annuloplasty for, *119-120*
   aortic regurgitation in, *120, 121*
   bicuspid mimicking tricuspid aortic
     valve, *119, 120*
   bicuspid with raphe, *119*
   cusp separation in, *120*
   with hole in right coronary cusp, *121*
   prolapse into left ventricular outflow
     tract, *118, 119*
   with significant regurgitation, *119, 120*
   versus vegetation or echo, 103
 redundant right coronary cusp, *117*
 regurgitation from, 103, *115-116*
 replacement of
   complications of, 182
   in descending thoracic dissection, *159*
   hematoma following, *486, 487*
   for stenosis and left ventricular septal
     myomectomy, *113*

stenosis of, 103, *105-113*, 349, *349-350*
systolic flutter of, *117*
thickening of, *114*
unicuspid
  unicommisural, 347, *347*, 348, *348*
vegetation
  as tumor mimic, *462*
vegetation on, *99*, *126-127*, *129*, *130-131*
Aortic valve prolapse
  in left ventricular outflow tract
    in aortic endocarditis, *92*, *93*
Aortic valve regurgitation
  from ascending aortic aneurysm, *132*, *133*
  from flail aortic valve
    in systemic lupus erythematosus, *124*
  from prolapse of aortic valve vegetation, *126*
  severe
    in aortic dissection, *143*
Aortic valve vegetation, 125-127, *125-127*, *129*, *129-131*, *129-131*, *130*, *131*
  with abscess formation, *127*
  gross specimen of, *126*
  involvement in aortic valve leaflet, *126*
  movement from left ventricular outflow track and back to aortic root, *125*
  prolapse into the outflow tract, *126*
Aortic valvuloplasty
  assessment in
    of residual regurgitation, *182*
    of site of repair, *182*
Aortopulmonary communication, 391, *391-395*, *392-395*
  in 7-month-old infant with truncus arteriosus, 391, *391*
  postoperative study, *391*, *392*
  in 1-year-old child
    with tetralogy of Fallot and complete atrioventricular septal defect, 393, *393*
  in 4-year-old patient
    with transposition of great vessels and pulmonary atresia, 393, *393*
  in 10-year-old patient
    with double outlet right ventricle and pulmonary artery banding, 395 *395*
    with tetralogy of Fallot, pulmonary atresia, nonconfluent pulmonary arteries, 394, *394*
Aortopulmonary fistula
  with Medtronic-Hall prosthesis, *226*, *227*
Aortopulmonary window, 430, *430*
Apical hypertrophic cardiomyopathy, 286, *286*
Artery(ies)
  common carotid, *11*, *12*
  coronary. *(see)* Coronary artery(ies)
  great. *(see)* Transposition of the great vessels
  intercostal
    normal anatomy of, *48-51*

lobar, *16*
pulmonary, *(see)* Pulmonary artery(ies)
renal, *58*, *59*
splenic, *58-59*
subclavian, *11*, *12*, *13*
transesophageal echocardiography of, *2*
Artifacts
  electrocautery-induced, 500, *500*
  next to descending thoracic aorta, *48*, *49*
  in vascular structure
    on transverse plane examination, *10*
Ascending aorta
  aneurysm of, 132-134, *132-134*
    short axis view of, *133*
  aortic root and
    longitudinal plane examination of, *27*
  atherosclerosis of, *162*, *165*
  dissection flap in, *147*
  on examination of right ventricle and pulmonary valve, *34*, *35*
  on longitudinal plane examination, *11*
  normal anatomy of, 17
  and pulmonary artery, 17-18
    longitudinal plane examination of, *17-18*
    transverse plane examination of, *17*
  transesophageal echocardiography of, *2*
  transgastric view of, *57*
  transverse plane examination of, *8*, 10, *10*
Ascending thoracic aorta
  aortic dissection extension into, *145*, *146*
Atherosclerosis
  aortic, 104, 161-166, *161-166*
    in descending aorta, *161*
    peripheral embolization from, *161*
  aortic dissection from, *146*
  in ascending aorta, *162*
Atria. *(see also)* Left atrium; Right atrium
  five-chamber view of, *39*
  four-chamber view of, *41-42*
    hemodynamics during cardiac cycle, *41*, *42*
Atrial appendages. *(see also named, e.g., Situs inversus)*
  juxtaposition of
    left, 404, *404*
    right, 404, *404*
    septal defect association with, *404*
    transesophageal features of, *404*
    in transesophageal sequential analysis, 404, *404*
Atrial baffle
  postoperative function of, *413*, 413-414
Atrial isomerism
  in transesophageal sequential analysis, 402-403
    left, 402, 403, *403*
    left persistent superior vena cava in, 403, *403*
    levoisomerism and, 403
    right, 402, 403, *403*

right superior vena cava abnormalities and, 402
  transverse axis imaging versus transthoracic in, 403
Atrial septal aneurysm, 305, *305-306*
  biplane study of, *305*
  bulge into left atrium, *305*
  mimic of left atrial cyst, *306*
  pericardial effusion with, 305, *306*
  relation to right ascending artery, *305*
Atrial septal defect(s), 295
  association with juxtaposition of atrial appendages, 404
  with double outlet right ventricle, 376, *376*
  mitral stenosis and, 71
  in mitral valve valvuloplasty, 64
  ostium primum type, 295
  post-balloon mitral valvuloplasty, 74
  septum secundum, 295, 302, *302-304*
    with Ebstein's anomaly, 365, *365*, 368, *368*
    tricuspid atresia with, *368*
  shunt volume estimation in, 302
  sinus venosus, 295, 309, *309-312*, 310, 312
    with associated left superior vena cava, *311*
    flow between right and left atria, *309*
    gross specimen of, *309*
    left-to-right shunting in, *312*
    patch closing, *309*
    right superior pulmonary vein opening into right atrium in, *311*
    in superior portion of atrial septum, *310*
    superior portion of atrial septum, *311*
  transesophageal echocardiography of
    diameter and area in, 420
    dimensions in, 420
    estimation of mixed shunts in, 420
    fossa ovalis, *420*
    indications for, 419
    lipomatous hypertrophy, 421
    location in
      with multiplane images, 420
    movement of interatrial septum in, 421, *421*
    ostium primum, 419
    ostium secundum, 419, 420
    patent foramen ovale, 419, *419*
    shunt variations in, *420*
    sinus venosus, 419, *419*, 420, *420*
    two-dimensional recordings from, 419
    types of, 419
    ventricular septal defect associated with, 330, *330*
Atrial septum
  lipomatous hypertrophy of, 472, *472*
  mitral regurgitation impacting, *175*
  myxoma on, *446*
  tricuspid regurgitation impacting, *175*

Atrial situs
  in transesophageal sequential analysis
    atrial isomerism, 402-403, *403*
    identification of, 399
    situs inversus, 401-402, *402*
    situs solitus, 399-401, *400-401*
    variants of, 399
Atrioventricular connection(s)
  absence of, 408-409
    characterization of, 408
    of right (tricuspid atresia), 408-409, *408-409*
  ambiguous, 406-407
    atrial appendages in, *406*
    criteria for, 405-406
    identification of ventricular morphology in, 407
    univentricular versus biventricular, 407
  concordant, 404-405
  crossed, 409-410
    color Doppler in, 409-410, *410*
    mode of connection in, 410
  discordant, 405-406
    reversal of ventricles in, 405, *405*
    with situs inversus, *406*
    with situs solitus, *406*
  double inlet ventricle, 407, 407-408, *408*
  in transesophageal sequential analysis, 404-411
    modes of, 399
    variants of, 399
Atrioventricular septal (canal) defect, 296
  complete, 362, *362*
    aortopulmonary communication in, 393, *393*
    in elderly woman and two other patients, 362, *362*
    left-to-right shunt in, *307, 308*, 362, *362*
  partial, 307, *307-308*
  patch closure of, *307*
  patent foramen ovale with, *307*
  schematic of, 307, *308*
Atrioventricular valves
  left-sided
    Ebstein's malformation of, 367, *367*
  opening into single ventricle, 377, *377*
Azygous vein
  hemiazygous vein joining to, *48, 50*
  normal anatomy of, 48
  opacification of
    in sclerosing mediastinitis, *481*
  versus other veins, 48, *50-51*
  pulsed Doppler interrogation of, *48, 50*
  relation to right superior vena cava and right pulmonary artery, *48, 50*
  schematic of, *48, 49*

Bicuspid valve(s)
  aortic
    coarctation of the aorta associated with, 354, *354*

five-chamber view of, *344*
    redundant, 343, *343*, 351, *351-352*
    unicommissural unicuspid mimic of, 347, *347*, 348, *348*
    in 60-year-old woman, 344, *344*
  pulmonary, 360, *360*
    in transposition of the great arteries, single ventricle, 378, *379*
Bioprosthetic valves, 181
  mitral cusp rupture with, *182*
Bjork-Shiley prosthesis(es), 181
  aortic, 220, *220-221*
    abscess with, *220-221*
    suture dehiscence with, *220*
    thrombosed, *220*
  mitral, 192, *192-195*
    pannus on, *192, 194*
    suture dehiscence in, *195*
    thrombus with, *192-194*
Brockenbrough needle
  in percutaneous mitral balloon valvuloplasty, *72*
Bronchial artery
  relationship to descending thoracic artery and left pulmonary artery, *48, 51*

Cabrol artery
  of ascending aorta, *151*
Calcification
  in left atrial free wall
    mimicking tumor, *452*
CarboMedics prosthesis(es)
  aortic, 181, 218, *218-219*
    for aortic stenosis, *105-106*
    normal, *218*
    paravalvular regurgitation with, *219*
  mitral, 181, 189, *189-191*, 191
    and dehiscence of left atrial wall, *191*
    four-chamber view of, *189*
    and left atrial pseudoaneurysm, *191-192*
    normal, 189, *189-190*
    schematics of, *189*
    valvular regurgitation with, *190*
  tricuspid, *248*
Cardiac rupture
  after acute myocardial infarction, *261*
    gross specimen, *261*
    transgastric views, *261*
Cardiomyopathy
  dilated, 275, *287-289*
  hypertrophic, 275, *276-277, 276-286, 279-286*. (*see also*) Hypertrophic cardiomyopathy
Cardioplegia needle/catheter
  image in ascending aorta, *502*
Cardioplegia solution
  contrast echoes from, 502, *502*
  cross aortic valve into left ventricular outflow tract, *502*

Cardiovascular segment(s)
  sequential analysis of
    after Mustard procedure, 411-413
    after Senning procedure, 411-413
    atrial situs, 399-404
    atrioventricular connection, 404-411
    in congenitally corrected transposition, 414-418
    in ventricular identification, 404
    ventriculoarterial connections, 411-413
Carpentier ring
  in mitral position
    gross specimen of, *199*
  in replacement
    of tricuspid valve prosthesis and ring, *248*
Carpentier-Edwards heterograft
  in mitral valve vegetation, 95, *96*
Chiari network, 46, *46, 47*, 296
Chordae tendineae
  anomalous insertion in interventricular septum, 437, *437*
  of anterior and posterior mitral leaflets
    rupture of, 84, *85*
  mitral
    rupture of, 80-85, *80-85*
    transgastric view, *52*
  in mitral prolapse, *67*
  in mitral stenosis, *66*
  of posterior mitral leaflet
    rupture of, *80*
    severe prolapse of, *81*
  in posterior mitral leaflet prolapse, *82*
  prolapse of
    into the left atrium, *81*
  ruptured
    echo posterior to mitral valve in M-mode study of, *83*
    mitral annuloplasty ring and, *202*
  in mitral valve endocarditis, *97*
Coarctation of the aorta, 296, 353, *353-356, 354-355*, 432-433, *433*
  associated with bicuspid aortic valve and subaortic membranous stenosis, 354, *354*
    in 23-year-old woman, 354, *354*
  collateral vessels in, 353, *353*, 355, *355*
  descending thoracic aorta proximal to, 355, *355*
  gross specimen of, 356, *356*
  intercostal artery carrying blood into descending thoracic aorta, *353*
  longitudinal examination of, 354-355, *354-355*
  schematic of longitudinal plane, *353*
  transverse examination of, 355, *355*
    in 17-year-old female, 355, *355*
Common atrioventricular canal
  atrioventricular valve anatomy and, 426
  Rastelli's classification of, 427

transesophageal echocardiography of, 426-427, *426-427*
  in infants and children, 426
  intraoperative use of, 427
  morphology on, 426, *426*
  in Rastelli type A, 426, *426*
Common carotid arteries
  on longitudinal plane examination, *11, 12*
Congenital heart disease. *(see also named, e.g., Aortic stenosis)*
  aortic stenosis, *105-113*
    subvalvular, 295-296
  atrial septal defects
    septum secundum, 295, *302-304*
    sinus venosus, 295, *309-312*
  atrioventricular canal defect, 296, *307-308, 363*
  coarctation of the aorta, 296, *353-356, 433*
  cor triatriatum, 295, *336-337*
  coronary artery abnormalities, *140, 156-158, 252-255, 296, 387*
  Ebstein's anomaly, 296, *363-368*
  infundibular stenosis, 296, *358*
  mitral stenosis
    congenital, *65-71, 295-296, 338*
  patent ductus arteriosus, 295, *332-334*
  patent foramen ovale, 296, *297-300*
  pulmonary stenosis, 295-296, *360, 440*
  septum secundum defect, 295, *302-304*
  sinus of Valsalva aneurysm, 296, *380-381*
  tetralogy of Fallot, 296, *370-371*
  transesophageal echocardiography versus transthoracic, 295
  transposition of great vessels, 296, *372-375*
  tricuspid atresia, 296, *368, 408*
  ventricular septal defects, 295, *327-331, 424-426*
Congenitally corrected transposition
  atrioventricular discordance in, 414
  defects associated with, 414
    left-sided Ebstein's anomaly, 414, *415*
    valvular, 414
    ventricular septal, 414
  double outlet right ventricle, 415-417
    posterior vessel overriding interventricular septum in, 415, *415, 416*
    pulmonary artery and artery connection to right ventricle in, 416, *416*
    and pulmonary stenosis, *416*
    side-to-side relationship of great arteries in, 416, *416*
    tricuspid regurgitation and ventricular septal defect in, 416, *416*
    truncus arteriosus in, 416-417, *417*
  pulmonary atresia with ventricular septal defect
    truncus arteriosus in, *417*, 417-418, *418*

transesophageal sequential analysis of, 414-418
  right ventricular function in, 415
  versus transthoracic study, 414
  tricuspid regurgitation in, 414, *415*
  ventriculoarterial discordance in, 414, *414*
Cooley-Cutter porcine mitral valve, 181, *196*
  stenosis of, 196, *196*
Cor triatriatum, 295, 336, 437-438
  abnormal insertion of mitral chordae tendineae, *437*
  in adult patient, 336-337
  appearance of membrane as extension of "Q-tip," 336-337
  four-chamber image, *438*
  schematic of, *336*
  in second adult patient, *337*
  spontaneous echo contrast in, *438*
  transverse plane, *438*
    with color Doppler and spectral analysis, *438*
Coronary artery fistula, 431-432, *431-432*
Coronary artery(ies). *(see also named, e.g., Left anterior descending coronary artery)*
  abnormalities of, 296
  dissection of, *140*
  left anterior descending
    aneurysm of, 387, *387*
    normal anatomy of, *25*
    right coronary artery origination from, 386, *386*
  left ascending
    in dilated cardiomyopathy, *287*
    normal anatomy of, *43, 52, 54*
    pectinate muscles versus thrombus in, *68*
  left circumflex
    anomalous origin of, 384-385, *384-385*
    fistula to coronary sinus, *389-390*, 398-390
    normal anatomy of, *22, 22-23, 25*
  left main
    aneurysm of, 387, *387*
    anomalous right coronary artery from, 347, *347*
    in aortic dissection, *135, 136, 141, 145*
    dehiscence of, *156-158*
    graft attachment to, *151*
    normal anatomy of, 22, *22*
  normal anatomy of, 22, *22-25, 24*
  origination of, 386, *386*
  right
    aneurysm of, 387, *387*
    anomalous, 347
    in aortic dissection, 143
    dissection of, *140*
    fistula to coronary sinus, 388, *388*
    normal anatomy of, 22, *23*
    origination of, *385-386, 385-386*
  stenosis of, *252-255*

Coronary lesion(s), 252-255
  atherosclerotic plaque, *252*
  contrast echocardiography of, *254*
  left main disease, *252*
  saphenous vein graft for, 252, *255*
  stenosis
    left anterior descending, 253, *254-255*
    left circumflex, *253*
    left main ostial, *252*
    mid-left main, *253*
    right coronary, *254*
Coronary sinus
  drainage into right atrium, 400, *400*
  enlarged
    from anomalous draining of left-sided superior vena cava, 324, *324*
    entering right atrium, *321*
    with left-sided superior vena cava drainage, 321, *321, 323, 323*
    relationship to left circumflex coronary artery, 319, *320*
    inferior vena cava entering, 323, *323*
    left circumflex coronary artery and fistula to, 25, 389, *389*
    relation to, *25*
    left-sided superior vena cava and connection to, 319, *320*
    draining into, 318, *318*
    entering in pulmonary atresia, 323, *323*
  pulsed Doppler interrogation of, 46, *47*
Critikon catheter
  in mitral valve orifice, 72

Denver peritoneovenous shunt
  thrombus from, *496*
Descending aorta
  atherosclerosis of, *161, 166*
  intra-aortic balloon pump in, 505, *505*
Descending thoracic aorta, 48-50
  aneurysm/thrombus of, 134, *134*
  aortic dissection extension into, *141, 142*
  dissection of, *135, 137*
  intercostal artery feeding into, *353*
  leiomyosarcoma on, *463*
    versus hematoma, *463-464*
  normal anatomy of, 48
  pleural effusion behind, *493*
  schematic of, *48, 49*
Dilated cardiomyopathy
  gross specimens of, *288*
  identification of, 275
  left and right ventricles in, *288*
  left ventricular function in, *287*
  right atrium free wall in hypertrophy and trabeculation of, *288*
  right ventricular assist device in, *289*
Dissection. *(see also)* Aortic dissection
  aortic, 104, *135-138, 141-160*
  of ascending aorta, *135*
  of descending thoracic aorta, *135, 137*
  of left sinus of Valsalva, *139*

Dissection—*Continued*
of right coronary artery, *140*
extension into aortic root, *140*
Double aortic arch, 433, *433*
M-mode and two dimensional longitudinal imaging, 434, *434*
Double inlet ventricle
in transesophageal sequential analysis
characterization of, 407
four-chamber imaging, *408*
mitral regurgitation in, *408*
transgastric transverse plane with
color Doppler, 407, *407*
Double outlet right ventricle, 375-376,
375-376
aortopulmonary communication in,
395 *395*
ventricular septal defect and secundum
atrial septal defects in, 376, *376*
in 10-year-old boy, 376, *376*
Double-chambered right ventricle,
357, *357*
Ductal carcinoma of breast
mediastinal metastasis from,
479, *479*
Duran ring, 203
dehiscence of, *203*
in mitral annuloplasty, 87
dehiscence of, *203*
obstruction from, *203*
thrombus from, *203*
in mitral position, *199*
thrombosed, *203*

Ebstein's anomaly, 296, 363, *363-368*,
364-366, 368, 438-440, *439*
anterior and posterior tricuspid leaflet
in, 363, *363*
characterization of, 438-439
color Doppler
evaluation of tricuspid regurgitation,
439, *439*
diagnosis of
two-dimensional echocardiography
in, 439
longitudinal and transverse examinations of, 366, *366*
longitudinal image of, *440*
with color Doppler, *440*
with secundum atrial septal defect, 365,
365, 368, *368*
transverse image, *439*
tricuspid replacement in
valvuloplasty for, 440
valvuloplasty for
transesophageal echocardiography
in, 440
in 17-year-old male, 366, *366*
transgastric examination in,
366, *366*
in 24-year-old man, 363, *363*

in 72-year-old woman
anterior and posterior tricuspid
leaflets in, 364, *364*
Embolization
peripheral
from aortic atherosclerosis, *161*
Embolus
impending paradoxic
right atrial, *469*
Endocarditis. (*see also*) Abscess(es)
of aortic homograft, *239, 241, 243*
of aortic valve, 91, *91-92*, 98, *98-99*
five-chamber view of, *92-93*
four-chamber view of, *92*
of mitral and aortic valves
perforation of anterior mitral leaflet
in, *91*
with perforation of valves, *92-93*
regurgitation in, *91*
vegetations in, *130, 131*
of mitral leaflet, 97
of mitral valve, 91, *91-94*, 92-94, 97,
97-99, 98-99
of right heart pacer, *499*
tricuspid, 177, *177*
Eustachian valve, 296
on examination of right ventricle and
pulmonary valve, 34, *35*
at junction of inferior vena cava-right
atrium, *44-45*
normal anatomy of, 44, 46
at right atrium inferior vena cava junction, 46, *47*

Fibroelastoma(s), 445
aortic valve, 460, *461*
papillary
of tricuspid valve, 473, *473*
schematic of, *461*
Fibroelastosis
in patient with aortic stenosis, *112*
Fistula(s)
aortic root-right ventricular
homograft aortic prosthesis and,
241-242, 243
aortic-right ventricular
in aortic dissection, *156, 158*
coronary artery
longitudinal images of, *431*,
431-432, *432*
transverse images of, 431, *431*
left circumflex coronary artery to coronary sinus, 389-390, *389-390*
with porcine aortic prosthesis,
235-236, 242
right coronary artery to coronary sinus,
388, *388*
postoperative findings, *388*

Five-chamber view
normal anatomy in, 39, *39-40*

Flail valve(s)
aortic, 122, *122-124*, 124
diastolic fluttering in, *122*
with hypertrophic cardiomyopathy,
122-123
right coronary cusp prolapse into left
ventricular outflow tract, *122*
in systemic lupus erythematosus, *124*
mitral
myxomatous degeneration of, *90*
Fontan-type surgery
description of, 410
transesophageal echocardiography in,
410-411
adjunctive in follow-up, 411
for connection sites of pulmonary
veins, 411
for integrity of tunnel wall, 410, *410*
for intracavitary thrombi, 411, *411*
for patch in total cavopulmonary
connections, 410, *411*
protocol and procedure for, 410
for thrombosis of prosthetic conduits,
411, *411*
Foramen ovale
normal anatomy of, 44
valve of, 41, *42*
four-chamber view of, *41, 42*
visualization of, *44-45*
Four-chamber view
normal anatomy in, 41, *41-42*

Graft(s)
aortic, *151, 156-158, 160*
homograft, *239-245*
Carpentier-Edwards, *95-96*
Hemashield interposition, *141, 142*
intraluminal tube, *151-155, 217*
pulmonary autograft, *246, 247, 434, 434*
saphenous vein, *252, 255*
Great vessels. (*see also*) Transposition of
the great vessels
identification of
transesophageal echocardiography
in, 411
Hemashield interposition graft
in resection of ascending aorta,
141, 142
Hematoma
behind ascending aorta and arch, *165*
versus extracardiac tumors, 445
in left sinus of Valsalva dissection
cavity, *139*
posterior to Medtronic-Hall prosthesis, *225*
right atrium compression by, *486, 487*
Hemiazygous vein
intercostal vein draining into, *48, 50*
joining azygous vein
on transverse examination, *48, 50*
normal anatomy of, 48

opacification of
  in sclerosing mediastinitis, *481*
  posterior to descending thoracic aorta, *48, 50*
  pulsed Doppler interrogation of, *48, 50*
  schematic of, *48, 49*
Hepatic veins
  transgastric view of, *58, 59*
Hepatopulmonary syndrome
  right-to-left shunt in, 301, *301*
Homograft, 181
  aortic, 239, *239-245, 243, 245*
    abscess of, 239, *241*
      subaortic obstruction with, *245*
    cusp prolapse of, 239, *240*
    degeneration of, 239, *240*
    dehiscence of, 239, *241*
    endocarditis of, 239, *240-241*
      with regurgitation, *244*
    fistula from aorta to right ventricle and, *243*
    fistula from aortic root to right ventricle and, *241-242*
    prolapse of
      into aortic root, 239, *240*
      into left ventricular outflow tract, 239, *240*
    pseudoaneurysm with, 239, *241*
    regurgitation from, 239-240, *241, 243, 244*
    stenosis of, *239*
    vegetation on
      prolapse of, 239, *240*
Hypertrophic cardiomyopathy
  aortic valve in
    preclosure of, *276*
    stenosis of, 103
  apical, *286*
    postoperative, *286*
  characterization of, 275
  flail aortic valve-associated
    left ventricular outflow tract turbulence in, *122-123*
  gross specimens of, *285*
  left upper pulmonary vein in, 283, *285*
  left ventricular, *284*
    post myectomy, 284, *285*
  left ventricular free wall, *286*
  mitral regurgitation in, *279*
  porcine aortic prosthesis and, *238*
  systolic anterior motion in, *284*
    of anterior and posterior mitral leaflets, 275, *277-278*
    of anterior mitral leaflet, *280*
    anterior mitral leaflet touching ventricular septum, *282*
    of mitral leaflets, 275, 276, *282*
    of mitral valve, *283*
  systolic flow in left ventricular outflow tract, *281*

ventricular septum in
  hypertrophy of, *280*
  myectomy of, *282*

Imaging planes, 7
  longitudinal, 7
  transverse, 7
Inferior vena cava
  draining into coronary sinus, 323, *323*
  on examination of right ventricle and pulmonary valve, *34, 35*
  hepatic veins entering, *58, 59*
  junction with right atrium
    eustachian valve at, *44-45*
  leiomyoma on, 465-466, *465-466*
    protrusion into left atrium and, *465*
    resected, *466*
  and superior vena cava
    schematic of, *44*
    simultaneous image of, *44, 45*
Infundibular stenosis, 358, *358*
  patient with tetralogy of Fallot and, 370, *370*
  right ventricular outflow tract narrowing in, 358-359, *358-359*
Innominate artery
  on longitudinal plane examination, *11, 12, 13*
  transesophageal echocardiography of, 2
Innominate vein
  aortic arch relation to, *10, 11, 11*
  on longitudinal plane examination, *12*
  transesophageal echocardiography of, 2
  in transverse plane examination, *9*
Intercostal arteries
  adjacent to descending thoracic artery, *48, 51*
  adjacent to hemiazygous veins, *48, 50*
  normal anatomy of, 48
Intercostal vein
  draining into hemiazygous vein, *48, 50*
  normal anatomy of, 48
  posterior
    joining left azygous vein posterior to descending aorta, 321, *322*
Intra-aortic balloon pump
  in descending aorta, 505, *505*
Intraluminal tube graft
  aortic, *217*
  at coronary anastomoses and pseudoaneurysm rupture in right atrium, *152-153*
  dehiscence of
    aortic dissection from, *152-153*
Intramyocardial coronary vessels
  on color Doppler system, *52, 55*
Intrarenal artery
  transgastric view of, *58, 59*

Ionescu-Shiley porcine prosthesis
  aortic regurgitation with, *238*
  prolapse/abscess/regurgitation with, *237-238*
Ischemic heart disease
  cardiac rupture following acute myocardial infarction, 261, *261*
  coronary stenosis, 252-255
  left ventricular
    apical aneurysm, 258, *258-259*
    dysfunction, 256, *256-257*
    pseudoaneurysm, 260, *260*
  left ventricular papillary muscle rupture, 266-273, *266-273*
  mechanical complications of, 251
  mitral regurgitation from, *256*
  pseudoaneurysm
    and septal rupture, 262, *262*
  ventricular septal rupture
    after acute anterior myocardial infarction, 263-265, *263-265*

Lambl's excrescence
  on aortic valve imaging, 27-28
  linear echoes versus
    in mitral prolapse, 63
Left anterior descending coronary artery, *24, 25*
  aneurysm of, 387, *387*
  anterior interventricular vein and, *25*
  circumflex branch of, *25*
  ramus branch of, *25*
  right coronary artery origination from, 386, *386*
Left ascending artery
  pectinate muscles versus thrombus in, *68*
  pericardial effusion around, *490*
  thrombus in
    in dilated cardiomyopathy, *287*
  transgastric view of, *52, 54*
  on two-chamber view, *43*
Left atrial appendage
  bilobed, *20*
  dysfunction of, *20*
  left-sided superior vena cava relationship to, 321, *321*
  in mitral stenosis, 67
    with atrial fibrillation, 67
  multiplane probe imaging of, *20*
  normal anatomy of, 20
  pectinate muscles and, *20*
  pulsed Doppler interrogation of, *20*
  separation from left upper pulmonary vein, *21*
  in situs solitus
    normal morphology in, 400, *400*
  thrombus at
    Bjork-Shiley mitral prosthesis-associated, *193*
  transgastric view of, *52, 54*
  tumor of, *452*

Left atrium
  aneurysm of, 79
  cusp rupture into
    with porcine mitral prosthesis, 211
  left-sided superior vena cava relation-
    ship to, 325, 325
  mitral prolapse into, 76, 84
  mitral regurgitation into, 75
  myxomas on, 445-446, 446-450, 447-448
  normal anatomy of, 34
  protrusion of inferior vena cava leiomy-
    oma into, 465
  spontaneous contrast echoes in, 503, 503
  thrombus in, 68, 69
    in mitral stenosis, 36, 37
    with porcine mitral prosthesis, 206
    tumor mimicking, 451, 453
  tumor on, 453
Left azygous artery
  entrance into left-sided superior vena
    cava, 319, 320
  relationship to cardiac structures,
    319, 320
Left azygous vein
  entering left-sided superior vena cava,
    321, 322
  joining with left-sided superior vena
    cava, 323, 323
Left circumflex coronary artery
  anatomic position of, 25
  anomalous origin of
    from right sinus of Valsalva, 385, 385
    from separate ostium in left coronary
      sinus, 384, 384
    fistula to coronary sinus, 389-390,
      389-390
      postoperative, 390
      in 53-year-old woman, 390
  normal anatomy of, 22, 22-23
Left heart
  air bubbles in, 504, 504
Left lower pulmonary vein
  longitudinal examination of, 29, 30
  normal anatomy of, 29
Left main coronary artery
  aneurysm of, 387, 387
  anomalous right coronary artery from,
    347, 347
  between aorta and right ventricular out-
    flow tract/main pulmonary artery,
    347, 347
  aortic dissection and, 141
    extension into, 135, 136
    flap extension into, 145
  dehiscence of, 156, 158
  graft attachment to, 151
  normal anatomy of, 22, 22
Left pulmonary artery
  branches of, 16
    Doppler interrogation of, 16
    lobar arteries, 16

left-sided superior vena cava and
  anterior to, 319, 320, 321, 321
  posterior to, 321, 322
Left pulmonary vein(s)
  lower and upper, 29, 31-32
    simultaneous examination of, 29, 31
  obstruction of
    postoperative study of, 335, 335
    in 9-year-old boy, 335, 335
Left upper pulmonary vein
  backflow into, 81, 84, 86
  isolated anomalous
    drainage of, 313, 313
    shunt flow estimation in, 313
  left-sided superior vena cava relation-
    ship to, 321, 321, 325, 325
  longitudinal examination of, 29, 30
  mitral regurgitation into, 70, 86
  normal anatomy of, 29, 29, 30
  transgastric view of, 52, 54
  transverse examination of, 29, 30
Left ventricle
  apical aneurysm of, 258, 258-259
    gross specimens of, 258, 259
    thrombus-containing, 258, 259
  artifacts obscuring, 500
  compression by pericardial hydatid cyst,
    491-492
  dilated, 288
  diverticulum of, 396, 396
  dysfunction of, 256, 256-257
  hypertrophy of
    aortic stenosis-associated, 112
  left atrial line mirror image mimicking
    catheter, 501
  lipoma on, 458, 458-459
  myxoma on, 456, 456-457
  pseudoaneurysm of, 260, 260
  thrombus in, 460
    in dilated cardiomyopathy, 288
  transgastric view, 52, 53
    in diastole and systole, 52, 54
  on two-chamber view, 43
Left ventricular outflow tract
  aortic valve abscess communication
    with, 128
  aortic vegetation prolapse into, 89
  flail coronary cusp prolapse into, 122
  in hypertrophic cardiomyopathy, 280,
    281, 282, 284, 285
  obstruction of
    in hypertrophic cardiomyopathy, 275
Left ventricular papillary muscle(s)
  multiple, 396, 396
  rupture of, 265-270, 265-273, 272-273
    of anterior, 266, 268
    with backflow into right upper pul-
      monary vein, 269
    five-chamber view, 268
    gross specimen of, 272
    of head, 267

into left atrium, 272
  movement between left ventricle and
    left atrium, 269, 270-271
  muscle head without prolapse into
    left atrium, 272
  of posterior, 266, 269
  in right atrium, 273
  site of rupture, 270
  transgastric view, 267, 268, 273
Left-sided superior vena cava
  anomalous drainage of, 324, 324
  anterior to left atrium, 317
  contrast signals after IV injection of
    normal saline, 317
  draining into coronary sinus, 317, 317-
    325, 318-319, 321, 323-325
    anterior to left pulmonary artery,
      320, 322
    diagrammatic representation of, 318
    enlarged coronary sinus entering
      right atrium, 321
    enlarged coronary sinus-left circum-
      flex artery relationship in, 319
    five-chamber view, transverse
      plane, 319
    four-chamber view, 321
    left azygous vein entrance into,
      320, 322
    left azygous vein-descending thoracic
      aorta relationship in, 320
    longitudinal plane, two-chamber
      view, 322
    pericardial effusion in, 320
    posterior intercostal vein-left azygous
      vein posterior to descending aorta,
      322
    posterior to left pulmonary artery
      and near aorta, 322
    relationship to adjacent coronary
      structures, 319, 320
    relationship to left pulmonary artery,
      320
    transverse plane, 321
    two-chamber, longitudinal plane, 319
    in 40-year-old woman, 321, 321-322
  entering coronary sinus
    in 20-year-old man with tetralogy of
      Fallot and pulmonary atresia, 323,
      323
  relationship to left upper pulmonary
    vein and left atrium, 325, 325
Left-to-right shunt
  in atrioventricular (canal) defect, 307,
    307
  with malpositioned Thoratec assist de-
    vice, 292, 293
  in patent foramen ovale, 297, 299
  in secundum atrial septal defect, 302, 303
  in sinus venosus atrial septal defect,
    312, 312
  in tetralogy of Fallot, 370, 370

Left-upper-pulmonary vein
  right-to-left shunting into, 297, *300*
Leiomyoma, 445
  of inferior vena cava, 465, *465*
    surgically resected, *466*
Leiomyosarcoma, 445
  aortic, 463, *463-464*
  left atrial, 448, *449-450*
    and invasion of mediastinum, *450*
Levoisomerism, 403
Lipoma
  left ventricular, *458-459*
  versus myxoma, 445
Lipomatous hypertrophy
  of atrial septum, 472, *472*
Lobar arteries, 16
Longitudinal imaging planes, 7, *7*
Longitudinal plane examination
  in identification of aortic vessels, *11-13*
Lung transplantation
  obstruction of right upper pulmonary
    vein following, 480, *480*

Main pulmonary artery
  normal systolic flow from, *56*
Mechanical assist device(s), 289-293,
  289-293
  biplane imaging of, *289*
  biventricular, 289-290, *289-290*
  right ventricular
    in dilated cardiomyopathy, *290*
    malpositioned Thoratec, *291*
  single plane imaging of, *290*
  Teflon conduit
    attachment to ascending aorta, *290*
Mechanical grafts
  versus bioprostheses, 181
Mediastinitis
  sclerosing, 445
    histology of biopsy tissue in, *485*
    infiltration of left atrium by, *482*
    obstruction in superior vena cava, *484*
    obstruction of right lower and upper
      pulmonary veins in, *483*
    opacification of azygous and hemi-
      azygous veins in, *481*
    single case, 481-485, *481-485*
Mediastinum
  aortic dissection rupture into, *150*
  leiomyosarcoma in, *448*
  metastatic mass in, 479, *479*
Medtronic-Hall prosthesis, 224, *224-227*,
  226
  abscess with, *224*, *225*, *226-227*
  aortic regurgitation with, *224*, *226*
  aortopulmonary fistula with, *226*, *227*
  paravalvular leak with, *224*
  regurgitation with
    paravalvular and valvular, *226*
Melanoma, metastatic
  of right ventricle, 475, *475-476*

Mitral annuloplasty
  mitral regurgitation following, 87, *87*
Mitral annuloplasty rings, 199-203,
  199-203
  Carpentier, *199*
  dehiscence of, *203*
  Duran, *199*, 199, *203*
  obstruction of, *203*
  postoperative residual mitral regurgita-
    tion with, *201*
  pre- and postoperative, *200*
  with ruptured chordae, *202*
  thrombosed, *203*
Mitral endocarditis
  with aneurysm of annulus fibrosis, *98*
  perforation of anterior mitral leaflet
    in, *91*
Mitral leaflet(s)
  anterior
    perforation in endocarditis, *91*
  flail posterior
    prolapse into left atrium, *84*
  myxomatous degeneration of, *77*
  papillary muscle insertion into, 338, *338*
  redundancy of, *77*
Mitral prosthesis(es), 181. *(see also)*
  Porcine mitral prosthesis
  Bjork-Shiley, *192-195*
  CarboMedics, *189-191*
  porcine, 204-209, *204-215*, 211, *214-215*
  St. Jude, *183-188*
Mitral regurgitation
  in aortic valve endocarditis, *91*
  in aortic valve vegetation with abscess
    formation, *127*
  assessment of, 63
    Nyquist limit in, 63
  in coronary artery disease, *78*
  from dilated mitral annulus, *78*
  in double inlet ventricle
    on transesophageal sequential analy-
      sis, *408*
  in endocarditis of posterior mitral
    leaflet, *97*
  in hypertrophic cardiomyopathy, *279*
  in ischemic heart disease, *256*
  into left ascending artery, *86*
  in left atrial aneurysm, *79*
  into left atrium, *75*
  into left upper pulmonary vein and left
    ascending artery extension, *86*
  in mitral valve endocarditis, *91*, *92*
  with porcine mitral prosthesis
    paravalvular, *208*
    valvular, *208*, *209*
  post mitral annuloplasty, 87, *87*, *201*
  post annuloplasty, *86*, 87, *87*
  prosthetic
    assessment of, 181
  small jet, *78*
  through anterior mitral leaflet, *75*

Mitral stenosis, 65-68, *65-71*, 70-71
  aortic stenosis and, *70*
  atrial septal defect and, *71*
  calcific and noncalcific, *65*
  calcified leaflets with thickened sub-
    valvular apparatus, *66*
  congenital, 295, 338, *338*
  gross specimen of fused chordae with
    nodular leaflet calcification, *66*
  left atrial appendage flow in, *67*
  with prolapse, *67*
  and regurgitation, *70*
  severe
    pathology specimens of, *65*
  spontaneous contrast echoes and
    thrombus, *68-69*
  subvalvular thickening, *66*
  transthoracic echocardiography
    for, *63*
Mitral valve, 63-64. *(see also* Prosthetic
  valve(s), mitral
  abscess of, 64, 93, *93*
  congenital malformations of,
    434-436
  duplication of orifice, 436, *436-437*
    anteroposterior relationship of ori-
      fices, *436*
    multiplane transesophageal
      study, *436*
    transesophageal study with color
      Doppler, *436*, *437*
    transgastric study, *436*
    with ventricular septal defect, *436*
  from esophageal-gastric junction, *48*
  flail
    myxomatous degeneration of, *90*
    posterior leaflet prolapse into
      left atrium and, *90*
  gross specimen of
    in systemic lupus erythemato-
      sus, *124*
  left circumflex coronary artery relation
    to, *25*
  myxoma on, 453, *453*
  myxomatous changes in, 90, *90*
  normal anatomy of, *48*
  percutaneous balloon valvuloplasty of,
    72, *72*
    atrial septal defect following, *74*
    rupture following, 72, *74*
  prolapse of, 63, 76, *76-77*
  regurgitation from, 63, 75, *75*,
    78, *86*
  replacement of
    transesophageal and transthoracic
      examinations of, *182*
  stenosis of, 63, *63-71*, 65
  thrombus/myxomatous degeneration of,
    454, *454-455*
  transesophageal versus transthoracic ap-
    proach to, 63

Mitral valve—*Continued*
  vegetation in, 95, *95-96, 129, 130, 131*
    Carpentier-Edwards heterograft for, *95, 96*
    four-chamber and two-chamber views of, *95*
    intraoperative study before debridement, *95*
    postoperative, *95*
    recurrence on prosthetic valve, *95, 96*
  vegetations in, 64, 95, *95*
    transesophageal versus transthoracic echocardiography of, 64
Mitral valve endocarditis, 91, *91-94, 92-94, 97, 97-99, 98-99*
  chordae infection in, *94*
  four-chamber view of postoperative, *92*
  with perforation of valve
    five-chamber view, *92*
    four-chamber view, *92*
  of posterior mitral leaflet, *97*
  vegetation and abscess in, *94*
Mitral valve leaflet(s)
  anterior
    from esophageal-gastric junction, *48*
    perforation of, *73*
  calcification of, *66*
  and chordae tendineae
    transgastric view, *52*
  four-chamber view of, *41, 42*
  posterior, *48*
Mitral valve prolapse, 63, 76-77, *76-77*
  of anterior and posterior leaflets severe, *76*
  from chordae tendineae rupture, 63
  into left atrium, *76*
  of posterior mitral leaflet into left atrium, *83*
  transgastric short-axis views, *77*
Mitral valvuloplasty
  transesophageal echocardiography in, 64
Mullins sheath
  in percutaneous mitral balloon valvuloplasty, *72*
Mustard procedure
  transesophageal sequential analysis of atrial baffle function following, *413, 413-414*
Myectomy of ventricular septum
  in hypertrophic cardiomyopathy, *282, 283*
Myxoma
  characterization of, 445
  left atrial, 446, *446-450, 447-448*
    calcification in, *448*
    dilation of right upper pulmonary vein, *450*
    gross specimen of, *449*
    invasion from right upper pulmonary vein, *450*
    lobulated, *449*

    obstruction of mitral orifice, *447, 449*
    postoperative study of, *446*
  left ventricular, 456, *457*
    attachment of, *456*
    identification as two masses, *457*
    origin at apex, *457*
  mitral valve, *453*
  multiple blood vessels within, *450*
  right atrial, 467, *467, 468*
  of tricuspid valve, *474*
Myxomatous degeneration, 90, *90*
  of aortic valve, 345, *345*
  of mitral leaflets, 77
  of mitral valve, 90, *90, 455*

Nyquist limit
  in aortic regurgitation
    assessment of, 104, *115, 116*
  change of
    effect on aortic regurgitation, *115, 116*
  in mitral regurgitation
    assessment of, 63

Obstruction(s)
  from Duran ring, 203
  of left pulmonary veins, 335, *335*
    postoperative study of, 335, *335*
  of left ventricular outflow tract
    in hypertrophic cardiomyopathy, 275
  of mitral annuloplasty rings, 203
  of mitral orifice
    myxoma in, 447, *449*
  in pulmonary valve stenosis
    subvalvular, 441
  of right lower and upper pulmonary veins
    in sclerosing mediastinitis, 483
  of right pulmonary vein
    post lung transplantation, 480
  from stenosis
    discrete subaortic membranous, 342, *342*

Pacer
  endocarditis of, *499*
Pacer lead
  vegetation on, 498, *498*
Pannus
  Bjork-Shiley mitral prosthesis-associated, *194*
  on tricuspid prosthesis and ring, *248*
Papillary muscle(s)
  insertion of
    abnormal, 338, *338*
  left ventricular
    multiple, 396, *396*
    rupture of, 266
  normal anatomy transgastric view of, *52-53*
  right ventricular
    rupture of, 273

Parachute mitral valve, 434-436, *435, 436*
Partial anomalous pulmonary venous connection, 421-422, *421-422*
  secondary dilatation of right heart cavities and tricuspid regurgitation, *422*
  transesophageal echocardiography of postoperative study, *421*
  of pulmonary veins
    drainage into inferior vena cava, *422*
    to right atrium, 421, *422*
  transesophageal echocardiogram with contrast, *422*
  transverse imaging of, 421-422, *422-423*
Patent ductus arteriosus, 295, 332, *332-334*, 417-431
  connection with main pulmonary artery, 332, *332, 333*
  flow from aorta into pulmonary artery, 334, *334*
  gross specimen of, 334, *334*
  infective endarteritis in, 428, *429*
  longitudinal imaging of, *428*
    with color Doppler and spectral analysis, 428, *428*
  postoperative views, 332, *332-333*
  with pulmonary hypertension, 428, *429*
  schematic of, 332, *333*
  transesophageal echocardiography of applications of, 427-428
    for detection of pulmonary artery vegetations, 428, *429*
    in diagnosis of, 427, *427-428, 429*
    in management of complications, 428
    transverse imaging, great arteries level, *429*
  with turbulent flow
    in adult patient, 332, *332*
  two-dimensional and color M-mode images of, 427, *427*
Patent foramen ovale, 296, 297, *297-300*
  with atrial septum bulge into left atrium, *298*
  with atrioventricular septal (canal) defect, 307, *307*
  diagnosis of, 297
  elderly female: right-to-left shunt in, *300*
  left-to-right shunt in, *298*
  post acute inferior myocardial infarction, 297
  right-to-left shunt in, 298, *299*
  two-dimensional image of, *299*
Pectinate muscles
  in left atrial appendage
    patient with aortic dissection, *21*
  versus thrombus
    in left ascending artery, *68*
Percutaneous mitral balloon valvuloplasty, 72, *72*

Pericardial effusion, 490, *490*
   around left ascending artery, *490*
   in ascending aorta examination
      on transverse plane, *17*
   with atrial septal aneurysm, 305, *306*
   behind right ventricle, *490*
Pericardial hydatid cyst, 491
   compression of right ventricle by,
      491-492
   compression of left ventricle by,
      491-492
   scolices in, *492*
Pleural effusion
   aortic dissection-associated, *148*
   behind descending thoracic aorta,
      493, *493*
   behind thoracic aorta, *48, 49*
   with descending thoracic aortic
      aneurysm, *134*
   right and left, *493*
   in sclerosing mediastinitis, *481*
   on transverse examination of pulmonary
      veins, *29, 30*
Porcine aortic prosthesis, 228-237, *229,
   229-238, 232-233, 235, 237-238*
   abscess/fistula with, *235-236*
   coronary cusp rupture of, *234*
   cusp rupture with, *211-213*
   cusp rupture with prolapse into left
      ventricle outflow tract, *233*
   degeneration of, *210, 229, 229, 230,
      230, 231*
   gross specimen of, *228, 233*
   hypertrophic cardiomyopathy with, *238*
   Ionescu-Shiley, 237, *237-238*
   left atrial pseudoaneurysm with, *214*
   normal, *228*
   paravalvular regurgitation from, *232*
   postoperative hematoma with, *487*
   prolapse of, *229, 230, 231*
   regurgitation from, *229, 233*
      paravalvular, *234*
   with tear of right coronary cusp, *234*
   valvular regurgitation from, *229,
      230, 232*
Porcine mitral prosthesis, 204-209,
   204-215, 211, 214-215
   cusp rupture with
      eccentric regurgitation and, *212*
      valvular and paravalvular regurgita-
         tion from, *213*
   mitral, *204-208, 210-215*
   normal, *204*
   regurgitation from, *205*
      paravalvular, *207, 208*
      valvular, *205, 208, 215*
   stenotic, *205*
   stents in left ventricle and, *204*
   and thrombus in left atrium, *206*
Posterior descending coronary artery
   transgastric approach to, *26*

Posterior mitral leaflet
   prolapse of, *76*
   redundancy of, *77*
Probe(s), 6
   biplane, *6*
   monoplane, *6*
   multiplane, *6*
   pediatric, *6*
Prosthetic valve(s)
   aortic
      Bjork-Shiley, *220-221*
      CarboMedics, *218-219*
      Cooley-Cutter, *196*
      homograft, *239-245*
      Inonescu-Shiley, *237-238*
      porcine, *215, 228-237, 232-233, 235,
         237-238*
      St. Jude, *216*
      Starr-Edwards, *222-223*
   mitral
      Bjork-Shiley, *92-195, 192*
      CarboMedics, 189, *189-191*, 191
      Medtronic-Hall, *224-227*
      porcine, 204-209, *204-215, 211,
         214-215*
      St. Jude, *183-188*
      Starr-Edwards, 197-198, *197-198*
   regurgitation with, 181
   short-axis view of, 182
Pseudoaneurysm
   definition of, 251
   left atrial
      CarboMedics mitral prosthesis and,
         191-192
      with porcine mitral prosthesis, *214*
   versus true aneurysm, 260. *260*
   and ventricular septal rupture, *262*
Pulmonary arteries. *(see also)* Left pulmonary artery; Main pulmonary artery;
   Right pulmonary artery
   aortic arch relation to, *10*
   ascending aorta and, *17-18*
   banding of
      aortopulmonary communication in,
         395 *395*
   idiopathic dilation of, 361, *361*
   on longitudinal plane examination,
      11, 12
   nonconfluent
      aortopulmonary communication and,
         394, *394*
   normal anatomy of, 17
   transverse plane examination of, *8*
   from upper esophagus, *14*
   vegetations on
      detection of, 428, *429*
Pulmonary atresia
   aortopulmonary communication in,
      393, *393, 394, 394*
   and left-sided superior vena cava enter-
      ing coronary sinus, 323, *323*

   with ventricular septal defect
      characterization of, 417
      transesophageal sequential analysis
         of, 417-418, *418*
Pulmonary autograft in aortic position
   with homograft pulmonary valve
      valvular and paravalvular regurgita-
         tion and, *246*
   with homograft replacement of pul-
      monary valve
      paravalvular leak in, *246, 247*
      prolapse in, *246*
      suture dehiscence in, *246, 247*
Pulmonary regurgitation, 177, *177, 246*
Pulmonary stenosis, 295
   with atrioventricular or ventricular sep-
      tal defects, 296
   congenital, 296
Pulmonary valve
   bicuspid, 360, *360*
   homograft replacement of
      in pulmonary autograft in aortic posi-
         tion, 246
   leaflets of
      in diastole and systole, *22*
      normal anatomy of, 22, *22*
      prolapse of, 169, 178, *178-179*
         pulmonic regurgitation with, *178-179*
      regurgitation from, 169, 177, *177, 246*
   right ventricle and, *34-35*
   stenosis of, 360, *360*
Pulmonary valve leaflets
   vegetations on, 428, *429*
Pulmonary valve prosthesis, 249, *249*
   regurgitation with
      pulmonary and aortic, *249*
Pulmonary valve stenosis, 360, *360,
   440, 440*
   bicuspid
      association with corrected transposi-
         tion of great arteries, 361, *361*
      levotransposition-associated, 361, *361*
      of right ventricular infundibulum, *441*
      subvalvular pulmonary obstructions
         in, *441*
   in 14-year-old boy, 361, *361*
Pulmonary vein(s)
   normal anatomy of, 29, *29, 30*
   in relation to heart
      diagrammatic representation of,
         29, 30
   right upper and lower
      separate and simultaneous examina-
         tion of, 29, *31*
      simultaneous visualization of, 29, *32*
   stenosis of, 295
   total anomalous connection of, 422-
      424, *423-424*
   upper and lower
      transverse and longitudinal examina-
         tion of, 29, *30*

Pulmonary venous return
    isolated right-sided anomalous into
        right atrium
            biplane examination of, *314*
            inferior vena cava in, *315*
            left superior pulmonary vein in left
                atrium, *315*
            longitudinal examination of, *314, 315*
            single case, 314, *314-316,* 315-316
            transverse plane, *316*

Quadricuspid aortic valve, 344, *344-347,*
    345-347
    infected
        anomalous origin of right coronary
            artery from left main coronary
            artery and, 347, *347*
        aortic regurgitation with, *346*
        saccular aneurysm of noncoronary
            sinus of Valsalva and, *346*
    mimic of, 345, *345*

Regurgitation
    aortic. *(see)* Aortic regurgitation
    mitral. *(see)* Mitral regurgitation
    paravalvular, 181
    thrombotic, 181
    tricuspid, regurgitation from. *(see)*
        Tricuspid valve
    valvular
        assessment of, 181
Renal arteries
    transgastric view of, 58, *59*
Right atrial appendage
    in aortic dissection, *155*
    normal anatomy of, 46
    pericardial effusion behind, *46*
    in situs solitus
        normal morphology of, 400, *400*
    and tricuspid valve, 46-47
    schematic of, *46*
Right atrium
    aortic valve abscess extension into, *128*
    atrial septum bulge into, *41, 42*
    isolated right-sided anomalous pulmo-
        nary venous return into, isolated
        right-sided. *(see)* Pulmonary venous
        return
    myxoma on, *467, 468*
    normal anatomy of, 34
    pseudoaneurysm rupture into
        from intraluminal tube graft dehis-
            cence, *154-155*
    superior vena cava and
        crista terminalis and, *36*
        on longitudinal examination, *36-38*
    thrombus on, *469-470, 471*
        right heart catheter-induced, *497*
    trabeculation in, *36, 37*
    tricuspid regurgitation into, *175*

Right coronary artery
    aneurysm of, 387, *387*
    anomalous origin of
        from left descending artery, 386, *386*
        from left main coronary artery,
            347, *347*
    aortic dissection extension into, *135, 136*
    aortic dissection flap extension into, *145*
    dissection of
        extension into aortic root, *140*
        fistula to coronary sinus, 388, *388*
        postoperative, *388*
    involvement in aortic dissection, *143*
    normal anatomy of, 22, *23*
    origin of, 26
        from left sinus of Valsalva, 385, *385*
        from right sinus of Valsalva, 385, *385*
    pulsed Doppler examination of, 26
Right heart catheter, 494-495, *494-495*
    thrombus from, *495*
Right pulmonary artery
    with IV injection of normal saline in
        superior vena cava, 36, *37*
    right superior vena cava relationship to,
        319, *320*
    thrombus of, *477*
Right pulmonary vein(s)
    lower
        longitudinal examination of, 29, *30*
        normal anatomy of, 29
        transverse examination of, 29, *30*
    transverse plane examination of, 29,
        32-33
    upper
        adjacent to right pulmonary artery,
            29, *32*
        longitudinal examination of, 29, *30*
        mediastinal mass on, *479*
        next to superior vena cava, 29, *32*
        normal anatomy of, 29
        obstruction following lung transplan-
            tation, *480*
        transverse examination of, 29, *30*
Right ventricle
    aortic dissection rupture into, *150*
    compression by pericardial cyst, *491*
    dilated, *288*
    double outlet, 375, *375*
    double-chambered, 357, *357*
    melanoma of
        metastatic, 475, *475-476*
    pacer lead in, 498, *498*
    pericardial effusion behind, *490*
    and pulmonary valve, 34-35
    thrombus in, *475-476*
        in dilated cardiomyopathy, *287*
    trabeculation in, 356, *356*
Right ventricular assist device
    malpositioned
        Thoratec, 291, 292, 293

Right ventricular outflow tract
    on five-chamber view
        with IV injection of normal saline,
            39, *40*
    pulmonic regurgitation into
        trabeculations in, 356, *356*
Right ventricular papillary muscles
    rupture of
        into the right atrium, *273*
        tricuspid regurgitation with, *273*
Right-sided superior vena cava
    relationship of right pulmonary artery,
        319, *320*
Right-to-left shunt
    in hepatopulmonary syndrome, 301, *301*
    with malpositioned Thoratec assist de-
        vice, *291*
    in patent foramen ovale, 297, 298,
        299, 300
Ross procedure, 246, *246*
    definition of, 181

Sclerosis. *(see)* Mediastinitis, sclerosing
Secundum atrial septal defect, 302,
    302-304
    associated with transposition of the
        great vessels, 378, *379*
    gross specimen of, *302*
    left-to-right shunt in, *303*
    schematic of, *302*
    with tricuspid regurgitation into left
        atrium, *303*
    two defects in, *304*
Senning procedure
    transesophageal sequential analysis of
        atrial baffle function following, *413,*
        413-414
Shunt(s)
    estimation of volume in, 302
    left-to-right. *(see)* Left-to-right shunt
    right-to-left. *(see)* Right-to-left shunt
Single ventricle, 377, *377*
    atrioventricular valves opening into,
        377, *377*
    in transposition of the great vessels,
        378, *378-379*
Sinuses of Valsalva
    aneurysm of, 296, 381, *381*
        with rupture into right ventricle, 382,
            382, 383, 383
    on aortic valve imaging, 27
    dilatation of, 380, *380-381*
    left
        dissection of, *139*
    right
        anomalous origin of left circumflex
            artery from, 385, *385*
Sinus venosus atrial septal defect
    examination of right pulmonary veins
        in, 29, *31*

Situs inversus
  with discordant atrioventricular con-
    nection, *406*
  in transesophageal sequential analysis,
    401-402, *402*
    atrioventricular discordance and,
      401, *402*
    characterization of, 401
    contrast study of, *402*
    mirror image in, 402
    transgastric recordings in, 401-402
    transverse imaging of, *402*
Situs solitus
  with discordant atrioventricular con-
    nection, *406*
  in transesophageal sequential analysis,
    399-401, *400-401*
    connection of right pulmonary vein
      to left atrium in, 400-401, *401*
    coronary sinus draining into right
      atrium in, 400, *400*
    left atrial appendage normal mor-
      phology in, 400, *400*
    left upper pulmonary vein connection
      with left atrium, 400-401, *401*
    right atrial appendage normal mor-
      phology of, 400, *400*
    superior vena cava connection to
      right atrium in, 400, *400*
Splenic artery
  transgastric view of, *58, 59*
Splenic vein
  transgastric view of, *58, 59*
St. Jude aortic prosthesis, 181, *216-217*
  normal, *216*
  paravalvular leak with, *217*
St. Jude mitral prosthesis, 181, *183-188*
  ectopic position for, 188, *188*
  normal, *183-184*, 183
  regurgitation from
    paravalvular, 187, *187-188*
    from suture dehiscence, *188*
  regurgitation from, periprosthetic
    with tricuspid regurgitation, *188*
  thrombosed, 185, *185-186*
Starr-Edwards prosthesis(es), 181
  aortic
    normal, *222*
    paravalvular regurgitation with, *223*
  mitral
    dehiscence of, 198, *198*
    normal, 197, *197*
Stenosis
  aortic, 105, *105-113*, 107, 109-113. *(see
    also)* Aortic stenosis
  of Cooley-Cutter mitral prosthesis, *196*
  discrete subaortic membranous, 339,
    339-342, 340, 341, 342
    attachment to anterior mitral leaflet,
      340, 341

attachment to base of aortic cusp,
  340, *340*
  gross specimen of, 342, *342*
  obstruction from, 342, *342*
  post modified Konno's operation,
    342, *342*
  postoperative study of, *339*, 340
  separation from aortic valve
    cusps, *341*
  identification of, 251
  infundibular, 358-359, *358-359*, 370, *370*
  mitral. *See* Mitral stenosis
  subaortic membranous
    coarctation of the aorta associated
      with, 354, *354*
  subvalvular, 295-296
Stomach
  transgastric view of, *60*
Subclavian artery
  on longitudinal plane examination, *11,
    12, 13*
Subvalvular aortic stenosis, 295-296, 434,
  434-435
Superior vena cava
  connection to right atrium
    in situs solitus, 400, *400*
  and inferior vena cava
    schematic of, *44*
    simultaneous image of, *44, 45*
  IV injection of saline in
    and right atrium filling, 36, *37*
  left-sided, *317-325*. *(see also)* Left-sided
    superior vena cava
  normal anatomy of, 34, 44
  right
    azygous vein entering, 36, *37-38*
    and right atrium, *36-38*
  transesophageal echocardiography of, *2*
Suture dehiscence
  with Bjork-Shiley mitral prosthesis,
    195, 220
  with pulmonary autograft in aortic
    position and homograft replace-
    ment of pulmonary valve, 246,
    247
  with St. Jude mitral prosthesis
    regurgitation from, *188*
  suspected
    in abdominal aortic aneurysm graft
      replacement, *160*
Swann-Ganz catheter
  in right heart, *494*
Systemic lupus erythematosus, 124
  flail aortic valve in, *124*
  gross specimen of aortic and mitral
    valves in, *124*
  mitral and aortic valvulitis in, *124*
Systolic anterior motion
  in hypertrophic cardiomyopathy, 275,
    276, 277-278

Tetralogy of Fallot, 296, 370, *370-371*,
  440-442
  aorta overrides ventricular septum,
    441, *441*
  aortopulmonary communication in,
    393-394, *393-394*
  applications of, 441
  characterization of, 440-441
  gross specimen of, *371*
  inpatient with pulmonary atresia 442, *442*
  and left-sided superior vena cava enter-
    ing coronary sinus, 323, *323*
  in patient with ventricular septal defect
    and infundibular stenosis, 370, *370*
  in patient with ventricular septal defect
    and infundibular stenosis
    patch to close defect, *370*
  pulmonary stenosis
    subvalvular or mixed, 441-442
  stenosis of ventricular infundibulum,
    441, *441*
Thebesian valve
  at coronary sinus-right atrium junction,
    46, 47
Thoratec right ventricular assist device
  malpositioned in left atrium, *291,
    292, 293*
Thrombus
  in aortic arch aneurysm, *134*
  Bjork-Shiley mitral prosthesis-
    associated, *192-193*, 220
    gross specimen of, *194*
  Denver peritoneovenous shunt-
    induced, *496*
  in descending thoracic aortic aneu-
    rysm, *134*
  in dilated cardiomyopathy
    in left ascending artery, *287*
    left ventricular, *287*
  Duran ring-induced
    in mitral annuloplasty, *203*
  in false lumen
    in aortic dissection, 141, *142*
  formation of
    in aortic dissection, 135, *138*
    in descending aorta, *144*
  gross specimen of surgically re-
    sected, *470*
  heart catheter-induced, *495*
  in left ascending artery
    in mitral stenosis, *68*
    nonspecific thickening versus, *68, 69*
  left atrial, *68, 69*, 452
    with porcine mitral prosthesis, *206*
  left ventricular, 460, *460*
  left ventricular apical
    on left ventricle examination, *289*
  in left ventricular apical aneurysm, 258,
    259
  mimic of left atrial tumor, *451*

Thrombus—*Continued*
mitral valve, *454*
right atrial, 469, *469-471*
elongated, *471*
gross specimen of, *497*
paradoxic embolus impending, *469-470*
right heart catheter-induced, *497*
of right pulmonary artery, 477, *477*
in right coronary artery aneurysm, 387, *387*
right ventricular, *476*
versus tumor, 445
valvular regurgitation with, 181
Total anomalous connection of pulmonary veins
sites of, 423
transesophageal echocardiography of, 422-424, *423-424*
at cardiac level, 423
dilation of coronary sinus on, 423, *423*
four-chamber view, 423, *423*
infracardiac, 424, *424*
to right atrium, 424, *424*
supracardiac, 423
types of, 422
Transesophageal echocardiography
anesthesia and sedation for, 4
antibiotic prophylaxis for, 3
complications of, 3
contraindications to, 3
examination procedure in, 1-2
five-chamber view, *39-40*
four-chamber view, 41, *41-42*
indications for, 2-3
in intubated patient, 4
performance of, 3-4
for postoperative results, 442
post-procedure
monitoring, 4
patient precautions, 4-5
preparation for, 3-4
procedure in, 4
procedure room set up for, 3
for transoperative results, 442
Transgastric view(s)
of abdominal structures, 58, *59*
anterior angulation
of aortic root, *56*
of left kidney
longitudinal and transverse, 58, *59*
long axis
of aortic root and ascending aorta, *57*
of normal anatomy, 52, *52-60*, *57*, *58*
of mitral valve leaflets and chordae tendineae, *52*
schematic, *52*

of stomach, *60*
of superior mesenteric and renal vessels, *58-59*
schematic of, *58*
transverse plane imaging, *58*
transverse plane
of pancreas, 58, *59*
Transposition of the great vessels, 296, 372, *372-375*, *374*
aortopulmonary communication in, 393, *393*
corrected
with Ebstein's malformation of left-sided atrioventricular valve, 367, *367*
gross specimens of, *372*
post-Mustard procedure, *373*
pulmonary artery posterior to aorta, *372*
pulmonary artery posterior to aortic root, *372*
single ventricle in, 378, *378-379*
associated secundum atrial septal defect in, *379*
bicuspid pulmonary valve in, *379*
in 14-year-old boy, 374, *374-375*
secundum atrial septal defect in, *375*
Transthoracic echocardiography
for mitral stenosis, 63
Transverse imaging planes, 7, *7*
Transverse sections, 7
Tricuspid aortic valve
as mimic of quadricuspid, 345, *345*
Tricuspid atresia, 296
with atrial and septal defects, 368, *368*
schematic of, *368*
in transesophageal sequential analysis
biplanar and transgastric recordings, 408, *408*
malalignment of interatrial and interventricular septa in, 408, *409*
mitral regurgitation with color Doppler, 409, *409*
secundum atrial septal defect with right-to-left shunting, 407, *409*
transverse image, *408*
Tricuspid leaflet(s)
anterior, *34*, *35*
vegetation on, *177*
in Ebstein's anomaly, 363-366, *365-366*
on examination of right ventricle and pulmonary valve, *34*, *35*
four-chamber view of, *41*, *42*
inferior posterior, *34*, *35*
in mitral stenosis and atrial septal defects, *71*
normal anatomy of, 34
transgastric view of, *57*
Tricuspid prosthesis and ring
CarboMedics, *248*
pannus in, *248*
regurgitation in, *248*

Tricuspid regurgitation, 169, 170, *170*, 175-176, *175-176*
eccentric along septal leaflet into atrial septum, *176*
impacting atrial septum, *175*
mild, *170*
mitral regurgitation with, *176*
moderate, *170*
post-balloon mitral valvuloplasty, *74*
into right atrium, *175*
severe, *170*, *171*, *176*
transgastric view, *170*
Tricuspid valve
endocarditis of, *177*
fibroelastoma on
papillary, *473*
myxoma of, *474*
porcine replacement of, *176*
prolapse of, 169, 172, *172-174*
anterior and septal leaflets in, *172*, *173-174*
four-chamber view of, *172*
longitudinal plane, *173*, *174*
with myxomatous degeneration, *172*, *174*
posterior leaflet in, *173-174*
regurgitation from, 169
double outlet right ventricle, 416, *416*
stenosis of, 169
straddling ventricular septum, 377, *377*
in systole, *57*
visualization of, *44-45*
Truncus arteriosus
in double outlet right ventricle, 416-417, *417*
in 7-month-old infant
aortopulmonary communication in, 391, *391*
with aortopulmonary window, 392, *392*
Tumor(s). (*see also* named, e.g., *Fibroelastoma*)
calcification mimicking, *452*
extracardiac
posterior to aortic root, *478*
fibroelastoma, 445, 460, 462, 473, *473*
leiomyoma, 445, 465, *465*, *466*
leiomyosarcoma, 445, *449-450*, *463-464*
lipoma, 445, *458-459*
myxoma. (*see*) Myxoma
right-sided versus normal structures, 445
Two-chamber view
of left ascending artery, *43*
of left ventricle, *43*

Unicuspid aortic valve
unicommissural, 347-348, *347-348*

Valvuloplasty. (*see also*) Percutaneous mitral balloon valvuloplasty aortic, 182
mitral, 64, 72, *72-74*, *73-74*

Vegetation
aortic, *89, 99, 126-127, 129,
    130-131*
    as tumor mimic, *462*
on chordae tendineae
    on mitral leaflets, *88*
on flail posterior leaflet, *89*
mitral, 88-89, *88-89, 88-89*, 95-96,
    95-96
    on anterior leaflet, *89*
    gross specimen of, *89*
    on leaflets, *88, 89*
    on posterior leaflet, *94*
    regurgitation and, *88*
at mitral-aortic junction, *130*
on tricuspid leaflet, *177*
Vein(s). *(see also named, e.g., Azygous veins)*
azygous, *36-38*, 48, *48-51*, 321, *322*
connection sites of, *411*
drainage of, *422*
hemiazygous, 48, *48-50*, 481
hepatic, *58, 59*
innominate, *10*, 11, *11*
intercostal, 48, *48, 50-51*, 321, *322*
normal anatomy of, 29, *29-32*
obstruction of, *483*
splenic, *58-59*
stenosis of, *295*
total anomalous connection of, 422-424,
    423-424
Ventricles, 39. *(see also)* Left ventricle;
    Right ventricle
four-chamber view of, *41, 42*
identification of
    criteria for, 404
    in transesophageal sequential analy-
        sis, 404, *405*
    transverse transgastric study
        of, *405*
    tricuspid septal leaflet insertion in
        interventricular septum in, *405*

normal anatomy of, 39, *39*
reversal of
    in discordant atrioventricular connec-
        tion, *406*
septum of
    tricuspid valve straddling, 377, *377*
in transesophageal sequential analysis
    identification of, 399
Ventricular assist device(s), 275
right, 289
    Thoratec, *291-293*
Ventricular septal aneurysm, 326, *326*
trabecular, 326, *326*
Ventricular septal defect(s), 295, 327, *327-*
331, 328, 330, 331
atrial septal defect-associated, 330, *330*
with double outlet right ventricle,
    376, *376*
mimic of, 331, *331*
patient with tetralogy of Fallot and,
    370, *370*
perimembranous, *327*, 328-329
    below tricuspid and aortic valves, *328*
    with left-to-right shunt, *328-329*
    schematics of, *329*
trabecular, 327
transesophageal echocardiography of,
    424-426, *424-426*
    aortic regurgitation in, *425,*
        425-426, 426
    four-chamber view, 424, *424*
    infective vegetations involving tricus-
        pid valve, 425, *425*
    of infundibular or outlet septum, 425
    intraoperative, 426
    of membranous septum, 424, *424*
    multiple, *425*
    of posterior of inlet septum, 424-425
    of trabecular septum, 425, *425*
tricuspid atresia with, 368, *368-369*, 369
in ventriculoarterial connections, 413

Ventricular septal hypertrophy
    in hypertrophic cardiomyopathy, *280*
Ventricular septal rupture
    after acute myocardial infarction, 263
        apical five-chamber view, *263*
        four-chamber view, *265*
        longitudinal plane, *264*
        right-to-left shunt and, *264*
        transgastric approach, *265*
        transgastric views, *264*
        transverse plane, *264*
    pseudoaneurysm and, 262, *262*
Ventricular septum
    in hypertrophic cardiomyopathy, *282*
    myectomy of, 282, *283*
    in tetralogy of Fallot, 441, *441*
    tricuspid valve straddling, 377, *377*
Ventriculoarterial connection(s)
    concordant, 411-412
    discordant
        characterization of, 412
        four-chamber image in, 413, *413*
        longitudinal image of, 412-413, *413*
        subvalvular pulmonary obstruction
            and stenosis in, 412, *412*
        transposition of the great arteries,
            412, *412, 413*
        transverse image of, 412, *412*
        ventricular septal defect in, 413
    in transesophageal sequential analysis,
        411-413
        identification of great vessels, 399
        mode of, 399
        variants of, 399

Wall motion abnormality(ies), 251
dyskinesis
    of anterior wall, 256, *257*
hypokinesis
    of anterior and inferior walls, 256
    of anterior septum, 256

STRENGTHEN YOUR *Cardiology* REFERENCE LIBRARY

Pearls & Pitfalls in Electrocardiography Pithy, Practical Pointers, Second Edition

Henry J. L. Marriott, MD, FACP, FACC
Tackle even the toughest ECGs with this strategic manual from leading diagnostician Henry Marriott.
Nov. 1997/198 pages/249 illustrations/0-683-30170-5

Pediatric Cardiac Intensive Care

Anthony C. Chang, MD; Frank L. Hanley, MD; Gil Wernovsky, MD, and David L. Wessel, MD
Leading intensivists explore recent advances in ultrasound technology and pharmacology.
1998/about 512 pages/0-683-01508-7

Clinical Synopsis of Moss and Adams' Heart Disease in Children

George C. Emmanouilides, MD; Thomas A. Riemenschneider, MD; Hugh D. Allen, MD; and Howard P. Gutgesell, MD
This concise summary of the benchmark parent text highlights essential clinical information on diagnosis and management.
1998/about 600 pages/0-683-18003-7

Science and Practice of Pediatric Cardiology, Second Edition

Arthur Garson, Jr., MD; J. Timothy Bricker, MD; David J. Fisher, MD; and Steven R. Neish, MD
Master the remarkable breakthroughs in pediatric cardiology with this innovative reference for both basic and clinical science issues.
November 1997/2,600 pages/0-683-03417-0

Heart Disease in Primary Care Primary Care Series

Michael L. Hess, MD and Andrea Hastillo, MD
Cardiovascular disease is covered for primary care practitioners, with specific recommendations for prevention, diagnostic methods, treatment, and follow-up care.
1998/about 400 pages/0-683-03988-1

VISIT US ON THE INTERNET!

E-mail:	custserv@wwilkins.com
Home page:	http://www.wwilkins.com

Clinical Hypertension Seventh Edition

Norman M. Kaplan, MD
Count on world-renowned authority Dr. Norman Kaplan for impeccable guidelines to evaluating and managing your hypertensive patients.
Oct. 1997/500 pages/110 illustrations/0-683-30132-2

Diagnostic and Therapeutic Cardiac Catheterization, Third Edition

Edited by Carl J. Pepine, MD; James A Hill, MD; and Charles R. Lambert, MD
Harness the vast diagnostic and treatment implications of catheterization with this unified look at all promising procedures.
Dec. 1997/1,329 pages/520 illustrations/0-683-30125-X

Practical Electrocardiography CD-ROM

Galen S. Wagner, MD; Robert Waugh, MD; and David Lawson
Enjoy instant access to the acclaimed 9th edition of Marriott's Practical Electrocardiography with this powerful CD-ROM.
March 1998/0-683-08617-0

Multimedia Textbook of Coronary Arteriography and Interventions

John D. Carroll, MD
Using text, graphics, case studies, digital cine video, and interactive features, the Multimedia Textbook CD-ROM helps you develop clinical problem-solving skills.
1997/0-683-30056-3

We invite you to preview these texts for a full month. If you're not completely satisfied, return them to us within 30 days at no further obligation (US and Canada only). Phone orders accepted 24 hours a day, 7 days a week (US only). Prices subject to change without notice.

From the US: Call: 1-800-638-0672
          Fax: 1-800-447-8438

From Canada: Call: 1-800-665-1148

From outside the US and Canada Fax: 410-528-8550